# Ethnopharmacology

# Ethnopharmacology

Edited by

**Michael Heinrich**
*Centre for Pharmacognosy and Phytotherapy/Research Cluster Biodiversity and Medicines, UCL School of Pharmacy*
*University of London*
*UK*

**Anna K. Jäger**
*Department of Drug Design and Pharmacology*
*Faculty of Health and Medicinal Sciences*
*University of Copenhagen*
*Denmark*

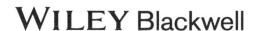

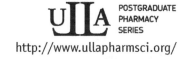

POSTGRADUATE
PHARMACY
SERIES

http://www.ullapharmsci.org/

*Library of Congress Cataloging-in-Publication Data applied for.*

ISBN: 9781118930748

A catalogue record for this book is available from the British Library.

Wiley also publishes its books in a variety of electronic formats. Some content that appears in print may not be available in electronic books.

Typeset in 10/12pt TimesTenLTStd by SPi Global, Chennai, India

1   2015

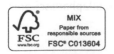

# Contents

## 7   NMR-based Metabolomics and Hyphenated NMR Techniques: A Perfect Match in Natural Products Research                                          63

*Joachim Møllesøe Vinther, Sileshi Gizachew Wubshet and Dan Staerk*

## 8   New Medicines Based On Traditional Knowledge: Indigenous and Intellectual Property Rights from an Ethnopharmacological Perspective          75

*Michael Heinrich*

## 9   Ethnopharmacology and Intellectual Property Rights                      87

*Alan Hesketh*

## The Pharmacological Angle

## Ethnopharmacology: Regional Perspectives

### 23 Ethnopharmacology in Sub-Sahara Africa: Current Trends and Future Perspectives 265

*Mack Moyo, Adeyemi O. Aremu and Johannes van Staden*

### 24 Ethnopharmacology and Integrative Medicine: An Indian Perspective 279

*Pulok K. Mukherjee, Sushil K. Chaudhary, Shiv Bahadur and Pratip K. Debnath*

# Contributors

**Christian Agyare** Department of Pharmaceutics, Faculty of Pharmacy and Pharmaceutical Sciences, College of Health Sciences, Kwame Nkrumah University of Science and Technology, Ghana

**Pravit Akarasereenont** Department of Pharmacology, Faculty of Medicine Siriraj Hospital, Mahidol University, Thailand, and Center of Applied Thai Traditional Medicine, Faculty of Medicine Siriraj Hospital, Mahidol University, Thailand.

**Adolfo Andrade-Cetto** Department of Cell Biology, School of Sciences, National Autonomous University of Mexico, Mexico

**Adeyemi O. Aremu** Research Centre for Plant Growth and Development, School of Life Sciences, University of KwaZulu-Natal, South Africa

**Alex Asase** Department of Botany, University of Ghana, Ghana

**Shiv Bahadur** School of Natural Product Studies, Department of Pharmaceutical Technology, Jadavpur University, India

**Maíra Bidart de Macedo** Laboratory of Microbiology, Parasitology and Hygiene, Faculty of Pharmaceutical, Biomedical and Veterinary Sciences, University of Antwerp, Belgium

**Anthony Booker** Research Cluster 'Biodiversity and Medicines', UCL School of Pharmacy, UK

**Eric Brand** School of Chinese Medicine, Hong Kong Baptist University, China

**Robert Bye** Jardín Botánico del Instituto de Biología, Universidad Nacional Autónoma de México, Mexico

**Salvador Cañigueral** Unitat de Farmacologia i Farmacognòsia, Facultat de Farmàcia, Universitat de Barcelona, Spain

**Sushil K. Chaudhary** School of Natural Product Studies, Department of Pharmaceutical Technology, Jadavpur University, India

**Sofie Clais** Laboratory of Microbiology, Parasitology and Hygiene, Faculty of Pharmaceutical, Biomedical and Veterinary Sciences, University of Antwerp, Belgium

**Geoffrey A. Cordell** Natural Products Inc., USA

**Paul Cos** Laboratory of Microbiology, Parasitology and Hygiene, Faculty of Pharmaceutical, Biomedical and Veterinary Sciences, University of Antwerp, Belgium

**Marianne J. Datiles** Centre for Pharmacognosy and Phytotherapy/Research Cluster Biodiversity and Medicines, UCL School of Pharmacy, UK

**Hugo de Boer** Naturalis Biodiversity Center, Leiden University, The Netherlands, and Department of Organismal Biology, Uppsala University, Sweden, and The Natural History Museum, University of Oslo, Norway

**Pratip K. Debnath** Gananath Sen Institute of Ayurveda and Research, India

**Gunter P. Eckert** Goethe-University, Campus Riedberg, Department of Pharmacology, Germany

**Thomas Efferth** Department of Pharmaceutical Biology, Institute of Pharmacy and Biochemistry, Johannes Gutenberg University, Germany

**Elaine Elisabetsky** Labratório de Etnofarmacologia, Universidade Federal do Rio Grande do Sul, Brazil

**José Fajardo** Instituto Botánico, Jardín Botánico de Castilla La Mancha, Spain, and Universidad Popular, Spain

**Jorge García-Alvarez** Department of Cell Biology, School of Sciences, National Autonomous University of Mexico, Mexico

**Bertrand Graz** Social and Preventive Medicine, University of Lausanne, Switzerland

**Andreas Hensel** Institute of Pharmaceutical Biology and Phytochemistry, University of Münster, Germany

**Henry J. Greten** Abel Salazar Biomedical Sciences Institute, University of Porto, Portugal, and Heidelberg School of Chinese Medicine, Germany

**Ping Guo** School of Chinese Medicine, Hong Kong Baptist University, China

**Michael Heinrich** Centre for Pharmacognosy and Phytotherapy/Research Cluster Biodiversity and Medicines, UCL School of Pharmacy, University of London, London, UK

**Alan Hesketh** Indigena Biodiversity Limited, London, UK

**Vernon H. Heywood** School of Biological Sciences, University of Reading, UK

**Peter J. Houghton** Department of Pharmacy and Forensic Science, Institute of Pharmaceutical Sciences, King's College London, London, UK.

**Anna K. Jäger** Department of Drug Design and Pharmacology, Faculty of Health and Medicinal Sciences, University of Copenhagen, Denmark

**Emelia Kisseih** Institute of Pharmaceutical Biology and Phytochemistry, University of Münster, Germany

**Ellen Lanckacker** Laboratory of Microbiology, Parasitology and Hygiene, Faculty of Pharmaceutical, Biomedical and Veterinary Sciences, University of Antwerp, Belgium

**Andreas Lardos** Research Cluster Biodiversity and Medicines/Centre for Pharmacognosy and Phytotherapy, UCL School of Pharmacy, London, UK

**Marco Leonti** Department of Biomedical Sciences, University of Cagliari, Italy

**Matthias Lechtenberg** Institute of Pharmaceutical Biology and Phytochemistry, University of Münster, Germany

**Graham Lloyd Jones** Pharmaceuticals and Nutraceuticals Group, Centre for Bioactive Discovery in Health and Ageing, University of New England Armidale, Australia

**Emerson Silva Lima** Faculdade de Ciências Farmacêuticas, Universidade Federal do Amazonas, Brasil

**Edelmira Linares** Jardín Botánico del Instituto de Biología, Universidad Nacional Autónoma de México, Mexico

**Natchagorn Lumlerdkij** Center of Applied Thai Traditional Medicine, Faculty of Medicine Siriraj Hospital, Mahidol University, Thailand, and Centre for Pharmacognosy and Phytotherapy/Research Cluster Biodiversity and Medicines, UCL School of Pharmacy, London, UK

**Louis Maes** Laboratory of Microbiology, Parasitology and Hygiene, Faculty of Pharmaceutical, Biomedical and Veterinary Sciences, University of Antwerp, Belgium

**Daniel E. Moerman** William E Stirton Emeritus Professor of Anthropology, University of Michigan-Dearborn, USA

**Mack Moyo** Research Centre for Plant Growth and Development, School of Life Sciences, University of KwaZulu-Natal, South Africa

**Pulok K Mukherjee** School of Natural Product Studies, Department of Pharmaceutical Technology, Jadavpur University, India

**Concepción Obón** Depto. de Biología Aplicada, Escuela Politécnica Superior de Orihuela. Universidad Miguel Hernández, Spain

**Manuel Pardo-de-Santayana** Departamento de Biología (Botánica). Universidad Autónoma de Madrid, Spain

**Frank Petereit** Institute of Pharmaceutical Biology and Phytochemistry, University of Münster, Germany

**Andrea Pieroni** University of Gastronomic Sciences, Italy

**Jose M. Prieto** Centre for Pharmacognosy and Phytotherapy/Research Cluster Biodiversity and Medicines, UCL School of Pharmacy, London, UK

**Cassandra L. Quave** Center for the Study of Human Health, Emory University, USA, and Department of Dermatology, Emory University School of Medicine, USA

**Diego Rivera** Depto. Biología Vegetal, Fac. Biología, Universidad de Murcia, Spain

**Jaume Sanz-Biset** Unitat de Farmacologia i Farmacognòsia, Facultat de Farmàcia, Universitat de Barcelona, Spain

**Nicholas J. Sadgrove** Pharmaceuticals and Nutraceuticals Group, Centre for Bioactive Discovery in Health and Ageing, University of New England Armidale, Australia

**Ean-Jeong Seo** Department of Pharmaceutical Biology, Institute of Pharmacy and Biochemistry, Johannes Gutenberg University, Germany

**Renata Sõukand** Estonian Literary Museum, Estonia

**Dan Staerk** Department of Drug Design and Pharmacology, Faculty of Health and Medical Sciences, University of Copenhagen, Denmark

**Alexandra Towns** Naturalis Biodiversity Center, Leiden University, The Netherlands

**Arturo Valdés** Instituto Botánico, Jardín Botánico de Castilla La Mancha, Spain

**José Ramón Vallejo** Depto. de Terapéutica Médico-Quirúrgica, Fac. de Medicina, Universidad de Extremadura, Spain

**Tinde van Andel** Naturalis Biodiversity Center, Leiden University, The Netherlands

**Johannes van Staden** Research Centre for Plant Growth and Development, School of Life Sciences, University of KwaZulu-Natal, Pietermaritzburg, Scottsville 3209, South Africa

**Ina Vandebroek** Matthew Calbraith Perry Assistant Curator of Economic Botany and Caribbean Program Director, The New York Botanical Garden, Bronx, New York, USA

**Alonso Verde** Instituto Los Olmos, Albacete. Spain, and Instituto Botánico, Jardín Botánico de Castilla La Mancha, Spain

**Joachim Møllesøe Vinther** Department of Drug Design and Pharmacology, Faculty of Health and Medical Sciences, University of Copenhagen, Denmark

**Caroline S. Weckerle** Institute of Systematic Botany, University of Zürich, Switzerland

**Merlin Willcox** Nuffield Department of Primary Care Health Sciences, University of Oxford, UK

**Elizabeth M. Williamson** The School of Pharmacy, University of Reading, UK

**Colin W. Wright** Bradford School of Pharmacy, University of Bradford, UK

**Ching-Fen Wu** Department of Pharmaceutical Biology, Institute of Pharmacy and Biochemistry, Johannes Gutenberg University, Germany

**Sileshi Gizachew Wubshet** Department of Drug Design and Pharmacology, Faculty of Health and Medical Sciences, University of Copenhagen, Denmark

**Harisun Yaakob** Institute of Bioproduct Development, Universiti Teknologi Malaysia, Malaysia

**Erdem Yesilada** Yeditepe University, Faculty of Pharmacy, Turkey

**Zhongzhen Zhao** School of Chinese Medicine, Hong Kong Baptist University, China

# Series Foreword

## ULLA Pharmacy Series

The ULLA Pharmacy Series is an innovative series of introductory text books for postgraduate students and researchers in the pharmaceutical sciences.

This series is produced by the ULLA Consortium (European University Consortium for Pharmaceutical Sciences). The Consortium is a European academic collaboration in research and teaching of the pharmaceutical sciences that is constantly growing and expanding. The Consortium was founded in 1992 and consists of pharmacy departments and faculties from leading universities throughout Europe, namely:

- Faculty of Pharmacy, Uppsala University, Sweden
- UCL School of Pharmacy, London, UK
- Leiden/Amsterdam Academic Center for Drug Research, University of Leiden and Vrije Universiteit Amsterdam, The Netherlands
- Drug Research Academy, Faculty of Health and Medical Sciences, University of Copenhagen, Denmark
- Faculty of Pharmacy, University Paris-Sud, France
- Department of Pharmacy, University of Parma, Italy
- Faculty of Pharmaceutical Sciences, University of Leuven (KU Leuven), Belgium
- Faculty of Pharmacy, University of Helsinki, Finland

The editorial board for the ULLA series consists of several academics from these European Institutions who are all experts in their individual field of pharmaceutical science.

**Previous titles include:**

*Pharmaceutical Toxicology*
*Paediatric Drug Handling*
*Molecular Biopharmaceutics*
*International Research in Healthcare*
*Facilitating Learning in Healthcare*
*Biomedical and Pharmaceutical Polymers*
*Inhalation Drug Delivery*
*Global New Drug Development*

The ULLA Pharmacy Series includes state-of-the-art textbooks for students and researchers in pharmacy and the pharmaceutical sciences written or edited by world-reknown experts based within the ULLA Consortium.

The books provide an overview and critical appraisal of core areas within the fast developing fields of pharmacy and aim at setting standards in these fields. The books are tailored most importantly towards PhD students and other postgraduate students undertaking masters or diploma courses anywhere in the world. They are equally suited for undergraduates studying specific courses and for practising pharmaceutical scientists and community pharmacists.

Further information can be found at www.ullapharmsci.org.

# Preface

Ethnopharmacology is a fast-developing, dynamic area of research. Annually thousands of papers on ethnopharmacological topics are now published. Researchers with diverse backgrounds, including pharmaceutical scientists, pharmacologists, anthropologists, biologists, botanists, toxicologists and practitioners/researchers of the diverse medical traditions, are all involved in such research. Ethnopharmacological research is particularly flourishing in most of the so-called BRICS and MINT countries (Brazil, Russia, India, China, South Africa; México, Indonesia, Nigeria and Turkey), but also in many of the other emerging economies, like Thailand and Malaysia. However, so far there has been no comprehensive and critical assessment of the state of the art in this important field of research. With this book the editors and authors hope to fill this gap.

Ethnopharmacology is not a very concisely defined field. In fact this book contributes to a debate about what the core research foci of ethnopharmacology are and how these should be developed further. As one step of the discussion, we invited all contributors to this book to send us their short definition of ethnopharmacology – a few sent even more than one. In the following we summarize these definitions (based on emails received between July and December 2014):

- **Pravit Akarasereenont (Thailand):** A science dealing with the study of the pharmacology of traditional medicine and focusing on the active substances and their pharmacological action.
- **Tinde van Andel (the Netherlands):** Ethnopharmacology is the study of medicinal plant use by various ethnic groups, including indigenous peoples, and the relevance of these traditional medicines for pharmacology in general and for the health of the people using these plants.
- **Adolfo Andrade Cetto (México):** Ethnopharmacology is the study and selection of traditionally used, biologically active natural products, with the aim of understanding their therapeutic actions.
- **Tony Booker (UK):** The study of the historical and modern interactions between humans and flora, fauna and minerals, and how these substances, their extracts and the chemical compounds derived from them, may be utilized to prevent and treat ill-health in people and their dependent animals.
- **Robert Bye and Edelmira Linares (México):** Ethnopharmacology [is] the study of the interactions and relationships between humans and biological organisms along with their bioactive constituents that promote the well-being of humans over social and geographic spaces as well as biological, chronological and cultural times.

- **Paul Cos (Belgium):** Ethnopharmacology is the meeting of two sciences, i.e. ethnomedicine and pharmacology

- **Marianne Datiles (UK/USA):** Ethnopharmacology [is] the study of human knowledge and use of synthetic and natural medicines in the past, present and potential future. It is a highly interdisciplinary field that includes pharmacy, chemistry, botany, anthropology, history, nutrition, environmental sciences, public health, medicine and the medical humanities. Many definitions of the field appear to exclude human knowledge of medicines, but I would consider this to be an essential area of study within the field.

- **Thomas Efferth (Germany):** Ethnopharmacology focuses on research on efficacy, safety and modes of actions of traditional medicines with pharmacological methods.

- **Bertrand Graz (Switzerland):** Ethnopharmacology is the study of the drugs (or poisons) used by other people.

- **Ping Guo, Eric Brand and Zhongzhen Zhao (Hong Kong/China):** Ethnopharmacology refers to the interdisciplinary scientific study of potentially bioactive substances utilized by different ethnic or cultural groups.

- **Michael Heinrich (UK):** Ethnopharmacology is the transdisciplinary study of locally and traditionally used medicines, integrating approaches from social and natural sciences (and in some cases medicine), often with the goal of contributing to a better and safer use of these medicines. More and more it plays a role in helping to develop a more sustainable future for people in marginalized regions and as such is becoming even more essential in global health.

- **Alan Hesketh (UK):** The study of the use of plants and other genetic resources by ethnic groups, especially indigenous communities, and the application of that knowledge to develop new or improved health products.

- **Peter Houghton (UK):** The historical, biological, chemical and pharmacological study of natural substances used by human societies and cultures for medicinal or medicinally related purposes.

- **Anna Jäger (Denmark):** Ethnopharmacology is a strange word. Investigation of pharmacological effects and mode of action of traditional practises and medicines, and the active compounds therein.

- **Graham Jones (Australia):** Ethnopharmacology constituting a respectful marriage between modern science and ancient wisdom with much to be gained in both directions.

- **Andreas Lardos (Switzerland):** Ethnopharmacology is a multidisciplinary field of research focusing on the investigation of plants and other natural products used as medicine in present-day as well as historical local or indigenous knowledge systems.

- **Marco Leonti (Italy):** Ethnopharmacology may be seen as a transdisciplinary medical self-reflection trying to find a consensus between the emic and the etic perspective.

- **Natchagorn Lumlerdkij (UK/Thailand):** Ethnopharmacology is a research area that explores the pharmacological activity of herbal medicine with appreciation of indigenous wisdom.

- **Dan Moerman (USA):** Ethnopharmacology is the study of the way people use plants, informing us about the varying ways people create meaning about these living objects.

- **Pulok Mukherjee (India):** Ethnopharmacology is a multi-disciplinary study dealing with the observations and experimental investigations of the biological activities of plants and animals used in traditional medicines of past and present culture. [See also in his chapter: The concept and methods of ethnopharmacological research incorporate elements from diverse medical practices like Ayurveda and Siddha and scientific disciplines like ethnobotany/ethnomedicine, anthropology, chemistry, pharmacognosy, pharmacology, biochemistry, molecular biology, pharmacy etc.]

- **José Prieto (UK):** Ethnopharmacology: the study of pharmacological interventions in traditional medicinal systems. These interventions consist of the administration of natural drugs from any origin (animal, plant, mineral, fungal and/or microbial) usually orally or externally. However, associated traditional non-pharmacological interventions (such as acupuncture, chiropractic, massage, music and sounds, colours, etc.), and religious or magical rituals may greatly contribute to the putative effect of the pharmacological intervention.
- **Diego Rivera (Spain):** Ethnopharmacology is – despite its appearances – not ethnic pharmacology.
- **Diego Rivera (Spain):** Ethnopharmacology is the people's pharmacology, which usually blurs with increasing distance from the natural sources of medicinal resources and the increase in the complexity of systems of manufacture and distribution of medicines.
- **Diego Rivera (Spain):** Ethnopharmacology is part of the spontaneous response of a given individual, family or culture against different diseases and illnesses through the use of natural resources around them, which scientists tend to document, analyse and interpret.
- **Diego Rivera (Spain):** Ethnopharmacology is related to traditional knowledge and is often part of the TKS, but in itself is a complex of external influences, new practices and others that become extinct, with mainline traditions, all in reference to medicinal resources or *materia medica*.
- **Nicholas Sadgrove and Graham Jones (Australia):** Ethnopharmacology seeks to employ the modern scientific method to translate traditional therapeutic empiricism into a biological story that at first captivates us, then encourages us to experiment with its limitations, then finally persuades us to incorporate it into our accepted pharmacopoeia. The first people to tell this 'biological story' would no doubt be pleased that it has continued to be told for much longer and to a wider audience.
- **José Ramón Vallejo Villalobos (Spain):** Ethnopharmacology is the interdisciplinary science that focuses on the study of traditional uses of plants, animals and minerals as drugs in order to validate their physiological activity and discern the meaning of their cultural uses.
- **Alonso Verde, Diego Rivera, José Ramón Vallejo, José Fajardo, Concepción Obón and Arturo Valdés (Spain):** Ethnopharmacology is an interdisciplinary science focusing on the study of chemical composition, therapeutic activity, about natural drugs used by the local people and their cultural interpretations.
- **Liz Williamson (UK):** Ethnopharmacology is the study of natural medicines used by people of different cultures, and how those medicines may work.

We leave it to the reader to interpret these ideas and to draw conclusions from them. However, the field's inter- (or trans-) disciplinarity and its unique position at the interface of socio-cultural and natural sciences are two commonalities. This book shows both these unifying tendencies but also the great variety of ideas that contribute to modern ethnopharmacology.

The book is organized into three main sections. It begins with an overview of the subject, including a brief history, ethnopharmacological methods, the role of intellectual property protection, key analytical approaches, the role of ethnopharmacology in primary/secondary education, and links to biodiversity and ecological research. This part provides the *conceptual and methodological basis* for the book. Part two looks at *ethnopharmacological contributions to developing modern medicines* across a range of conditions, including CNS disorders, cancer, bone and joint health, and parasitic diseases. The final part is devoted to regional perspectives covering all continents, providing a *state-of-the-art assessment of the status of ethnopharmaco-logical research globally*, highlighting the diversity of perspectives on the five continents.

We as editors really want to and must thank all contributors. Contrary to other edited books, here the editors gave a very clear brief on what the main theme of each chapter should be and we are very grateful to the contributors for providing their perspectives on these topics.

The book also is part of the ULLA Pharmacy Series (www.ullapharmsci.org), which provides state-of-the-art, critical insights into a wide range of pharmaceutically relevant topics. ULLA is a European Consortium founded more than 20 years ago and includes nine leading schools of pharmacy at European universities in eight countries.

# Abbreviations

| | |
|---|---|
| 1D | one-dimensional |
| 2D | two-dimensional |
| AchE | acetylcholine esterase |
| AD | Alzheimer's disease |
| ADME | absorption, distribution, metabolism, and excretion (of a medicine) |
| AGI | α-glucosidase inhibitor |
| AHL | N-Acyl homoserine lactone |
| AI | autoinducer |
| AIDS | acquired immune deficiency syndrome |
| AIP | autoinducing peptide |
| ANVISA | Agência Nacional de Vigilância Sanitária (Brazil) |
| ART | artesunate |
| ART | anti-retroviral therapy |
| ATCC | American Type Culture Collection |
| ATM | African traditional medicine |
| AYUSH | Ayurveda, yoga & naturopathy, Unani, Siddha and homoeopathy |
| BFAD | Bureau of Food and Drugs |
| BP | blood pressure |
| CA | chlorogenic acid |
| CaCC | calcium-activated chloride channel |
| CAM | Complementary and Alternative Medicine |
| CBD | Convention on Biological Diversity |
| CET | cephalotaxine |
| CEMAT | Mesoamerican Centre of Appropriate Technology Studies (Guatemala) |
| CFDA | China Food and Drug Administration |
| CFTR | cystic fibrosis transmembrane conductance regulator |
| CHM | Chinese herbal medicine |
| CHMP | Chinese herbal medicinal product |
| CITES | Convention on International Trade in Endangered Species of Wild Flora and Fauna |
| CM | Chinese medicine |
| CNS | central nervous system |
| COPD | chronic obstructive pulmonary disease |

| | |
|---|---|
| COX | cyclooxygenase |
| COX-2 | cyclooxygenase-2 |
| CPD | continuing professional development |
| CSA | constitutive salicylic acid |
| CSIR | Council for Scientific and Industrial Research |
| CT | computed tomography |
| CVD | cardiovascular disease |
| D-IBS | diarrhoea-prominent irritable bowel syndrome |
| DMSO | Dimethylsulfoxide |
| DOH | Department of Health of the Philippines |
| DPD | 4,5-dihydroxy-2,3-pentadione |
| ECOWAS | Economic Community of West African States |
| EFSA | European Food Safety Authority |
| EGFR | epidermal growth factor receptor |
| EMA | European Medicines Agency |
| ESCOP | European Scientific Cooperative on Phytotherapy |
| FDA | Food and Drug Administration |
| FFA | free fatty acid |
| FRLHT | Foundation for the Revitalization of Local Health Traditions |
| GACP | good agricultural and collection practice |
| GBM | glioblastoma multiforme |
| GC | gas chromatography |
| GIP | glucose-dependent insulinotropic polypeptide |
| GLP | good laboratory practice |
| GMP | good manufacturing practice |
| HDL | high-density lipoprotein |
| HER | human epidermal growth factor receptor |
| HHT | homoharringtonine |
| HIV | human immunodeficiency virus |
| HMP | herbal medicinal product |
| HMPC | Committee for Herbal Medicinal Products |
| HPLC | high-performance liquid chromatography |
| HPLC-MS-SPE-NMR | high-performance liquid chromatography-mass spectrometry-solid-phase extraction-nuclear magnetic resonance |
| HRMS | high resolution mass spectrometry |
| HSV | herpes simplex virus |
| HTS | high throughput screening |
| ICBG | International Cooperative Biodiversity Group |
| ICH | International Conference on Harmonization (of Technical Requirements for Registration of Pharmaceuticals for Human Use) |
| IDF | International Diabetes Federation |
| IgE | immunoglobulin E |
| IGF | insulin growth factor |
| IGT | impaired glucose tolerance |
| IKK | IkB kinase |
| IL-1$\beta$ | interleukin-1$\beta$ |
| IMSS | Instituto Mexicano de Seguro Social |

| iNOS | inducible nitric oxide synthase |
|------|-------------------------------|
| IP | intellectual property |
| ISCED | International Standard Classification of Education |
| ISM&H | Department of Indian Systems of Medicines and Homeopathy |
| IUCN | International Union for the Conservancy of Nature |
| LC-MS | liquid chromatography-mass spectrometry |
| LOX-5 | lipoxygenase-5 |
| MAP | medicinal and aromatic plant |
| MCP | monocyte chemo-attractant protein |
| MDR | multidrug resistance |
| MHRA | Medicines and Healthcare Products Regulatory Agency |
| MIC | minimal inhibitory concentration |
| MIP | migration inhibitory protein |
| MRSA | methicillin-resistant *Staphylococcus aureus* |
| MS | mass spectrometry |
| MS | metabolic syndrome |
| MTT | 3-(4,5-dimethylthiazol-2-yl)-2,5-diphenyltetrazolium bromide |
| MVDA | multivariate data analysis |
| NDM-1 | New Delhi metallo-$\beta$-lactamase-1 |
| NF-kB | kappa-light-chain-enhancer B cells |
| NGO | non-governmental organisation |
| NIH | National Institutes of Health |
| NIHM | National Institutes of Herbal Medicine |
| NK | natural killer |
| NMDA | N-methyl-D-aspartate |
| NMPB | National Medicinal Plant Board |
| NMR | nuclear magnetic resonance |
| NSAID | non-steroidal anti-inflammatory drug |
| NSCLC | non-small cell lung carcinoma |
| OTC | over-the-counter |
| PBP | penicillin-binding protein |
| PCA | principal component analysis |
| PCR | polymerase chain reaction |
| PG | prostaglandin |
| PGE2 | prostaglandin E2 |
| PITAHC | traditional and alternative health care |
| PKC | protein kinase C |
| Pp1 | first Philippine pharmacopoeia |
| QS | quorum sensing |
| QSEC | quality, safe, efficacious and consistent |
| R&D | research and development |
| RCT | randomized controlled trial |
| RMA | resistance-modifying agent |
| RTO | retrospective treatment-outcome |
| SAHG | South African Hoodia Growers |
| SCLC | small cell lung carcinoma |
| SERM | selective oestrogen receptor modulator |
| SI | selectivity index |

| SPE | solid-phase extraction |
|-----|------------------------|
| SSRI | selective serotonin reuptake inhibitors |
| STI | sexually transmitted infection |
| T2D | type 2 diabetes |
| TB | tuberculosis |
| TCM | traditional Chinese medicine |
| THMP | traditional herbal medicinal products |
| THR | Traditional Herbal Regulation (of the European Union) |
| TK | traditional knowledge |
| TKDL | traditional knowledge digital library |
| TLR | toll-like receptor |
| TM | traditional medicine |
| TNF | tumour necrosis factor |
| TNFα | tumour necrosis factor α |
| TOCSY | total correlation spectroscopy |
| TRAMIL | Traditional Medicine in the Islands |
| TRIPS | trade-related aspects of intellectual property rights |
| TRPV1 | vanilloid type 1 protein |
| TTM | Thai traditional medicine |
| TTSS | type III secretion system |
| UNAM | Universidad Nacional Autónoma de México |
| UTI | urinary tract infection |
| VEGF | vascular endothelial growth factor |
| WHO | World Health Organization |
| WIMSA | Working Group of Indigenous Minorities in Southern Africa |
| WIPO | World Intellectual Property Organization |
| WTO | World Trade Organization |

# Ethnopharmacology: The Fundamental Challenges

# 1

# Ethnopharmacology: A Short History of a Multidisciplinary Field of Research

Michael Heinrich

*Centre for Pharmacognosy and Phytotherapy, UCL School of Pharmacy, University of London, London*

## 1.1 Introduction

Ethnopharmacology is an interdisciplinary field of research and as such it is defined by it concepts (its frame of reference) derived from a range of disciplines and the methodologies used. There can be no doubt that it is a fast-developing and thriving discipline. Confusingly, a large number of terms are used to describe research, which often uses relatively similar methods and concepts. However, each of these is distinguished by being placed in a certain tradition of research. Such terms include

- pharmacognosy, first used in 1811 by Johann Adam Schmidt and used very widely to describe the field of medicinal plant and natural product research
- phytotherapy research, derived from the French concept 'phytotherapie' introduced by Henri Leclerq in 1913 and used in various editions of his *Précis de Phytothérapie*
- phytomedicine, a term introduced much more recently and less well established internationally.

In addition there is a wide range of more descriptive terms, including medicinal plant research or natural product research, and there exists a considerable overlap between these and related terms. Phytotherapy research, for example, focuses on plant-based forms of treatment within a science-based medical practice and thus distinguishes what has also been called 'rational phytotherapy' from other more traditional approaches like medical herbalism,

*Ethnopharmacology*, First Edition. Edited by Michael Heinrich and Anna K. Jäger.
© 2015 John Wiley & Sons, Ltd. Published 2015 by John Wiley & Sons, Ltd.

which relies on an empirical appreciation of 'medicinal herbs'. Phytotherapy research is best described as a *science* embedded in the medical (and pharmaceutical) field (Heinrich, 2013). Contrary to this, at least in a part of the scholarly output, ethnopharmacology incorporates sociocultural concepts and methods.

In the broadest sense ethnopharmacology is based on approaches from the sociocultural sciences and the natural sciences/medicine. As such any historical overview will have to be based on the development of this scientific approach. However, written accounts of using herbal medicines and of the wider medical practice are of course available from many cultures (cf. Leonti, 2011). Importantly, this definition excludes the daily medical practice and the practitioners' observations associated with it. Such descriptions of medicines, as well as reflections about their usefulness, are very much part of traditions like Ayurveda, Kampo, Unnani, Arabic medicine, TCM, Aztec medicine, European herbalism or any other regionally or culturally defined medical practice. Clearly many of these original descriptions do not survive, and as a consequence today we often only have a few pieces of what was a much larger puzzle.

Compared to medical practice (be it in the context of its usage within biomedicine or one of the regional traditions as exemplified above), in ethnopharmacology there is an added focus on an empirical scientific (e.g. pharmacological, phytochemical, toxicological) evaluation of such therapeutic uses. In very general terms any form of empirical use and 'medical testing' of a plant for novel uses may be considered an ethnopharmacological approach. The physician William Withering (1741–1799) systematically explored the medical properties of foxglove (*Digitalis purpurea* L., Scrophulariaceae), which reportedly was used by an English housewife to treat dropsy. He used the orally transmitted knowledge of British herbalism to develop a medicine used by medical doctors. Prior to such studies, herbalism was more of a clinical practice interested in the patient's welfare and less of a systematic study of the virtues and chemical properties of medicinal plants.

Juerg Gertsch (2009) provided a short and concise definition: ethnopharmacology uses an approach where 'anecdotal efficacy of medicinal plants is put to test in the laboratory. The ethnopharmacologist tries to understand the pharmacological basis of culturally important plants.' Similarly, Daniel Moerman (University of Michigan, Dearborn) argued: 'Essentially ethnopharmacology is the examination of non-Western (not mine) medicinal plant use in terms of Western (my) plant use.' (Moerman, pers. comm.). Both definitions imply that ethnopharmacology has been a clearly defined field of research certainly since the quest of the 'unknown other' through Europeans and their descendants started with the explorations of missionaries, conquerors and explorers. Particularly in the 19th century, many researchers were involved in colonial explorations. This period is considered by Gertsch (2009) to be the golden age of ethnopharmacology. Without doubt these travellers in the broadest sense tried to grasp the essence of what 'other' people use and how it can be transformed into a useful commodity.

Ethnopharmacology investigates the pharmacological and toxicological activities of any preparation used by humans that has – in the very broadest sense – some beneficial or toxic or other direct pharmacological effects. This field of research is therefore not an exclusively descriptive field of research (i.e. describing local or traditional uses or medical practices), but about the combined anthropological (in a broad sense) and pharmacological–toxicological study of these preparations. Today, studies describing the use of medicinal and other useful plants are included within ethnopharmacological research, but these are generally conducted with the goal that they lead to an experimental study of some of these botanical drugs (cf. Heinrich *et al.*, 2009). At the same time ethnopharmacology is not focused on the description of medical effects in the content of a treatment (or medical case histories), but here again incorporates bioscientific research. The definition used here is therefore somewhat more focused and highlights the integration of experimental research on the effects of a local or traditional medicine with sociocultural approaches.

A classic example of ethnopharmacological research that has led to new medicines is the 'discovery' of curare. The study of the botanical origin of the arrow poison curare, its physiological (as well as toxic) effects and the compound responsible for these provides a fascinating example of an early ethnopharmacological approach. Curare was used by 'certain wild tribes in South America for poisoning their arrows' (von Humboldt, 1997). Many other explorers documented this usage and the poison fascinated both researchers and the wider public. Particularly well known are the detailed descriptions of the process used by Alexander von Humboldt (1769–1859) in 1800 to prepare poisoned arrows in Venezuela. There, von Humboldt met a group of indigenous people who were celebrating their return from an expedition to obtain the raw material for making the poison. Von Humboldt describes the 'chemical laboratory' used:

'He [an old Indian] was the chemist of the community. With him we saw large cooking pots (Siedekessel) made out of clay, to be used for boiling the plant sap; plainer containers, which speed up the evaporation process because of their large surface; banana leaves, rolled to form a cone-shaped bag [and] used to filter the liquid which may contain varying amounts of fibres. This hut transformed into a laboratory was very tidy and clean.'

(von Humboldt, 1997, p. 88)

And he too faced one of the classical problems of ethnopharmacology:

'We are unable to make a botanical identification because this tree [which produces the raw material for the production of curare] only grows at quite some distance from Esmeralda and because [it] did not have flowers and fruit. I had mentioned this type of misfortune previously, that the most noteworthy plants cannot be examined by the traveler, while others whose chemical activities are not known [i.e. which are not used locally] are found covered with thousands of flowers and fruit.'

In a later step *Chondrodendron tomentosum* Ruiz et Pavon was identified as being the botanical source of tube curare (named because of the Graminaeous tubes used as storage containers). Other species of the Menispermaceae (*Chondrodendron* spp., *Curarea* spp. and *Abuta* spp.) and species of the Loganiaceae (*Strychnos* spp.) have also been used in the production of curares.

However, this did not provide any understanding of the pharmacological effects of this poison. The French physiologist Claude Bernard (1813–1878) is recognized as being the first to have conducted such research. For example; he provides the following description of the pharmacological effects of curare in some detail: 'If curare is applied into a living tissue via an arrow or a poisoned instrument, it results in death more quickly if it gets into the blood vessels more rapidly. Therefore death occurs more rapidly if one uses dissolved curare instead of the dried toxin.' (Bernard, 1966, p. 92 [orig. 1864]). 'One of the facts noted by all those who reported on curare is the lack of toxicity of the poison in the gastrointestinal tract. The Indians indeed use curare as a poison and as a remedy for the stomach' (Bernard, 1966, p. 93). He showed that the animals did not show any nervousness and any sign of pain. Instead, the main sign of death induced by curare is muscular paralysis. If the blood flow in the hind leg of a frog is interrupted using a ligature, but without interrupting the innervation, and it is poisoned via an injury of the hind leg, it retains its mobility and the animal does not die from curare poisoning (Bernard, 1966, p. 115). These and subsequent studies allowed a detailed understanding of the pharmacological effects of curare in causing respiratory paralysis. Later on the main secondary metabolite responsible for this activity was isolated for the first time from *C. tomentosum*, and in 1947 the structure of the bisbenzylisoquinoline alkaloid d-tubocurarine was established. Finally, tubocurarine's structure was established unequivocally using nuclear magnetic resonance (NMR) in the 1970s (Heinrich, 2001, 2010).

This account describes a sequence of research activities, which in their totality clearly may today be labelled ethnopharmacogical research. However, at the time it was simply one of the many explorations of the unknown followed by the pharmacological investigation of the botanical drug and later on the identification of the active principles. In essence it was just normal state-of-the-art pharmacological research using new 'leads'. In other words it had no specific claim to be an activity different from mainstream (or normal) pharmacology (in a Thomas S. Kuhnian sense). In fact discoveries in the chemistry and pharmacology of natural products are generally linked to species that are of major importance as a medicine or toxin (Heinrich *et al.*, 2012). However 'Phantastica' (Holmstedt, 1967) and toxins certainly attracted the attention of 19th century researchers (and many before and after them). Terms used to describe this research in the 19th and early 20th century include 'Pharmakoëthnologie' used by Tschirch (1910) in his classic *Handbuch der Pharmakognosie* and 'pharmacoetnologia'. Other terms used include 'ethnobotany' and 'aboriginal botany' (both conceptually much broader terms dealing with useful plants in general). However, all these terms in essence focused on the description of indigenous medicinal plant use and not so much on their pharmacological investigation.

A paradigm shift in pharmacology, drug development and more broadly in the biosciences and medicine resulted from the serendipitous discovery of the first antibiotics derived from the fungus *Penicillum notatum* by Alexander Fleming (1881–1955) in 1928 at St Mary's Hospital (London), which were soon afterwards identified as benzylpenicillin and introduced into clinical practice by a team involving, most importantly, Howard Florey (1898–1968) and Ernst B. Chain (1906–1979). These fungal metabolites changed forever the perception and use of plant-derived metabolites as medicines by both scientists and the lay public. Of similar importance was the advent of synthetic chemistry in the field of pharmacy and its use in the development of new medicines (which started well before the discovery of the penicillins). In 1891 Paul Ehrlich in Germany (1854–1915) for the first time used a synthetic compound as a chemotherapeutic agent – methylene blue in the treatment of mild forms of malaria. Both developments proved that there were diverse and newer avenues to discover new medicines (Heinrich *et al.*, 2012) and revolutionized drug development during and after the Second World War. At the same time there can be no doubt that this resulted in a decline in an interest in the classical approaches as described above.

None of the research activities discussed in the previous paragraphs were labelled 'ethnopharmacology'. This term was – to the best of our knowledge – only formally introduced in 1967 by Efron *et al.*, who used it in the title of a book on hallucinogens: *Ethnopharmacological Search for Psychoactive Drugs* (Efron *et al.*, 1970; Holmstedt, 1967). This is much later than, for example, the term 'ethnobotany', which in 1896 was coined by the American botanist William Harshberger describing the study of human plant use. Both ethnopharmacology and ethnobotany investigate the relationship between humans and plants in all its complexity. However, interestingly, in the early years of its usage the term 'ethnopharmacology' was very much associated with the study of hallucinogenic plants used by indigenous people throughout the world. Along a similar vein of argument, 19th-century research into phantastica and other hallucinogenic substances played a crucial role in developing the field of psychopharmacology/neuropharmacology (cf. Holmstedt, 1967). Bo Holmstedt (1919–2002), who had a keen interest in toxicology, neuropharmacology and neurotoxicology as well as in analytical aspects of medicinal plant research, has to be credited with being one of the first to develop a perspective on what ethnopharmacology can contribute to science. However, his role and contribution has not been researched in detail from the perspective of the history of science.

In the context of modern ethnopharmacology the focus has moved to understanding the benefits and risks of commonly used local and traditional plants with the goal of contributing to better and safer uses of such resources (e.g. Heinrich, 2006; Heinrich *et al.*, 2009). As in the 19th century it requires an integration of pharmacological (or other natural science) approaches with research on local and traditional uses. After its initial use in the context of hallucinogenic plants the term was only used occasionally until 1979, when the *Journal of Ethnopharmacology* was founded by Laurent Rivier and Jan Bruhn. Here the scope was broadened to 'a multi-disciplinary area of research concerned with the observation, description, and experimental investigation of indigenous drugs and their biological activity' (Rivier and Bruhn, 1979).

Today, research which claims to use an ethnopharmacological approach is commonly conducted in the fast-emerging economies of Asia (India, China, where it is often seen as specific research on traditional Chinese medicine (TCM), and South Korea), America south of the Rio Grande (Brazil and Mexico) and Africa (South Africa). The classical research-active countries of the West (USA, UK, Spain, France, Germany and Italy) also have some research-active groups (data based on an analysis of the source items documented in Scopus). The overall research output has also skyrocketed, with a dramatic increase in the number of papers published since the first paper was published in 1967. A detailed content analysis of what is published in the field is beyond the scope of this overview, but if one takes the more than 2000 source items that include the term 'ethnopharmacology' in the keywords, abstract or title, the two therapeutic areas most commonly included are the anti-inflammatory and anti-cancer effects of locally and traditionally used plants, which are included in a third and a quarter of these studies, respectively. Gastrointestinal, respiratory and dermatological conditions are addressed in about 10% each of these studies, with veterinary ethnopharmacology accounting for a similar share. All others are of lesser importance and interestingly only about 5% of all studies incorporate central nervous system (CNS) activities (and even fewer studies include hallucinogenic effects (<2%). As one would expect, questions relating to the toxicity of local and traditional medicines are addressed in a quite a few studies (about a quarter). Even though this is a very crude measure, it highlights the main trends and interests in ethnopharmacology and demonstrates how the current focus has moved away from the interests that were the main focus in the 19th century and the 1960s and 1970s. Recent years have also seen an increasing awareness of basic conceptual and methodological standards in the field, an aspect addressed not only by many of the authors cited above but also in a series of critical reviews trying to define good practice as it relates to specific methodological and conceptual foundations of the field (Verspohl, 2002; Cos *et al.*, 2006; Chan *et al.*, 2012; Sheridan *et al.*, 2012; Uzuner *et al.*, 2012; Bennett and Balick, 2014; Rivera *et al.*, 2014).

This brief historical sketch identifies some major developments of a field of research that is not a clearly defined discipline, a point highlighted by Nina Etkin and Elaine Elisabetsky (2005, p. 23):

'A primary difficulty in defining and projecting a future for ethnopharmacology is to identify the objectives of a largely virtual field whose self-identified membership represents, in addition to commercial entities, a diverse suite of academic and applied disciplines.'

(Etkin and Elisabetsky, 2005).

In their analysis they identify key areas of relevance in the future, but most importantly they see the need to build theoretical capacity in ethnopharmacology (Etkin and Elisabetsky, 2005, p. 26). This is one foundation for developing more context-driven and critical approaches in ethnopharmacology (Etkin and Elisabetsky, 2005). As this overview shows, the historical development of the field was very much driven by interdisciplinary collaborations generally led by natural scientists. A more detailed historical analysis will provide a basis to build up the 'theoretical capacity' the Etkin and Elisabetsky call for.

## Acknowledgements

The history of the field has been an ongoing interest of mine and the ideas presented here have developed over many years. Some were discussed in more detail previously (especially in Heinrich, 2014; Heinrich *et al.*, 2012) and this work presents a new synthesis of these concepts. The history of ethnopharmacology has received relatively little attention and a more detailed study of the developments since the mid-1960s would certainly be highly desirable. I am grateful to all the colleagues who responded to my query about the field's history, most importantly Lars Bohlin (Sweden), Jan G. Bruhn (Sweden), Elaine Elisabetsky (Brazil), Anna Jäger (Denmark), Marco Leonti (Italy), J. David Phillipson (UK), Laurent Rivier (Switzerland), Dan E. Moerman (Michigan, USA), Gunnar Samuelsson (Sweden) Peter A.G.M. de Smet (the Netherlands) and Caroline Weckerle (Switzerland).

## References

Bennett, B.C. and Balick, M.J. (2014) Does the name really matter? The importance of botanical nomenclature and plant taxonomy in biomedical research. *Journal of Ethnopharmacology*, **152**, 387–392.

Bernard, C. (1966) Physiologische Untersuchungen über einige amerikanische Gifte. Das Curare, in *Ausgewählte physiologische Schriften* (eds C. Bernard and N. Mani), Huber Verlag. Bern. [French original. 1864], pp. 84–133.

Chan, K., Shaw, D., Simmonds, M.S.J., *et al.* (2012). Good practice in reviewing and publishing studies on herbal medicine, with special emphasis on traditional Chinese medicine and Chinese materia medica. *Journal of Ethnopharmacology*, **140**, 469–475.

Cos, P., Vlietinck, A.J., Berghe, D.V. and Maes, L. (2006) Anti-infective potential of natural products: How to develop a stronger in vitro 'proof-of-concept. *Journal of Ethnopharmacology*, **106**, 290–302.

Efron, D., Holmstedt, B. and Kline, N.L. (1970) *Ethnopharmacologic Search for Psychoactive Drugs*, Government Printing Office, Public Health Service Publications No. 1645 (original 1967), Reprint, Washington, D.C.

Etkin, N.L. and Elisabetsky, E. (2005) Seeking a transdisciplinary and culturally germane science: The future of ethnopharmacology. *Journal of Ethnopharmacology*, **100** (1–2), 23–26.

Gertsch, J. (2009) How scientific is the science in ethnopharmacology? Historical perspectives and epistemological problems. *Journal of Ethnopharmacology*, **122**, 177–183.

Heinrich, M. (2001) *Ethnobotanik und Ethnopharmazie,* Eine Einführung, Stuttgart, Wissenschaftliche Verlagsgesellschaft.

Heinrich, M. (2006) La Etnofarmacología – 'quo vadis? *BLACPMA* [Boletín Latinoamericana y del Caribe de plantas medicinales y aromáticas, ISSN 0717 7917], **5** (1), 7.

Heinrich, M. (2010) Ethnopharmacology and drug development, in *Comprehensive Natural Products II, Chemistry and Biology*, Vol. **3** (eds L. Mander and H.-W. Lui), Elsevier, Oxford, pp. 351–381.

Heinrich, M. (2013) Phytotherapy, in *Encyclopedia Britannica*, http://www.britannica.com/EBchecked/topic/1936369/phytotherapy.

Heinrich, M. (2014) Ethnopharmacology – quo vadis? Challenges for the future. *Revista Brasileira de Farmacognosia* **24**, 99–102.

Heinrich, M., Edwards, S., Moerman, D.E. and Leonti, M. (2009) Ethnopharmacological Field Studies: A Critical Assessment of their Conceptual Basis and Methods. *Journal of Ethnopharmacology*, **124**, 1–17.

Heinrich, M., Barnes, J., Gibbons, S. and Williamson, E.M. (2012) *Fundamentals of Pharmacognosy and Phytotherapy*, 2nd edn, Churchill Livingston (Elsevier), Edinburgh & London.

Holmstedt, B. (1967) An overview of ethnopharmacology. Historical survey. *Psychopharmacology Bulletin*, **4** (3), 2–3.

Leonti, M. (2011) The future is written: impact of scripts on the cognition, selection, knowledge and transmission of medicinal plant use and its implications for ethnobotany and ethnopharmacology. *Journal of* Ethnopharmacology, **134** (3), 542–555.

Rivera, D., Allkin, R., Obón, C., *et al.* (2014) What is in a name? The need for accurate scientific nomenclature for plants. *Journal of Ethnopharmacology*, **152**, 393–402.

Rivier, L. and Bruhn, J.G. (1979) *Editorial. Journal of Ethnopharmacology*, **1** (1), 1.

Sheridan, H., Krenn, L., Jiang, R., *et al.* (2012) The potential of metabolic fingerprinting as a tool for the modernisation of TCM preparations. *Journal of Ethnopharmacology*, **140**, 482–491.

Tschirch, A. (1910) *Handbuch der Pharmakognosie*. 2. Abteilung (Die Hilfswissenschaften der Pharmakognosie), 1. Auflage, C.H. Tachnitz, Leipzig.

Uzuner, H., Bauer, R., Fan, T.-P., *et al.* (2012) Traditional Chinese medicine research in the post-genomic era: Good practice, priorities, challenges and opportunities. *Journal of Ethnopharmacology*, **140** (3), 458–468.

Verspohl, E.J. (2002) Recommended testing in diabetes research. *Planta Medica*, **68** (7), 581–590.

von Humboldt, A. (1997) *Die Forschungsreise in den Tropen Amerikas* (Hrsg. H. Beck), Wissenschaftliche Buchgesellschaft, Darmstadt.

# 2

# Medicinal Plant Research: A Reflection on Translational Tasks

Anna K Jäger

*Department of Drug Design and Pharmacology, Faculty of Health and Medicinal Sciences, University of Copenhagen, Denmark*

## 2.1  Introduction

Allopathic medicine is based on the underlying principle that drugs and treatments have been objectively and scientifically evaluated, whereas traditional medicine systems are based on a 'holistic' approach integrating medicinal and psychological therapies. In traditional practice, the psychological, spiritual and social aspects play an important role, exploiting the power of the mind of the patient. This holistic treatment can to some degree make up for plant medicines not being as effective as allopathic biomedicine.

Traditional medicine, which is closely linked with peoples' cultures, is therefore not going to vanish if and when allopathic health care becomes available. A study from Kenya showed that patients chose to visit a health clinic for some diseases, but preferred a traditional healer in other cases (van der Geest, 1997). In South Africa, traditional healers are flourishing in urban areas alongside allopathic health care (Mander *et al.*, 1997), thus traditional healing practice is not dying out 'when the young flock to the city and forget their culture', as has been predicted.

Despite allopathic and traditional healing systems having a common goal in helping patients, the two systems are fundamentally too divergent in their views for any meaningful integration. Healers might say that their ancestors guide them, that they know all there is to be known, but I believe there is still place for new knowledge that can be accepted by traditional healers. We as scientists cannot meddle with the non-scientific aspects of traditional medicine, our role must be to work on improving the medicinal aspect, the usage of medicinal plants.

*Ethnopharmacology*, First Edition. Edited by Michael Heinrich and Anna K. Jäger.
© 2015 John Wiley & Sons, Ltd. Published 2015 by John Wiley & Sons, Ltd.

In recent years, 'back-translation' has become a buzz word in pharmacological research. However, the good old discipline of ethnopharmacology is and has always been back-translation. Ethnopharmacology is centred around the patient, observing diagnosis, treatment and treatment outcomes, and then taking these observations back to the laboratory to investigate the (plant-based) medicines involved. This might lead both to new drugs and to identifying new targets, but most importantly it develops an evidence base for such preparations.

If the aim is not a new drug lead or, even better, a new target, but improvement of traditional medicines, what then is our task? Whether we aim at a traditional commercial product or a situation where the healer or patient prepares the remedy, the initial preclinical procedures are the same. A key assumption underlying this chapter and the other chapters in this book is that we need evidence-based, safe traditional medicines and medical practice.

## 2.2   Translational research: preclinical research

Traditional medicine consists of plant, animal and mineral materials. As plant material constitutes the major part of traditional medicine, I refer only to plants in this text, but the principles are the same for animal-derived materials, and to a degree for minerals.

Translational research spans over several disciplines connecting preclinical and clinical work. In our field we first do back-translation from patient to the laboratory, then forward translation through preclinical work, including *in vitro* methods for elucidating mode of action, *in vivo* studies, ADME, toxicology and clinical studies, to finally get the medicine (or knowledge on the medicine) to the patient.

The very first step in the forward translation, and in a way the most crucial, is the test material. The identity of the material has to be certain and to be documented. It is required that the species investigated are precisely defined using a fully taxonomically validated nomenclature, which includes the current systematic binominal name and authority. It requires botanical expertise to ensure that a particular plant is determined to the right species and 'converted' from an old name (synonym) to the current name (currently, the best practice is to use www.theplantlist.org for checking botanical names and families). There ought not to be an issue with documentation, it should to be a normal part of good laboratory practice (GLP), but sadly as a reviewer for many journals I recurrently find problems with the botanical documentation in the form of vouchers. When authors are requested to provide documentation, voucher numbers are then provided; I honestly sometime wonder if these vouchers really exist. I would recommend that scientific journals request a photograph of the voucher submitted as supplementary material; *Journal of Ethnopharmacology* is now recommending this practice (Heinrich and Verpoorte, 2014).

Where preclinical work on a synthetic compound may have issues with contaminants from the manufacturing processes, in case of plant extracts we deal with a very complicated, mostly ill-defined matrix. The plant material used for traditional medicine will in most cases vary in concentration of active constituents from batch to batch due to the biological variation in the material. The variation is due to geographical factors, climatic variations and genetic factors. Ideally, it would be good to make a broad sampling of material to compare the variation before any preclinical work commences. By opting for a NMR-based technique, which measures all constituents, it is possible to see patterns of similarity in cases where the active constituent(s) are unknown. With modern NMR-based multivariate analysis it is possible to ascertain outliers, so a batch can be chosen that is representative of the general sampling. The results then have a better chance of being representative of the species under investigation.

While clinical trials and *in vivo* experiments are under strict regulation by authorities, the *in vitro* area is not. This has resulted in a situation where many methods are applied. My students recently wanted to compare some antibacterial results with published literature. This proved difficult. The studies used different inoculum sizes, did not state the concentration of ethanol or dimethyl sulfoxide used to dissolve the extracts, used different numbers of replicates, used different volumes of reactants, incubated for different times, determined inhibition in different ways, and, of course, different test bacteria were used. This highlights the problem we have in our field with a lack of standard methods. It should be possible to perform something as simple as an antibacterial test in the same way in laboratories all over the world.

If we look to a younger research field such as molecular biology, they have benefitted enormously from having standard methods that everyone uses. Commercial companies have developed kits for these methods, further ensuring comparable results. Such results can then be compiled in world-wide databases, for example GeneBank. Of course, contrary to genes, which are made up of the same few components in all living organisms, the variation in the plant matrix is so great that it would be difficult to apply standard methods for extraction – or would it? Are we just too anarchistic or sloppy to make our extracts in the same way? If we return to *in vitro* testing, here we are beyond the differences in the plant matrix, we have a test substance and it is possible to test it by adhering to the same protocols all over the world. The *Journal of Ethnopharmacology* has taken the lead with publishing a series of Setting Standard papers. The series includes the topics of ethnopharmacological field studies (Heinrich *et al.*, 2009), anti-infective agents (Cos *et al.*, 2006), diagnostic procedures in experimental diabetes research (Matteucci and Giampietro, 2008) and animal models in diabetes (Froede and Medeiros, 2008). This covers only a fraction of the methods in this wide field, so herewith is a call to anyone who can contribute an adequate setting standard paper to write it.

Toxicology is the Achilles' heel of ethnopharmacology. We all want to promote efficient and *safe* traditional medicines, but toxicological aspects of local and traditional medicinal plants are sorely under investigated. It is relatively clear what the task is, the WHO (2000) has guidelines for toxicology testing of traditional medicine and many regulatory authorities have precise descriptions of what is required for registering herbal products – the same level should be what we want for traditional medicines. Most regulatory authorities require tests for acute and chronic toxicity, mutagenicity and teratogenicity. Of equal importance is the purity of the herbal substances used medicinally. Assessment of potential interactions of herbal medicines with other medicines is also an important field.

A recent book reviews methods in toxicology testing of medicinal plants and gives an overview of the toxicology of African medicinal plants (Kuerte, 2014).

Toxicological testing is costly, tenacious and does not make a high-impact journal article. Most of the laboratories undertaking preclinical work on medicinal plants are not geared to perform toxicology testing and academic research institutions do not have the funds to out-source toxicology testing to laboratories running on a commercial basis. I have a dream that one day a centre will open that will perform toxicology testing on all the major medicinal plants from all over the world.

## 2.3  Translational research: clinical research

When reading articles in journals in the medicinal plant field, one often reads in the conclusion claims along the lines of 'these data support the use of this plant in traditional medicine'. Sadly, these claims are often very broad and are, in fact, not substantiated by the data presented. The data might lend support for a pharmacological use for the plant, but it is mostly only a very small part of the picture and it would not be possible to make any recommendations for use in patients.

Maybe it would be a good exercise to ask yourself, if you put money into a clinical trial, what preclinical evidence would you want to see as a minimum? Assessing such data, one learns all too often that the research in general is scattered and not sufficient. There needs to be much more focused research to provide the necessary preclinical evidence for medicinal plants.

When a good case has been built on preclinical data and a safe toxicology profile, the next stumbling block is moving to a clinical trial. Most of the preclinical work on medicinal plants is today done in academic laboratories by non-medical staff. The laboratory-based researchers involved have little contact with clinical trial scientists, the link in the translational chain is missing. It is imperative that scientists designing and running clinical trials have the proper training. Clinical trials on traditional medicine must meet the scientific standards set for clinical trials of allopathic drugs. In order to ascertain that a clinical trial has an impact, one must ensure that the research is of a good quality. Far too often meta-analyses of clinical trials on herbal products come to the conclusion that the clinical trials are not of sufficient quality and do not provide new insights. This is tainting herbal medicine. We need to get better at bridging this step from preclinical work to clinical trial. We have a problem in persuading allopathic-trained medical scientists experienced in clinical trials to conduct trials on traditional medicines. Part of the solution is to raise the quality of the preclinical work. It is encouraging to see that around the world several programmes have been initiated to train clinical scientists to specifically run trials on traditional medicine (Wilcox *et al.*, 2012).

For clinical trials, the production of the trial medicine under conditions acceptable to the regulatory medicines agency, which must grant permission to perform the clinical trial, might be another problem. In some countries it might be difficult to find places that are geared to handle extractions of larger quantities of plant materials under full good manufacturing practice (GMP). It is essential that all botanical material used for the trial medicine is authenticated and that chemical profiles for the final product are available.

## 2.4   Reaching the patient

The final part of the translational process is to get the medicine – now with evidence for efficacy and safety – to the patients who need it. If a commercial traditional product is being produced, the marketing rests with the producer, who can be expected to be effective as financial interests are involved. The situation is different where the preclinical and clinical work has been done with no aim of producing a commercial product, maybe by an academic institution. Indigenous knowledge, patenting and licensing of patents are addressed by Alan Hesketh (see Chapter 9). How will the knowledge on medicinal plants reach healers and patients? In countries with functional traditional healers' associations it might be possible to disseminate scientific results via their networks. Otherwise, we stand with an immense problem, which we as a discipline have not been able to solve in the past (Jäger, 2005). Maybe some clever mobile phone/internet-based app that distributes information on how to prepare safe and effective herbal medicines could be a way forward?

## 2.5   A 'developed' traditional medicine system

Although there is not an even distribution of medicinal plants among the geographical areas of our planet, there is a striking difference in the number of medicinal plants that have

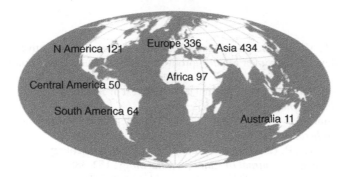

**Figure 2.1**  Estimate of continental origin of commercialized medicinal plants. (Source: Adapted from van Wyk and Wink 2004.)

been developed commercially from the different continents (Figure 2.1). The historical and economic reasons for this situation are many, but it also points to unharvested potentials.

In 1998, just over half of all medicinal plants in the *European Pharmacopoeia* came from the northern temperate zone (Heinrich and Leimkugel, 1999). In recent years, the section on plant monographs in the *European Pharmacopeia* has expanded rapidly. A very large percentage of these new monographs are on Chinese traditional medicine plants. Very few new monographs are on plants originating in Africa or South America.

A peculiar aspect about Europe, especially northern Europe, is that it has mostly lost its traditional healing practice. I always like to say that the knowledge 'went up in smoke' with the burning of our witches, though not all were burned and it was other and later developments that lead to the move away from 'folk' medical systems – herbal medicine was also the only medicine available to trained medical doctors at that time. Scientific developments such as the isolation of the first alkaloid, morphine, in 1804, developed new paradigms and a tremendous push in research interest. It planted the idea of using a single compound rather than a plant-based preparation. The industrial revolution formed the basis for a pharmaceutical industry, which from the beginning of the 20th century focused on synthetic drugs. The new synthetic drugs totally outcompeted the old plant-based medicines.

Although the traditional healers largely disappeared, the knowledge of the plants survived, partly due to well-written records on how to use such preparations.

Europe had the expertise and production facilities that could be used for the production of herbal products, and a tradition for legal regulation. These factors facilitated the transformation of traditional medicine into regulated commercialized phytomedicines and food supplements, with appropriate quality assurance and often as standardized products. Today new 'traditional healers' are in place, called phytotherapists or naturopaths and operating within the alternative and complementary healthcare systems. They undergo training that is more or less regulated (in many cases by competent authorities) and have associations that recognize qualified members.

In this way Europe has managed to create a (alternative) health system where the healers are trained to a certain level of qualifications, where the herbal medicine is safe, effective and standardised. The European situation shows this is achievable and could serve as a model for the development of traditional medicine that is in line with the recommendations of WHO's new Traditional Medicine Strategy: 2014–2023 (WHO, 2013).

# References

Cos, P., Vlietinck, A.J., Vanden Berghe, D. and Maes, L. (2006) Anti-infective potential of natural products: how to develop a stronger *in vitro* 'proof-of-concept'. *Journal of Ethnopharmacology*, **106**, 290–302.

Froede, T.S.A. and Medeiros, Y.S. (2008) Animal models to test drugs with potential antidiabetic activity. *Journal of Ethnopharmacology*, **115**, 173–183.

Heinrich, M. and Leimkugel, J. (1999) Arzneidrogen im deutschen und europäischen Arzneibuch. *Zeitschrift für Phytotherapie*, **20**, 264–267.

Heinrich, M. and Verpoorte, R. (2014) Good practice in ethnopharmacology and other sciences relying on taxonomic nomenclature. *Journal of Ethnopharmacology*, **152**, 385–386.

Heinrich, M., Edwards, S., Moerman, D.E. and Leonti, M. (2009) Ethnopharmacological field studies: a critical assessment of their conceptual basis and methods. *Journal of Ethnopharmacology*, **124**, 1–17.

Jäger, A.K. (2005) Is traditional medicine better off 25 years later? *Journal of Ethnopharmacology*, **100**, 3–4.

Kuerte, V. (2014) *Toxicological Survey of African Medicinal Plants*, Elsevier, London. ISBN 9780128000182.

Mander, J., Quinn, N.W. and Mander, M. (1997) Trade in Wildlife Medicinals in South Africa, Investigational Report Number 157, Institute of Natural Resources, Pietermaritzburg.

Matteucci, E. and Giampietro, O. (2008) Proposal open for discussion: defining agreed diagnostic procedures in experimental diabetes research. *Journal of Ethnopharmacology*, **115**, 163–172.

van der Geest, S. (1997) Is there a role for traditional medicine in basic health services in Africa? A plea for a community perspective. *Tropical Medicine and International Health*, **2**, 903–911.

van Wyk, B.E. and Wink, M. (2004) *Medicinal Plants of the World*, Briza Publications, Pretoria.

WHO (2000) General Guidelines for Methodologies on Research and Evaluation of Traditional Medicine, WHO/EDM/TRM/2000.1.

WHO (2013) WHO traditional medicine strategy: 2014–2023, WHO Press, World Health Organization, Switzerland ISBN 978-92-4-150609-0, http://apps.who.int/iris/bitstream/10665/92455/1/978924150609 0_eng.pdf?ua=1.

Willcox, M., Siegfried, N. and Johnson, Q. (2012) Capacity for clinical research on herbal medicine in Africa. *Journal of Alternative and Complementary Medicine*, **18**, 622–688.

# 3

# The Anthropology of Ethnopharmacology

Ina Vandebroek[1] and Daniel E. Moerman[2]

[1]*Matthew Calbraith Perry Assistant Curator of Economic Botany and Caribbean Program Director, The New York Botanical Garden, Bronx, New York, USA*
[2]*William E Stirton Emeritus Professor of Anthropology, University of Michigan-Dearborn, USA*

## 3.1   Introduction

Ten years ago, Nina Etkin and Elaine Elisabetsky, in the 100th issue of *Journal of Ethnopharmacology*, argued for a multidisciplinary ethnopharmacology of equal parts, they said: 'ethno- (Gr., culture or people) [and] pharmacology (Gr., drug) … a transdisciplinary exploration that spans the biological and social sciences' (Etkin and Elisabetsky, 2005). They also noted that a number of analyses done over time looking closely at the flagship journal of the field showed that *Journal of Ethnopharmacology* was nearly fully populated by articles that were purely pharmacology or pharmacognosy; only 4–6% of articles, they noted, were multidisciplinary in nature. Surely this is still true today.

Moreover, much research in ethnopharmacology to this day trumpets the ideal of finding the cures for cancer and Aids (or other high-profile diseases) in the tropical forest; see, for example, Albuquerque *et al.* (2012) or Saslis-Lagoudakis *et al.* (2012) or Leitão *et al.* (2013) to mention only a few.

This remains a popular cry even though the record of the past 50 years is very thin indeed: the Vinca alkaloids (Wani and Horwitz, 2014), Taxol from *Taxus brevifolia* Nutt. (Suffness, 1993)[1] and perhaps artemisinin from *Artemisia annua* L. (Miller and Su, 2011). These cases show that it is possible, but the rise and fall of Shaman Pharmaceuticals (Clapp and Crook, 2002), for example, and the sad history of Paul Cox's prostratin (probably the best ethnobotanical lead of all times (Gustafson *et al.*, 1992; Cox, 2001), which could probably cure both AIDS and

---

[1] Taxol was originally identified in a random screen; the plant had been in use by many north-western native Americans and First Nations people, often for skin irritations (Moerman, 1998).

---

*Ethnopharmacology*, First Edition. Edited by Michael Heinrich and Anna K. Jäger.
© 2015 John Wiley & Sons, Ltd. Published 2015 by John Wiley & Sons, Ltd.

ebola, and 15 years later it still isn't approved for use) all point to the difficulties inherent in this enterprise.

By contrast, there is much satisfaction to be obtained from pursuing a richly multidisciplinary approach to the relationships between plants and the people who know, or think about, or care for them. We give one longer and several shorter examples of this, operating on dramatically different scales.

## 3.2   Primary example: Traditional medicine in New York City

*Botánicas* in New York City are Hispanic/Latino-Afro-Caribbean stores that sell statues, beads and potions for spiritual well-being and often also herbal remedies (Viladrich, 2006) (Figures 3.1, 3.2 and 3.3). During a visit to one of these *botánicas*, I (IV) met a middle-aged woman from the Dominican Republic who was purchasing a *botella* (a herbal mixture; Vandebroek *et al.*, 2010) prepared by the store owner. I asked her about her health complaint and she told me she had been diagnosed with ovarian cysts. She explained that she had gone to the hospital to find out what she was suffering from. As soon as she got her diagnosis, she knew exactly what treatment to choose. I asked her why she had chosen a *botella*. The answer she gave was without hesitation: she had faith in the *botánica* owner and in his remedies. The Dominican community in New York City is tight knit and easily exchanges information about health, and the *botánica* owner is well-known for successfully treating ovarian cysts

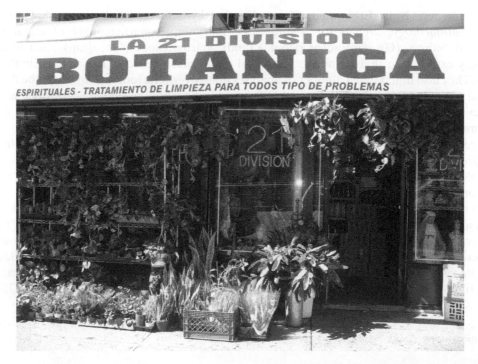

**Figure 3.1**   Storefront of a *botánica* in New York City. Banner reads: 'Cleansing treatment for all kinds of problems'.

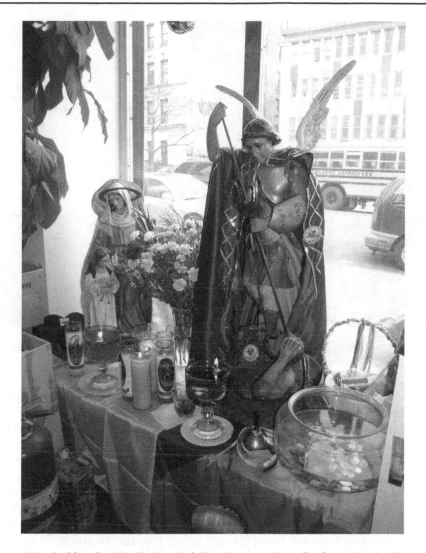

**Figure 3.2**   Inside a *botánica* in New York City. Statues and candles for spiritual well-being.

with his own recipes. Thus, it did not come as a surprise that the *botánica* was exactly where the woman went for help.

This is not an isolated story and it reveals three issues of relevance to ethnopharmacology as a scientific discipline.

## 3.2.1   Missing out on cultural context

The first issue is that the full picture may not be seen if culture is not included in research into the pharmacological effects of plants. Culture is at the heart of plant meaning. Understanding the use of medicinal plants without detailed knowledge of their cultural context is like watching a movie in a language you do not understand. Much as you might misinterpret the images of a foreign movie without subtitles, you may come to incorrect conclusions about plant use if you

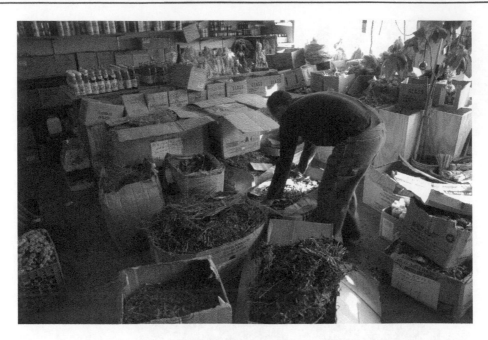

**Figure 3.3**   Inside a *botánica* in New York City. Boxes of dried medicinal plants for health care.

only take into account your own scientific understanding of the pharmacology of plants. Thus, important pieces of information may be missed. That information is cultural. For example, in the Dominican community there is a shared cultural belief that plants with bitter properties 'burn sugar in the blood', which renders them useful medicines for treating diabetes (Vandebroek *et al.*, 2007). In Jamaican culture, bitter plants are believed to cleanse the blood and thereby rid the body of skin rashes and other skin problems (Payne-Jackson and Alleyne, 2004). According to Italian traditional knowledge, bitter edible greens are perceived as being particularly beneficial for the liver and for cleansing the blood (Nebel *et al.*, 2006). Cultural meaning can also include the belief that for a plant medicine to work properly, it should be able to expel something from the body, through either vomiting or stools. In the Dominican community, the shared belief exists that pharmaceuticals hide the pain of the disease but do not cure it because nothing is expelled; in contrast people use plants that are able to promote this desired physiological effect. These cultural observations may be of importance to the ethnopharmacological evaluation of the efficacies of different groups of plant chemicals, as well as their toxicities. This kind of information can enrich laboratory data in complementary ways, and may even lead to testing new mechanisms of action. For example, do all 'bitter' plant species used for a similar ethnobotanical purpose, even those belonging to different plant families, show a similar mechanism of action when tested in the laboratory?

### 3.2.2   People change plants due to availability

The second issue is that culture influences the dynamics of plant knowledge and use. In an urban context, immigrants from the Dominican Republic who move to New York City substitute plants with others that are more easily available in their new environment (Ososki *et al.*, 2007). Examples of this include the use of cat's claw (*Uncaria tomentosa* DC.,

Rubiaceae) and cranberry (*Vaccinium macrocarpon* Aiton, Ericaceae) for treating uterine fibroids. Dominicans also adapt their plant pharmacopoeias to better match and respond to the epidemiological context of New York City. For example, in the Dominican Republic *botellas* are used more often to treat genitourinary disorders, whereas in New York City they become more popular for treating respiratory disorders (Vandebroek *et al.*, 2007).

### 3.2.3 The spiritual component

The third issue is that a plant medicine usually has more than one meaning. Its physiological effect cannot be separated from its anticipated other meanings – emotional or spiritual – by the people who use or sell the plant. Another *botánica*-related story illustrates this. A Puerto Rican man in his 50s has been a needle user for about 20 years. He has been in and out of different drug programmes and travels back and forth to Puerto Rico to detox. When he comes back to New York City, he often relapses. He regularly visits a *botánica,* usually once or twice a day, to drink a herbal tea remedy prepared by the *botánica* owner. The owner claims it helps him deal with the anxiety associated with his substance abuse problem. The tea consists of half an ounce of *sándalo* (mint, *Mentha* sp., Lamiaceae) mixed with *perejil* (parsley, *Petroselinum crispum* (Mill.) Fuss, Apiaceae) and one branch of *ruda* (rue, *Ruta* spp., Rutaceae). The owner prepares the remedy in advance in bulk and stores it in the refrigerator, so that when the patient drops in he can get immediate assistance. While explaining the use of medicinal plants, the *botánica* owner stressed the importance of the spiritual component of healing. He reiterated that whereas medicinal plants assist in alleviating a biomedical problem, healing also has a spiritual component. It prepares the patient mentally in the healing process. Spiritual healing can be achieved through cleansing ('*limpieza*'), bathing, faith and spiritual consultations. This supposedly 'cuts off' the negative energy that a patient has been accumulating. It is important to note here that it is not the issue whether or not a spiritual component is effective, but that this component is relevant to both traditional healthcare provider and patient. It contributes to the realm of healing, and as such merits its place as a subject of scientific inquiry.

The needle user's story unravels the many often complex layers of traditional medicine, entwining physical, cultural, emotional and spiritual dimensions. The richness of the cultural context clearly goes beyond utilitarian knowledge about plants. This multidimensionality is not restricted to isolated rural areas, nor is it something from the past. It exists within urban and even transnational environments, for example in New York City, and it is used today for conditions as 'modern' as substance abuse and ovarian cysts.

The aspiring ethnopharmacologist might wonder if this complexity in traditional medicine is something he or she should take on as a research task. How relevant is culture in the face of the evaluation of the pharmacological properties of plants in the laboratory? Perhaps the question can be rephrased as follows: should ethnopharmacologists focus only on that part of culture that is associated with the utilitarian aspect of plants? Do we take culture into account when we want to obtain data on local plant uses, but not when it relates to other types of knowledge linked to plants, the kind that is psycho-social or spiritual in nature? An easy answer would be 'I cannot do it all.' Or 'the funding agency I am applying for does not support these kinds of musings'. Nevertheless, generating a rich, inclusive dataset to develop a comprehensive plant monograph can be indispensable to understand (cultural patterns of) plant knowledge, as opposed to a reductionist (and inevitably incomplete) approach. It also serves the added benefit that it can help preserve the integrity of cultural heritage. The psycho-social, religious or spiritual components of plant knowledge contain a lot of meaning for conservation of useful plant species at the community level since unfragmented stories associated with plants have direct cultural relevance to keep knowledge about plants (and their uses) alive. It has been argued before that to 'deprive a people of their language, culture and spiritual values [makes them] lose all sense of direction and purpose' (Posey, 1999).

As an ethnobotanist educated in and trained from a botanical perspective, I became increasingly aware of the overarching importance of culture during fieldwork. The more I studied medicinal plants, the more I began to understand that culture shapes everything, including plant knowledge. After all, biomedicine is a cultural construct too, which is elegantly demonstrated by Miner (1956) in his influential article about the Nacirema. Furthermore, anthropology has highlighted the importance of cultural relativism, the view that beliefs, customs and ethics vary from culture to culture and that all are equally valid; no one system is 'better' than another (Spiro, 1986). Spiro writes: 'In short all science is ethnoscience. Hence, since modern science is western science, its truth claims (and canons of proof) are no less culturally relative than those of any other ethnoscience.' Other scholars have gone as far as to bring up the notion that traditional medicine needs to be evaluated within its own cultural framework rather than approved and subdued by the rules of biological (western) medicine (Gorn and Sugiyama, 2004). Finally, Lynn Payer's compelling work *Culture & Medicine: Varieties of Treatment in the United States, England, West Germany and France* (Payer, 1996) shows in a compelling way how even contemporary western cultures differ, sometimes dramatically, in the ways in which they construct scientific medicine.

The key to improving healthcare in an increasingly globalized world may lie in integrating different cultural dimensions of healthcare, or at least in keeping an open mind about different ways in which other cultures think about, experience and respond to health and healthcare. In that regard, it would be useful to adopt the term 'culturally competent healthcare' systems (Anderson *et al.*, 2003), which take into account the cultural knowledge, beliefs and practices of patients as well as physicians. Ethnopharmacology can be at the forefront of building bridges between these different systems of healthcare by embracing culture as the indispensable link between a plant and a medicine.

## 3.3   An example from ancient Roman architecture

A paper on Roman architecture shows how the most minor architectural details refer to a number of big ideas in the culture of ancient Rome (Caneva *et al.*, 2014). The Ara Pacis Augustae in Rome is an elaborate monument – an altar to the worship of Pax, the goddess of peace – built between 13 and 9 BCE to celebrate the victories of the Roman Emperor Augustus in his campaigns in Gaul and Spain. After very close observations of the altar, the authors of the paper were able to identify about 100 species of plants in the various carvings and other representations. For example, one of the most common plants was *Acanthus mollis* L. (bear's britches). 'In the Mediterranean region, this perennial has a seasonally specific form and phenology: it appears dead in the summer, but starts to grow again at the beginning of autumn. *Acanthus* is frequently represented in classical sculptures as a symbol of rebirth … [in this case it] represents Rome's rebirth and prosperity' (ibid., p112) after the external rebellions and internal struggles that started with the murder of Julius Caesar in 44 BCE. The authors note that *Acanthus* is only shown in association with the founding of Rome (with Romulus and Remus, the twin boys raised by a wolf who founded Rome) and with images representing the time of the triumphant Augustus.

These representations can be complex. One of them displays not only an emerging *Pteridium aquilinum* [L.] Kohn (bracken fern) but also a flying eagle; note that bracken fern is also known as eagle fern, and that the specific epithet is based on the Latin *aquila*, meaning 'eagle'.

The symbol, the authors assert, represents simultaneously the idea of 'the world soul … and ideas of imperial power and conquest'. While these representations provide rich insights into the power and richness of decoration with plants, and of the world of meaning of ancient Romans, there is no mention of pharmacological leads.

## 3.4 An example from native North America

Among the 49 American species of crane's-bill, or wild or hardy geranium, the one most favoured as a medicine by native peoples was *Geranium maculatum* L., the spotted crane's-bill (Figure 3.4). A favourite of a number of Midwestern tribes – Menominee, Meskwaki and Ojibwa used it for diarrhoea, sore gums and toothache – its use by the Iroquois shows us some important elements in the medical thinking of non-western peoples (Herrick and Snow, 1995). As it goes to seed, *Geranium maculatum* develops a series of very distinctive hooks from its pistil which hold newly formed seeds (Figure 3.5). These hooks, for the Iroquois, were distinctive and important, putting it in a special category of plants with 'hook-like or ensnaring features' (Herrick and Snow, 1995), along with a number of other plants like *Anemone canadensis* L. (Canadian anemone), which has spiky hooks on its seeds, as does *Geum rivale* L. (purple avens) and a number of other species.

Most of these are utilized by the Iroquois for conditions of eversion, looseness or escape, like cold sores or diarrhoea. Their idea is that the hook-like, ensnaring quality of the plant will engage, grab or capture the looseness and pull it back, and so a tea of the roots is used to wash a chancre sore and a poultice of dried root is applied to the unhealed navel of an infant. The ethnopharmacologists are happy when they find that the geranium root contains substantial quantities of tannin, which is a strong astringent, hence validating this usage.

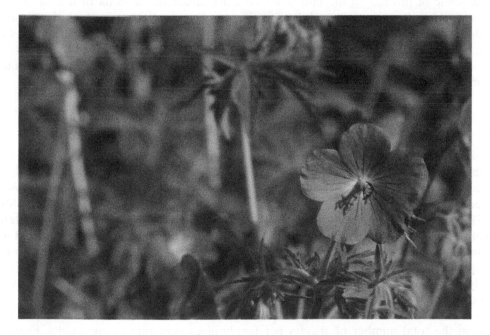

**Figure 3.4** *Geranium maculatum* L. Wild geranium or crane's bill in flower.

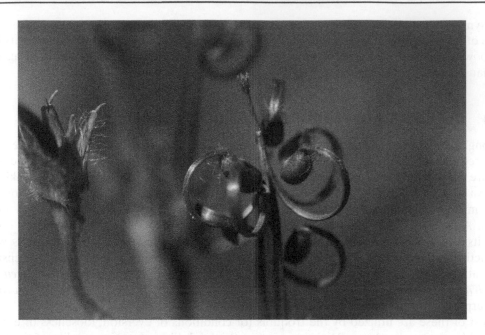

**Figure 3.5**   Wild geranium seeds, with 'hooks'.

The wild geranium, however, has more uses than that. Suppose a wife was suspected of having a flirtation with another man. Putting a bit of geranium root or flower in her food or drink might capture her and bring her back. Similarly, when fishing it would be a good idea to sprinkle some of this tea on the bait to entice a fish closer to the hook or it could be used to bring a rabbit closer to a snare. Likewise, when trying to sell some baskets, they could be sprinkled with geranium root tea to ensnare a buyer (and I (DM) can attest that books with drawings of wild geraniums included in them sell better than ones that don't). There is more to medicine than chemistry (Moerman, 2002). In addition, no garden is complete without an assortment of wild geraniums.

## 3.5   Comparative ethnobotany

It is also possible to learn a great deal about people and the plants they use on a much larger scale than is evident in the preceding examples from Dominicans in New York, ancient Roman architecture or geraniums for the Iroquois. Having worked with very large scale analyses of the medicinal uses of plants by native American and First Nations peoples of Canada (Moerman, 1998), I (DM) have also, with colleagues, done comparisons of such uses elsewhere in the world (Moerman *et al.*, 1999). In those studies, and others, it commonly happens that some plant families are far more likely to be utilized for medicines than others. Most authors use a technique similar to one I developed in the 1970s (Moerman, 1979) using regression analysis; recently other authors have developed more complex approaches, for example using Bayesian statistics, which ordinarily come to essentially similar results (cf. Weckerle *et al.*, 2011).

In the North American case, a regression analysis of the number of medicinal species per family on the total number of species per family gives very interesting results. Figure 3.6 displays a graph of the relationship.

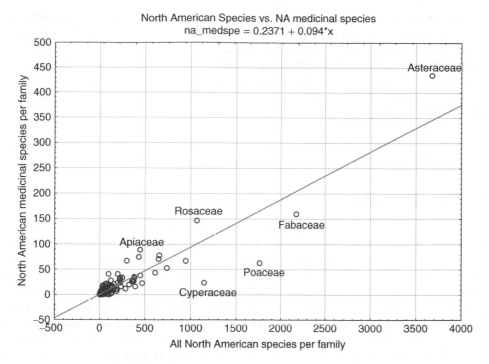

**Figure 3.6** Regression analysis of native North American medicinal plants (by family) on all North American plants.

Compare two families, the Asteraceae and the Poaceae, which are both very large. The Asteraceae (sunflowers) have about 3600 species in North America (north of Mexico), of which 427 are used as medicines. The Poaceae (grasses) have nearly 1800 species, of which only 63 are used medicinally. In a regression analysis, the line shown is the one line that is 'closest' to all the points in the graph. The vertical distance between the line and each point is called the residual, which is positive if it is above the line and negative below the line. In such an analysis, if you add all the residuals together the result is zero. In this situation, the families listed above the line are ones used more often than chance; they are positively selected for use. Families below the line are less utilized as medicines. The residual in Figure 3.6 for Asteraceae is about 80; the residual for Poaceae is about –100. Asteraceae is far more useful as a source of drugs than is Poaceae. This result has been shown many times; in the northern hemisphere, it seems always to be true. Note that Poaceae is neglected as a source of medicines, but not as a source of foods. Our major food grains – wheat, barley, rice, millet, oats, rye, and corn or maize – are all members of the Poaceae family. One reason that plants are medicinal at all is that they often contain chemicals toxic to insects. Such biologically active substances – like the opium in poppies or nicotine in tobacco – are often toxic in large doses, but in smaller ones can be useful in varying ways, in these cases as narcotic analgesics or as satisfying mood altering drugs. The Poaceae family rarely produces such toxic substances to protect against browsers so it is a useful source of food plants.

Some families are rather in the middle of this. Most famous is the Solanaceae family, which produces some very toxic plants (like nightshade, *Solanum* spp.) but also some very important food plants, like potatoes, tomatoes, eggplants, peppers and tobacco. It seems clear that these generalizations are true for large areas of the planet, including almost all of the northern part of the globe, and some places in Africa as far south as Namibia. By contrast, in the Amazon region, with probably the richest flora in the world, it seems that tropical peoples each follow their own paths and select medicinal floras dramatically different from those in the north, and also significantly different from each other. For a compelling example, see Glenn Shepard's comparison of two peoples living on opposite sides of the same river in eastern Ecuador, who select very different plants from the very same flora (Shepard, 2004). This kind of an analysis, only touched on here, can provide rich detail about the lives of human beings all over the world as they interact with the plants that are the basis of their foods, drugs, dyes, fibres and the flowers in their hair.

## 3.6   Conclusions

The study of people and the plants that they use, grow, forage, think about and imagine is a rich way to more fully understand the ways that people enact their humanness. This is not to say that the study of plants and people is more important or valuable than the study of people and birds (Hage and Miller, 1976), or any other aspect of ethnobiology (Anderson *et al.*, 2012), but it is unlikely that many other areas in the human sciences will pass the majesty of, say, Nancy Turner's *Ancient pathways, ancestral knowledge: Ethnobotany and ecological wisdom of indigenous peoples of northwestern North America* (Turner, 2014). Anthropology has shown us that human beings 'operate in an environment as they *perceive* it, not as it *is*' (Brookfield 1969, cited in Cotton, 1996). Research has come a long way from Harshberger's definition of ethnobotany more than 100 years ago, which emphasized the utilitarian aspects of plants, towards a discipline that has embraced peoples' perception and management of the natural world, in addition to their use of those natural resources. In order to understand why and how people use and manage plants, we need to understand first how they perceive their environment. There are many ways to learn about how plants are culturally perceived. The most obvious way is first-hand experience in the field, but even the use of information sources less conventionally accessed by ethnopharmacologists, for example Shakespeare, has something to teach us. In King Henry IV, Part I, Act II, Scene IV, Shakespeare writes about his observation of the ecological resilience of chamomile: ' … for though the chamomile, the more it is trodden the faster it grows, yet youth, the more it is wasted the sooner it wears'. In Othello, Act III, Scene III, Shakespeare refers to the narcotic effect of the poppy: ' … Not poppy, nor mandragora / Nor all the drowsy syrups of the world / Shall ever medicine thee to that sweet sleep / Which thou ow'dst' yesterday'. In Romeo and Juliet, Act II, Scene III, the poisonous and medicinal plant belladonna features: 'Within the infant rind of this weak flower / Poison hath residence, and medicine power / For this, being smelt, with that part cheers each part / Being tasted, slays all senses with the heart'.

Sources such as these show that detailed cultural and contextual information about plants as observed by the keen human eye can be found everywhere we are willing to look. Hopefully, ethnobotanists and ethnopharmacologists alike may continue to find joy and scientific wisdom in exploring the diverse array of ethno-related knowledge, beliefs and practices, both from conventional and non-conventional sources, with an open mind. After all, has it not been said repeatedly that local people's science is good science? Shakespeare's observation of plants stems from his life as a countryman, not as a botanist, yet his descriptions faithfully report what he observed about the English plant species that surrounded him.

# References

Albuquerque, U.P., Ramos, M.A. and Melo, J.G. (2012) New strategies for drug discovery in tropical forests based on ethnobotanical and chemical ecological studies. *Journal of Ethnopharmacology*, **140**, 197–201.

Anderson, L.M., Scrimshaw, S.C., Fullilove, M.T., *et al.* (2003) Culturally competent healthcare systems: a systematic review. *American Journal of Preventive Medicine*, **24**, 68–79.

Anderson, E.N., Pearsall, D., Hunn, E. and Turner, N. (2012) *Ethnobiology*, John Wiley & Sons, Ltd, Chichester.

Brookfield, H.C. (1969) On the environment as perceived. *Progress in Geology*, **1**, 51–80.

Caneva, G., Savo, V. and Kumbaric, A. (2014) Big Messages in Small Details: Nature in Roman Archaeology. *Economic Botany*, **68**, 109–115.

Clapp, R.A. and Crook, C. (2002) Drowning in the magic well: Shaman Pharmaceuticals and the elusive value of traditional knowledge. *Journal of Environment & Development*, **11**, 79–102.

Cotton, C.M. (1996) *Ethnobotany: Principles and Applications,* John Wiley & Sons.

Cox, P.A. (2001) Ensuring equitable benefits: The Falealupo covenant and the isolation of anti-viral drug prostratin from a Samoan medicinal plant. *Pharmaceutical Biology*, **39**, 33–40.

Etkin, N.L. and Elisabetsky, E. (2005) Seeking a transdisciplinary and culturally germane science: the future of ethnopharmacology. *Journal of Ethnopharmacology*, **100**, 23–26.

Gorn, S.B. and Sugiyama, E.I. (2004) Between traditional and scientific medicine: a research strategy for the study of the pathways to treatment followed by a group of Mexican patients with emotional disorders, *Forum Qualitative Sozialforschung/Forum: Qualitative Social Research*, **5**, Issue 2.

Gustafson, K.R., Cardellina, J.H., McMahon, J.B., *et al.* (1992) A nonpromoting phorbol from the samoan medicinal plant Homalanthus nutans inhibits cell killing by HIV-1. *Journal of Medicinal Chemistry*, **35**, 1978–1986.

Hage, P. and Miller, W.R. (1976) 'eagle' = 'bird': a note on the structure and evolution of Shoshoni ethnoornithological nomenclature 1. *American Ethnologist*, **3**, 481–488.

Herrick, J.W. and Snow, D.R. (1995) *Iroquois Medical Botany*, 1st edn, Syracuse University Press, Syracuse, NY.

Leitão, F., Leitão, S.G., de Almeida, M.Z., *et al.* (2013) Medicinal plants from open-air markets in the State of Rio de Janeiro, Brazil as a potential source of new antimycobacterial agents. *Journal of Ethnopharmacology*, **149**, 513–521.

Miller, L.H. and Su, X. (2011) Artemisinin: discovery from the Chinese herbal garden. *Cell*, **146**, 855–858.

Miner, H. (1956) Body Ritual of the Nacirema. *American Anthropologist*, **58**, 503–507.

Moerman, D.E. (1979) Symbols and selectivity: a statistical analysis of native American medical ethnobotany. *Journal of Ethnopharmacology*, **1**, 111–119.

Moerman, D.E. (1998) *Native American Ethnobotany*. Timber Press, Portland, OR.

Moerman, D.E. (2002) *Meaning, Medicine, and the 'Placebo Effect'*. Cambridge University Press, Cambridge.

Moerman, D.E., Pemberton, R.W., Kiefer, D. and Berlin, B. (1999) A comparative analysis of five medicinal floras. *Journal of Ethnobiology*, **19**, 46–67.

Nebel, S., Pieroni, A. and Heinrich, M. (2006) Ta chòrta: Wild edible greens used in the Graecanic area in Calabria, Southern Italy. *Appetite*, **47**, 333–342.

Ososki, A.L., Balick, M.J. and Daly, D.C. (2007) Medicinal plants and cultural variation across Dominican rural, urban, and transnational landscapes, in *Traveling Cultures and Plants: The Ethnobiology and Ethnopharmacy of Migrations* (eds A. Pieroni and I. Vandebroek), Berghahn Books, New York, pp. 14–38.

Payer, L. (1996) Medicine and Culture, *An Owl Book*, Henry Holt and Company, New York.

Payne-Jackson, A. and Alleyne, M.C. (2004) *Jamaican Folk Medicine: A Source of Healing*, University of West Indies Press, Kingston.

Posey, D.A. (1999) *Cultural and Spiritual Values of Biodiversity: A Complementary Contribution to the Global Biodiversity Assessment*. Intermediate Technmology Publications.

Saslis-Lagoudakis, C.H., Savolainen, V., Williamson, E.M., *et al.* (2012) Phylogenies reveal predictive power of traditional medicine in bioprospecting. *Proceedings of the National Academy of Sciences*, **109**, 15835–15840.

Shepard, G.H. (2004) A sensory ecology of medicinal plant therapy in two Amazonian societies. *American Anthropologist*, **106**, 252–266.

Spiro, M.E. (1986) Cultural relativism and the future of anthropology. *Cultural Anthropology*, **1**, 259–286.

Suffness, M. (1993) Taxol: From discovery to therapeutic use. *Annual Reports in Medicinal Chemistry*, **28**, 305–314.

Turner, N. (2014) *Ancient Pathways, Ancestral Knowledge: Ethnobotany and Ecological Wisdom of Indigenous Peoples of Northwestern North America*, McGill-Queen's Press.

Vandebroek, I., Balick, M.J., Yukes, J., *et al.* (2007) Use of medicinal plants by Dominican immigrants in New York City for the treatment of common health conditions. A comparative analysis with literature data from the Dominican Republic, in *Traveling Cultures and Plants: The Ethnobiology and Ethnopharmacy of Human Migrations* (eds A. Pierone and I. Vandebroek), Berghahn Books, New York, pp. 39–64.

Vandebroek, I., Balick, M.J., Ososki, A., *et al.* (2010) The importance of botellas and other plant mixtures in Dominican traditional medicine. *Journal of Ethnopharmacology*, **128**, 20–41.

Viladrich, A. (2006) Botánicas in America's backyard: Uncovering the world of Latino healers' herb-healing practices in New York City. *Human Organization*, **65,** 407–419.

Wani, M.C. and Horwitz, S.B. (2014) Nature as a remarkable chemist: a personal story of the discovery and development of Taxol. *Anti-cancer Drugs*, **25**, 482–487.

Weckerle, C.S., Cabras, S., Castellanos, M.E. and Leonti, M. (2011) Quantitative methods in ethnobotany and ethnopharmacology: Considering the overall flora—hypothesis testing for over-and underused plant families with the Bayesian approach. *Journal of Ethnopharmacology*, **137**, 837–843.

# 4
# Quantitative and Comparative Methods in Ethnopharmacology

Marco Leonti[1] and Caroline S. Weckerle[2]

[1] *Department of Biomedical Sciences, University of Cagliari, Italy*
[2] *Institute of Systematic Botany, University of Zürich, Switzerland*

## 4.1 Introduction

### 4.1.1 Materia medica and cultural consensus

The world's cultures can be conceived as a cultural landscape that may be described in terms of a geographical map showing abysses, foul grounds, ditches, plateaus, hills and peaks of cultural consensus, variation, dissension and vacancies. This dynamic cultural topography can be described, compared and analysed to find local and universal patterns. Ethnopharmacology focuses on a specific cultural realm, the *materia medica* (also called ethnopharmacopoeia) and its use by different peoples. It investigates the local use of pharmaceutical agents, the mode of preparation, application, and associated therapeutical believes and knowledge. Usually, the focus is on plants, generally the most numerous part of any *materia medica*. The term 'medicinal flora' is thus used to subsume the medicinal plants of a specific area or community.

A local *materia medica* is the product of a consensus among the local community and its local and/or traditional healthcare practitioners on what to use to prevent, diagnose and cure diseases and illnesses, and how to sustain and promote emotional and spiritual well-being. Local *materia medica* is shaped by community-internal as well as external factors, such as local and cross-cultural knowledge exchange, globalization and resulting syncretism. A generally accepted theory is that among humans the search for food and edible greens, especially after the transition from a nomadic to a sedentary agriculturalist lifestyle, promoted the exchange and consensus on the physiological and therapeutical properties of plants (Johns, 1990; Logan and Dixon, 1994). People continuously modify their medicinal flora to adapt to new diseases and epidemics, and also to socio-economic changes. Belief systems related to medicine may be adapted to new social hegemonies or the *materia medica* may be abandoned and/or substituted by newly introduced remedies (Bye *et al.*, 1995). The transmission of knowledge through scripts, books and other media also exerts a powerful influence on the consensus of medicinal plant use. Today, global economy and advertisement progressively influence the selection of medicines and the perception of their therapeutical effectiveness as well as socio-economic values of local medicines (Leonti and Casu, 2013).

## 4.1.2 The intent of ethnopharmacological projects: Basic and applied research

As in other academic disciplines, ethnopharmacological research projects have either an applied or a basic research character or may combine both aspects in a single project. Applied research projects usually focus on an urgent 'real-world problem' brought up by local stakeholders or governmental bodies. However, they may also be a response to market demands. Applied ethnopharmacological projects are typically found in the fields of development (Graz *et al.*, 2010) or bioprospecting (Soejarto *et al.*, 2012). They may focus on issues related to primary healthcare and try to validate and integrate local medicinal plants and medicinal practices into official governmental healthcare policies, or they may aim to develop new drug leads based on traditional knowledge. In the latter case the search for promising bioactive substances or extracts as well as insights into pharmacological interactions is the main interest (Heinrich, 2010).

Basic research is primarily interested in the generation of insights and knowledge out of curiosity. Basic ethnopharmacological research projects span a wide range of topics revolving around the question of why specific agents are used as medicine and how *materia medica* evolve (Leonti and Casu, 2013). They largely overlap with basic ethnobotanical or ethnomedical research and may form the basis for applied projects. Basic ethnopharmacological research projects, for example, are interested in plant use and knowledge transfer within a specific community or focus on the historical development of medicinal plant knowledge or the question of how environment and culture influence the use of *materia medica* and health-seeking behaviour (e.g. Gesler, 1992; Etkin, 1993; Heinrich *et al.*, 2009). Most commonly, the objectives of the project define it as applied or basic, and much less so its content, structure or methods. Most ethnopharmacological projects, whether basic or applied, follow a similar structure. They start from field research among a local community and aim at finding a consensus on local disease concepts and the use of specific medicinal plants. They document modes of preparation and administration of the plants for the treatment of specific health conditions. The emic perception, i.e. the perspective of the local people of disease and illness, is at this stage of major interest (for a detailed discussion on the emic and etic perspective see below). In a second step the documented ethnomedical conditions are usually translated into biomedical disease concepts as far as possible, which allows for a comparison with other medical and knowledge systems (i.e. the etic view; Berlin *et al.*, 1993). This includes analysing converging and diverging domains between the scientific and indigenous perspectives. Finally, pharmacological studies may shed light on the role of chemical substances in the use of specific plants (Browner *et al.*, 1988; Etkin, 2001; Gertsch, 2009).

## 4.1.3 Ethnopharmacology as cross-cultural endeavour and the concept of emic and etic

Ethnopharmacological studies can be described as cross-cultural. The meaning of cross-cultural can vary considerably. In the scientific world it is usually applied to comparative studies among different cultures aiming to find universal and general patterns of human culture in space and time (e.g. Moerman *et al.*, 1999; Ember and Ember, 2001). Cross-cultural studies therefore also help to understand unique cultural characteristics, as 'either way of looking – for uniqueness or similarity – is comparative' (Ember and Ember, 2001). 'Cross-cultural' may also stand for transdisciplinary approaches bridging different cultures and knowledge systems with the aim of developing new perspectives based on an equal exchange (Davis, 2010). For ethnopharmacological projects both the comparative and the multidisciplinary approaches are relevant, especially if they include questions on why and how the local perception of *materia medica* has come about. However, ethnopharmacology itself may also be described as cross-cultural in nature since it combines the emic perceptions of local people with the etic perception of the researcher and the applied scientific methods. Generally, cross-cultural approaches aim to contextualize local data and results within a global perspective. For cross-cultural research, Bernard (2006) and Ember and Ember (2001), for instance, provide well-structured introductions into anthropological concepts and methods, which are also relevant to ethnopharmacological studies.

While cross-cultural studies are driven by an etic perspective (outside view), field research, which stands at the beginning of every cross-cultural analysis, is very much interested in the emic perspective (inside view) of local communities. The anthropological research concept of the 'emic' and 'etic' perspectives originates in linguistics and in 1954 was introduced by Pike (Headland, 1990). The interpretation and definition of the now well-established concept is, however, not consistent across disciplines and sub-disciplines (Headland, 1990). Generally, the emic viewpoint is understood to come from within a culture, while the etic perspective is that of the researcher as an outsider, coming from another culture. The researcher looks through his/her own 'cultural lens' as well as a 'scientific lens' and, for example, compares the ethnographic data with ethnological baseline data. However, emic and etic can be stretched further and finally come close to the 'self' and the 'other' or the 'known' and the 'unknown'. In every single communication between two persons an emic (inside, self, known) component and an etic (outside, other, unknown) component are involved. The concept of emic and etic helps the researcher to become aware of his/her own cultural and scientific filters through which she/he looks at the world and more specifically at the research topic. Through these filters perception becomes a selective process, which tends to be accompanied by various levels of conscious and unconscious judgments. In fact, Hickerson (1992) proposed to use 'emic' and 'etic' not as strictly opposed or dichotomous terms but as 'stages in a dialectic process'. Such a conceptual transition of perspectives, from the emic to the etic, is a crucial component of every well-conceived ethnopharmacological study, as it helps to broaden the perception without judging prematurely. A couple of methods and concepts, including the above, thus aim at evading our own filters as far as possible.

The ongoing urbanization and global migration intermingle cultures, resulting in numerous subcultures existing side by side on small scales. Not surprisingly, recent ethnopharmacological studies are also conducted in urban settings or within the researcher's own 'cultural background'. However, neither methodologically nor philosophically is poking your nose into your neighbour's garden the same thing as coping with a completely different cultural setting and crossing a cultural barrier. The transition from the emic to the etic perspective is much more challenging in one's own cultural background, as the setting supports the feeling of familiarity, and becoming aware of one's own filters is very difficult in this context.

## 4.2 Research questions

At the beginning of every research project stands a research question. We differentiate here between descriptive questions and relational questions, based on the approach of Ember and Ember (2001) for cross-cultural research.

## 4.2.1    Descriptive questions

Descriptive questions are 'what' questions as they are interested in what is out there. Usually they deal with the prevalence or the frequency of a specific trait. Most ethnopharmacological field studies fall within this category and they usually provide Latin binomial lists of medicinal plant species together with their local name, use, plant parts used and mode of administration (for a critical discussion of this see Heinrich *et al.*, 2009). Typical descriptive questions are:

- What kind of health care is available to the local people and how do they make use of it (e.g. biomedical outposts, hospital, traditional healers, self-medication)?
- How many different medicinal specialists exist in a community and what is their medicinal specialty and knowledge? How do they (clinicians, health workers, local healers, bone-setters, herbalists, ritual specialists, midwives) collaborate?
- What kind of specialists do people visit for their perceived health conditions and ailments, and what kind of medicine do they use (e.g. Boulogne *et al.*, 2011)?
- How common is the use of medicinal plants and what kinds of species are employed for which health condition?
- Which are the most common illnesses and what are the most often used medicinal plants?
- How common is the use of medicinal plant books and modern media for acquiring medicinal plant knowledge?

## 4.2.2    Relational questions

Relational questions focus on how things or traits are related to each other. What are the causes and what are the effects of a specific trait or a custom? How does something change over time? Typical ethnopharmacological questions falling into this category are:

- Why do certain communities rely on specific plant-based therapies (e.g. Flores and Quinlan, 2014)?
- What are the ecological and historical factors exerting an influence on regional medicinal plant use?
- Is there a relationship between plants selected for medicine and their taxonomy (e.g. Moerman and Estabrook, 2003)?
- Are the most salient and cross-culturally employed remedies also the most efficacious (e.g. Trotter and Logan, 1986)?
- What is the relationship between medicinal plant knowledge and gender? Do men and women with the same cultural background know and use different kinds of herbal remedies?
- How do people adjust their medicinal flora to (abrupt) social and economic change? Do people, for example, continue to use the same medicinal plants (continuity, maintenance), do they use the same species but adapt the ethnomedical beliefs to the new context and concepts (disjunction), do they abandon herbal medicine (discontinuity) or do they substitute and adapt their pharmacopoeia (synchronism, syncretism; e.g. Bye *et al.*, 1995; Giovannini *et al.*, 2011; Monigatti *et al.*, 2013)?

It always makes sense to search for the hidden assumptions and beliefs behind the research questions, and to spell out the implicit and explicit ideas behind them. This helps to clarify the theories on which the research is based. In a next step, the following questions need to be addressed (see also Ember and Ember, 2001):

- How does the research question fit into the state of the art of the scientific community?
- Is the research question scientifically relevant and can it really help to close gaps in our understanding of a cultural context or are we repeating what has already been shown?
- Do we have a sufficiently large number of cases and collaborate with enough knowledgeable persons with respect to the range of intra-cultural variation?
- Have we considered all influential parameters in order to thoroughly answer our research questions?

By answering these basic questions, the specific methods can be selected, the methodology designed and the sample size approximated. In general, the important characteristics of cross-cultural comparisons are (Ember and Ember 2001): (i) their geographical scale (worldwide, regional, local), (ii) their sample size (number of included cultures, individual informants), (iii) the use of primary or secondary data (field research data vs published data) and (iv) the time frame (synchronic comparison or diachronic comparison).

## 4.3 Field research

Usually, ethnopharmacological research starts with field research, which draws on ethnographic methods such as participant observation (also participative observation) and an array of questionnaire techniques, as well as botanical methods including plant vouchering and the preparation of herbarium specimens. Since ethnopharmacology is characterized by multi- and interdisciplinary research and since it relies on concepts and methodologies from the humanities as well as the natural sciences, it is important to define the basic methodological standards to make sure that ethnopharmacological field data are valid and can be compared cross-culturally (for details see Heinrich *et al.* (2009), general methods manuals like Martin (1995) or Alexiades (1996), for anthropological methods and especially the development of interviews see Bernard (2006) and for botanical aspects see, for example, Liesner (no date) and Bussmann (2015)).

### 4.3.1 Data sampling

For the collection of data, ethnopharmacological field research largely relies on interviews conducted with informants, but how many informants should be interviewed and how do we choose the informants? Since a census is generally not feasible, we have to interview a sub-sample of the population, which represents the cultural (therapeutical) knowledge. What determines the population depends on our research focus, which can either be directed towards the average local medical knowledge and thus to an ideally unbiased sample of the entire population or towards the knowledge of specialists in local herbal medicine (expert knowledge). This differentiation is crucial because research strategies and sampling methods differ (cf. Bernard, 2006). If the research focus is on the general knowledge of a community about medicinal plant use, or the general importance of self-medication and therapeutic choices, a sufficiently large, randomly selected and unbiased sample is necessary ('probability sampling' or 'random sampling', see Bernard, 2006). Usually, however, ethnopharmacological field studies focus on expert knowledge and to this end informants need to be chosen carefully (Heinrich *et al.*, 2009). Bernard (2006) refers to such specialist knowledge as 'cultural data' and describes the required sampling method as 'non-probability sampling'. Non-probability sampling is usually identical to chain referral methods and what ethnopharmacologists and ethnobotanists generally call snowball sampling or respondent-driven sampling. In this sampling approach, an expert indicates colleague experts and thereby guides the way to other informants for the same knowledge domain, leading to the virtual visualization of a network of specialists within a community. Snowball sampling, however, does not produce representative samples if the overall population is relatively large (Bernard, 2006).

It is essential to make sure that the whole research process is reproducible, which is a basic requirement of any scientific endeavour. In general, all the plants mentioned in the interviews need to be documented and validated with taxonomic keys and herbarium specimens. Every plant name in the data needs to be connected to a specific voucher. Often the voucher is also necessary to identify the correct scientific name of the plant. Voucher specimens need to be deposited at an internationally recognized herbarium.

Although field researchers try their best to get reliable data, to choose knowledgeable and culturally representative informants, and to transcribe the information as accurately as possible, any ethnographic data is afflicted with a margin of error (Romney *et al.*, 1986). According to Weller (2007) the reliability of an informant as well as his/her cultural competence can be estimated by comparing his/her responses with that of the other respondents assessing the level of agreement. By triangulation, the resulting consensus may be cross-verified by participant observation in order to understand if informants really do what they say. The more informants provide the same information about a certain topic, the higher is the probability of getting a culturally valid picture.

A clear picture of the cultural consensus is not only important for scientific communication, but also for local dissemination. Researchers often share their results with the local population, for example in the form of medicinal plant booklets. If such booklets contain the information and consensus of only a handful of informants from a single location but are distributed to households over a wider geographic area, it can be assumed that such information stemming from few individuals will shape and homogenize the consensus of a whole population, which might not have the effect anticipated by the researchers.

## 4.4   Analyzing the data

### 4.4.1   Use-reports for quantification

In order to identify similarity and uniqueness within and between cultures or communities, a scale has to be developed that allows for comparison and to decide whether one case differs from another. Basically, measurements can be either qualitative or quantitative. Whether or not parameters are quantified depends on the research focus and the research question. Documentation and detailed description of local medicinal knowledge constitutes the basis of any ethnopharmacological enquiry. To quantify medicinal knowledge so-called use-reports are used widely. They are defined as a plant (or animal or mineral) taxon or part of it, mentioned by an individual healer for a specific use. With use-reports it can easily be shown how frequently specific plants, plant parts, preparations or diseases have been mentioned. If we assume that culturally important needs (e.g. remedies, diseases) are mentioned more frequently, the number of use-reports can be taken as a proxy for the cultural importance of a specific plant remedy for the treatment of a specific health condition.

To get reliable data representing the overall pattern, it is important to respect the so-called 'law of the large numbers'. This means that the researcher has to work as thoroughly as possible with as many knowledgeable informants as possible, in order to get as much culturally representative data as possible. The more single-point data we have, the smaller the sampling error will be and the more accurate, and also statistically significant, the results are. The absolute number of use-reports provided in relation to the number of total informants that have been interviewed provides comparable and transparent data, which can be used for cross-cultural comparisons. Counting of use-reports is also a recommended tool to select species as candidates for phytochemical and pharmacological analysis (Trotter and Logan, 1986; Berlin and Berlin, 2005; Heinrich *et al.*, 2009). High proportions of use-reports are found for taxa which are used frequently in populations and communities, and which are therefore interesting candidates for experimental analyses. Beside use-report numbers, which are a transparent and straightforward approach for quantification and comparability, various indices can be found in the ethnobotanical and ethnopharmacological literature. The added value of many of these indices, especially for comparisons, is questionable (Collins *et al.*, 2006) and we only refer here to one of the indices introduced early by Trotter and Logan (1986): the informant agreement ratio or informant consensus factor, used to assess intra-cultural consensus with respect to the remedies used for a specific ailment category. It is based on the following calculation and ranges from 0 to 1, where 1 indicates high agreement:

$$F = n_{ur} - n_{spp.used}/n_{ur} - 1$$

where $n_{ur}$ is the number of use-reports per category of use and $n_{spp.used}$ is the number of species used per category of use.

The cultural consensus factor, however, does not reflect the distribution of use-reports and the individual cultural importance of the taxa. For example, if three species are used for an ailment with 30 use-reports, the consensus factor is the same whether one species has 28 use-reports and the remaining two only have one each, or all three species have 10 use-reports. This consensus factor may also be applied for cross-cultural comparisons if the use-categories correspond between the cultures (Heinrich *et al.*, 1998).

## 4.5 Pharmacological research

As ethnopharmacology seeks to understand the pharmacological basis of culturally important plants they may also include laboratory experiments and clinical trials (Rivier and Bruhn, 1979; Gertsch, 2009). First the biomedical understanding of the disease symptoms as well as the aetiology are compared to the ethnomedical condition, trying to identify converging and diverging aspects between the two perspectives (Berlin *et al.*, 1993). A specific medicinal plant may have many different uses in a specific culture and even more between cultures, an aspect often underestimated by ethnobotanists and ethnopharmacologists alike.

Plant species collected for pharmacological analyses need to be documented with a herbarium specimen from the same plant or plant population from which the material for the experiments comes[1]. The species needs to be identified with its current taxonomically valid Latin binomial according to international botanical standards (Bennett and Balick, 2014). For pharmacological testing usually less plant material is needed than for phytochemical analyses (e.g. 0.1–10 g of crude drug for *in vitro* tests). Considerably more material is needed for *in vivo* studies.

The solvent used to extract the crude drug should reflect the preparation method observed and described in the local *materia medica*, and in most cases this would thus be water. If animal models are used it is crucial to administer the extract or the drug preparation in the same

---

[1] We presuppose that legal requirements and intellectual property rights issues have been cleared and that the Convention on Biological Diversity (CBD) is followed.

way as observed in the field. The selection of an appropriate biological test system is a crucial step and is often determined by the financial and institutional possibilities. In any case results obtained from single-test systems should not be over-estimated. *In vitro* tests are often too simplistic and reductionistic: an extract able to inhibit the growth of *Plasmodium* sp. *in vitro* should be labelled 'anti-plasmodial' and not 'anti-malarial', as the extract might be ineffective *in vivo* (Houghton *et al.*, 2007). Similarly, a plant extract able to kill cancer cells *in vitro* should be referred to as cytotoxic and not as having antitumour or anticancer properties because cancer is a pathological state observed *in vivo* (Gertsch, 2009). Houghton *et al.* (2007) recommend the use of different test systems physiologically related to the disease state, and Gertsch (2009), referencing Paracelsus (1492–1541), points out that in pharmacology concentration determines pharmacological effects and that far too often exceedingly high concentration of extracts are applied to bioassays in order to elicit a measurable response. The same problem was addressed by Cos *et al.* (2006), who criticized the unrealistically high doses applied to antimicrobial *in vitro* tests often without conducting cytotoxicity screens, which would help to discern non-specific cell toxicity. Pure isolated compounds found to be particularly active (for a review on isolation procedures see Sticher (2008)) should be cross-screened in a set of different assays in order to generate data on how selective the compound actually is (Heinrich *et al.*, 2004). Usually pharmacologists and medicinal chemists prefer highly selective compounds instead of ubiquitous and frequent 'hitters' such as flavonoids. However, herbal medicines and whole extracts are complex mixtures of substances potentially exerting synergistic and antagonistic polypharmacological molecular interactions. Since *in vitro* tests are not able to detect pharmacological networks, systems biology, *in vivo* tests, gathering clinical data and comparing effectiveness and treatment outcomes as well as clinical studies are the proposed alternatives (e.g. Verpoorte *et al.*, 2005; Wagner and Ulrich-Merzenich, 2009; Graz *et al.*, 2010; Witt, 2013).

## 4.6   Contextualization

A general objective of many ethnopharmacological surveys is to compare the primary data gathered in the field with data from the literature looking for consensus, variation or uniqueness. For such a comparison, a systematic approach with a clear pharmacological and toxicological focus as well as a defined geographical (space) or historical (time) scale together with a reproducible methodology is essential. In order to make the comparison, contextualization and the conclusions transparent, the inclusion criteria of the literature to which the primary data is compared have to be given. Particularly in Europe, including the Mediterranean region with its neighbouring countries and regions such as Turkey, the Levant, Near East and Northern Africa, an extremely rich written tradition dealing with *materia medica* exists besides the oral tradition. As discovering hitherto neglected or unknown plant uses are often the goal of comparisons, it is important to consider not only the standard books on herbal medicine but also historical sources and therapeutical indications reported in popular books and brochures. If new plant uses are highlighted and recommended for further investigation their use should be consensus based and related to an emic perception of effectiveness (Trotter and Logan, 1986; Berlin and Berlin, 2005; Heinrich *et al.*, 2009). The relevance of only one or a few use-reports describing a particular therapeutical plant use is questionable. As already mentioned, statements and replies collected during field interviews should be treated as probabilistic in nature and there is a real possibility that the data contains wrong information (Romney *et al.*, 1986). Of course it is problematic to speak of culturally 'wrong' data because deviant answers might also be culturally characteristic. However, cultural consensus occurs at the point where answers converge.

Descriptive cross-cultural comparisons in Europe and adjacent regions generally show a high overlap of local medicinal plant use and medicinal floras (e.g. Leporatti and Ivancheva, 2003; Pieroni and Quave, 2005). Moreover, the overlapping plant species as well as those used most commonly tend to be best represented in historic textbooks on *materia medica* (Leonti *et al.*, 2009, 2010). The relatively high consensus between inventories of medicinal plants and popular pharmacopoeias in Europe and the Mediterranean can be explained by the common cultural heritage, including the divulgence of knowledge through scripts, trade and the migration of people, which have homogenized the knowledge of these regions. Cross-cultural comparisons help to contextualize the data and when entire medicinal floras are compared cross-culturally Venn diagrams are an appropriate and commonly used tool to visualize consensus (number of shared species and use-reports) and variation (number of uniquely used species and use-reports) in one figure (Leonti *et al.*, 2006, 2009). What can nicely be shown through comparisons within the same geographical and historical context is that species receiving high intracultural consensus also have high intercultural consensus (Leonti *et al.*, 2009).

In regions of the world where due to remoteness the processes and mechanisms of globalization are delayed, the situation can be quite different. In the Amazon, for example, a cross-cultural comparison of the medicinal flora between the Matsigenka and the Yora living in adjacent habitats in south-eastern Peru showed moderate similarity in terms of shared species, as well as largely different selection criteria and local principles of plant use (Shepard, 2004).

However, only if we consider what is available for selection can we really appreciate the cultural selection and local use of plant-based remedies. A cross-cultural comparison of medicinal plant use benefits from an analysis in the context of the available flora overall (Moerman *et al.*, 1999). Moerman and colleagues have shown that medicinal plant selection among different indigenous communities is generally biased in favour of specific taxa, especially families such as Asteraceae and Lamiaceae, while others are generally neglected, such as Cyperaceae, Poaceae and Orchidaceae. The question is to what extent this general picture is influenced by a common knowledge background due to knowledge transmission, the distribution and availability of taxa, the meaning response or the biological effectiveness (Moerman, 2007). Double or triple cross-over comparisons taking the overall flora and the uses of the medicinal flora into account are able to point out consensus and variation quite clearly and can help to better characterize local particularities (Leonti *et al.*, 2009, 2010; Weckerle *et al.*, 2011). Such approaches can contextualize ecological constraints and biogeographical parameters with medicinal plant selection processes and may lead to interesting new hypotheses.

## 4.7  Conclusion

Ethnopharmacology can be seen as a transdisciplinary and intercultural medical self-reflectory science and therefore it is important that appropriate methods and concepts developed in the socio-cultural as well as natural sciences are applied.

## References

Alexiades, M.N. (1996) Collecting ethnobotanical data: An introduction to basic concepts and techniques, in *Selected Guidelines for Ethnobotanical Research: A Field Manual* (eds M.N. Alexiades and J.W. Sheldon), Advances in Economic Botany, New York Botanical Garden Bronx, New York, pp. 53–94.

Bennett, B.C. and Balick, M.J. (2014) Does the name really matter? The importance of botanical nomenclature and plant taxonomy in biomedical research. *Journal of Ethnopharmacology*, **152**, 387–392.

Berlin, E.A. and Berlin, B. (2005) Some field methods in medical ethnobiology. *Field Methods*, **17**, 235–268.

Berlin, E.A., Jara, V.M., Berlin, B., *et al.* (1993) Me' winik: discovery of the biomedical equivalence for a Maya ethnomedical syndrome. *Social Science and Medicine*, **37**, 671–678.

Bernard, H.R. (2006) *Research Methods in Anthropology – Qualitative and Quantitative Approaches*, Altamira Press, New York.

Boulogne, I., Germosén-Robineau, L., Ozier-Lafontaine, H., *et al.* (2011) TRAMIL ethnopharmalogical survey in Les Saintes (Guadeloupe, French West Indies): a comparative study. *Journal of Ethnopharmacology*, **133**, 1039–1050.

Browner, C.H., De Montellano, B.R.O. and Rubel, A.J. (1988) A methodology for cross-cultural ethnomedical research. *Current Anthropology*, **29**, 681–702.

Bussmann, R.W. (2015) Taxonomy – an irreplaceable tool for validation of herbal medicine, in *Evidence-Based Validation of Herbal Medicines. Farm to Pharma*, (ed. P. Mukherjee), Elsevier, pp. 87–118.

Bye, R., Linares, E. and Estrada, E. (1995) Biological diversity of medicinal plants in Mexico, in *Phytochemistry of Medicinal Plants* (eds J.T. Arnason, R. Mata, and J.T. Romeo), Plenum Press, New York, pp. 65–82.

Collins S., Martins, X., Mitchell, A., *et al.* (2006) Quantitative ethnobotany in two East Timorese cultures. *Economic Botany*, **60**, 347–361.

Cos, P., Vlietinck, A.J., Berghe, D.V. and Maes, L. (2006) Anti-infective potential of natural products: how to develop a stronger in vitro 'proof-of-concept'. *Journal of Ethnopharmacology*, **106**, 290–302.

Davis, W. (2010) Last of their kind. *Scientific American*, **303**, 60–67.

Ember, C.R. and Ember, M. (2001) *Cross-Cultural Research Methods*, AltaMira Press, Lanham, MD.

Etkin, N.L. (1993) Anthropological methods in ethnopharmacology. *Journal of Ethnopharmacology*, **38**, 93–104.

Etkin, N.L. (2001) Perspectives in ethnopharmacology: forging a closer link between bioscience and traditional empirical knowledge. *Journal of Ethnopharmacology*, **76**, 177–182.

Flores, K.E. and Quinlan, M.B. (2014) Ethnomedicine of menstruation in rural Dominica, West Indies. *Journal of Ethnopharmacology*, **153**, 624–634.

Gertsch, J. (2009) How scientific is the science in ethnopharmacology? Historical perspectives and epistemological problems. *Journal of Ethnopharmacology*, **122**, 177–183.

Gesler, W.M. (1992) Therapeutic landscapes: Medical issues in light of the new cultural geography. *Social Science and Medicine*, **34**, 735–746.

Giovannini, P., Reyes-García, V., Waldstein, A. and Heinrich, M. (2011) Do pharmaceuticals displace local knowledge and use of medicinal plants? Estimates from a cross-sectional study in a rural indigenous community, Mexico. *Social Science and Medicine*, **72**, 928–936.

Graz, B., Falquet, J. and Elisabetsky, E. (2010). Ethnopharmacology, sustainable development and cooperation: The importance of gathering clinical data during field surveys. *Journal of Ethnopharmacology*, **130**, 635–638.

Headland, N.H. (1990) Introduction: A dialogue between Kenneth Pike and Marvin Harris on emics and etics, in *Emics and Etics: The Insider/Outsider Debate* (eds T. Headland, K. Pike and H. Harris), Sage, Newbury Park, pp. 13–27.

Heinrich, M. (2010) Ethnopharmacology and drug discovery, in *Comprehensive Natural Products II Chemistry and Biology*, *Vol.* **3** (eds L. Mander and H.-W. Lui), Elsevier, Oxford, pp. 351–381.

Heinrich, M., Ankli, A., Frei, B., Weimann, C. and Sticher, O. (1998) Medicinal plants in Mexico: healers' consensus and cultural importance. *Social Science and Medicine*, **47**, 1863–1875.

Heinrich, M., Barnes, J., Gibbons, S. and Williamson, E.M. (2004) *Fundamentals of Pharmacognosy and Phytotherapy*, Churchill Livingstone, London.

Heinrich, M., Edwards, S., Moerman, D.E. and Leonti, M. (2009) Ethnopharmacological field studies: a critical assessment of their conceptual basis and methods. *Journal of Ethnopharmacology*, **124**, 1–17.

Hickerson, N. (1992) Emics and etics: The insider/outsider debate. *American Anthropologist*, **94**, 186–187.

Houghton, P.J., Howes, M.J., Lee, C.C. and Steventon, G. (2007) Uses and abuses of in vitro tests in ethnopharmacology: visualizing an elephant. *Journal of Ethnopharmacology*, **110**, 391–400.

Johns, T. (1990) *With Bitter Herbs They Shall Eat it: Chemical Ecology and the Origins of Human Diet and Medicine*, University of Arizona Press, Tucson.

Leonti, M. and Casu, L. (2013) Traditional medicines and globalization: current and future perspectives in ethnopharmacology. *Frontiers in Pharmacology*, **4**, 92.

Leonti, M., Nebel, S., Rivera, D. and Heinrich, M. (2006) Wild gathered food plants in the European Mediterranean: A comparative analysis. *Economic Botany*, **60**, 130–142.

Leonti, M., Casu, L., Sanna, F. and Bonsignore, L. (2009) A comparison of medicinal plant use in Sardinia and Sicily – *De Materia Medica* revisited? *Journal of Ethnopharmacology*, **121**, 255–267.

Leonti, M., Cabras, S., Weckerle, C.S., *et al.* (2010) The causal dependence of present plant knowledge on herbals – contemporary medicinal plant use in Campania (Italy) compared to Matthioli (1568). *Journal of Ethnopharmacology*, **130**, 379–391.

Leporatti, M.L. and Ivancheva, S. (2003) Preliminary comparative analysis of medicinal plants used in the traditional medicine of Bulgaria and Italy. *Journal of Ethnopharmacology*, **87**, 123–142.

Liesner, R. (no date) Field techniques used by Missouri Botanical Garden. PDF in English, French and Spanish, http://www.mobot.org/MOBOT/molib/fieldtechbook/welcome.shtml.

Logan, M.H. and Dixon, A.R. (1994) Agriculture and the acquisition of medicinal plant knowledge, in *Eating on the Wild Side*, (ed. N.L. Etkin), University of Arizona Press, Tucson, pp. 25–45.

Martin, G.M. (1995) *Ethnobotany*, Chapman and Hall, London.

Moerman, D.E. (2007) Agreement and meaning: rethinking consensus analysis. *Journal of Ethnopharmacology*, **112**, 451–460.

Moerman, D.E. and Estabrook, G.F. (2003) Native Americans' choice of species for medicinal use is dependent on plant family: confirmation with meta-significance analysis. *Journal of Ethnopharmacology*, **87**, 51–59.

Moerman, D.E., Pemberton, R.W., Kiefer, D. and Berlin, B. (1999) A comparative analysis of five medicinal floras. *Journal of Ethnobiology*, **19**, 49–67.

Monigatti, M., Bussmann, R.W. and Weckerle, C.S. (2013) Medicinal plant use in two Andean communities located at different altitudes in the Bolívar Province, Peru. *Journal of Ethnopharmacology*, **145**, 450–464.

Pieroni, A. and Quave, C.L. (2005) Traditional pharmacopoeias and medicines among Albanians and Italians in southern Italy: a comparison. *Journal of Ethnopharmacology*, **101**, 258–270.

Rivier, L. and Bruhn, J.G. (1979) Editorial. *Journal of Ethnopharmacology*, **1**, 1.

Romney, A.K., Weller, S. and Batchelder, W. (1986) Culture as consensus: A theory of culture and informant accuracy. *American Anthropologist*, **88**, 313–338.

Shepard, G. (2004) A sensory ecology of medicinal plant therapy in two Amazonian societies. *American Anthropologist*, **106**, 252–266.

Soejarto, D.D., Gyllenhaal, C., Kadushin, M.R., *et al.* (2012) An ethnobotanical survey of medicinal plants of Laos toward the discovery of bioactive compounds as potential candidates for pharmaceutical development. *Pharmaceutical Biology*, **50**, 42–60.

Sticher, O. (2008) Natural product isolation. *Natural Product Reports*, **25**, 517–554.

Trotter, R. and Logan, M. (1986) Informant consensus, a new approach for identifying potentially effective medicinal plants, in *Plants in Indigenous Medicine and Diet, Biobehavioural Approaches* (ed. N.L. Etkin), Redgrave Publishers, Bedford Hills, NY, pp. 91–112.

Verpoorte, R., Choi, Y.H. and Kim, H.K. (2005) Ethnopharmacology and systems biology: a perfect holistic match. *Journal of Ethnopharmacology*, **100**, 53–56.

Wagner, H. and Ulrich-Merzenich, G. (2009) Synergy research: Approaching a new generation of phytopharmaceuticals. *Phytomedicine*, **16**, 97–110.

Weckerle, C.S., Cabras, S., Castellanos, M.E. and Leonti, M. (2011) Quantitative methods in ethnobotany and ethnopharmacology: considering the overall flora – hypothesis testing for over- and underused plant families with the Bayesian approach. *Journal of Ethnopharmacology*, **137**, 837–843.

Weller, S.C. (2007) Cultural consensus theory: Applications and frequently asked questions. *Field Methods*, **19**, 339–368.

Witt, C.M. (2013) Clinical research on traditional drugs and food items – the potential of comparative effectiveness research for interdisciplinary research. *Journal of Ethnopharmacology*, **147**, 254–258.

# 5
# Biodiversity, Conservation and Ethnopharmacology

Vernon H. Heywood

*School of Biological Sciences, University of Reading, Whiteknights, UK*

## 5.1   Introduction

'Work in ethnobiology and ethnomedicine, including ethnobotany, ethnozoology, and ethnoecology, necessarily entails meticulous and rigorous systematic observation of the myriad ways indigenous and local communities cognize, utilize, and classify the floral and faunal resources on which they depend for survival.'

Nolan and Pieroni (2013)

Ultimately, the raw material of ethnopharmacology is the vast diversity of plants, animals and microorganisms (both terrestrial and marine) that grow and live on our planet in natural or semi-natural ecosystems, which are or may potentially be exploited for medicine and the indigenous knowledge about their use. Today, that resource base is increasingly under threat, mainly from habitat loss or degradation, overexploitation, growth in the human population and the impacts of invasive alien species, but its conservation and sustainable use has attracted too little attention from ethnopharmacologists.

Although the central goal of ethnopharmacology is to investigate 'the anthropological rationale and the pharmacological basis of the medicinal use of plants, animals, fungi, microorganisms, and minerals by human cultures' (Leonti and Casu, 2013), it is increasingly becoming a multidisciplinary field of inquiry. In particular, the linkages between ethnopharmacology, food and nutrition are increasingly being recognized. As has been argued elsewhere (Arnason, 2005; Heywood, 2011, 2013), ethnopharmacology, biodiversity, agriculture, food and nutrition are inextricably linked but suffer from compartmentalization and a lack of communication which have to be overcome if progress is to be made. Consequently, ethnopharmacology has to extend its remit beyond medicinal uses and take into consideration the food and nutritional aspects of the many species used in traditional agricultural and forestry societies. Indeed the distinction between food and medicine is difficult to maintain and the title of one of Nina Etkin's influential books is *Edible Medicines. An ethnopharmacology of food* (Etkin, 2007). In this book she describes the interface between diet, medicine and natural products. As she points out, '... virtually all societies use plants and animals in more than one way, as food, medicine, and cosmetics'.

## 5.2    Changing attitudes to the ownership of biodiversity

The collection of wild plants and animals for medicines or food goes back to the beginning of human habitation of the planet. The use of plants as medicines has been recorded from ancient civilizations such as those of Mesopotamia, Egypt, China and Greece (for a historical overview see Dias *et al.*, 2012). Until 30 years ago, there were few restrictions on the freedom of individuals, organizations or companies to collect, evaluate and exploit biodiversity, mainly plants and animals, from around the world as sources of potential drugs or medicines or as new food, fibre, oil or energy crops. In addition to local use, the exploitation of wild plants by people not indigenous to the region where they grow is a long-standing tradition that dates back to the expedition to Punt (probably today's Somalia) sent by Queen Hatshepsut of Egypt in 1495 BC to bring back trees with fragrant resin. Later, naturalists, biologists and others engaged in sampling the natural world for plants and animals that could be exploited, either in the country concerned or by bringing them back to their own country for introduction to cultivation or domestication. This was an important part of the colonial process and under various guises persists to the present day. During parts of the 20th century some pharmaceutical companies and others invested heavily in plant exploration to seek out new sources of natural products that might have potential for the development of new drugs and large numbers of species were screened for this purpose.

The situation changed dramatically with the coming into force of the Convention on Biological Diversity (CBD) in 1993. Prior to the CBD, the world's diversity of plants, animals and microorganisms was regarded as the 'common heritage of mankind' and there to be exploited more or less at will. During the negotiations leading up to the CBD, it was forcibly stated that such an attitude was completely unacceptable and on the contrary the position that countries have sovereignty over the biodiversity and genetic resources within their own frontiers was enshrined within the CBD. It specifically mentions species of medicinal value in the indicative list of categories of the components of biological diversity to be identified and monitored (CBD, 1994). It also calls for measures to respect, preserve and maintain the knowledge, innovations and practices of indigenous and local communities for conserving and sustainably using biodiversity. Following the agreement of the Bonn guidelines on access to genetic resources and the fair and equitable sharing of the benefits arising from their utilization in 2002, the CBD adopted the Nagoya Protocol in 2010 which 'aims at sharing the benefits arising from the utilization of genetic resources in a fair and equitable way, including by appropriate access to genetic resources and by appropriate transfer of relevant technologies, taking into account all rights over those resources and to technologies, and by appropriate funding, thereby contributing to the conservation of biological diversity and the sustainable use of its components' (CBD, 2011).

The exploitation of biodiversity, including medicinal plants, is now much more strictly controlled as a result of both national and international legislation and instruments such as the CBD and the Convention on International Trade in Endangered Species of Wild Flora and Fauna (CITES). CITES is the only international instrument for listing species of plants and animals whose numbers are considered to be endangered to the extent that commercial trade must either be monitored and controlled or prohibited. However, the number of medicinal or aromatic species listed in Appendix I (which prohibits commercial trade) is some 200 plus (Schippmann, 2001) while a few are listed under Appendix II (which requires the presentation of export permits). A growing number of countries have legislation dealing specifically with medicinal plants and some countries have restrictions on the commercial collection of medicinal plants.

Although the consequences of these various legal instruments have generally been beneficial in creating an ethical regime within which natural products research can be undertaken, the levels of regulation have been exploited by some countries in such a way as to prevent access by outside workers or are so onerous as to have serious consequences for medicinal plant exploration and research (see discussions in Cordell, 2012 and Kingston, 2011).

In addition to international conventions and national legislation, there are various 'soft law' approaches such as guidelines on the conservation of medicinal and aromatic plants. These include the WHO, IUCN, WWF Guidelines (Heywood and Synge, 1993), currently under revision, the WHO (2003) Guidelines on Good Agricultural and Collection Practices (GACP) for Medicinal Plants, the International Standard for Sustainable Wild Collection of Medicinal and Aromatic Plants (ISSC-MAP) Version 1.0 Bundesamt für Naturschutz (2007) and the FairWild Standard version 2 (FairWild, 2010; Kathe *et al.*, 2010; Kathe, 2011).

Today's ethnopharmacologists need to be cognisant not only of the ethical, legal, ecological, sociocultural and sociopolitical context and implications of their work (Etkin, 2007) but of the relentless threats to biodiversity and the need for sustainable use and to conserve it for future generations. As has been noted (Heywood, 2011), although some ethnopharmacologists have expressed concern at the loss of biodiversity, there has been little direct involvement and it is perhaps now time to consider a more proactive role in determining the actions needed to assess, monitor and conserve the resource base. Another, more recent, concern is the need to assess the implications of global change on the resource base of ethnopharmacology.

# 5.3 Medicinal and aromatic plants as resources

' ... much of Nature's "treasure trove of small molecules" remains to be explored, particularly from the marine and microbial environments' (Newman and Cragg, 2012)

It is only in the last few decades that medicinal plants have been regarded as resources and an important and highly valuable component of biodiversity (Heywood, 1999). When regarded in this light, medicinal and aromatic plants may be viewed from quite different perspectives. For the hundreds of millions[1] who depend on them as a major part of their healthcare delivery system they are a vital local resource and their usage often depends on various kinds of practitioner.

In South Africa, for example, about 10% (2062 species) of the native flora has been recorded as being used for traditional medicine (Williams *et al.*, 2013) and an estimated 27 million people make regular use of the services of the country's 200 000 traditional healthcare practitioners, all of whom apply indigenous and exotic plants in their remedies. This number excludes the people who purchase medicinal plants solely from informal markets. It has been estimated

---

[1] The much cited estimate by WHO that '80% of the population living in rural areas in developing countries depend on traditional medicine for their health care needs' does not appear to have a sound factual basis (cf. http://africacheck.org/reports/do-80-of-s-africans-regularly-consult-traditional-healers-the-claim-is-false/#sthash.E52Ss3Px.dpuf).

that the local trade in medicinal plants, representing 574 species, amounts to 20 000 t per annum (Wentzel and van Ginkel, 2012), and is worth €200 million (R2.9 billion) per annum, which is 5.6% of the South African National Health budget (Mander *et al.*, 2011).

On the other hand, for western societies and pharmaceutical companies there has been a tendency to regard the diversity of wild organisms as a cornucopia to be enjoyed, with little regard for the people and cultures in the countries where they occur. As Cordell (2012) rightly points out, the remarkable advances in the past 100 years and the huge investment in drug discovery and development by major pharmaceutical companies has provided us with an array of drugs that have transformed our health and life expectancy but has done little to benefit those who rely on or choose to depend partly on plant-based phytotherapeuticals or dietary supplements as the basis of their primary health care: 'Those billions of people, many of them living close to or below the poverty line, have seen little or no improvement in the quality and delivery of their medicinal agents, usually wild-crafted plants. With selected exceptions, there has been no well-funded, science-based activity which would assure them, quite simply, of a quality assured product that worked.' In the closely related field of plant genetic resources of plants of agriculture, one can detect a paradigm shift in participatory approaches to collecting traditional knowledge from extracting knowledge for scientific use to a focus on how local communities can benefit from working with scientists (Quek and Friis-Hansen, 2011; Heywood, 2013). The challenge for ethnopharmacology and ethnobiology is to ensure a similar change in emphasis so that local communities are the primary or at least co-equal beneficiaries.

## 5.4   How many species?

The number of species of plants, animals and microorganisms used in ethnomedicine cannot be stated with any degree of accuracy and depends partly on how medicinal plants are defined.[2] No comprehensive global database exists although a Global Checklist of Medicinal Plants is under preparation by the Medicinal Plant Specialist Group of the IUCN Species Survival Commission (Leaman, 2012) and includes more than 28,000 species of plants with well-documented medicinal uses, based on a variety of sources, including the NAPRALERT®[3] database which, since its launch in 1975, provides a compendium of published information about natural products, including ethnomedical information on more than 20,000 species of plants (University of Illinois Board of Trustees, 2012).

A list prepared by WHO contained 21,000 names and Farnsworth and Soejarto (1991) suggested that 14–28% of the world's plant species have been used ethnomedically, an estimate based on an extrapolation from the NAPRALERT database. This would indicate a figure of between 65,000 and 118,000 depending on the total number of plant species believed to exist. In another extrapolation, from the proportion of national floras included in 15 national pharmacopoeias, Schippmann *et al.* (2006) estimated that 50,000–70,000 species of higher plants are used as medicines worldwide.

So far, plants have provided many more active compounds used in medicines than have animals, although marine organisms are increasingly proving to be an important source. Likewise, microorganisms are not only key in the production of antibiotics but, as pointed out by

---

[2] If a narrow definition is adopted – that the term 'medicinal' applied to a plant indicates that it contains a substance or substances which modulate beneficially the physiology of sick mammals, and that has been used by humans for that purpose – the number of species will be much smaller than if the more widely framed definition of say, Srivavasta *et al.* (1996): 'those that are commonly used treating and preventing specific ailments and diseases, and that are generally considered to play a beneficial role in health care' is applied.

[3] Acronym of NAtural PRoducts ALERT.

Newman and Cragg (2012) in their review of natural products as sources of drugs from 1981 to 2010, it is becoming clear that as regards the role of microbes as sources of novel bioactive entities there are molecules whose production depends on the interaction with organisms from similar or occasionally widely different taxa. They cite the case of the activations of natural product biosynthesis in *Streptomyces* by mycolic acid-containing bacteria (Onaka *et al.*, 2011).

## 5.5 Chemical diversity

The chemical diversity and the underlying genetic diversity found in natural populations is of particular importance when dealing with medicinal and aromatic plants, where it is precisely their chemical features, such as alkaloids, essential oils, etc., that are the characteristics for which they are valued.

However, in the assessment and conservation of plant biodiversity, with its organismic, ecological and genetic components, the last of these are the least studied. Likewise in research on medicinal plants, the genetic aspect is also seriously neglected, in contrast with the enormous amount of effort that has gone into isolating and characterizing these chemical constituents from the limited samples that are traditionally used in phytochemical studies.

It is worth noting that although combinatorial chemistry coupled with high throughput screening (HTS) since the 1990s has allowed the generation and screening of libraries of hundreds of thousands of compounds, and led to the diversion of resources away from natural product screening, it has had very limited success in developing *de novo* combinatorial compounds – only one has been approved as a drug in the period 1981–2010 (Kingston, 2011; Newman and Cragg, 2012).

Probably less than 10% of the world's biodiversity has been evaluated for potential biological activity so it is likely that a large number of useful natural lead compounds await discovery, especially from plants, marine organisms and microorganisms. Accessing this vast library of natural chemical diversity will pose many technical scientific, social and legal challenges (Cragg and Newman, 2005; Kingston, 2011) but it is also critical that steps are taken to maintain the continued availability of this diversity through appropriate and effective conservation measures in the face of the persistent threats facing biodiversity across the globe.

## 5.6 Wild harvesting and over-collection

The great majority of medicinal and aromatic plant (MAP) species used today are collected from the wild. The type of wild harvesting or gathering of medicinal and aromatic plants that is a cause of concern in the context of biodiversity conservation is where parts of the target species – leaves, stems, bark, roots, flowers, fruits, seeds or whole plants – are collected, often destructively, in some quantity for medicinal purposes, either as part of traditional medicine systems or for commercial exploitation by national or international pharmaceutical companies. The concern stems from the possible effects of wild harvesting on the regeneration or even survival of the populations of the species that are sampled.

As the collectors are usually paid very low prices for this wild-harvested material, with prices maintained at artificially low levels by small groups of traders acting as a monopoly, this may have the effect of encouraging over-harvesting so that the collectors get sufficient reward for their work. Of course, such low prices do not allow for the costs involved in managing or replacing the resources, and little attention is paid to these aspects by importing companies that require the collection of large quantities of wild material.

Specific examples of serious over-collecting have been reported, as in the case of *Voacanga africana* Scott-Elliot (Apocynaceae) where Cunningham and Mbenkum (1993) reported that 900 tonnes of the seed, used for the industrial production of the alkaloid tabersonine, a depressor of the central nervous system activity in geriatric patients, were exported from Cameroon to France between 1985 and 1991, and 11,537 tonnes of the bark of *Prunus africana* (Hook.f.) Kalkman (Rosaceae) (red stinkwood), used to treat prostatitis, in the same period. In fact, some important medicinal plant species are already considered extinct outside protected areas as in KwaZulu-Natal, for example, where the wild ginger (*Siphonochilus aethiopicus* (Schweinf.) B.L.Burtt, Zingberaceae), the pepper bark tree (*Warburgia salutaris* (G.Bertol.) Chiov., Canellaceae) and the black stinkwood (*Ocotea bullata* (Burch.) E. Meyer, Lauraceae) are no longer found outside reserves and parks (Mander, 1999). One approach to sustainable utilisation of wild populations of medicinal plants is to establish holding nurseries on a regional scale where local traditional health practitioners and plant gatherers can obtain stock that they can propagate themselves. Emphasis should be placed on the training of traditional health practitioners and plant gatherers to enable them to propagate their own medicinal plants

## 5.7 Medicinal plant conservation

Until the 1980s, medicinal plant conservation was a largely neglected and underappreciated field. A key milestone was the International Consultation on the Conservation of Medicinal Plants WHO-IUCN-WWF in Chiang Mai, Thailand in 1988 and the Chiang Mai Declaration issued by the Consultation that affirmed the importance of medicinal plants and called upon the UN and its agencies and other international organizations to take action and support countries to ensure the conservation of medicinal plants. A draft set of guidelines for the conservation and sustainable use of medicinal plants was approved and subsequently revised and published (Heywood and Synge, 1993). The proceedings of the meeting were also published (Akerele *et al.*, 1991).

## 5.8 Conservation approaches

The conservation of medicinal plants and animals presents a series of intractable problems, including:

- the potentially very large numbers of species involved
- lack of information on the conservation status of the majority of the species and on the detailed nature of the threats to them
- the threats from over-collecting
- the need to sample adequately the genetic variation responsible for the chemical diversity in the targeted secondary metabolites found in populations
- the need to conserve not just the organisms but the indigenous traditional knowledge associated with them
- the legal complexities under ABS regimes and issues such as ownership of intellectual property rights
- a reluctance on the part of many governments and agencies to become involved and invest in conservation of these species.

## 5.9    Protected areas

The generally accepted paradigm for effective conservation of biodiversity is *in situ* through maintenance of the ecosystems in which it occurs, by setting aside protected areas. Protected areas do not necessarily ensure the maintenance of particular component target species (such as medicinal plants) nor of the genetic and chemical diversity that they contain without specific management intervention to ensure their survival (Heywood, 2014). A drawback is that the distribution and abundance of medicinal plant species is generally poorly known, thus making it difficult to evaluate their presence in protected areas (Leaman *et al.*, 1999). Moreover, the distribution of protected areas does not match that of many of the species that are most threatened and requires considerable targeted expansion (Pimm *et al.*, 2014; Venter *et al.*, 2014) and in the case of widespread species medicinal species may not cover sufficiently the occurrence of all the chemically significant populations. A study on genetic diversity within tea tree (*Melaleuca alternifolia* (Maiden and Betche) Cheel, Myrtaceae), which is harvested from natural stands and plantations for production of Australian tea-tree oil, showed that although there is considerable genetic variation across the species, the majority of the variation occurs within single populations, some of which may be quite localized (Rossetto *et al.*, 1999).

## 5.10    Community conservation

Various forms of community conservation are often adopted for medicinally important species in traditional societies. Although often lacking legal recognition or government support, community-based approaches are increasingly receiving support from non-governmental organisations (NGOs) and are useful in combining both local and formal systems of medicine (Shukla and Gardner, 2006). Culturally protected forest patches or sacred groves are examples of community conservation (for other examples see Hawkins, 2008). As Hamilton (2004) notes, 'The special significance of medicinal plants in conservation stems from the major cultural, livelihood or economic roles that they play in many people's lives.' He argues that most work by conservationists on medicinal plants should be with those people who own, manage or make use of these species, or else own or manage the land on which they grow and 'the significance of medicinal plants to people can be sufficiently great that arrangements made for the conservation and sustainable use of medicinal plants can lay important foundations for the conservation of natural habitats and ecological services more generally'.

## 5.11    Genetic conservation

Structured scientific approaches to the conservation of medicinal and aromatic plants, such as genetic conservation, have developed significantly in the past 20–30 years. In particular, the *in situ* conservation of target species within ecosystems can be a complex and difficult process (Heywood and Dulloo, 2005; Iriondo *et al.*, 2008; Hunter and Heywood, 2011; Heywood, 2014) and has been attempted so far for only a very small number of medicinal plants. As with agricultural plants, including wild food plants and crop wild relatives, the focus is on the genetic variation (hence the term 'genetic conservation') that is responsible for providing the desired characteristics — in the case of medicinal plants, the secondary metabolites that are exploited. Genetic conservation involves technical procedures such as ecogeographical surveying, population sampling and analytical techniques for determining genetic variation, and socio-economic issues such as wild harvesting and sustainable use of these resources, bioprospecting agreements and the role of local communities and intellectual property rights.

Particular attention has to be paid in sampling of populations for genetic conservation to the variation in the constituents, such as essential oils, which may be affected by many factors. Infraspecific variation can occur as a result of differing soil conditions, altitude, climatic conditions, seasonal factors and other environmental features, leading in some cases to the evolution of different chemical variants or chemotypes. This significant chemical variation occurring in plants, especially those with prominent chemical components such as terpenoids, alkaloids, etc., has attracted considerable attention and an extensive literature has developed.

The *ex situ* conservation of germplasm of medicinal plants in seedbanks, living collections in botanic gardens, field genebanks, tissue and cell culture is an important complement to *in situ* approaches. Many seed banks do contain samples of some medicinal plants, but they are not generally the result of deliberate sampling campaigns. Botanic gardens have occupied an important role in the study of medicinal plants for the past 500 years (Heywood, 1987) and recommendations for medicinal plant conservation have been made by Heywood (1991) and Hawkins (2008). A review of the techniques used to preserve germplasm for ethnobiology is given by Dierig *et al.* (2014).

In practice both *in situ* and *ex situ* approaches are complementary. An example is the network of 55 conservation sites that has been established for the conservation of medicinal plant diversity in southern India by the Foundation for the Revitalization of Local Health Traditions (FRLHT). These include 30 *in situ* areas, 15 *ex situ* centres and 10 *in situ* medicinal plant development areas in cooperation with the local community (Tandon, 1996).

## 5.12   Cultivation

Bringing widely used medical plant species into cultivation may take the pressure off their wild populations by reducing the amounts that need to be harvested. It also permits better species identification, improved quality control and increased prospects for genetic improvements. On the other hand, it can be argued that cultivation of medicinal plants may also in some cases lead to a loss of wild habitat and reduce incentives to conserve and manage wild populations (Dulloo *et al.*, 2014). According to Mulliken and Inskipp (2006) the number of medicinal plant species in trade that are cultivated is probably less than 1000.

## 5.13   Conclusions

Wild biodiversity has been exploited by humans as a resource for thousands of years but the greater part of it stills remains to be described and assessed. In the case of medicinal plants, animals and microorganisms, ethnopharmacology has so far utilized only a small percentage of the world's biodiversity – in the case of plants, of the world's 350,000–400,000 species, only about 4–5% have been reported on ethnomedically and of these more than half have not been studied biologically or chemically, while for other groups such as marine organisms, exploration is in its infancy. Much of this resource base and the traditional knowledge on its use is at risk because of anthropogenic change and urgently needs conservation action to ensure its continued availability for present and future generations. Given the large numbers of species involved and the very limited resources available, action is needed to establish priorities at national, regional and global levels. It is essential that local communities should be closely involved in these decisions and in the conservation actions that ensue.

# References

Akerele, O., Heywood, V. and Synge, H. (eds) (1991) *Conservation of Medicinal Plants*, Cambridge University Press, Cambridge.

Arnason, J.T. (ed.) (2005) *Biodiversity and Health*, Volume 46332 of NRCC publication, National Research Council of Canada, NRC Research Press.

CBD (1994) *Convention on Biological Diversity, Text and Annexes*, Interim Secretariat of the Convention on Biological Diversity, Geneva.

CBD (2011) *Nagoya Protocol on Access to Genetic Resources and the Fair and Equitable Sharing of Benefits Arising from their Utilization to the Convention on Biological Diversity: text and annex*, Secretariat of the Convention on Biological Diversity, Montreal.

Cordell, G.A. (2012) New strategies for traditional medicine, in *Medicinal Plants: Biodiversity and Drugs* (eds M.K. Rai, G.A. Cordell, J.L. Martinez, M. Marinoff and L. Rastrelli), CRC Press, Boca Raton, FL, pp. 1–45.

Cragg, G.M. and Newman, D.J. (2005) Biodiversity: A continuing source of novel drug leads. *Pure and Appled Chemistry*, **77**, 7–24.

Cunningham, A.B. and Mbenkum, F.T. (1993) *Sustainability of harvesting* Prunus africana *bark in Cameroon: a medicinal plant in international trade*, People and Plants Working Paper 2, UNESCO, Paris.

Dias, D.A., Urban, S. and Roessner, U. (2012) A historical overview of natural products in drug discovery. *Metabolites*, **2**, 303–336, doi:10.3390/metabo2020303.

Dierig, D., Blackburn, H., Ellis, H. and Nesbitt, N. (2014) Curating seeds and other genetic resources foe wthnobiologu, in *Curating Biocultural Collections: A Handbook* (eds J. Salick, K. Konchar and M. Nesbitt), Kew Publications, Richmond.

Dulloo, E., Hunter D. and Leaman, D. (2014) Plant diversity in addressing food, nutrition and medicinal needs, in *Novel Plant Bioresources: Applications in Food, Medicine and Cosmetics* (ed. A. Gurib-Fakim), Wiley Blackwell, Chichester.

Etkin, N.L. (2007) *Edible Medicines. An ethnopharmacology of food*, University of Arizona Press, Tucson.

FairWild (2010) Fair Wild Standard: Version 2.0. FairWild Foundation, Weinfelden, Switzerland.

Farnsworth, N.R. and Soejarto, D.D. (1991) Global importance of medicinal plants, in *The Conservation of Medicinal Plants* (eds O. Akerele, V. Heywood and H. Synge), Cambridge University Press, Cambridge, pp. 25–27.

Hamilton, A.C. (2004) Medicinal plants, conservation and livelihoods. *Biodiversity and Conservation*, **13**, 1477–1517.

Hawkins, B. (2008) *Plants for Life: Medicinal Plant Conservation and Botanic Gardens*, Botanic Gardens Conservation International, Richmond.

Heywood, V.H. (1987) The changing rôle of the botanic gardens, in *Botanic Gardens and the World Conservation Strategy* (eds D. Bramwell *et al.*), Academic Press, London, pp. 3–18.

Heywood, V. (1991) Botanic gardens and the conservation of medicinal plants, in *Conservation of Medicinal Plants* (eds O. Akerele, V. Heywood and H. Synge), Cambridge University Press, Cambridge, pp. 213–228.

Heywood, V. (1999) Medicinal and aromatic plants as global resources, in *Proceedings of the Second World Congress on Medicinal and Aromatic Plants WOCMAP-2*, Acta Horticulturae No. 500, pp. 21–29.

Heywood, V.H. (2011) Ethnopharmacology, food production, nutrition and biodiversity conservation: towards a sustainable future for indigenous peoples. *Journal of Ethnopharmacology*, **137**, 1–15, doi:10.1016/j.jep.2011.05.027.

Heywood, V.H. (2013) Overview of agricultural biodiversity and its importance to nutrition and Health, in *Diversifying Food and Diets: Using Agricultural Biodiversity to Improve Nutrition and Health* (eds J. Fanzo, D. Hunter, T. Borelli and F. Mattei), Earthscan/Routledge, London.

Heywood, V.H. (2014) An overview of *in situ* conservation of plant species in the Medterranean. *Flora Mediterranea*, **24**, 5–24, doi: 10 7320/FlMedit24.000.

Heywood, V.H. and Dulloo, M.E. (2005) In Situ *Conservation of Wild Plant Species – A Critical Global Review of Good Practices*, IPGRI Technical Bulletin, No 11, FAO and IPGRI, IPGRI, Rome, Italy.

Heywood, V.H. and Synge, H. (eds) (1993) *Guidelines on the Conservation of Medicinal Plants*, WHO, IUCN, WWF, Gland, vii + 50 pp.

Hunter, D. and Heywood, V. (eds) (2011) *Crop Wild Relatives. A Manual of* in situ *Conservation. Earthscan*, London.

Iriondo, J.M., Dulloo, E. and Maxted, N. (eds) (2008) *Conserving Plant Genetic Diversity in Protected Areas: Population Management of Crop Wild Relatives*, CAB International Publishing, Wallingford.

Kathe, W., Pätzold, B., Leaman, D., *et al.* (2010) Wild for a cure: ground-truthing a standard for sustainable management of wild plants in the field, TRAFFIC International, Cambridge, pp. 44

Kathe, W. (2011) The new FairWild standard – a tool to ensure sustainable wild-collection of Plants. *Medicinal plant conservation. Newsletter of the Medicinal Plant Specialist Group of the IUCN Species Survival Commission*, **14**, 14–17.

Kingston, D.G.I. (2011) Modern natural products drug discovery and its relevance to biodiversity conservation. *Journal of Natural Products*, **74** (3), 496–511, doi: 10.2021/np100550t.

Leaman, D.J. (2012) Medicinal plant conservation. *Newsletter of the Medicinal Plant Specialist Group of the IUCN Species Survival Commission*, **15**, 3.

Leaman, D.J., Fassil, H. and Thormann, I. (1999) Conserving medicinal and aromatic plant species: identifying the contributions of the International Plant Genetic Resources Institute (IPGRI), IPGRI, Rome.Leonti, M. and Casu, L. (2013) Traditional medicines and globalization: current and future perspectives in ethnopharmacology. *Frontiers in Pharmacology*, **4**, 92 (published online 25 July 2013). doi: 10.3389/fphar.2013.00092.

Mander, M. (1999) Marketing of Indigenous Medicinal Plants in South Africa : A Case Study in KwaZulu-Natal: Summary of Findings, *Food and Agricultural Organisation of the United Nations*, Forest Products Division, FAO, Rome.

Mander, M., Ntulii, L., Diederichsi, N. and Mavundlai, K. (2011) *Economics of the Traditional Medicine Trade in South Africa*, www.hst.org.za/uploads/files/chap13_07.pdf, accessed 28 June 2014.

Mulliken, T. and Inskipp, C. (2006) Medicinal plant cultivation – scope, scale and diversity: results from an initial analysis, in *Proceedings of the 1st IFOAM International Conference on Organic Wild Production, Teslic, Bosnia and Herzegovina, May 2006*, International Federation of Organic Agricultural Movements (IFOAM), Bonn.

Newman, D.J. and Cragg, G.M. (2012) Natural Products as Sources of New Drugs over the 30 Years from 1981 to 2010. *Journal of Natural Products*, **75** (3): 311–335. Published online 8 February 2012, doi: 10.1021/np200906s.

Nolan, J. and Pieroni, P. (2013) Recollections, reflections, and revelations: ethnobiologists and their 'First Time' in the field. *Journal of Ethnobiology and Ethnomedicine*, **9**, 12, http://www.ethnobiomed.com/content/9/1/12, doi:10.1186/1746-4269-9-12.

Onaka, H., Mori, Y., Igarashi, Y. and Furumai, T. (2011) Mycolic acid-containing bacteria induce natural-product biosynthesis in Streptomyces species. *Applied and Environmental Microbiology*, **77** (2), 400–406, doi: 10.1128/AEM.01337-10, Epub 19 November 2010.

Pimm, S.L., Jenkins, C.N., Abell, R., *et al.* (2014) The biodiversity of species and their rates of extinction, distribution, and protection. *Science*, **344** (6187), doi: 10.1126/science.1246752.

Quek, P. and Friis-Hansen, E. (2011) Collecting plant genetic resources and documenting associated indigenous knowledge in the field: a participatory approach, in *Collecting Plant Genetic Diversity:Technical guidelines − 2011 update* (eds L. Guarino, V. Ramanatha Rao and E. Goldberg), Bioversity International, Rome, http://cropgenebank.sgrp.cgiar.org/images/file/procedures/collecting2011/Chapter18-2011.pdf.

Rossetto, M., Slade, R.W., Baverstock, P.R., *et al.* (1999) Microsatellite variation and assessment of genetic structure in tea tree (*Melaleuca alternifolia* – Myrtaceae). *Molecular Ecology*, **8**, 633–643.

Schippmann, U., Leaman, D. and Cunningham, A.B. (2006) Cultivation and wild collection of medicinal and aromatic plants under sustainability aspects, in *Medicinal and Aromatic Plants: Agricultural, Commercial, Ecological, Legal, Pharmacological and Social Aspects* (eds R.J. Bogers, L.E. Craker and D. Lange), Springer, Dordrecht.

Shukla, S. and Gardner, J. (2006) Local knowledge in community-based approaches to medicinal plant conservation: lessons from India. *Journal of Ethnobiology and Ethnomedicine*, **2**, 20, doi: 10.1186/1746-4269-2-20.

Tandon, V. (1996) Medicinal plant diversity and its conservation in southern India, in *Floristic Characteristics and Diversity of East Asian Plants* (eds Z. Aoluo and W. Sugong), China Higher Education Press, Beijing and Springer-Verlag, Berlin, pp. 461–471.

University of Illinois Board of Trustees (2012) *NAPRALERT. Program for collaborative research in the pharmaceutical sciences*, College of Pharmacy, University of Illinois at Chicago, www.napralert.org, accessed 28 June 2014.

Venter, O., Fuller, R.A., Segan, D.B., *et al.* (2014) Targeting global protected area expansion for imperiled biodiversity. *PLOS Biology*, **12**, (6), e1001891.

Wentzel, J. and van Ginkel, C.E. (2012) *Distribution, use and ecological roles of the medicinal plants confined to freshwater ecosystems in South Africa*, WRC Report No. KV 300/12, Water Research Commision Gezira, South Africa.

WHO (2003) *WHO guidelines on good agricultural and collection practices (GACP) for medicinal plants*, World Health Organization, Geneva.

Williams, V.L., Victor, J.E. and Crouch, N.R. (2013) Red listed medicinal plants of South Africa: Status, trends, and assessment challenges. *South African Journal of Botany*, **86**, 23–35.

# 6
# Ecopharmacognosy

Geoffrey A. Cordell

*Natural Products Inc., Evanston, Illinois, USA; College of Pharmacy, University of Florida, Gainesville, Florida, USA*

## 6.1   Introduction

In series of previous articles (Cordell, 1987a, 1987b, 1990, 1993, 1995, 2000, 2001, 2004, 2007, 2008, 2009, 2011a–c, 2012, 2014a,b; Cordell and Colvard, 2005, 2007, 2012) this author and a colleague discussed various aspects of 'pharmacognosy' in terms of its burgeoning role in society, its renaissance, the need for diversification of the research parameters, the importance in establishing an evidence base for traditional medicine and that it used technology at the cutting edges of several sciences. At an early point in these discussions, a new definition of pharmacognosy was proposed: 'pharmacognosy is the study of biologically active natural products' (Cordell, 1993). This definition was designed, deliberately, to be broad. It embraces many different aspects of natural product research without specifying, in a limiting manner, the source (plant, marine, microbial, mammalian, etc.) of the studied material or indeed the nature of the research (botanical, chemical, analytical, biosynthetic, biological, pharmacological, clinical, economic, legal, etc.). In the intervening 22 years, the fundamental importance of pharmacognosy in society has intensified, while another aspect of pharmacognosy has become apparent. That aspect involves sustainability.

All human health systems are based, in part, on drugs. In an age when the world has been challenged by numerous groups at the national and international levels to examine sustainability, any discussion regarding the future of medicinal agents must begin with the question: 'How green is your medicine?' This is an enormous topic which spans both the synthetic and the natural origins of drugs in all forms. Here, only a very limited discussion will be presented of how the concept of sustainability can impact the plant-based approaches to drug discovery and traditional medicine in order to deliver a quality, safe, efficacious and consistent (QSEC) product.

Research related to any and all aspects of pharmacognosy is based on a fundamental assumption: that the organism of interest will be available now, and in the future. In general terms, that is a false assumption, which can only be ameliorated through monitoring, conservation

*Ethnopharmacology*, First Edition. Edited by Michael Heinrich and Anna K. Jäger.
© 2015 John Wiley & Sons, Ltd. Published 2015 by John Wiley & Sons, Ltd.

and scientific efforts (WHO, 2002, 2012, 2014). Accepting this realization clarified the need for a new philosophy for practical applications of biologically active natural products, and the evolution of the term 'ecopharmacognosy'.

The requirement for medicinal plants is firmly established in all global societies. Given the rapidly rising cost of allopathic medicines, and the limited breadth of drug discovery programmes in the major pharmaceutical companies (Jarvis, 2010; Cordell and Colvard, 2012), the reliance on plants as medicinal agents will be a global challenge. Given a burgeoning population projected to reach 10 billion by 2040, how can accessibility, which embraces both availability and affordability, be maintained (Cordell and Colvard, 2012)? At a time of globalization of traditional medicine systems, and the development of new phytotherapeuticals and dietary supplements, together with the tremendous increase in the e-commerce of totally unregulated medicinal agents, continuing the availability of the required medicinal plant materials becomes a challenge to be met, not ignored. An additional concerning factor is that because most traditional medicines are wild-crafted, they are disappearing from their respective habitats to the point of local extinction (Schippmann *et al.*, 2006).

## 6.2   Sustainable medicines and pharmacognosy

Several years ago, this author began to discuss the need to consider all medicinal agents, whether naturally or totally synthetic-based, as sustainable medicines (Cordell and Michel, 2007; Cordell, 2008, 2009, 2011a–c, 2012; Cordell and Colvard, 2012). With respect to plant-based drugs, the assessment of medicinal plant distribution, conservation and active monitoring are therefore crucial for the long-term availability of plant-based medicinal agents to patients. In addition, there is the aspect of how medicinal plants are prescribed, processed and delivered as medicinal agents in a manner which minimizes use and optimizes safety and efficacy. Overarching these considerations of medicinal plant utilization is a broad, yet basic question: How can pharmacognosy think and act in more sustainable terms?

In the early 1990s, the concept of 'green chemistry' was launched by the US Environmental Protection Agency (Anastas and Warner, 1998; Anastas and Kirchoff, 2002; Anastas and Eghbali, 2010), which, when considering medicinal agents, can be offered as six practical principles (Cordell *et al.*, 2007; Cordell and Michel, 2007; Cordell, 2011b). These principles are: (i) recyclable and safer solvents, (ii) more energy-efficient processes (temperature and time), (iii) recyclable reagents, (iv) renewable feedstocks, (v) avoiding unnecessary process steps and (vi) having environmentally friendly by-products.

How has pharmacognosy responded in the past 15 years to these green chemistry principles? Have the strategies of pharmacognosy research changed? Has thinking through the common processes of our research changed? Are more or fewer resources being used for a given isolation or structure elucidation, or biological testing process? How much effort is made to recycle solvents and other materials? Or has pharmacognosy ignored green chemistry? Do we think we are already green enough? Are we also working on the basis of the same assumption that whatever resources are needed, they will be there? More succinctly, has green chemistry changed our philosophy about the directions of pharmacognosy for the future?

We should not lose sight of the maintenance of those resources which constitute the underlying means through which those agents are made accessible. At the same time, it was also pointed out that most sourcing of the plants (and some animal parts) used in systems of traditional medicine in the world is not sustainable. Overall, only minimal efforts have been made to transform this forest economy to a field economy. The financial and social reasons for this situation in various countries of the world are numerous and complex. All of these considerations, bound together by sustainability and practicality (is the goal reasonable?), lead to a new consciousness regarding natural product development, and a new term with a new definition, 'ecopharmacognosy' [1] .

## 6.3  Ecopharmacognosy: background

Ecopharmacognosy is about environmental pharmacognosy; it stresses the importance of environmental considerations in pharmacognosy research. This author believes that the term should be defined as 'the study of sustainable biologically active natural products'. In this application, 'eco' indicates 'sustainable' and inherently poses the question, does the research embrace both sustainable practices and outcomes? In other words, if, as one example, a goal is the development of a new medicinal agent or the evaluation of a traditional medicine, it is pertinent to ask how that material would be resourced, long term and in a sustainable manner, at an early stage in the subsequent discovery and development process. It also poses the question of whether the steps involved in the study of the plant for its active principles are being conducted in a green manner. The term is thus a fundamental philosophical perspective of natural product research in terms of long-term environmental impact and resourcing, and a practical aid in guiding where research priorities and research practices should be focused. The result is a challenging question: How can pharmacognosy research become more eco-centric? An old example will illustrate the point.

In the 1980s, the diterpene polyester derivative taxol had generated exceptional interest as a clinically significant antitumour agent, and several kilograms were needed for a large clinical trial. However, taxol was being isolated in 0.0007% yield (2 kg from 27,000 kg) from the (non-sustainable) bark of *Taxus brevifolia* Nutt. (Taxaceae), the Pacific yew, native to the northwestern USA. When the Food and Drug Administration (FDA) developed an environmental impact statement, it was estimated that two to three million trees would need to be harvested to treat the 60,000 patients contracting ovarian and breast cancer each year in the USA alone (see Croom, 1995). Fortunately, a renewable source (the leaves of a related species) for a derivative which could be transformed straightforwardly into taxol was found, and taxol became a 'blockbuster' drug.

Estimates are in the range of 70–85% for the wild-crafting of medicinal plants. As a result, at least 9000 medicinal plants are in the threatened status of the International Union for the Conservancy of Nature (IUCN) (Lange, 2004). A recent ethnopharmacological study in Bosnia and Herzegovina showed that of the 238 species currently used in 34 locations, 173 (72.7%) were wild-crafted, while the rest were cultivated (Šarić-Kundalić *et al.*, 2010). A study of the 1543 species of plant materials sold in Germany showed that only 3–6% were cultivated (Lange and Schippmann, 1997). Of the 1000 or so commonly used plants in TCM, about 10–20% are cultivated (He and Sheng, 1997) and in India of the 400 most widely used plants, fewer than 20 are cultivated (Uniyal *et al.*, 2000).

## 6.4  Ecopharmacognosy practices

With this background, what are some ecopharmacognosy practices that can be promoted in the future for the sustainable development of traditional medicines, phytotherapeuticals, and for

---

[1] This term was first used in a lecture presented by the author at the 8th International Symposium on the Chromatography of Natural Products meeting held in Lubin, Poland in May, 2012.

drug discovery? Some of these aspects of pharmacognosy are well known, others are arising as the field develops.

## 6.4.1 Replacement plant parts

Root and bark plant materials are not sustainable plant parts for the development of traditional medicines or for drug discovery. On the other hand, the leaves, flowers, seeds and fruits are. Thus, when efforts are made regarding the quality control standards, the safety and the efficacy of traditional medicines, if the traditional plant part used is a root or bark, efforts should be directed towards establishing the safety and the standardization of sustainable plant parts, with a view to using them as a replacement. It is recognized that this may not always be possible, given the anticipated differences in metabolic profile of the plant parts involved. However, the important initial aspect is to consider the sustainability of the plant parts being examined for standardization and projected use as commercial medicinal agents.

## 6.4.2 Vegetables as chemical reagents

Can the metabolic processes deployed naturally for the formation of secondary metabolites be utilized for the total and semi-synthesis of desired medicinal agents? The use of microbial systems for effecting specific chemical transformations has been well known for almost 50 years as a way to access chemically unreactive sites in steroids (Eppstein *et al.*, 1956; Mahato and Garai, 1997; Fernandes *et al.*, 2003; Kristan and Rižner, 2012) and for producing new compounds of various classes for exploration of new biologically active compounds (Donova and Egorova, 2012). In addition, the use of cloned and expressed enzymes derived from plants for effecting chemical reactions has been well discussed (González-Sabín *et al.*, 2011; Hollmann *et al.*, 2011; Drauz *et al.*, 2012). More interestingly, limited attention has also been paid to the use of plants, particularly cheap vegetables, as chiral reagents for the formation of alcohols from ketones (Cordell *et al.*, 2007), an area of sustainable organic synthesis which began in 2000 with studies using whole carrots (Baldassarre *et al.*, 2000). Since whole vegetable systems are used, enzyme isolation and purification are not a prerequisite. Compared with the use of expensive chiral heavy metal or borohydride reagents, which are used once and discarded, cheap vegetables offer significant ecological, as well as exceptional financial, advantages. The synthesis of alcohols from ketones with other vegetable reagents, such as manihot (Sousa *et al.*, 2006), cane sugar (Assunção *et al.*, 2008) and coconut juice (Fonseca *et al.*, 2009), typically proceeds in <97% yield and <97% enantiomeric excess at room temperature, over three days, with minimal work-up required, and with a reagent that can be lyophilized and re-used up to seven times without major loss of effectiveness (Sousa *et al.*, 2006). Can this be accomplished for other important chemical reactions, both achiral and chiral, using whole-plant materials? In addition to plants, other intact, fast-growing organisms, such as insects, earthworms, various larvae, and the ascomycota and basidomycetes, also need to be examined for their ability to conduct important chemical transformations.

## 6.4.3 The 'Medicine Man' approach and remote sensing

In the traditional screening approach to the study of biologically active natural products from plant resources, material is collected, dried and brought back to the laboratory for extraction, biological evaluation and, if activity is demonstrated, phytochemical analysis. In ecopharmacognosy terms, this approach is inefficient, and from a resources perspective ecologically inappropriate, unless the long-term goal is to establish an extract library for long-term biological screening initiatives. The Sean Connery movie 'Medicine Man' (1992) provided an example of a very different approach to anticancer drug discovery from plants. Instead of taking the field (the plant materials) to the laboratory, take the laboratory to the field. This idea has been proposed in the form of 'pharmacognosy in a suitcase' and some of the relevant technologies discussed (Cordell, 2007, 2009, 2011b, 2011c, 2012, 2014a; Cordell and Colvard, 2012). The development of such selectively integrated technologies, using currently available hand-held instruments (NIR, Raman, AA, etc.), would also allow for the evaluation of cultivated, or perhaps even wild-crafted, traditional medicines prior to harvesting, and for preliminary biological determinations to be made *in situ*. From an ecopharmacognosy perspective, minimum plant material is being accessed for maximum purpose, and can reflect both local plant use as well as the evaluation of only sustainable plant samples.

## 6.4.4 Dereplication

Biologically active compounds from plants frequently occur in more than one plant, thus an alkaloid such as berberine, which has multiple significant activities, occurs in numerous plant species in at least four plant families (Berberidaceae, Menispermaceae, Papaveraceae and Ranunculaceae). Given that in classical drug discovery from plants one is looking for both biological activity and novelty of structure, finding a known active compound is not of interest (unless it is mechanistically novel), and from an ecopharmacognosy perspective the isolation process for such a known metabolite is a waste of resources (plant, human and fiscal). This same situation in the microbial world led to the development of dereplication for detecting known, biologically active metabolites at an early purification stage (Cordell and Shin, 1999).

Two strategies were developed over time; one involving a chemical approach, in which a mycelial extract was evaluated chromatographically for specific known compounds. A second approach was developed by the National Cancer Institute in their screening of natural extracts where the profile of biological activity against 63 cell lines was used to assess the mechanism of action of a cytotoxic agent. If no match was made, the extract was deemed to be of high priority for isolation (Cordell and Shin, 1999). In a National Collaborative Drug Discovery Grant programme at the University of Illinois at Chicago, it was decided to combine these approaches. A method was needed to prioritize for fractionation to optimize the chances of obtaining novel bioactive metabolites. The result was a high-performance liquid chromatography (HPLC) system for separation into two streams for 96-well plates, one for mass spectrometry and another for biological evaluation. An individual well therefore represents a mass (or series of masses) whose fragmentation can be viewed, and a time-equivalent, biological response that can be correlated. Database comparisons with known compounds having that biological activity then gave an indication of potential novelty and therefore a priority for isolation (Cordell and Shin, 1999).

## 6.4.5 *In silico* evaluation of natural products

*In silico* evaluation does not require that an actual compound be at hand in order to conduct the screening for potential bioactivity (enzyme inhibition), and fits with the philosophy of ecopharmacognosy. Firstly, no plants or other biological materials are collected unnecessarily, and no compounds are isolated unless there is good reason to determine an *in vitro* or *in vivo* activity. In addition, it may be possible to select compounds for testing and synthetic development which are derived from a readily sustainable resource. For example, an *in silico* study of a small selected group of diverse alkaloid structures for inhibition at the active site of the trypanothione reductase of *Trypanosma cruzi*, the parasite causing Chagas' disease, afforded a number of potent alkaloids. Three were chosen for further development, derived from commonly occurring plants, for functional group modification to potentiate the theoretical activity (Argüelles *et al.*, unpublished results). As a result a very limited number of exceptionally active derivatives have been targeted for synthesis and assessment of their biological activity.

## 6.4.6   Biosynthesis of secondary metabolites

How nature produces secondary metabolites has been of interest for many years, and significant progress has been made in elucidating the biosynthetic pathways at the gene level for microbial metabolites, less so for plant metabolites and very little progress for marine metabolites. The key issue from a medicinal agent perspective, whether the organism is microbial, a terrestrial plant or from the marine environment, is control of the secondary metabolic processes. The need is clearly to enhance (optimize) the production of the desired metabolites and minimize the production of undesired (such as toxic and inactive, closely related) metabolites. Optimizing the production of whole plants or microbial systems under controlled conditions permits the potential development of a more available and more highly standardized product with less plant material being used. Thus targeted cultivation of selected strains of important medicinal plants, especially those where the active principles are known, and which are still being wild-crafted, is an important focus for ecopharmacognosy.

All of the biosynthetic investigations, from understanding even simple precursor relationships which may enhance product yields to the isolation and cloning of whole gene sequences for selective metabolite production into fast-growing systems, are aspects of ecopharmacognosy. Efforts have begun, once a complete gene system has been obtained, to identify those genes in a cluster which are the responsible 'gates' in the pathway, which control the formation and availability of precursors at various biosynthetic steps. Because of the dispersed nature of the genes for the biosynthesis of plant secondary metabolites, directed and predictable control of the production of these metabolites by a reconstituted gene cluster will be significantly more challenging. The need is for the ability to stitch together the genes of fragmented pathways, possibly from different sources, into a single unit which can function *in vitro* in a manner similar to that of a microbial system or which can be inserted into a fast-growing yeast or insect cell system.

## 6.4.7   Complex traditional medicines

Many traditional medicines used in various systems around the world are composed of multiple plants. Whether all of the plants are needed in a particular preparation is a valid question that has to be explored and justified on an evidentiary basis as a core issue in optimizing sustainable plant use. In other words, how do each of these individual plants contribute to the efficacy of the traditional medicine? What are the synergisms (and antagonisms) that are evident as the functions of these plants and their metabolites are examined? If only four plants in a ten-component mixture are required for safety and effectiveness, can the other plants be omitted, thereby enhancing the sustainability of the overall preparation by conserving plant use? Clearly, network pharmacology (see next section) will be of major importance as the diverse impact of individual compounds at the gene level becomes more widely known.

## 6.4.8 Network pharmacology

The term 'network pharmacology' has become an important facet of traditional Chinese medicine. The term was first introduced by Hopkins in 2007 (Hopkins, 2007, 2008) in response to studies (Yildirim *et al.*, 2007) which examined the polypharmacology of single drugs. The philosophy changes the 'one target, one drug' approach (sometimes called 'magic bullet') to a 'network target, multiple components' approach. It reflects that a network target will be unique to a disease, and provides a way to define, at the genome level, the mechanistic impact of drugs, and allows the examination of overlap with other disease networks. Based on such an approach, a traditional medicine may be predicted to treat more than one disease. Construction of the genome maps of selected compounds, and their development into databases (Li and Zhang, 2013; Zhang *et al.*, 2013) has allowed correlations to be made, looking for uniqueness and overlap of genome targets, and hence the mapping of diseases which can then be mapped to specific traditional medicines. This permits commentary on the relevance of the bioactive constituents in the plant materials to the recommended uses, possibly providing a rationale for the philosophy of use.

Some applications of the approach include (i) the identification of active ingredients and their respective role in complex mixtures of plants, (ii) the detection of synergistic effects when the effect is more pronounced than predicted because of multiple interactions at a node, (iii) possibly an examination of the validity of the TCM syndrome approach, (iv) explanations of the toxicities or possible adverse reactions of specific plant and (v) the identification of new biological activities of known compounds and new medicinal plant combinations with new uses (Zhang *et al.*, 2013). If the number of plants in a traditional medicine can lead to more selective and sustainable approaches, then new pathways for established plants may allow for the development of new recommendations for potential pharmacological and clinical experimentation, leading to new formulations to tackle specific disease states, which may also reduce the possibility of drug resistance.

## 6.4.9 Can ecopharmacognosy change the dark side of traditional medicine?

Of the 252 essential medicines on the WHO list, 11.1% are plant-derived and 8.7% come from animals; about 18% of US prescription drugs are also animal-derived (Alves and Rosa, 2005). Certain traditional medicine practices in various parts of the world cast a dark cloud on the whole field of medicinal agents derived from natural resources because threatened or endangered species are involved in the trade. Ecopharmacognosy must be on the appropriate side of that phenomenon, the ethical side of conservation and preservation of species that are not sustainably developed for traditional medicine usage, and promote the development of sustainable alternatives. The trading in rare and threatened animal parts, such as rhino horn, tiger bone, bear bile, bear paw, etc., must be dramatically reduced and, if necessary, alternatives found. Governments which allow trading in these animal parts need to be much more proactive globally about the trading and use of those materials as an approved medical practice. In general terms, the utilization of animal parts in traditional medicine systems around the globe requires more scientific study in order to determine if there is useful biological activity, and if there is, whether a sustainable replacement can be found and introduced into commerce following a more multidimensional approach in line with the philosophies of ecopharmacognosy.

## 6.5   Conclusions

Ecopharmacognosy adds and integrates the concept of sustainability to the study of biologically active natural products. It calls for considerations of sustainable development of natural products in healthcare, cosmeceuticals and agriculture at an early stage in the development process, and suggests that the diverse natural product sciences are now at a point where such considerations can be brought specifically to the area of traditional medicine to minimize the use of non-sustainable plant parts and of wild-crafted plant and other biological materials generally. It offers challenges for the processing of plants under conditions which require lower energy consumption and for the development of alternative strategies for organic synthesis involving common plants and vegetables. It also supports the *in silico* evaluation of known compounds prior to *in vitro* testing to conserve resources and valuable compounds. Finally, ecopharmacognosy offers an alternative pathway, only partially trodden thus far, for rethinking how pharmacognosy, in all its breadth and depth, can contribute to the global call for sustainable initiatives.

## Acknowledgements

The author appreciates the feedback from numerous friends and colleagues around the world who have supported the philosophy and concepts that are outlined in this chapter.

## References

Alves, R.R.N. and Rosa, I.L. (2005) Why study the use of animal products in traditional medicines? *Journal of Ethnobiology and Ethnomedicine*, **1**, 5.

Anastas, P. and Eghbali, N. (2010) Green chemistry: principles and practice. *Chemical Society Reviews*, **39**, 301–312.

Anastas, P.T. and Kirchhoff, M.M. (2002) Origins, current status, and future challenges of green chemistry. *Accounts of Chemical Research*, **35**, 686–694.

Anastas, P.T. and Warner, J.C. (1998) *Green Chemistry: Theory and Practice*, Oxford University Press, New York.

Assunção, J.C.C., Machado, L.L., Lemos, T.L.G., *et al.* (2008) Sugar cane juice for the reduction of carbonyl compounds. *Journal of Molecular Catalysis B: Enzymatic*, **52–53**, 194–198.

Baldassarre, F., Bertoni, G., Chiappe, C. and Marioni, F. (2000) Preparative synthesis of chiral alcohols by enantioselective reduction with *Daucus carota* root as biocatalyst. *Journal of Molecular Catalysis B: Enzymatic*, **11**, 55–58.

Cordell, G.A. (1987a) Pharmacognosy: far from dead. *American Druggist*, March, 96–98.

Cordell, G.A. (1987b) Pharmacognosy: far from dead. *Thai Journal of Pharmaceutical Sciences*, **12**, 221–224.

Cordell, G.A. (1990) Pharmacognosy – a high-tech pharmaceutical science. *Pharmacia*, **30**, 169–181.

Cordell, G.A. (1993) Pharmacognosy – new roots for an old science, in *Studies in Natural Products Chemistry, Volume 13* (eds Atta-ur-Rahman and F.Z. Basha), Bioactive Natural Products (Part A), Elsevier, Amsterdam, pp. 629–675.

Cordell, G.A. (1995) Changing strategies in natural products chemistry. *Phytochemistry*, **40**, 1585–1612.

Cordell, G.A. (2000) Biodiversity and drug discovery – a symbiotic relationship. *Phytochemistry*, **55**, 463–480.

Cordell, G.A. (2001) The yin and yang of natural products in the new millennium. *Acta Manilana*, **49**, 1–4.

Cordell, G.A. (2004) Accessing our gifts from nature, now and in the future. Part III. *Revista Quimica*, **19**, 33–41.

Cordell, G.A. (2007) A vision for medicinal plants. *BLACPMA*, **6**, 89–91.

Cordell, G.A. (2008) Natural products research – a view through the looking glass. *Science and Culture*, **74**, 11–16.

Cordell, G.A. (2009) Sustainable drugs and global health care. *Quimica Nova*, **32**, 1356–1364.

Cordell, G.A. (2011a) Plant medicines key to global health. *Chemical and Engineering News, June* **27**, 52–56.

Cordell, G.A. (2011b) Sustainable medicines and global health care. *Planta Medica*, **77**, 1129–1138.

Cordell, G.A. (2011c) Phytochemistry and traditional medicine – a revolution in process. *Phytochemistry Letters*, **4**, 391–398.

Cordell, G.A. (2012) New strategies in traditional medicine, in *Medicinal Plants: Diversity and Drugs* (eds M. Rai, G.A. Cordell, J.L. Martinez, M. Marinoff and L. Rastrelli), CRC Press, Boca Raton, pp. 1–45.

Cordell, G.A. (2014a) Ecopharmacognosy: exploring the chemical and biological potential of nature for human health. *Journal of Biological and Medicinal Natural Product Chemistry*, **4**, 1–21.

Cordell, G.A. (2014b) Phytochemistry and traditional medicine – the revolution continues. *Phytochemisry Letters*, **10**, 28–40.

Cordell, G.A. and Colvard, M.D. (2005) Some thoughts on the future of ethnopharmacology. *Journal of Ethnopharmacology*, **100**, 5–14.

Cordell, G.A. and Colvard, M.D. (2007) Natural products in a world out-of-balance. *Arkivoc*, **vii**, 97–115.

Cordell, G.A. and Colvard, M.D. (2012) Natural products and traditional medicine – turning on a paradigm. *Journal of Natural Products*, **75**, 514–525.

Cordell, G.A. and Michel, J. (2007) Sustainable drugs and women's health, in *Proceedings of the Third Women's Health and Asian Traditional Medicine Conference and Exhibition* (ed. A.N. Rao), Kuala Lumpur, Malaysia, pp. 15–27.

Cordell, G.A. and Shin, Y.G. (1999) Finding the needle in the haystack. The dereplication of natural product extracts. *Pure and Applied Chemistry*, **71**, 1089–1094.

Cordell, G.A., Lemos, T.L.G., Monte, F.J.Q. and de Mattos, M.C. (2007) Vegetables as chemical reagents. *Journal of Natural Products*, **70**, 478–492.

Croom, Jr., E.M. (1995) *Taxus* for taxol and toxoids, in *Taxol* (ed. M. Suffness), CRC Press, Boca Raton, pp. 37–70.

Donova, M.V. and Egorova, O.V. (2012) Microbial steroid transformations: current state and prospects. *Applied Microbiology and Biotechnology*, **94**, 1423–1447.

Drauz, K., Gröger, H. and May, O. (2012) *Enzyme Catalysis in Organic Synthesis: a Comprehensive Handbook*, 2nd edn, John Wiley & Sons Ltd, New York.

Eppstein, S.H., Meister, P.D., Murray, H.C. and Peterson, D.H. (1956) Microbiological transformations of steroids and their applications to the synthesis of hormones. *Vitamins and Hormones*, **14**, 359–432.

Fernandes, P., Cruz, A., Angelova, B., *et al.* (2003) Microbial conversion of steroid compounds: recent developments. *Enzyme and Microbial Technology*, **32**, 688–705.

Fonseca, A.M., Monte, F.J.Q., Braz-Filho, R., *et al.* (2009) Coconut juice (*Cocos nucifera*) – a new biocatalyst system for organic synthesis. *Journal of Molecular Catalysis B: Enzymatic*, **57**, 78–82.

González-Sabín, J., Morán-Ramallal, R. and Rebolledo, F. (2011) Regioselective enzymatic acylation of complex natural products: expanding molecular diversity. *Chemical Society Reviews*, **40**, 5321–5335.

He, S.A. and Sheng, N. (1997) Utilization and conservation of medicinal plants in China. *Medicinal Plants for Conservation and Health Care*, **11**, 109.

Hollmann, F., Arends, I.W.C.E. and Holtmann, D. (2011) Enzymatic reductions for the chemist. *Green Chemistry*, **13**, 2285–2314.

Hopkins, A.L. (2007) Network pharmacology. *Nature Biotechnology*, **23**, 1110–1111.

Hopkins, A.L. (2008) Network pharmacology: the next paradigm in drug discovery. *Nature Chemical Biology*, **4**, 682–690.

Jarvis, L.M. (2010) Research recalibrated. *Chemical and Engineering News, June* **7**, 13–18.

Kristan, K. and Rižner, T.L. (2012) Steroid-transforming enzymes in fungi. *Journal of Steroid Biochemistry and Molecular Biology*, **129**, 79–91.

Lange, D. (2004) Medicinal and aromatic plants: trade, production and management of botanical resources. *Acta Horticulturae*, **629**, 177–197.

Li, S. and Zhang, B. (2013) Traditional Chinese medicine network pharmacology: theory, methodology and application. *Chinese Journal of Natural Medicines*, **11**, 110–120.

Mahato, S.B. and Garai. S. (1997) Advances in microbial steroid biotransformation. *Steroids*, **62**, 332–345.

Šarić-Kundalić, B., Dobeš, C., Klatte-Asselmeyer, V. and Saukel, J. (2010) Ethnobotanical study on medicinal use of wild and cultivated plants in middle, south and west Bosnia and Herzegovina. *Journal of Ethnopharmacology*, **131**, 33–55.

Schippmann, U.W.E., Leaman, D. and Cunningham, A.B. (2006) A comparison of cultivation and wild collection of medicinal and aromatic plants under sustainability aspects. *Frontis*, **17**, 75–95.

Sousa, J.S.N., Machado, L.L., de Mattos, M.C., *et al.* (2006) Bioreduction of aromatic aldehydes and ketones using *Manihot* species. *Phytochemistry*, **67**, 1637–1643.

Uniyal, R.C., Uniyal, M.R. and Jain, P. (2000) *Cultivation of medicinal plants in India: a reference book*, TRAFFIC.

WHO (2002) WHO Traditional Medicine Strategy 2002–2005, WHO, Geneva, 74 pp, http://apps.who.int/medicinedocs/en/d/Js2297e/, accessed 3 August 2014.

WHO (2012) The Regional Strategy for Traditional Medicine in the Western Pacific (2011–2020), WHO, Regional Office for the Western Pacific, Manila, 71 pp.

WHO (2014) WHO Traditional Medicine Strategy 2014–2023, WHO, Geneva, 71 pp, http://apps.who.int/iris/bitstream/10665/92455/1/9789241506090_eng.pdf, accessed 3 August 2014.

Yildirim, M.A., Goh, K.-I., Cusick, M.E., *et al.* (2007) Drug – target network. *Nature Biotechnology*, **25**, 1119–1126.

Zhang, G.-B., Li, Q.-Y., Chen, Q.-L. and Su, S.-B. (2013) Network pharmacology: a new approach to Chinese herbal medicine research. *Evidence-Based Complementary and Alternative Medicine*, id: 621423.

# 7

# NMR-based Metabolomics and Hyphenated NMR Techniques: A Perfect Match in Natural Products Research

Joachim Møllesøe Vinther[1], Sileshi Gizachew Wubshet[1] and Dan Staerk[1]

*Department of Drug Design and Pharmacology, Faculty of Health and Medical Sciences, University of Copenhagen, Denmark*

## 7.1   Introduction

Nature has a long history of providing bioactive constituents, both as single compounds serving as drug leads for the development of new chemical entities in modern western medicine (Newman and Cragg, 2012) and as mixtures of bioactive constituents in plants used as traditional medicines or herbal preparations (Benzie and Wachtel-Galor, 2011). Identifying bioactive constituents in complex mixtures like plant extracts is a challenging task – whether in a targeted drug lead discovery approach or in a holistic ethnopharmacological approach – and bioactivity-guided fractionation has been the preferred method for many years. Similarly, phytochemical studies aiming at (i) exploring biosynthetic pathways, (ii) assessing variation in metabolite profiles or (iii) monitoring distribution of bioactive constituents across plant species, genera or families are challenging tasks. In all instances, scientific landmarks have been spurred by new technology providing, for example, improved separation of analytes in complex mixtures, lowered detection limits and improved response factors in detection devices, hyphenation and/or integration of technologies, and improved software control, data management and data processing. In this chapter we will deal with two new technologies that have proven very successful in natural products research (i.e. the broad term for ethnopharmacology, phytochemistry, medicinal plant research and medicinal food research) in recent years. The first is metabolomics – a data-driven approach based on multivariate data analysis

*Ethnopharmacology*, First Edition. Edited by Michael Heinrich and Anna K. Jäger.
© 2015 John Wiley & Sons, Ltd. Published 2015 by John Wiley & Sons, Ltd.

of chemical fingerprints of complex metabolomics mixtures like plant extracts. The second is hyphenated nuclear magnetic resonance (NMR) techniques – a technology that allows separation and structure elucidation of individual constituents from complex metabolomics mixtures. Most interesting, however, is the combination of the two technologies, i.e. the use of hyphenated NMR techniques for biomarker identification in metabolomics studies. We hope that this chapter will give the reader an idea of the possibilities for using NMR-based metabolomics and hyphenated NMR techniques in ethnopharmacology, and that this may serve as inspiration for the use of these technologies in their own research.

## 7.2   Metabolomics

The entire assembly of low-molecular-weight molecules in an organism (cell, organ, tissue, etc.) is defined as the metabolome, i.e. the equivalent to the genome and the proteome. The metabolome can be considered as the biological end-point of the genome and the proteome, and metabolomics is therefore an important technique for assessing the state of an organism (cell, organ, tissue, etc.). There are two terminologies describing the discipline of exploring the metabolome, i.e. metabonomics and metabolomics. Metabonomics was originally defined in 1999 by Jeremy K. Nicholson, John Lindon and Elaine Holmes from Imperial College (Nicholson *et al.*, 1999):

‘the quantitative measurement of the dynamic multiparametric metabolic response of living systems to pathophysiological stimuli or genetic modification’

This definition was based on their work with the multivariate data analysis of mainly NMR data of biofluids for understanding biochemistry and disease models. A few years later, Oliver Fiehn proposed the following definition of metabolomics (Fiehn, 2002):

‘a comprehensive analysis in which all the metabolites of a biological system are identified and quantified’

Fiehns’ definition was based on his work with multivariate data analysis of mass spectrometry (MS) data for understanding the plant metabolome, and for this reason metabolomics has been the preferred terminology for scientists working within plant science. However,

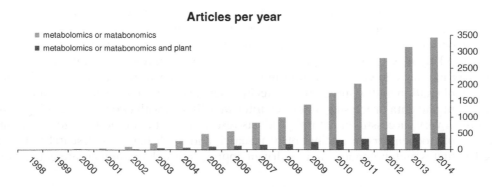

**Figure 7.1**   Total number of publications employing metabolomics/metabonomics (gray bars) and publications employing metabolomics/metabonomics for investigation of plant extracts (black bars).

metabolomics and metabonomics cover the same underlying discipline, i.e. exploring differences and/or similarities in the metabolome by using multivariate data analysis of chemical fingerprints based on MS, NMR, liquid chromatography-mass spectrometry (LC-MS), etc.

Metabolomics has become increasingly popular since its introduction at the beginning of the millennium. Figure 7.1 shows a steadily increasing number of publications within the field of metabolomics (SciFinder Search 26 May 2015). Studies related to plant metabolomics have also increased steadily, and there are now 500 papers published each year using metabolomics for investigating the plant metabolome.

## 7.3   Principles of NMR-based metabolomics

In this chapter we will restrict our discussion to studies employing metabolomics based on NMR data, i.e. NMR-based metabolomics. Metabolomics is a data-driven approach and the overall workflow in metabolomics studies is shown in Figure 7.2.

Owing to the physical characteristics of the chemical shift measured, NMR spectroscopy is very reproducible. This is a clear advantage over other techniques, for example LC-MS, which are also used for metabolomics. Furthermore, the intensity of the resonances in one-dimensional (1D) $^1$H NMR constitutes quantitative measures of all $^1$H-containing compounds in the sample. In addition, the structural information obtained from NMR spectra is unsurpassed relative to any other spectroscopic technique.

For plant metabolomics, the sample preparation consists of collection/harvesting, grinding, extraction (directly into deuterated solvent, otherwise evaporation and reconstitution in deuterated solvent) and transfer to NMR tubes. The next step is acquisition of high-quality 1D $^1$H NMR spectra or other kinds of NMR data, *vide infra*. Having obtained the spectra, the data analysis constitutes the central part of a metabolomics study, which, in the successful case, pinpoints the spectral features inherited from the intersample differences and eventually explains the assayed variations such as bioactivity, as discussed in the last section of this chapter. A thorough review of the procedures is given in Kim *et al.* (2010) and the following description will be restricted to the data analysis only. Using principal component analysis (PCA) as an example, the generic procedure is schematically depicted in Figure 7.3.

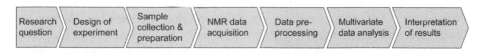

**Figure 7.2**   Workflow in metabolomics studies.

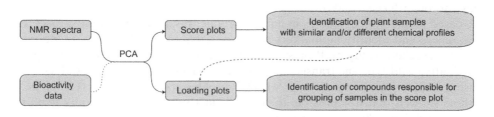

**Figure 7.3**   Diagram showing the procedures for PCA in NMR-based metabolomics.

PCA (Eriksson *et al.*, 2001; Trygg and Lundstedt 2007) is the most commonly used algorithm for unsupervised multivariate analysis. Prior to the statistical analysis, preprocessing of the NMR data is needed. This includes removal of unwanted signals and artefacts (e.g. remaining solvent resonances), and alignment of spectra. Secondly, the data set needs to be pretreated to adjust for concentration differences between high and low abundant metabolites. This can be done by scaling all resonances to the same weight, i.e. unit variance scaling, by subtracting the average spectrum of the data set from the individual spectrum, i.e. mean centring or the in-between choice pareto-scaling (Eriksson *et al.*, 2001). Thirdly, the spectra are binned, i.e. integrated in discrete regions, in order to decrease the size of the data set. A benefit from this procedure is the possibility to adjust the binning in order to suppress uninteresting influences of small shifts and disturbances of the resonances. The preprocessed data are subsequently analysed by PCA, from which score plots and the loading plots can be obtained. The score plots show each spectrum as a point in the space spanned by the principal components, and in the successful case grouping of spectra will reveal the intersample differences and similarities. The loading plots correlate each principal component to spectral features, and the grouping in the score plots is correlated to these features. In favourable cases it might be possible to assign the features to resonances of known compounds. However, in many cases additional analytical techniques, for example LC-MS or high-performance liquid chromatography-mass spectrometry-solid-phase extraction-nuclear magnetic resonance (HPLC-SPE-NMR) (*vide infra*), are needed before conclusive identification of individual constituents can be made.

Excluded from the presentation above are several other statistical algorithms, of which the most prominent is the supervised counterpart to PCA: partial least squares discriminant analysis (PLS-DA), which is intended to reveal the differentiating spectral features between pre-grouped samples (Eriksson *et al.*, 2001).

## 7.4   NMR-based metabolomics in natural products research

NMR spectroscopy has been the method of choice for metabolite profiling in natural product research. This is due to major advantages of NMR, such as relatively simple sample preparation requirements and non-discriminative response to a wide range of molecules. The majority of NMR-based metabolomics studies of natural products are based on the use of 1D $^1$H NMR spectra. Because of the relatively high sensitivity of the $^1$H nuclei and simplicity of the pulse sequence, 1D $^1$H NMR profiling is regarded as a rapid and robust method. NMR-based metabolomics is also a versatile technique in terms of applications within natural products research. Thus, NMR-based metabolomics have been used to successfully address important biological questions in matrices ranging from higher plants (Agnolet *et al.*, 2010) to pathogenic microbes (Boroujerdi *et al.*, 2009).

NMR-based metabolomics studies in natural product research aim, in most cases, to highlight differences and identify biomarkers within pharmaceutical, botanical or nutraceutical research. An excellent study by Professor Verpoorte and coworkers showed the possibility of discriminating wild-type and transgenic constitutive salicylic acid (CSA) producing tobacco plants using multivariate data analysis of $^1$H NMR profiles of crude extracts (Choi *et al.*, 2004). The authors showed that it is possible to see a distinct separation using only two principal components explaining 89.6% of the variation (Figure 7.4). The corresponding loading plot

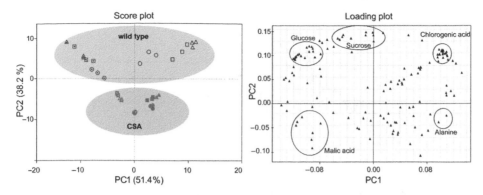

**Figure 7.4** Score and loading plot from $^1$H NMR-based PCA of aqueous methanol extracts of wild-type and CSA-line transgenic tobacco. (Source: Choi *et al.* 2004. Reproduced with permission of Elsevier.)

showed the resonances of metabolites responsible for the variation between the wild-type and transgenic samples. These metabolites were later identified as glucose, sucrose, malic acid, alanine and chlorogenic acid by comparing chemical shifts with known tobacco metabolites. Furthermore, the sub-grouping observed in the score plot could be ascribed to (i) sampling (leaf and vein) and (ii) a viral infection systematically introduced to a selected set of samples in order to highlight the differences in connection with metabolic pathways related to the defence response.

In most cases, identification of biomarkers, underlining a given variation in a set of samples, is facilitated by authentic reference spectra acquired either separately as pure compounds or together with the biological sample through spiking experiments. However, this limits the study to a comparison of known biomarkers whereas unknown or novel compounds will remain unassigned. The need for a rapid identification method is therefore undoubtable. Professor Staerk and coworkers presented an approach based on the combined use of $^1$H NMR-based metabolomics and hyphenated NMR (specifically HPLC-PDA-MS-SPE-NMR, *vide infra*) for comprehensive characterization of the global composition of standardized *Ginkgo biloba* preparations (Agnolet *et al.*, 2010). This study highlighted principal differences within 16 commercial *G. biloba* preparations from four different countries using PCA for the study of 1D $^1$H NMR profiles. Moreover, the authors were able to identify fortification by quercetin and detect a potentially harmful phenolic lipid.

Insufficient chemical shift dispersion is one of the common challenges when dealing with 1D $^1$H NMR profiles of natural products. To some extent this has been addressed by development of high field strength NMR magnets. However, $^1$H NMR of complex biological matrices such as raw plant extracts yields spectra with a high degree of overlapping $^1$H resonances. In such instances resolution can be gained by using multidimensional NMR data. In addition to the significant gain in resolution, investigations of crude mixtures using multidimensional NMR data provide additional structural information. Robinette *et al.* used two-dimensional (2D) total correlation spectroscopy (TOCSY) based PCA of extracts from two nematode species, *Pristionchus pacificus* and *Panagrellus redivivus*, to differentiate the two species and identify species-specific metabolites (Figure 7.5). In the score plot presented in Figure 7.5b a clear distinction between the two species is observed along PC 1 (Robinette *et al.*, 2011). Similarly, Yilmaz *et al.* demonstrated application of 2D *J*-resolved experiments in metabolic profiling of *Crocus sativus* L. flowers (saffron) (Yilmaz *et al.*, 2011).

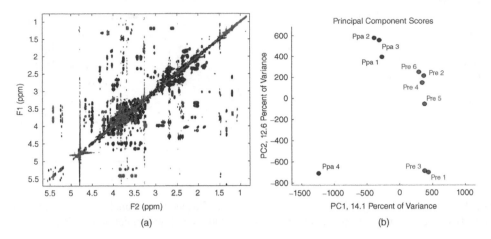

(a)                           (b)

**Figure 7.5**   Overlaid TOCSY spectra of nematodes *Pristionchus pacificus* (Ppa, light grey) and *Panagrellus redivivus* (Pre, dark grey) extracts (a) and the corresponding score plots (b) separating the two nematodes along principal component 1 based on their differing metabolome. (Source: Robinette *et al.* 2011. Reproduced with permission of American Chemical Society.)

## 7.5   Hyphenated NMR techniques

Hyphenation of efficient separation technologies like gas chromatography (GC) and high-performance liquid chromatography (HPLC) with sensitive detectors like photodiode array and mass spectrometry, e.g. GC-MS, HPLC-PDA and LC-HRMS, has for many years facilitated natural products research. However, neither PDA nor MS provide the detailed information needed for structure elucidation – including identification of regioisomerism or relative configuration – and especially for structure elucidation of new compounds NMR spectroscopy is an invaluable spectroscopic technique. Thus, the first direct hyphenation of HPLC with NMR (Watanabe and Niki, 1978; Bayer *et al.*, 1979), i.e. HPLC-NMR, started a transition towards hyphenated NMR as a useful technique in natural products research. Initially direct hyphenated NMR experiments were performed in the continuous-flow mode, stopped-flow mode or loop-storage mode, where the HPLC eluate was directed to an NMR flow cell while NMR experiments were performed with the eluate running continuously (applicable to 1D NMR experiments of major metabolites), the eluate stopped when peaks of interest were in the flow cell (applicable to 1D experiments of minor metabolites and 2D experiments) or the eluate parked in capillary loops for acquisition at a later stage, respectively. For further information about these direct HPLC-NMR modes, the reader is advised to read the excellent review by Professor Jaroszewski (Jaroszewski, 2005a,b) or the book chapter by Staerk *et al.* (2006). However, all these direct HPLC-NMR modes suffered from high running costs due to the use of deuterated water in the mobile phase as well as problems with efficient solvent suppression of non-deuterated acetonitrile and residual water solvent. It was therefore not until the introduction of commercial HPLC-SPE-NMR systems, i.e. the intervening of HPLC and NMR by an automated solid-phase extraction unit for trapping (adsorption on solid-phase extraction (SPE) cartridges) of metabolites, that hyphenated NMR became a versatile tool in natural products research (Seger and Sturm, 2007; Kesting *et al.*, 2011). HPLC-SPE-NMR has proven successful for full structure elucidation directly from crude extracts without any pre-purification (Sprogøe *et al.*, 2007; Staerk *et al.*, 2009; Johansen *et al.*, 2011). This includes HPLC-SPE-NMR in combination with circular dichroism for assignment of absolute configuration (Sprogøe *et al.*, 2008), and recently acquisition of direct-detected $^{13}$C NMR spectra has also been demonstrated (Wubshet *et al.*, 2012).

## 7.6   Principle of HPLC-SPE-NMR

HPLC-SPE-NMR is an indirect hyphenated NMR method (Jaroszewski, 2005b) because NMR experiments of analytes are not acquired directly in the HPLC eluate. A schematic presentation of the HPLC-HRMS-SPE-NMR operated in the tube-transfer mode is shown in Figure 7.6.

The above system includes PDA and HRMS as detectors for controlling trapping on SPE cartridges based on UV and/or MS thresholds. The HPLC eluate is diluted with a makeup flow of water, typically at a flow rate two times higher than the HPLC flow rate. This decreases the eluotropic strength of the eluate, and thereby allows automated trapping (adsorption) of individual analytes triggered by UV absorption or MS ion count thresholds. The HPLC separation can be repeated multiple times to increase the amount of analyte trapped on the SPE cartridges. The SPE cartridges are subsequently dried with a stream of nitrogen gas to remove any non-deuterated solvents from the HPLC eluate. Finally, the analytes are eluted into NMR tubes (in the tube-transfer mode typically into 1.7 mm tubes in 96-type tube racks for automated NMR acquisition afterwards) or directly into a NMR flow cell. There are several advantages of indirect HPLC-SPE-NMR compared to direct HPLC-NMR:

- the entire HPLC elution volume is concentrated in volume-matched NMR tubes or in a volume-matched NMR flow cell
- post-column water dilution allows trapping at high organic solvent ratios
- multiple trappings lead to increased sensitivity
- removal of HPLC solvent: SPE decouples NMR from chromatography
- use of deuterated solvent – better solvent suppression.

The increased sensitivity obtained by analyte focusing and multiple trappings have especially advanced the use of HPLC-SPE-NMR for full structure elucidation of even very complex metabolites. Thus, Jaroszewski and co-workers (Clarkson *et al.*, 2006a,b) identified 17 metabolites directly from crude extract of *Harpagophytum procumbens*, including a novel Diels–Alder dimer and novel unstable chinane-type tricyclic diterpenes.

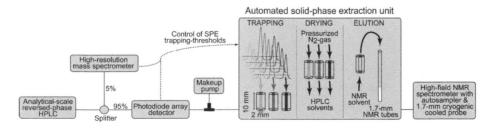

**Figure 7.6**   Schematic presentation of the HPLC-HRMS-SPE-NMR operated in the tube-transfer mode with 1.7-mm NMR tubes and cryogenically cooled probe.

## 7.7   High-resolution bioassay-coupled HPLC-SPE-NMR

A major disadvantage of the basic HPLC-SPE-NMR setup is the lack of information about the bioactivity of individual constituents in the crude extract. Thus, the recent coupling of microplate-based high-resolution (bio)assays with HPLC-SPE-NMR, i.e. high-resolution bioassay/HPLC-SPE-NMR, is the most promising new technology for identifying bioactive constituents directly from crude plant extracts (Agnolet *et al.*, 2012; Grosso *et al.*, 2013; Kongstad *et al.*, 2014) and plant-based food (Schmidt *et al.*, 2012; Wiese *et al.*, 2013; Wubshet *et al.*, 2013). The principle of high-resolution bioassay-coupled HPLC-SPE-NMR is shown in Figure 7.7.

The processes are as follows: (i) microfractionation into one or more 96-well microplates, (ii) bioassays performed for each well in the microplate(s) (HPLC solvent is evaporated before enzyme assays are performed), (iii) construction of a biochromatogram underlying the

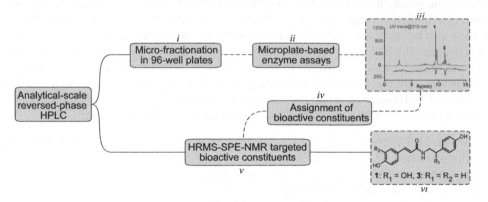

**Figure 7.7**   Principle of bioassay-coupled HPLC-HRMS-SPE-NMR. (Source: Schmidt *et al.* 2014. Reproduced with permission of Elsevier.)

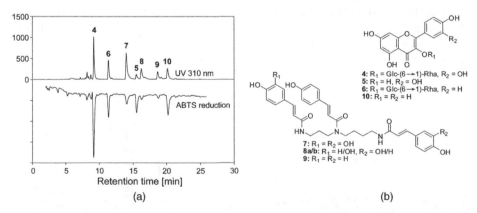

**Figure 7.8**   Analytical-scale HPLC chromatogram of caper bud extract (top) and the corresponding radical scavenging profile (bottom) (a). Compounds 4–10 identified using HPLC-SPE-NMR (b). (Source: Wiese *et al.* 2013. Reproduced with permission of Elsevier.)

HPLC chromatogram by plotting the results from bioassays against their respective retention times, (iv) assigning HPLC peaks correlating with peaks in the biochromatogram, (v) targeting HPLC-HRMS-SPE-NMR analysis towards bioactive peaks only and (vi) structure elucidation of bioactive constituents.

Bioassay-coupled HPLC-SPE-NMR has successfully been used for identifying radical scavengers in caper buds (Wiese *et al.*, 2013). The high-resolution radical scavenging/HPLC-SPE-NMR setup allowed separation of all major analytes on an analytical-scale HPLC column, and after microfractionation and radical scavenging assaying of each well the resulting radical scavenging profile allowed pin-pointing of peaks 4–10 as the major radical scavengers (Figure 7.8). The corresponding analytes 4–10 were identified as quercetin, kaempferol, rutin, kaempferol-3-*O*-β-rutinoside and $N^1,N^5,N^{10}$-triphenylpropenoyl spermidine amides.

## 7.8 Combining metabolomics and hyphenated NMR techniques

Especially interesting is the combination of NMR-based metabolomics with HPLC-HRMS-SPE-NMR. This was recently demonstrated by Professor Staerk and co-workers (Schmidt *et al.*, 2014) in a study where they used NMR- and MS-based metabolomics, high-resolution α-glucosidase profiling and HPLC-SPE-NMR for investigation of bioactive constituents in *Allium*. The experimental setup used in this study is shown in Figure 7.9.

The study included 30 different *Allium* species, and with different collection years and different drying methods this amounted to a total of 94 samples. They used α-glucosidase assays as well as NMR- and MS-based metabolomics of crude extracts for studying the overall composition of the different *Allium* species and for exploring the effect of different drying methods. This showed that oven as well as freeze drying of *Allium* causes deglycosylation of flavonoid glycosides. Furthermore, the metabolomics experiments showed that only garlic and elephant garlic contain allicin in traceable amounts. Based on these results, the number of samples for high-resolution α-glucosidase/HPLC-SPE-NMR could be reduced from 94 to 30, thereby diminishing the workload considerably. The high-resolution α-glucosidase/HPLC-SPE-NMR analysis led to identification of three α-glucosidase inhibitors, i.e. *N-p*-coumaroyloctopamine, *N-p*-coumaroyltyramine and quercetin, and based on the HPLC-ESI-HRMS experiments acquired for the MS-based metabolomics, a distribution plot of these three metabolites was prepared for all 94 samples included in the study.

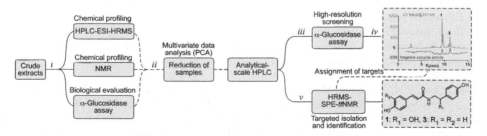

**Figure 7.9** Experimental setup for combined use of NMR- and MS-based metabolomics, high-resolution α-glucosidase profiling and HPLC-SPE-NMR for investigation of bioactive constituents in *Allium*. (Source: Schmidt *et al.* 2014. Reproduced with permission of Elsevier.)

# 7.9   Perspectives in ethnopharmacology

As shown above, NMR-based metabolomics and hyphenated NMR techniques provide solid technology platforms for investigating complex plant extracts – a challenge frequently encountered in the holistic and multifaceted approach needed for successful ethnopharmacological studies. Thus, high-resolution bioassays coupled with hyphenated NMR provide fast and reliable analyses of individual bioactive constituents in complex mixtures such as the extracts of plants used in traditional medicine. The speed and reliability of these analyses allows evidence-based ethnopharmacology to be performed with an unprecedented level of detail without performing lengthy and time-consuming preparative scale analyses. The metabolomics approach even enables identification of synergistic effects of compounds in preparation, a core challenge to ethnopharmacology (Heinrich, 2010). In addition, metabolomics allows evaluation of variation in the global composition of a large set of plant extracts of different origin before compound identification is initiated.

# 7.10   Conclusions

In conclusion, NMR-based metabolomics and HPLC-SPE-NMR – eventually in combination with high-resolution bioactivity profiling – have proven to be very strong analytical tools for the investigation of bioactive natural products from plants. Whether used alone or in combination, these techniques hold promise for providing fast and reliable analyses of even very complex mixtures, thereby providing the technological platform for a deeper understanding of the complex mechanisms underlying the successful use of plants for the treatment of human diseases among traditional practitioners as well as in western medicine.

# References

Agnolet, S., Jaroszewski, J.W., Verpoorte, R. and Staerk, D. (2010) [1]H NMR-based metabolomics combined with HPLC-PDA-MS-SPE-NMR for investigation of standardized *Ginkgo biloba* preparations. *Metabolomics*, **6**, 292–302.

Agnolet, S., Wiese, S., Verpoorte, R. and Staerk, D. (2012) Comprehensive analysis of commercial willow bark extracts by new technology platform: Combined use of metabolomics, high-performance liquid chromatography-solid-phase extraction-nuclear magnetic resonance spectroscopy and high-resolution radical scavenging assay. *Journal of Chromatography A*, **1262**, 130–137.

Bayer, E., Albert, K., Nieder, M., *et al.* (1979) On-line coupling of high-performance liquid chromatography and nuclear magnetic resonance. *Journal of Chromatography*, **186**, 497–507.

Benzie, I.F.F. and Wachtel-Galor, S. (2011) *Herbal Medicine,* Biomolecular and Clinical Aspects, CRC Press, Boca Raton, FL.

Boroujerdi, A.F., Vizcaino, M.I., Meyers, A., *et al.* (2009) NMR-based microbial metabolomics and the temperature-dependent coral pathogen *Vibrio coralliilyticus*. *Environmental Science and Technology*, **43**, 7658–7664.

Choi, H.-K., Choi, Y.H., Verberne, M., *et al.* (2004) Metabolic fingerprinting of wild type and transgenic tobacco plants by [1]H NMR and multivariate analysis technique. *Phytochemistry*, **65**, 857–864.

Clarkson, C., Stærk, D., Hansen, S.H., *et al.* (2006a) Identification of major and minor constituents of *Harpagophytum procumbens* (Devil's Claw) using HPLC-SPE-NMR and HPLC-ESIMS/APCIMS. *Journal of Natural Products*, **69**, 1280–1288.

Clarkson, C., Stærk, D., Hansen, S.H., *et al.* (2006b) Discovering new natural products directly from crude extracts by HPLC-SPE-NMR: chinane diterpenes in *Harpagophytum procumbens*. *Journal of Natural Products*, **69**, 527–530.

Eriksson, L., Johansson, E., Kettaneh-Wold, N. and Wold, S. (2001) *Multi- and Megavariate Data Analysis. Principles and Applications*, Umetrics AB, Umeå.

Fiehn, O. (2002) Metabolomics – the link between genotypes and fenotypes. *Plant Molecular Biology*, **48**, 155–171.

Grosso, C., Jäger, A.K. and Staerk, D. (2013) Coupling of a high-resolution monoamine oxidase-A inhibitor assay and HPLC-SPE-NMR for advanced bioactivity profiling of plant extracts. *Phytochemical Analysis*, **24**, 141–147.

Heinrich, M. (2010) Ethnopharmacology in the 21st Century – Grand Challenges. *Frontiers in Pharmacology*, **8**, 1–3.

Jaroszewski, J.W. (2005a) Hyphenated NMR methods in natural products research, part 1: direct hyphenation. *Planta Medica*, **71**, 691–700.

Jaroszewski, J.W. (2005b) Hyphenated NMR methods in natural products research, part 2: HPLC-SPE-NMR and other new trends in NMR hyphenation. *Planta Medica*, **71**, 795–802.

Johansen, K.T., Wubshet, S.G., Nyberg, N.T. and Jaroszewski, J.W. (2011) From retrospective assessment to prospective decisions in natural product isolation: HPLC-SPE-NMR analysis of *Carthamus oxyacantha*. *Journal of Natural Products*, **74**, 2454–2461.

Kesting, J.R., Johansen, K.T. and Jaroszewski, J.W. (2011) Hyphenated NMR techniques, in *Advances in Biomedical Spectroscopy, Vol.* **3** (eds A.J. Dingley and S.M. Pascal), IOS Press, Amsterdam, pp. 413–434.

Kim, H.K., Choi, Y.H. and Verpoorte, R. (2010) NMR-based metabolomics analysis of plants. *Nature Protocols*, **5**, 536–549.

Kongstad, K.T., Wubshet, S.G., Johannesen, A., *et al.* (2014) High-resolution screening combined with HPLC–HRMS–SPE–NMR for identification of fungal plasma membrane $H^+$-ATPase inhibitors from plants. *Journal of Agricultural and Food Chemistry*, **62**, 5595–5602.

Newman, D.J. and Cragg, G.M. (2012) Natural products as sources of new drugs over the 30 years from 1981 to 2010. *Journal of Natural Products*, **75**, 311–335.

Nicholson, J.K., Lindon, J. and Holmes, E. (1999) 'Metabonomics': understanding the metabolic responses of living systems to pathophysiological stimuli via multivariate statistical analysis of biological NMR spectroscopic data. *Xenobiotica*, **29**, 1181–1189.

Robinette, S.L., Ajredini R., Rasheed H., *et al.* (2011) Hierarchical alignment and full resolution pattern recognition of 2D NMR spectra: Application to nematode chemical ecology. *Analytical Chemistry*, **83**, 1649–1657.

Schmidt, J.S., Lauridsen, M.B., Dragsted, L.O., *et al.* (2012) Development of a bioassay-coupled HPLC-SPE-ttNMR platform for identification of α-glucosidase inhibitors in apple peel (*Malus* × *domestica* Borkh.). *Food Chemistry*, **135**, 1692–1699.

Schmidt, J.S., Nyberg, N.T. and Staerk, D. (2014) Assessment of constituents in *Allium* by multivariate data analysis, high-resolution α-glucosidase inhibition assay and HPLC-SPE-NMR. *Food Chemistry*, **161**, 192–198.

Seger, C. and Sturm, S. (2007) HPLC-SPE-NMR: A new hyphenation technique. *LC GC Europe*, **11**, 587–597.

Sprogøe, K., Stærk, D., Jäger, A.K., *et al.* (2007) Targeted natural product isolation guided by HPLC-SPE-NMR: Constituents of *Hubertia* species. *Journal of Natural Products*, **70**, 1472–1477.

Sprogøe, K., Stærk, D., Ziegler, H.L., *et al.* (2008) Combining HPLC-PDA-MS-SPE-NMR with circular dichroism for complete natural product characterization in crude extracts: Levorotatory gossypol in *Thespesia danis*. *Journal of Natural Products*, **71**, 516–519.

Stærk, D., Lambert, M. and Jaroszewski, J.W. (2006) HPLC-NMR techniques for plant extract analysis, in *Medicinal Plant Biotechnology. From Basic Research to Applications* (eds O. Kayser and W. Quax), Wiley-VCH, Weinheim, pp. 29–48.

Staerk, D., Kesting, J.R., Sairafianpour, M., *et al.* (2009) Accelerated dereplication of crude extracts using HPLC-PDA-MS-SPE-NMR: Quinolone alkaloids of *Haplophyllum acutifolium*. *Phytochemistry*, **70**, 1055–1061.

Trygg, J. and Lundstedt, T. (2007) Chemometrics techniques for metabonomics, in *The Handbook of Metabonomics and Metabolomics* (eds J.C. Lindon, J.K. Nicholson and E. Holmes), Elsevier, Amsterdam, pp. 171–200.

Watanabe, N. and Niki, E. (1978) Direct-coupling of FT-NMR to high-performance liquid chromatography. *Proceedings of the Japanese Academy Series B*, **54**, 194–199.

Wiese, S., Wubshet, S.G., Nielsen, J. and Staerk, D. (2013) Coupling HPLC-SPE-NMR with a microplate-based high-resolution antioxidant assay for efficient analysis of antioxidants in food – Validation and proof-of-concept study with caper buds. *Food Chemistry*, **141**, 4010–4018.

Wubshet, S.G., Johansen, K.T., Nyber,g N.T. and Jaroszewski, J.W. (2012) Direct [13]C NMR detection in HPLC hyphenation mode: Analysis of *Ganoderma lucidum* terpenoids. *Journal of Natural Products*, **75**, 876–882.

Wubshet, S.G., Schmidt, J.S., Wiese, S. and Staerk, D. (2013) High-resolution screening combined with HPLC–HRMS–SPE–NMR for identification of potential health-promoting constituents in sea aster and searocket – New Nordic food ingredients. *Journal of Agricultural and Food Chemistry*, **61**, 8616–8623.

Yilmaz, A., Nyberg, N.T. and Jaroszewski, J.W. (2011) Metabolic profiling based on two-dimensional *J*-Resolved [1]H NMR data and parallel factor analysis. *Analytical Chemistry*, **83**, 8278–8285.

# 8

# New Medicines Based On Traditional Knowledge: Indigenous and Intellectual Property Rights from an Ethnopharmacological Perspective

Michael Heinrich

*Centre for Pharmacognosy and Phytotherapy, UCL School of Pharmacy, University of London, London*

## 8.1   Introduction

From the perspective of the wider public, the media and the scientific communities, potential new high-value medicines are the most widely recognised and high profile 'benefit' of ethnopharmacological research. This has been expressed very poignantly by Cox (2008):

> 'Ethnobotanical approaches are the oldest, but perhaps most successful, techniques in discovering new pharmaceuticals from biodiversity.'
>
> (p. 272)

Similarly, Schmidt *et al.* (2007) argued:

> 'Indeed, bioprospecting combined with the utilization of indigenous and traditional medical knowledge has been central to the history of the discovery of botanical therapeutics.'

*Ethnopharmacology*, First Edition. Edited by Michael Heinrich and Anna K. Jäger.
© 2015 John Wiley & Sons, Ltd. Published 2015 by John Wiley & Sons, Ltd.

On the other hand, the use of indigenous and traditional knowledge in such projects has been criticised by a range of researchers, as exemplified by Isla (2007), who argues from what she calls an 'ecofeminist' perspective:

'This perspective understands the current triumphant neoliberal agenda as a continuation of a long history of capitalist, patriarchal, and racist colonization of women, peasants, indigenous peoples, land, and nature. So much of the accumulated capital was expropriated from these groups that a great deal of what counts as economic growth has been and continues today to be simply the transfer of local and communal wealth into external markets. Their subsistence production is both necessary to capital and necessary to their own survival and is taken through capitalist patriarchal violence.'

This critique has been embedded in a more fundamental critique of the legal and economic aspects of protecting intellectual property (e.g. Mgbeoji, 2006) as well as being based on a critique of the lack of respecting existing values recognized by local communities:

'The "decontextualization" of the "components" of biodiversity or culture results in the unauthorized extraction of inalienable information and materials. This ignores the "sacred balance" between all life, and violates the kinship relationships that indigenous and traditional peoples maintain with their "extended family" of all living things.'

(Posey, 2002a)

In essence there is no way to reconcile such fundamentally diverging views and this chapter will not try to achieve this. Instead it will look at the direct responsibilities of researchers in the context of ethnopharmacological and bioprospecting work, and discuss examples of compounds or extracts that have been developed up to a clinical level. The focus of this brief overview is therefore on the researchers' responsibilities in a context as it has been outlined by many, including, for example, Shiva (2007), who also takes a critical view and offers what fundamental requirements need to be fulfilled:

'The bioprospecting paradigm needs to be examined in the context of equity, specifically its effect on the donor community, potential recipient communities, and bioprospecting corporations. Even though bio-prospecting contracts are based on prior informed consent and compensation, unlike the case of biopiracy where no consent is taken and no compensation given, not all owners/carriers of an indigenous knowledge tradition are consulted or compensated. Not only does this lead to inequity and injustice but it also has the potential of pitting individual against individual within a community and community against community.'

## 8.2   The legal framework

Without doubt today's ethnobiological research and any other research involving the use of the biological resources of a country are based on agreements and permits, which in turn are based on international and bilateral treaties. The most important of these is the Convention of Rio or CBD, which provides a framework for research and development (R&D) based on biodiversity at an international level (Secretariat of the Convention on Biological Diversity, 2001):

'The objectives of this Convention, to be pursued in accordance with its relevant provisions, are the conservation of biological diversity, the sustainable use of its components and the fair and equitable sharing of the benefits arising out of the utilisation of genetic resources, including by appropriate access to genetic resources and by appropriate transfer of relevant technologies, taking into account all rights over those resources and to technologies, and by appropriate funding.'

(Secretariat of the Convention on Biological Diversity 2001)

This defines the rights of countries (i.e. internationally) and as such is directly relevant in the context of international R&D projects on biodiversity (including local and traditional knowledge). The rights of indigenous peoples and other keepers of local knowledge is clearly stated in article 8j:

> '(j) Subject to its national legislation, respect, preserve and maintain knowledge, innovations and practices of indigenous and local communities embodying traditional lifestyles relevant for the conservation and sustainable use of biological diversity and promote their wider application with the approval and involvement of the holders of such knowledge, innovations and practices and encourage the equitable sharing of the benefits arising from the utilization of such knowledge, innovations and practices.'
>
> (Secretariat of the Convention on Biological Diversity 2001)

This and the subsequent treaties significantly changed the basic conditions for ethnopharmacological and bioprospecting research. Countries that provide resources for natural product research and drug development have well-defined rights, which specifically include sharing benefits that may potentially arise from such research.

Numerous other agreements (including most recently the Nagoya Protocol of 2010, http://www.cbd.int/abs/about/, which aims to ascertain the 'fair and equitable sharing of benefits arising out of the utilization of genetic resources (Article 1)' or trade-related aspects of intellectual property rights (TRIPS), World Trade Organization (WTO) agreements, cf. www.wto.org) now form a complex framework of regulations and it is the general consensus in major academic circles that their implementation is an essential foundation of any form of ethnopharmacological and related research.

The debate about access rights and benefit sharing dates back to well before these international conventions and several learned societies played a crucial role in its development and later implementation. As pointed out many times, 'there is an inextricable link between cultural and biological diversity'. This principle was first formulated at the First International Congress on Ethnobiology in Belem in 1988. No generally agreed on standards have so far been accepted, but the importance of obtaining the informants' prior informed consent and ascertaining appropriate benefit-sharing agreements has been stressed by numerous authors (e.g. Posey, 2002b), even though the exact requirements of such arrangements sometimes remain contentious.

## 8.3   Industrial research in an ethnopharmacological context

While there is a fundamental academic consensus on the ethical foundations of research, research in the context of commercial development is both complex and driven by a wide range of stakeholders and factors. Firstly, while this chapter and the entire book focuses on the academic field of ethnopharmacology, the borderline to what is called 'bioprospecting' is blurred. Traditionally ethnopharmaoclogy is defined as a scientific approach that focuses on the 'exchange of information and understandings about people's use of plants, fungi, animals, microorganisms and minerals and their biological and pharmacological effects based on the principles established through international conventions' (*Journal of Ethnopharmacology* 2014). The goal is often seen to evaluate traditional and local medicines with the idea to contribute to a more evidence-based use of such medicines in the context of the respective cultures of origin (Verpoorte, 2012). On the other hand, the 'transformation of traditional medicines into modern drugs' (Corson and Crews, 2007) and into other higher value products directly targeted to the rich markets is a reality in an ever-increasing number of countries, including in Europe, North America, Australia/New Zealand and more recently in fast-growing markets in Asia, South America and Africa. While a lot of attention has been paid to new medicines, there also is a rising demand for new healthcare products like nutraceuticals, cosmetics and high-value foods.

Industrial R&D generally works on fundamentally different principles in terms of the key criteria used to develop a new product. The specific criteria vary in the various sectors of industry and between companies, but there is a set of common principles relevant in the industry that are used as decision points to decide whether a project (e.g. on a specific species) should be taken forward or not (so-called go/no go decisions):

- First and foremost, industrial R&D will always focus on projects that avoid any form of obstacles that may result in problems with the development of a product into a commodity. These problems range from problems with the long-term and large-scale supply of material (a common problem with natural products and less often of concern with synthetic compounds) and possible concerns about toxicity and other risks, to concerns about the acceptability of the final product. The supply problem may, for example, be due to problems associated with securing sufficient quantities of the starting material, but also pre-existing claims, for example based on local or traditional use.
- The protection of the intellectual property (IP) for the company is, of course, a central requirement for any industrial R&D project. Ideally this IP should be a new chemical entity with a new biological–pharmacological activity, but there are also weaker patent claims a company may want to consider (see chapter 9, A. Hesketh).
- An industrial drug or nutraceutical development is a unidirectional process, which, for example in case of medicine development, goes from early preclinical research to advanced studies focusing on safety and formulation science, and then into the various stages of clinical development (and is because of its unidirectionality often called a 'pipeline').
- Ideally such a new product should offer a unique selling point to the company which allows them to position themselves in a key market (see below).
- From an industrial perspective the demands of key markets result in a very different set of diseases, which are of primary relevance. In general terms chronic, degenerative conditions and diseases are more important than the acute diseases often at the centre of ethnopharmacological research.
- Any R&D activity for a product will have to fit into the wider strategy of a company for developing a certain sector of a market, therefore very potent pharmacological effects not relevant to the core economic areas of a company may well result in the ending of a project.
- Importantly, a specific local or traditional use of a species is generally *not* central to a company's strategy, aside from possibly at a later stage, for marketing purposes, especially in case of supplements and cosmetics (with a few exceptions of companies that consciously want to develop products based on local and traditional uses).

Relatively little is known about a specific industrial project prior to reaching the level of wider commercialisation. Commercial secrets generally cover all aspects relating to specific arrangements for benefit sharing and commercial development. This situation is made more complex by the fact that many of the R&D projects are managed or driven by small enterprises, which often are very reluctant to share information. The best approach is therefore to assess examples of natural products that either were brought to the market or got close to getting a full marketing authorisation.

# 8.4 Some case studies

Several examples of pure chemical entities (prostratine, peplin, galanthamine) and mixtures (Sangre de drago or *Croton lechleri* Müll.Arg. and Hoodia) are discussed in this section. The most famous example, artemisinin, obtained from Chinese *Artemisia annua* L., shows what can be achieved and this development has been reviewed and discussed widely (e.g. Hsu, 2006, 2010). Its development predates the CBD and is therefore not discussed here. This discussion is not about success in scientific and R&D terms, but the way indigenous and local intellectual rights were taken into account or not. Consequently, the focus is on:

- the evidence for links between local/traditional knowledge and drug development
- the mechanisms put in place to ascertain benefit sharing (if any)
- the benefits for local communities arising from it
- the problems and challenges.

Excluded are substances that were discovered as a part of a larger screening effort which did not incorporate an ethnopharmacological element, and drugs that were developed well before the implementation of the CBD. Consequently, there are only limited examples that can be used to analyse the success of ethnopharmacologically driven drug developments.

## 8.4.1 Pure natural products as drug leads

A promising lead derived from *Homalanthus nutans* (G.Forst.) Guill. (Euphorbiaceac), a small rainforest tree used by Samoan healers to treat hepatitis, is currently considered for clinical development in the treatment of HIV/AIDS. Its extracts exhibited potent *in vitro* anti-HIV activity. It yielded a unique non-tumor-promoting protein kinase C (PKC) activator, prostratin, a 12-deoxyphorbol ester, which showed strong anti-HIV-1 effects (Figure 8.1). The compound was first isolated and its structure reported in 1992 at the time of the implementation of the CBD. Prostratin effectively activates HIV gene expression in latently infected Jurkat cells and acts by stimulating IκB kinase (IKK)-dependent phosphorylation and degradation of IκBα, leading to the rapid nuclear translocation of NF-κB and activation of the HIV-1 long terminal repeat. Ultimately, it has been postulated that prostratin induces the HIV virus to leave cells and thus makes a silent virus accessible to other medication. Prostratin has been licensed to the NCI as a candidate drug for treating AIDS/HIV. The inventors made the commitment that

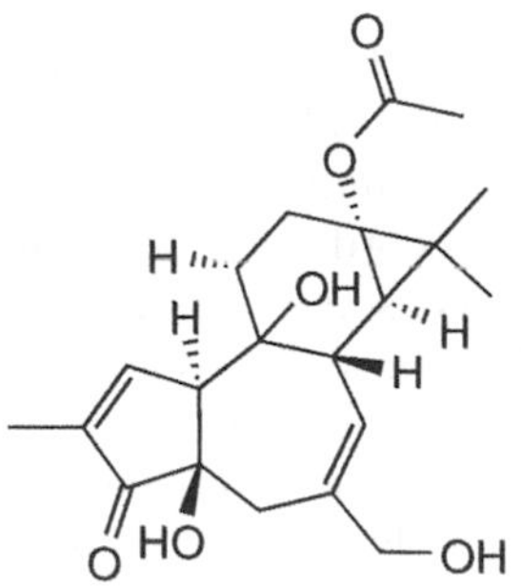

**Figure 8.1** Structure of prostatin.

20% of the potential license income shall be returned to the Samoan people if a product based on this compound reaches the market. Prior to such a marketing authorization funds were also made available to the community in order to support schools, medical clinics, water supplies, trails, an aerial rainforest canopy walkway and an endowment for the rainforest. However, the exact amount that became available in the region of origin is unknown and since the product has not reached the market it is likely to be low (Cox, 2001, 2008; Heinrich, 2013). To date no clinically used product has been developed and, therefore, no socioeconomic benefits have been derived from prostatin.

The second example offers fascinating insights into the complexity of ethnopharmacology-based drug discovery. In 2012, a gel containing 0.015% or 0.05% peplin or ingenol mebutate (Picato®), an unusual diterpene ester, isolated from *Euphorbia peplus* L., petty spurge (Euphorbiaceae), was licensed for use in actinic keratoses on the face, scalp, trunk and extremities. Clinical research into other cancers (bladder, intravesicular; leukemia, systemically) are ongoing. The research was started by an Australian company in Brisbane (Peplin Ltd), which in 2009 was bought by the Danish pharmaceutical company LeoPharma.

*E. peplus* is a weedy species native to Europe, where it is widely distributed and particularly common in gardens and other disturbed environments. As part of European migration it became a common weed in many temperate to warmer regions of the world. Local and traditional uses of the species in Europe, most notably in the treatment of warts and other skin conditions, have been well documented and span many centuries. In fact the species is included in many of the classical early 16th century herbals. However, the discovery of its medicinal potential goes back to uses of the species saps in the Brisbane region of Australia. During the 1970s and 1980s, members of the Australian public used the sap from *E. peplus* to treat skin cancers and solar keratosis (Green and Beardmore, 1988; Wheeton and Chick, 1976). This is based on only eight use reports from a total of 2095 respondents who returned the survey. However, this made *E. peplus* the second most popular plant within this survey with *Aloe vera* having 35 reports (Green and Beardmore, 1988) and a total of 164 persons indicating self-treating/ment of skin cancers and solar keratoses. Although this is a relatively small number, it clearly served as a starting point to investigate the species' medical effects (Ogbourne *et al.*, 2007), proving that this R&D project was clearly ethnopharmacologically driven. *In vitro* and *in vivo* evidence led to the establishment of a well-defined mechanism of action and clinical trials proved its effectiveness (Lebwohl *et al.*, 2012). Interestingly, in this case questions relating to the CBD and to benefit sharing were never raised and the author is not aware of any claims relating to the use of this species in the development of a medicine.

A third example, Galanthamine (syn. galantamine), is an anti-Alzheimer's drug developed in the 1990s and initially isolated from *Galanthus* and *Leucojum* species as well as other members of the Amaryllidaceae (Figure 8.2). Its history has been reviewed in detail (cf. Heinrich and Teoh 2004; Heinrich 2010). The initial idea for developing a medicine (in this case in the treatment of poliomyelitis) firstly from *Galanthus woronowii* Losinsk. seems to be based on the local use in far Eastern Europe. According to unconfirmed reports, in the 1950s the common snowdrop growing in the wild was used to ease nerve pain by rubbing it on the forehead, but without more ethnobotanical data these claims are impossible to assess.

The early development of galanthamine in Eastern Europe for use in the treatment of poliomyelitis started with the alkaloid's isolation from the garden snowdrop (*Galanthus* spp., most notably *G. woronowii*), but today the compound is obtained from other members of the same plant family, such as the daffodil (*Narcissus* spp.) and the snowflake (*Leucojum* spp., esp. *L. aestivum* L.), as well as, most importantly, being made synthetically.

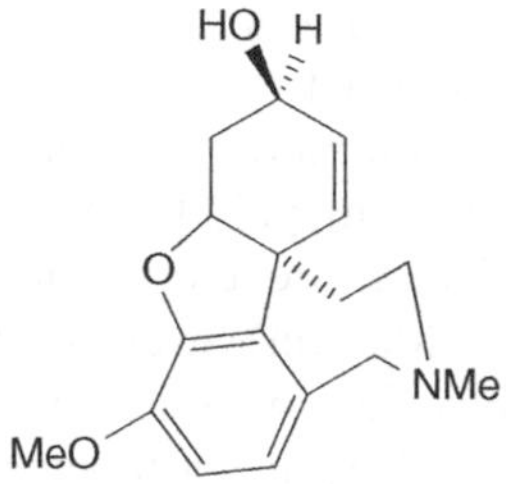

**6** Galanthamine

**Figure 8.2** Structure of galanthamine.

Based on unconfirmed reports, in the Caucasian mountains region snowdrops were used to treat poliomyelitis but no reference is made to the traditional use of snowdrop in the Caucasian region by the Russian authors who published the initial papers on this topic (Heinrich, 2010). However, all this is based on very few secondhand reports on the use of snowdrops prior to the development of galanthamine as a licensed medicine. Despite the lack of precise data on local and traditional uses of this species it is highly likely that this development process for a new antipoliomylitis drug is based on such information. It is therefore an example of the successful ethnobotany-driven development of a natural product into a clinically important drug. At the same time it throws a spotlight on the difficulties of establishing the link between local and traditional uses and drug development. The initial commercial R&D (in the 1950s in the Soviet Union and other Eastern Block countries) is focused on the drug's effect on the peripheral nervous system, while later research targeted similar enzymes in the CNS (acetylcholine esterase, AchE). Interestingly, local and traditional use gave an essential initial idea, but at this point the evidence for where the initial ethnobotanical information came from remains scanty, pointing to the need not only to fully record such knowledge, but also to make this information publicly available.

## 8.4.2 Extracts and partially purified preparations as drug leads

Most drug development programmes focus on pure compounds and the following examples highlight some of the specific challenges of industrial projects based on ethnopharmacological data. In 2012 a product based on *Croton lechleri* Muell. Arg., Sangre de drago (Euphorbiaceae), a Peruvian rainforest plant commonly used in its region of origin for a variety of diseases, including for the treatment of diarrhoea, was licensed as a medicine to treat HIV/AIDS-associated diarrhoea. In the Amazon this species is well known for treating gastrointestinal problems. A semi-purified proanthocyanidin oligomer mixture from *C. lechlerii* was initially shown to have broad activity against a variety of RNA and DNA viruses (Ubillas *et al.*, 1994). Later on it was shown to modulate chloride and fluid secretion in the gastrointestinal tract (Gabriel *et al.*, 1999; Cottreau *et al.*, 2010; Tradtrantip *et al.*, 2010). In terms of the R&D, there can be no doubt that the development of this medicine was based on local and traditional knowledge. Its development was initiated by Shaman Pharmaceuticals, a California-based small company dedicated to developing new medicines based on the principles of benefit sharing not only once a product is on the market but also during its development (Wells, 1998). The company was active from 1989 until 1999, when it stopped

R&D on new pharmaceutical entities and was taken over by Napo Pharmaceuticals, which in 2005 and 2008, respectively, licensed it to Glenmark Pharmaceuticals (India) and Salix Pharmaceuticals (USA) for exclusive commercialisation in in different countries. It remains unclear whether benefits are currently being paid to the countries or regions of origin.

A now classical example of a failure to develop a new high-value product is the Southern African species *Hoodia gordonii* (Masson) Sweet ex Decne (Apocynaceae), from which two hunger-suppressing pregnane glycosides were isolated and that was patented in 1998 (for details see Heinrich, 2013) (Figure 8.3). The appetite-suppressant effect of the plants extracts had already been established in 1983. At least since the 19th century it was known that this desert plant quenches thirst, e.g. as recorded for the Khoi-San people, but it seems to have been known also in other groups.

This research was initiated and driven by the Council for Scientific and Industrial Research (CSIR) of South Africa. A small British company (Phytopharm) obtained the rights and the extracts were investigated for hunger-suppressant and later antidiabetic effects. In 1998 clinical studies for treating obesity were started and the extract was licensed to Pfizer, with the goal of developing a fully licensed medicine on the basis of a characterized extract with a defined amount of the active metabolites for the treatment of obesity. After a considerable investment in clinical and preclinical research, in July 2003 Pfizer unexpectedly returned the license to Phytopharm. In late 2004, Unilever stepped in with the strategic goal of developing a slimming food but in 2008 this R&D was stopped, too. An important element in this decision

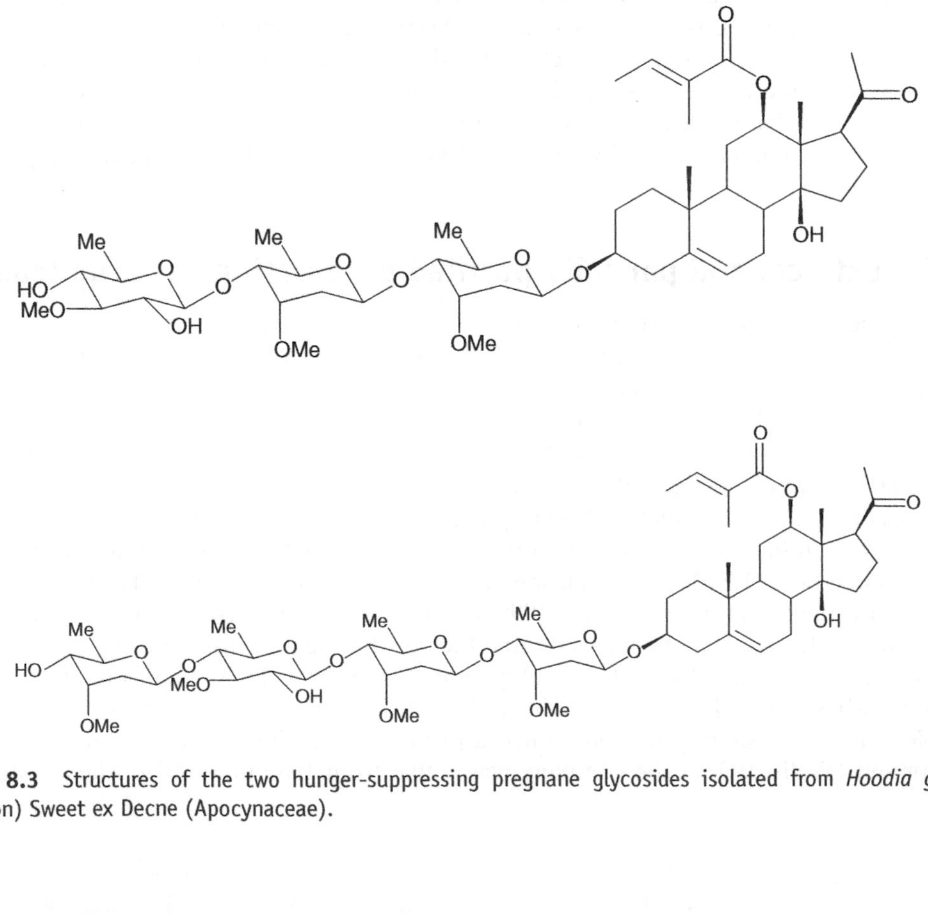

**Figure 8.3** Structures of the two hunger-suppressing pregnane glycosides isolated from *Hoodia gordonii* (Masson) Sweet ex Decne (Apocynaceae).

were concerns about the product's safety. Today only unlicensed products of very doubtful composition and quality are on the market. This is linked to the non-existent regulatory basis of these products, but also to problems with the supply of a wild-harvested slow-growing desert species.

Without doubt this development was driven by ethnpharmacological considerations, and, interestingly and worryingly, the IP had been patented and developed without the prior consent of the Khoi-San people. Only in 2004 was a benefit-sharing agreement signed between the Khoi-San and CSIR. This is one of the first benefit-sharing agreements and it would have given the Khoi-San a share of royalties derived from the sale of products containing the patented extract if a product would have been developed on the basis of this knowledge (see Heinrich, 2013).

## 8.5 Conclusions

While there certainly is a wide recognition that drug development based on ethnopharmacological studies possesses considerable potential, as in all other drug discovery programmes the chances for developing a new product that ultimately makes it to the market are very slim indeed (Amirkia and Heinrich, 2015). This is not only linked to the intrinsic challenges of the drug discovery process, but also to some very specific aspects of natural product and ethnopharmacological research:

- The supply of the starting material and the sustainable extraction of a compound depends on a multitude of factors and most successful programmes are focused on either widely distributed plants (weeds) or compounds for which an economically viable synthesis was developed.
- There is not necessarily a direct link between local/traditional uses and the key targets in drug discovery. It is well known that local/traditional medicines are commonly used for acute and often infectious conditions, while most of the commercial drug development activities are focused on diseases like diverse cancers or chronic, aging-related conditions.
- The multidisciplinary expertise required for such ethnopharmacology-driven drug development programmes and the willingness in the relevant industries to support commercial projects with an uncertain supply chain is lacking
- The advent of 'biologicals', i.e. pharmaceuticals derived from research in molecular biology and pharmacological biochemistry, offers an attractive alternative to such a 'classical' approach.

Ethnopharmacologically driven research generally has much more non-commercial, scientific and social benefits (Heinrich *et al.*, 2014) and these should be at the centre of attention. Not discussed in this context are food supplements and other healthcare products, which are developed under very different frameworks, especially in poorly regulated markets. Here concerns continue both about the products' quality and the risks of non-sustainable, often short-term product cycles. This chapter has focused on the period since about 1992 and highlighted that industrial development offers unique opportunities for ethically based drug development. It also shows that major debates continue about the benefits of such an approach. Clearly, in the long run the development of new medicines that is conducted in a highly regulated environment offers some opportunities for achieving sustainable partnerships and for improving health care.

# Note

The development of new medicines has been an ongoing interest of mine and the ideas presented here have developed over many years. Some were discussed in more detail previously (especially in Heinrich, 2013; Heinrich and Teoh, 2004) and this work presents a new synthesis of these concepts.

# References

Amirkia, V. and Heinrich, M. (2015) Alkaloids as Drug leads: A predictive structural and biodiversity-BASED Analysis. *Phytochemistry Letters*, **10**, 48–53. dx.doi.org/10.1016/j.phytol. 2014.06.015.

Corson, T.W. and Crews, C.M. (2007) Molecular understanding and modern application of traditional medicines: Triumphs and trials. *Cell*, **130**, 769–774.

Cottreau, J., Tucker, A., Crutchley, R. and Garey, K.W. (2012) Crofelemer for the treatment of secretory diarrhea. *Expert Reviews in Gastroenterology and Hepatology*, **6**, 17–23.

Cox, P.A. (2001) Ensuring equitable benefits: The Falealupo covenant and the isolation of anti-viral drug prostratin from a Samoan medicinal plant. *Pharmaceutical Biology*, **39** (Suppl.), 32–40.

Cox, P.A. (2008) Biodiversity and the search for new medicines, in *Biodiversity Change and Human Health: from Ecosystem Services to Spread of Disease* (eds O.E. Sala, L.A. Meyerson and C. Parmesan), SCOPE Report No. 69, Island Press, Washington, DC.

Gabriel, S.E., Davenport, S.E., Steagall, R.J., *et al.* (1999) A novel plant-derived inhibitor of cAMP-mediated fluid and chloride secretion. *American Journal of Physiology*, **276**, G58–G63.

Green, A.C. and Beardmore, G.L. (1988) Home treatment of skin cancer and solar keratoses. *Australasian Journal of Dermatology*, **29**, 127–130.

Heinrich, M. (2010) Galanthamine from galanthus and other amaryllidaceae – chemistry and biology based on traditional use. *The Alkaloids*, **68**, 157–165.

Heinrich, M. (2013) Ethnopharmacology and drug discovery, in *Elsevier Reference Module in Chemistry, Molecular Sciences and Chemical Engineering* (ed. J. Reedijk), Elsevier, Waltham, MA. doi: 10.1016/ B978-0-12-409547-2.02773-6.

Heinrich, M. and Teoh, H.L. (2004) Galanthamine from snowdrop – the development of a modern drug against Alzheimer's disease from local Caucasian knowledge. *Journal of Ethnopharmacology*, **92**, 147–162.

Heinrich, M., Leonti, M. and Frei-Haller, B. (2014) A perspective on natural products research and ethnopharmacology in México. The eagle and the serpent on the prickly pear cactus. *Journal of Natural Products*, dx.doi.org/10.1021/np4009927.

Hsu, E. (2006) The history of *qing hao* – 青蒿 in the Chinese *Materia Medica*. *Transactions of the Royal Society of Tropical Medicine and Hygiene*, **100**, 505–508.

Hsu, E. (2010) Qing hao – 青蒿 (Herba *Artemisiae annuae*) in the Chinese *Materia Medica*, in *Plants, Health and Healing: On the Interface of Ethnobotany and Medical Anthropology* (eds E. Hsu and St Harris), Berghahn, Oxford/New York, pp. 83–120.

Isla, A. (2007) An ecofeminist perspective on biopiracy in Latin America. *Signs*, **32**, 323–332.

*Journal of Ethnopharmacology* (2014) Aims and Scope. http://www.journals.elsevier.com/journal-of -ethnopharmacology.

Lebwohl, M., Swanson, N., Anderson, L.L., *et al.* (2012) Ingenol mebutate gel for actinic keratosis. *New England Journal of Medicine*, **366**, 1010–1019.

Mgbeoji, I. (2006) *Global Biopiracy*, Univerzity of Britsh Columbia Press, Vancouver.

Ogbourne, S., Hampson, M.P., Lord, J.M., *et al.* (2007) Antitumor activity of 3-ingenyl angelate: plasma membrane and mitochondrial disruption and necrotic cell death. *Anticancer Drugs*, **18**, 357–362.

Posey, D.A. (2002a) Commodification of the sacred through intellectual property rights. *Journal of Ethnopharmacology*, **83**, 3–12.

Posey, D.A. (2002b) Kayapó ethnoecology and culture, in *Studies in Environmental Anthropology, Vol.* **6** (ed. K. Plenderleith), Routledge, London and New York.

Schmidt, B.M., Ribnicky, D.M., Lipsky, P.E. and Raskin, I. (2007) Revisiting the ancient concept of botanical therapeutics. *Natural Chemistry and Biology*, **3**, 360–366.

Secretariat of the Convention on Biological Diversity (2001) *Handbook of the Convention on Biological Diversity*, Earthscan, London.

Shiva, V. (2007) Bioprospecting as sophisticated biopiracy. *Signs*, **32**, 307–313.

Tradtrantip, L., Namkung, W. and Verkman, A.S. (2010) Crofelemer, an antisecretory antidiarrheal proanthocyanidin oligomer extracted from *Croton lechleri*, targets two distinct intestinal chloride channels. *Molecular Pharmacology*, **77**, 69–78.

Ubillas, R., Jolad, S.D., Bruening, R.C., *et al.* (1994) SP-303, an antiviral oligomeric proanthocyanidin from the latex of *Croton lechleri* (Sangre de Drago). *Phytomedicine*, **1**, 77–106.

Verpoorte, R. (2012) Good practices: The basis for evidence-based medicines. *Journal of Ethnopharmacology*, **140**, 455–457.

Weedon, D. and Chick, J. (1976) Home treatment of basal cell carcinoma. *Medical Journal of Australia*, **1**, 928.

Wells, W.A. (1998) Rainforest remedies. Shaman Pharmaceuticals, Inc. *Chemistry & Biology*, **5**, R63–R64.

# 9
# Ethnopharmacology and Intellectual Property Rights

Alan Hesketh

*Indigena Biodiversity Limited*

## 9.1 Introduction

Ethnopharmacological studies can often provide the scientific basis for the commercial use of natural products and so allow the considerable value of genetic resources to be realized (Heywood, 2011), but scientific information alone is not sufficient to ensure successful commercialization. Can IP, in the broadest sense, be used to maximize the commercial potential of natural products, including plant extracts?

IP is generally thought of in terms of patents, trademarks and copyright. But IP is broader than those categories. It would include, for example, traditional knowledge of indigenous communities, and other rights of ownership of genetic resources provided by the Convention on Biological Diversity (CBD, 1992). The CBD was the first international treaty to deal with ownership of genetic resources. Its three objectives are:

1. the conservation of biological diversity
2. the sustainable use of its components
3. the fair and equitable sharing of the benefits arising out of the utilization of genetic resources.

Thus, the CBD envisages the commercial use of natural products and creates ownership rights in genetic resources to facilitate that use. Those rights can then be supplemented by other forms of IP, such as patents.

Not everyone agrees with the advantages of IP (Goodman, 1993). Other chapters of this book highlight the mixed views about whether commercial benefit should be derived from natural products, and whether IP is an asset to the world economy or a mechanism that can

*Ethnopharmacology*, First Edition. Edited by Michael Heinrich and Anna K. Jäger.
© 2015 John Wiley & Sons, Ltd. Published 2015 by John Wiley & Sons, Ltd.

be misused to encourage biopiracy. Although the opposing views in that debate seem to be intractable, many of the perceived issues could be resolved, or at least tempered, by an improved dialogue and culture of partnership and transparency.

Industry, however, has not always been supportive. Some companies have taken adversarial positions with respect to the ownership rights of natural products by countries of origin of genetic resources to protect perceived threats to conventional practices. That builds up barriers to partnership.

On the other hand, IP rights, and patents in particular, are often mistrusted by indigenous peoples on the basis that they have been used to legitimize misappropriation of local resources. However, patent protection can be valued (Lagrost *et al.*, 2010). Developing countries could actually gain from the mechanisms recognized by the western world, such as IP, to realize economic value. The important point to realize is that whoever owns the IP, the exclusivity adds value to the genetic resources, so that all parties will benefit, including the country of origin and the indigenous communities.

## 9.2   Indigenous community rights and traditional knowledge

Genetic resources represent the property of stakeholders in the country in which they exist in the natural habitat. These stakeholders can include local individuals, indigenous communities, landowners and governments. The CBD recognizes that property right by establishing a right to access genetic resources and requiring benefit deriving from their use to be shared with the country of origin. The provisions of the CBD also extend to traditional knowledge. Article 8(j) requires countries to promote the use of traditional knowledge only with the approval and involvement of its owners, including indigenous communities, and to encourage equitable sharing of the benefits from its utilization.

The rights of ownership under the CBD are reinforced by the more recent Nagoya Protocol (CBD, 2010). The Nagoya Protocol on ABS was adopted on 29 October 2010 in Nagoya, Japan. Importantly, the Protocol contains compliance provisions; Article 15 puts an obligation on all ratifying countries to ensure that natural products used in that country have been correctly accessed and mutually agreed terms have been established.

The ownership rights provided by the CBD and the Nagoya protocol gives stakeholders in the country of origin of genetic resources the ability to capture the wealth of their genetic resources and traditional knowledge, and to retain control of their use. It is important for any ethnopharmacological study to respect those rights, to be aware of any appropriate legislation or administrative systems in place in the countries of origin and, most importantly, to work within the spirit and the intentions of the CBD.

So, the legal framework is in place. But there are still hurdles and difficulties that arise in the process. Some are illustrated by the much publicised Hoodia example (Wynberg, 2008).

Hoodia is a genus of flowering plant, endemic to Africa, that has been used by successive generations of the indigenous San peoples of the Namib desert to stave off hunger. During the 1990s, the South African-based CSIR investigated Hoodia extracts and identified the active ingredient, a steroidal glycoside, responsible for Hoodia's properties. CSIR filed a patent application in 1997 relating to the extract and the compound for use as an appetite suppressant. Patents subsequently granted around the world, including European patent 973534, following an appeal. The patents were licensed to a British company, Phytopharm, and subsequently sub-licensed to Pfizer and then to Unilever (Vermaak *et al.*, 2011).

When the agreement with Phytopharm was being negotiated, CSIR did obtain consent from government authorities, but failed to approach the San, who held the traditional knowledge about the properties of Hoodia. It was only in 2001, following media pressure, that CSIR began to negotiate with the San, and a satisfactory benefit-sharing agreement was concluded. The first issue arising from the Hoodia example then, is the need to ensure that the holders of local traditional knowledge are part of the consultation process whenever interest is expressed in the commercial development of a genetic resource.

The second issue is the identification of *all* possible holders of traditional knowledge. Although a benefit-sharing agreement was in place with the San, concern was expressed that there were other non-San groups, such as the Nama, Damara and Topnaar, who had historically occupied areas where Hoodia grows. This led to the negotiation of a further benefit-sharing agreement with a broader group of indigenous peoples, negotiated in conjunction with another local organization, the Working Group of Indigenous Minorities in Southern Africa (WIMSA).

A third issue related to the *scope* of the benefit-sharing agreements. In the Hoodia case, both Pfizer and Unilever eventually abandoned plans to market the product, but another benefit stream had emerged, namely the growing and sale of Hoodia as a raw material, without any extraction process. Because that activity was not covered by the patent, it fell outside the CSIR agreement. The San were able to negotiate a third benefit-sharing agreement, with the South African Hoodia Growers (SAHG) company.

Although all the issues arising from the Hoodia case were eventually resolved after a series of related negotiations, the example illustrates some of the hurdles that can arise that could have been tackled at the outset of the project. It is contended that many of these hurdles can be avoided by an effective international partnership. What does that entail?

## 9.3   Identifying a partner

The CBD is an international treaty. It contemplates genetic resources being transferred from the country of origin to another country for research and ultimate commercialization, and the benefits passing back to stakeholders in the original country to help sustain biodiversity. The question, then, is how those country stakeholders can take full advantage of the ownership rights. It is clear that local indigenous communities, or private individuals, cannot achieve the CBD benefits alone. There has to be some international collaboration. To whom do the locals turn?

The local government is one good starting point. Governments will be aware of the country's priorities in terms of biodiversity, as well as having foreign contacts. However, it may be argued that indigenous communities cannot always rely on their governments to protect their interests against foreign corporations and potential users of their genetic resources and traditional knowledge. The Hoodia example above illustrates that point; although CSIR had gained government consent to export and develop Hoodia, the government made no effort to draw that fact to the attention of the San peoples. Representatives of indigenous peoples have consistently argued that their own customary laws should be respected (Alexander *et al.*, 2009). Here again, the Nagoya Protocol is helpful. Article 12 requires countries to:

'take into consideration indigenous and local communities' customary laws, community protocols and procedures, as applicable, with respect to traditional knowledge associated with genetic resources'

Although local government contacts are useful, it is nevertheless advantageous for country stakeholders to also work with foreign partners, with the aim of commercializing local genetic resources, if they are to benefit from the opportunities provided by the CBD. Why? Because not only does that treaty encourage international access and commercial use of genetic resources and traditional knowledge, it *relies* on that mechanism to achieve its objectives. The country-of-origin stakeholders will gain if they can build a partnership of trust. The foreign partnership may be with a university, a foreign government agency, a botanical garden or directly with a commercial partner. In addition, Sampath has pointed to the advantages of intermediary organizations or firms who 'have a reputation to safeguard since, on the one hand, they will indulge in repeated transactions with drug firms and, on the other hand, with source countries' (Sampath, 2005).

In considering potential foreign partners, their attitude towards local customs and practices is an important factor to assess.

## 9.3.1   The foreign partner's attitude

If any collaboration is to succeed, there has to be a mutual respect for each partner's priorities. A foreign partner must take care to respect the cultural identity of indigenous peoples and to bring value to the communities without conflicting with the local culture, or with the continuance of traditional practices. A high priority should be given to understanding their social structure and traditions.

One of the key factors in an effective partnership is to strive for open and transparent dialogue between the parties. Foreign industrial companies that attempt to access local genetic resources are often accused of biopiracy. Some of the difficulties arise because of a mismatch of expectations and lack of experience with industry, but it is not difficult to communicate openly, to understand the structure of the communities and to build up a partnership of trust and dialogue. It is helpful to provide clear explanations of how equitable benefit, deriving from the use of genetic resources, will flow back to countries of origin. Taking time to share objectives can often allay fears of biopiracy.

Part of the dialogue should be to manage expectations; not all discoveries and traditional knowledge will be susceptible to successful global commercialization, and financial returns from a commercial venture are not always predictable. It is important to be transparent about the process of selection and, for those projects that are progressed, to be realistic in estimates of the potential return.

## 9.3.2   The advantages of IP

A partnership has to be looked at from both sides. The collaboration will only work if local stakeholders, especially indigenous communities, also recognize the value that western commercial interests can add to their ownership rights of genetic resources. Nevertheless, licensing to global industry is a competitive business enterprise. Yes, industry is always seeking new opportunities to progress, but companies select only those which have the best potential to make good sales; company licensing executives are experienced in being able to select development candidates that have promise and a good probability of being successfully developed into a commercial product. That will usually mean that they look for some sort of exclusive position, such as IP rights.

Country stakeholders owning the genetic resources will increase the chances of successful commercialization if, together with their partner, they create an IP package that is attractive to industry.

# 9.4   Hurdles in considering IP

There is often a culture of resistance to patent rights in developing countries. Many indigenous communities believe that 'all knowledge and resources come from God, and hence cannot be owned by anyone' (Swiderska, 2006).

An objective of a close working relationship with local communities is to be able to point to the fact that their own rights to the genetic resources and traditional knowledge ensures that a product cannot be commercialized without their permission. A patent merely complements those rights to provide a stronger overall IP package. Patent protection – even owned by other parties – is in their interests. It will increase the global sales of any commercialization, and a portion of that increased revenue will flow back to the country and local communities.

So resistance can sometimes be weakened. Interestingly, the Hoodia example sheds light on this dilemma. The San, like many indigenous peoples, held the view described above that life cannot be patented. However, instead of challenging the CSIR patent they 'unashamedly chose the path of self-interest' (Chennells, 2003) and relied on the patent rights to earn benefit.

Even if the inherent resistance to patenting is overcome, there is the question of cost. Patenting is an expensive process. It is certainly a solid investment to help secure and enhance future income, but how can indigenous communities, or individuals, who make an invention in the country of origin find the investment to start the patenting process there? This is again when the right foreign partner can help. A business-minded partner, including some intermediary firms, may be willing to invest in the early stages of the patenting process in exchange for some percentage of future royalties if the product is successful.

Alternatively, if the foreign partner is a university or other research institute, further research may identify inventions that can be patented, starting in that country. In that case, the research partner would normally handle the patenting.

Patenting may not always be possible, for example if the intended commercial use of the genetic resource is fully contemplated by existing local traditional knowledge. In that case, a partner or intermediary may be able to invest in the legal protection of the rights provided by the CBD. The present author believes that legal agreements to authorize commercialization provide the most effective mechanism to protect ownership rights and traditional knowledge, secure their value and translate those rights into benefits for indigenous peoples. A legal agreement merely enshrines the ownership rights of a community in an enforceable instrument. Such agreements can be used as a means to participate in the international marketplace, they provide protection by legally defining authorized uses and they give a community the right to control use of its traditional knowledge. Exclusive agreements in particular will be more attractive to potential users and so increase their likelihood of gaining benefits. A legal contract is a means to capture the benefit-sharing rights which indigenous communities have under the CBD.

# 9.5   Building an effective IP portfolio

If the premise above is accepted, that IP rights greatly enhance the likelihood of successful licensing and therefore of realizing the commercial benefit from genetic resources, then it is important to realize that the competitive advantage is even greater if a professionally crafted, strong IP portfolio is constructed. To that end, it is worthwhile considering some of the subject matter that can be patented and the level of protection each affords. The objective is to maximize the value of the IP portfolio to best satisfy the needs of industry.

### 9.5.1   Requirements for patentability

There are three general requirements, common to most countries, for a patent to be granted. The invention must be:

- novel
- non-obvious
- useful.

The novelty requirement is universal, i.e. a disclosure in any one country destroys novelty worldwide. The disclosure may be any written or verbal material that becomes available to the public. Thus, as well as published literature, any verbal communication of an invention to a person not under an obligation of confidence will prevent a valid patent being granted on that invention. (Proof of such verbal disclosure can be provided by written evidence or testimony.) All the relevant disclosures that occur before the filing of a patent application are known collectively as 'prior art'.

Obviousness is a more subjective test. An assessment has to be made as to whether the alleged invention would be obvious to a person of average skill in the particular technical field, in the light of all relevant 'prior art'. That assessment is made by the national Patent Office or, subsequently, by national courts.

Usefulness, sometimes referred to as utility, means that a patented invention must have commercial applicability. Everything encompassed within the scope of the patent must achieve the results that the inventor promises.

### 9.5.2   The value of different types of patent protection

A patent can be obtained for anything that is an invention, as long as it complies with the requirements of novelty, non-obviousness and utility. Inventions can arise in a broad range of technical fields, such as mechanical, electrical, electronic, chemical, biotechnological etc. For research derived from ethnopharmacology, we are likely to see inventions in the field of chemistry. As well as reviewing whether subject matter is patentable, it is also important to consider how valuable the patent would be as part of a commercial portfolio. Typical subjects which can be considered for patenting in this field include the following:

(Note that the views expressed here are those of the present author, and are presented as general guidelines. The value of a particular patent is always dependent on the facts in that case.)

- *A chemical compound isolated from a plant or animal source*
    If research on a natural resource allows the chemical structure of an active ingredient to be identified, patenting the chemical compound provides the strongest form of protection because a molecular formula allows a very specific definition of the scope of the patent. That helps in clarifying both novelty – and hence obtaining a valid patent – and infringement, i.e. defining a clear boundary of what a patentee can prevent others from doing. Chemical compound patents provide a solid basis for potential licensing. The pharmaceutical industry, for example, relies heavily on patents relating to chemical compounds.
- *An extract from a natural source*
    This would include, for example, an aqueous extract or an alcoholic extract of a plant material, providing its properties are not obvious over the *known* properties of the plant. Such a patent is not as valuable as a compound patent, as it would not prevent someone from finding and using a different type of extract that could avoid the patent.

Also, consistency of the extract is important because the utility requirements for a patent are only satisfied if every extract as defined in the patent exhibits the promised activity. Nevertheless, if both of those issues are kept in mind when framing the scope of the patent, an extract can still provide the basis for a reasonable level of IP protection.

- *An extraction process*

  It is also possible to obtain a patent on an extraction process (as distinct from the extract *per se*, as mentioned above). However, a process patent can usually be avoided because of the likelihood of an alternative, non-infringing, process being devised. Thus, although there could be exceptional cases, in general an extraction process is unlikely to provide significant value in an IP portfolio.

- *A newly discovered use*

  It is possible to patent a new use of a plant, chemical compound or extract. Use patents can often provide valuable protection, even when the compound is known. The use must be previously undisclosed and not predictable from known uses of the compound or the plant from which it is derived. Use protection can often provide a broad protection, as the patent would prevent competitors from marketing a product identified for that use. One drawback, however, is that if the product is approved and on the market for other uses, the new use patent cannot prevent sale of the compound (or extract) indicated for those other uses. Customers/patients could then use the product for the patented utility. This is known in the pharmaceutical industry as 'off-label use'.

- *Formulations/compositions*

  Formulation patents vary considerably in their value. A very specific formulation containing ranges of ingredients is certainly patentable, but the patent is often too narrow to prevent competitors finding an alternative formulation and so avoiding your patent. On the other hand, there can be considerable value in a broad composition patent written in the form 'A composition comprising compound X'. Compound X may be known and the invention is based on the finding of the first use for that compound. Such a patent is probably second only to a compound patent in providing valuable protection for a commercial product.

- *Synergistic combinations*

  If two substances are combined, and the combination demonstrates properties that are advantageous compared to the two components used separately, then that combination may be patentable, even if the two components are known. In the natural product field, for example, a substance could be added to a natural product extract to enhance its effectiveness in some way. This type of patent is again close to a compound patent in terms of its effectiveness. A synergistic combination patent provides a valuable asset in a patent portfolio.

- *Chemical synthesis*

  As with the extraction processes mentioned above, a chemical process patent provides only limited protection for a commercial product as the patent can be circumvented if an alternative process is devised. However, process patents should not be ignored as part of an IP portfolio. If a process patent protects a commercially attractive synthesis, it can provide a competitive advantage over other, perhaps less efficient, production methods.

## 9.6  The patentability of products of nature

As mentioned above, obtaining a patent requires the subject matter to be both novel and inventive (i.e. not obvious). How do we deal with these concepts in terms of materials that already occur in nature? Suppose we have a chemical compound that is isolated from a plant source. To be patentable, the compound must be novel. How can something that exists naturally be novel?

## 9.6.1   Novelty

In Europe, and in most other developed countries, the situation is clear. A compound (or gene sequence) that is isolated from a natural source can be patentable, even if the structure is identical to that found in nature. The justification is that isolation and purification are 'techniques which human beings alone are capable of putting into practice and which nature is incapable of accomplishing itself' (European Guidelines, 2013).

One major exception to that principle is the situation in the USA. Although the USA has also, in the past, followed the principle that a compound isolated from nature can be patentable, that changed in 2013, when the US Supreme Court issued a decision in the Myriad case (Supreme Court, 2013) which held that a naturally occurring DNA segment is a product of nature and not patent eligible, even when isolated from its source. Since then, in March 2014, the US Patent Office issued a set of guidelines (US Patent Office Guidelines, 2014) which apply the facts of the Myriad case to all natural products. There is some controversy as to whether the US patent office has extended the principles of the Myriad decision beyond what the Supreme Court intended and it is still unclear exactly where the new boundary for patentability lies. The guidelines state that a patent must claim 'something significantly different' from the substance as found in nature. What does that mean? US patent attorneys say that the scope of what is patentable in this area will only become clear over years as case law develops as a result of litigation. A structurally different derivative of the natural product would certainly qualify. Furthermore, the guidelines suggest that if the invention comprises an additional non-natural ingredient or process step, which is not conventional or routine and amounts to a practical application of the natural product, then that could confer patentability. Overall, we should be aware that, although compounds isolated from nature are no longer patentable *per se* in the USA, there are options for protecting inventions made in the natural products field.

## 9.6.2   Novelty and traditional knowledge

Does traditional knowledge form part of the prior art over which a patent must be novel? In the patent laws of most countries, the concept of novelty is universal; that is, wherever knowledge is available to the public, and not secret, even in some remote corner of the world, that destroys novelty in all countries. It could be argued that if the knowledge is confined within a community then it is not known to the general public. However, it would be rare for a community to be able to implement sufficient safeguards to ensure that confidentiality is reliably retained. If our aim is to achieve valid and enforceable patents, a far better strategy is to accept that traditional knowledge is part of the information base over which our research results must be inventive. That does not exclude the ability to patent the achievements of research, but it is an issue that has to be taken into account when building a commercially valuable patent portfolio.

## 9.6.3   Obviousness

Novelty, however, is only the first hurdle. The question of obviousness also has to be considered. If we were investigating a plant material about which there is no existing knowledge in the public domain, then any use or activity we discover as a basis for a patent would not be obvious. However, in the field of ethnopharmacology, that is rarely the factual situation. The whole point of the type of investigations we are considering here is that they are based on local knowledge, which drives the course of research. For example, an extract of a plant that exhibits the same medicinal properties as those known locally in the country of origin will not provide a subject for patenting. However. the whole point of carrying out research is to find new discoveries, even if the direction of research was initially driven by local knowledge. Research, by its very nature, often leads to unexpected results. It is the application of those results which must be compared with the original starting point in order to assess patentability. For example, identification and isolation of a compound, or a specific fraction, can often remove the toxicity of other components of the natural product or lead to a more potent formulation. Alternatively, a new use could be identified that would not be suggested by previously known facts.

It may be that the local knowledge held in the country of origin is not always fully made available to researchers investigating a natural product. The above discussion demonstrates the importance for any researcher to make every effort to investigate all local knowledge before research is commenced, if commercialization – and therefore patent protection – is a factor in the project.

The issues of novelty and obviousness can provide a challenge when considering patentability for the outcome of ethnopharmacological research on natural products. However, with knowledge of the hurdles and good advice from patent experts, valuable patents can be achieved. The rich and unique opportunities with which nature provides us make the efforts worthwhile.

## 9.7 Conclusion

The CBD was established to tackle the issue of the world's loss of biodiversity by encouraging the commercial use of genetic resources. Ethnopharmacological studies can help to achieve success by that mechanism, although there are hurdles to overcome. An effective international partnership is essential and the creation of a strong IP portfolio can assist all parties in turning the CBD objectives into reality.

## References

Alexander, M., Hardison, P. and Ahren, M. (2009) *Study on compliance in relation to the customary law of indigenous and local communities, national law, across jurisdictions, and international law*, Document UNEP/CBD/WG-ABS/7/INF/5, Secretariat of the Convention on Biological Diversity, Montreal, https://www.cbd.int/doc/meetings/abs/abswg-09/information/abswg-09-abswg-07-inf-05-en.pdf.

CBD (1992) Text of the Convention on Biological Diversity, Secretariat of the Convention on Biological Diversity, Montreal, http://www.cbd.int/convention/text/default.shtml

CBD (2010) Text of the Nagoya Protocol, Secretariat of the Convention on Biological Diversity, Montreal, http://www.cbd.int/abs/text/default.shtml.

Chennells, R. (2003) *Ethics and practice in ethnobiology, and prior informed consent with indigenous peoples regarding genetic resources*, Paper presented at a conference on Biodiversity, Biotechnology and the Protection of Traditional Knowledge, St Louis 4–6 April 2003, https://law.wustl.edu/centeris/Papers/Biodiversity/PDFWrdDoc/ChennelFinalApril2003.pdf.

European Guidelines (2013) *Guidelines for Examination in the European Patent Office, September 2013*, Part G, Chapter II, page 16, http://www.epo.org/law-practice/legal-texts/guidelines.html.

Goodman, K. (1993) Intellectual property and control. *Academic Medicine*, **68** (9 Suppl), S88–S91.

Heywood, V. (2011) Ethnopharmacology, food production, nutrition and biodiversity conservation: Towards a sustainable future for indigenous peoples. *Journal of Ethnopharmacology*, **137** (1), 1–15.

Lagrost, C., Martin, D. Dubois, C. and Quazzotti, S. (2010) Intellectual property valuation: how to approach the selection of an appropriate valuation method. *Journal of Intellectual Capital*, **11** (4), 481–503.

Sampath, P.G. (2005) *Regulating Bioprospecting*, United Nations University Press, pp. 76–77.

Supreme Court (2013) Supreme Court Decision in Association for Molecular Pathology v. Myriad Genetics, Inc., US Supreme Court Decision case number 12-398, 13 June 2103, http://www.supremecourt.gov/opinions/12pdf/12-398_1b7d.pdf.

Swiderska, K. (2006) *Banishing the Biopirates: A new approach to Protecting Traditional Knowledge*, Gatekeeper Series 129, International Institute for Environment and Development, London, http://pubs.iied.org/pdfs/14537IIED.pdf.

US Patent Office Guidelines (2014) *Procedure for subject matter eligibility analysis of claims reciting or involving laws of nature, natural principles, natural phenomena, and/or natural products*, US Patent Office 4 March 2014, http://www.uspto.gov/patents/law/exam/myriad-mayo_guidance.pdf.

Vermaak, I., Hamman, J.H. and Viljoen, A.M. (2011) *Hoodia gordonii*: an up-to-date review of a commercially important anti-obesity plant. *Planta Medica*, **77**, 1149–1160.

Wynberg, R. (2008) *Access and Benefit-Sharing in Practice: Trends in Partnerships across Sectors*, Technical Series No. 38, Secretariat of the Convention on Biological Diversity, pp. 83–98.

# 10

# Ethnopharmacology in Elementary, Primary and Secondary Education: Current Perspectives and Future Prospects

Alonso Verde[1,5], Diego Rivera[2], José Ramón Vallejo[5], José Fajardo[4], Concepción Obón[3] and Arturo Valdés[4]

[1]Instituto Los Olmos, Albacete, Spain
[2]Depto. Biología Vegetal, Fac. Biología, Universidad de Murcia, Spain
[3]Depto. de Biología Aplicada, Escuela Politécnica Superior de Orihuela, Universidad Miguel Hernández, Orihuela, Alicante, Spain
[4]Instituto Botánico, Jardín Botánico de Castilla La Mancha, Albacete, Spain
[5]Depto. de Terapéutica Médico-Quirúrgica, Fac. de Medicina, Universidad de Extremadura, Badajoz, and Depto de Biología y Geología, Colegio Santa María Assumpta, Badajoz, Spain

## 10.1   Introduction

The concept of ethnopharmacology covers two distinct but closely interwoven aspects: *uses* and *knowledge*. These aspects appear to be part of the same thing but this is not the case. Uses are a matter of fact that can be documented through observation and respond to both traditional knowledge and recent short-term external factors. Traditional knowledge, on the other hand, may be fully operational or simply appear as a vague memory of a more or less happy past (Rivera and Obón, 1998). This distinction is particularly pertinent in an educational context because it is essential but not easy to determine what is substantial and what is merely accidental.

Traditional knowledge (TK), as far as it is related to biodiversity, merges both culture and nature, thus becoming part of natural and cultural heritage (Pardo de Santayana and Gómez, 2003). It represents a part of the intangible heritage that is not written in books, but

*Ethnopharmacology*, First Edition. Edited by Michael Heinrich and Anna K. Jäger.
© 2015 John Wiley & Sons, Ltd. Published 2015 by John Wiley & Sons, Ltd.

instead is in the collective memory of the community, orally transmitted from generation to generation (Fajardo *et al.*, 2008). Each TK system in its ethnobiological facet is local and unique. It aims to solve problems affecting the local community, although some are largely common to humankind. Each local community has its own way of adapting to its environment, and operating and managing its local resources, which is reflected cultural heritage linked to biodiversity and is of great importance and should be preserved (Pardo de Santayana *et al.*, 2012; Morales *et al.*, 2011).

At the beginning of the 21st century European rural populations are undergoing both erosion and loss of TK as a result of the disappearance of oral transmission systems of such knowledge, which in turn is linked to dramatic changes in lifestyles (Quave *et al.*, 2012). Technological progress, together with the abandonment of rural life over the past 50 years in Europe, has been beneficial for urban societies but nevertheless has brought about a process of transculturation. This has resulted in a sharp decline in rural customs and practices, and in the loss of the knowledge which is part of European (and any other) cultural and natural heritage. Currently, the direct transmission and the skills related to the traditional knowledge system (TKS), which for centuries were based on oral transmission and experience, are broken (Fajardo *et al.*, 2008; Verde *et al.*, 2009, 2010). This presents a challenge for different societies globally and for European ones specifically, which undoubtedly must react to the erosion and loss of this local knowledge. This knowledge, eminently practical, ecological and local, is condemned to immediate disappearance if not transmitted in an appropriate manner to the next generation. The transmission failure would entail an irreparable loss of biocultural diversity and potential resources to address new challenges, such as those derived from global change, mass migration and the emergence of resistance to current drugs.

At this point, it is important to remember that from the biomedical point of view, which is widely adopted in North America, Europe and some other countries as the healthcare model, knowledge and practices recorded in the context of ethnopharmacology are considered marginal. However, reality has set in, forcing western countries to create a new concept of alternative and complementary medicines, which can fit, even in the European urban world, the TK that we discussed earlier. This is part of what the European Medicines Agency named traditional herbal medicinal products (THMP), whose use is well-established in European markets (EMA, 2013), but, of course, only a part!

No doubt part of this knowledge already is no longer useful for our urban society, but some is practical, including the use as drugs of biological (plants, animals and fungi) and non-biological (minerals) materials, which are part of what is called traditional medicine and local popular medicine. Hence the responsibility to locally transmit those that are local knowledge systems and to globally transmit those that are global traditions.

While self-medication might not be widely promoted, it should be recognised that herbal medicines are more sustainable and less expensive than other pharmaceuticals. To provide access to these local resources as a complement to standard drugs that the official healthcare system makes available to citizens is in itself interesting from the point of view of sustainability and the conservation of TK, as well as improving overall community health status. Experiences in Latin America show the possibilities for the coexistence of both standard drugs and traditional medicines (Mignone *et al.*, 2007; Vanderbroek, 2013). In addition, there are complex links between the knowledge and use of medicinal plants and the concomitant use of pharmaceuticals (Giovannini *et al.*, 2011).

Information from global media such as TV, radio and the internet gives people a new way of treating certain diseases, especially chronic diseases and those involved in ageing

(Leonti and Casu, 2013). The need therefore arises to critically confront this torrent of information with directly transmitted (word and experience) practical knowledge. How can this be achieved? Which mechanism or transmission belt can replace the system of TK? Educational, humanitarian, social and healthcare NGOs who develop specific tasks in this regard can help to do this (Verde and Fajardo, 2014).

## 10.2  Ethnopharmacology: a multidisciplinary subject for education

Recent efforts to incorporate general ethnobiology and ethnobotany in the curriculum in higher levels of education have succeeded, most notably in graduate and postgraduate courses in European and American universities (Bennett, 2005; Rivera, 2008). However, ethnobotany has not yet been introduced at elementary and secondary levels (McClatchey and Bridges, 2014; OSN, 2014). It is worth highlighting the work developed in Ireland, where in the late 1930s the new Republic initiated a series of activities for school children to 'interview' their families. Fionna Shannon (Centre for Pharmacognosy and Phytotherapy, UCL School of Pharmacy, London) is working on the review of the formularies recorded during this period with a focus on medicinal plant uses. Between 1935 and 1970 the Irish Folklore Commission compiled information on diverse aspects of Irish TK, including 'folk medicine' (Briody, 2007). These data have been used also for dissemination books (see Allen and Hatfield, 2012).

However, different experiences occurred in different countries, and have been developed on the initiative of individual teachers and under very different approaches, for example education for health, environmental education, education for diversity, etc. (Verde *et al.*, 2004a, 2005; Vilá, 2014). This work was often linked to research projects within a framework of collaboration between universities and centres of secondary education (Verde and Fajardo, 2002, 2003a,2003b; Vallejo *et al.*, 2007; Valdés *et al.*, 2008; Pérez *et al.*, 2009) and in most cases was considered a transversal subject (Verde *et al.*, 2005, 2009). Occasionally these initiatives were part of international projects financially supported by the European Commission, for example the Local Food: Nutraceuticals in the 5th Framework Program (Verde *et al.*, 2004b). They often had the aim of raising awareness and bringing students into direct contact with their natural environment, and of showing the curricular, educational and behavioural benefits, for students and teachers, who may have to learn and teach through the world of plants from a different perspective outside the classroom (Blair, 2009; Ahmed *et al.*, 2011; Laaksoharj *et al.*, 2012; Ruíz-Gallardo *et al.*, 2013). These experiments were carried out primarily in urban areas, where the majority of the European population resides, and in the context of strong transculturation of younger European generations.

The need to recover and transmit traditional practical knowledge of medicinal plant uses (see above) leads one to ask what contents and subjects should be incorporated and taught at different educational levels (Table 10.1). Ethnopharmacology is a multidisciplinary form of learning about TK and biosciences (Etkin, 2001; Heinrich *et al.*, 2006; Reyes-Garcia, 2010), therefore it is possible to incorporate concepts ranging from chemistry (composition and characteristics of the active principles) to social sciences (history of medicinal plants) and biology (description and identification of the botanical or zoological species of medicinal use) and health. Furthermore, the possibilities for incorporating this discipline in the curriculum of formal education are extremely broad and range from local food, health and botany to chemistry, history and literature (Verde *et al*, 2004b; 2010).

**Table 10.1**  Proposal for basic knowledge and skills content (Figure 10.1) in the field of ethnopharmacology adjusted to different educational levels.

| Course objectives | Overlapping disciplines | Pre-primary and primary | Lower and upper secondary | Post-secondary vocational (health) | Tertiary (undergraduate/ graduate) |
|---|---|---|---|---|---|
| **Knowledge** | | | | | |
| Concept of ethnopharmacology | Ethnobiology, phytotherapy | – | Be | Be/m | Bm/d |
| History of medicinal plant (and other natural products) drug use | History, history of medicine and pharmacy | Te | Te | Be/m | Bm/d |
| Medicinal plants in different cultures | History, social | Te | Te | Be/m | Bm/d |
| Plant-based drugs in biomedicine | Pharmacognosy, pharmacology, pharmaceutical technology | – | Te | Bm/d | Bm/d |
| Systems of traditional knowledge | Anthropology, ethnobotany, social | Te | Te | Be/m | Bm/d |
| Systems of traditional medicine | Medical anthropology, ethnobotany, social | – | Te | Be/m | Bm/d |
| Ethical issues of plant drugs development and use | Bioethics, biology, social | – | Te | Be/m | Bm/d |
| **Skills** | | | | | |
| Field and laboratory methods | Biology, laboratory | Te | Te | Bm/d | Bm/d |
| Identification of medicinal plants (and other natural products) | Botany, science, technics, zoology | Te | Te | Bm/d | Bm/d |
| Recognition of local toxic plants and poisonous mushrooms and animals | Botany, science, zoology | Te | Te | Bm/d | Bm/d |
| Local food production and consumption within the framework of the Mediterranean diet | Food science and technology, nutrition, science, social | Te | Te | Bm/d | Bm/d |
| Traditional methods of collecting, processing and conserving medicinal plants | Biology, science, technics, pharmaceutical technology | Te | Te | Bm/d | Bm/d |
| Rational use of natural medicines | Biology, patient safety, social | Te | Te | Bm/d | Bm/d |
| Legal framework for ethnopharmacology | Pharmaceutical legislation, social | – | – | Bm/d | Bm/d |
| Applications to non-humans (veterinary, farming) | Chemotherapeutics, technics, veterinary | – | Te | Bm/d | Bm/d |

B, basic; d, deep; e, elementary; m, middle; T, transversal.

Ethnopharmacology courses are taught at various European and American universities (Gillespie, 1995; UIO, 2014) with a value of three to ten credits and including specific subjects such as:

- the concept and history of ethnopharmacology
- plant-based drugs used in western medicine that originated in traditional medicine
- professional and non-professional traditional medicine
- traditional healers and ethnic pharmacopoeias
- theories about chemical ecology
- human diets
- field and laboratory methods as well as ethical issues and IP rights
- medicinal plant conservation
- transculturation
- medicinal plants, natural products and their pharmacological effects.

Courses are usually part of biological and health education programmes, but are open to any students with adequate academic backgrounds. A general prerequisite or recommendation for attending ethnopharmacology graduate and undergraduate courses is a basic knowledge of botany, pharmacognosy and pharmaceutical chemistry.

## 10.3 Developing an ethnopharmacological curriculum: some strategies

Ethnopharmacology is a useful tool to assist students at different levels in a comprehensive training process, and can be incorporated in the curriculum using basic (unidisciplinary, interdisciplinary) or transversal approaches, as shown in the experience of developing such a curriculum in Spain (Table 10.1; Gillespie, 1995; Bennet, 2005; Vallejo *et al.*, 2006; Rivera, 2008; Valdés *et al.*, 2008; Pérez *et al.*, 2009; Verde *et al.*, 2009, 2010; González, 2014).

Educational programmes in Europe are structured into different levels (Eurostat, 2014a) according to International Standard Classification of Education (ISCED) fields and student age (UNESCO, 2014):

- Levels 0 and 1: Pre-primary and primary education for children aged 3–12 years.
- Levels 2 and 3: Lower and upper secondary education. The entrance age is 13 years and typical duration varies from 5 to 6 years.
- Level 4: Post-secondary non-tertiary/vocational education, which includes 16–20-year-old students. This broadens the knowledge of ISCED Level 3 graduates or prepares students for direct entry into the labour market.
- Levels 5 and 6: First and second stages of tertiary education, provided by universities and other higher education institutions to students aged usually over 18.

A key objective of all educational systems is to equip students with a wide range of skills and competences. This encompasses not only basic skills such as reading and mathematics, but also more transversal skills such as information and communications technology, entrepreneurship (Eurostat, 2014b) and health education (Verde *et al.*, 2010). This transversal set of skills and competences is acquired in different subjects, primarily focusing on basic skills. The degree of breadth, depth and detail in which the matter is addressed either in transversal or basic form at the different educational levels, leads to a distinction into elementary, intermediate and deep learning.

In countries such as Spain different educational reforms (LOGSE, 1990; LOCE, 2002; LOE, 2006; LOMCE, 2014) have not included changes to the curriculum to generate learning based on functional competencies. Thus, skills are mostly acquired outside the educational system. However, within secondary education an optional course of applied botany was developed (administrative resolution from 25 May 1994) that focuses on teaching–learning processes based on the study of economic plants and the relationships between humankind and plant communities. The contents includes biodiversity and numerous plants uses, such as industrial, food, construction and ornamental, medicine and pharmacy, and plant crops.

Currently the legislation in force, due to ideological, political and technical issues, has not left space for the specific development of ethnopharmacology in pre-primary, primary or secondary education as a basic subject. However, incorporating such a topic is possible through natural sciences such as biology and chemistry in primary, secondary and post-secondary education (including vocational). A great handicap for the implementation of ethnopharmacological contents within these subjects may be the already overloaded curriculum (Coll, 2007), the inappropriate distribution of schedules and the irrational assignation of relative relevance for different subjects. Each year teachers should consider only a selected repertory of contents and how to implement them, taking into account the differences between the official curriculum proposal and its translation into the classroom, and contrasted with other aspects such as the curriculum learned and the skills acquired by students (Duschl and Hamilton, 1992).

A very promising strategy to connect with local TK would be to work from the context of the students, from their own experience and thoughts, so that they can take positions on their ethnobiological or ethnopharmacological heritage. It is possible to introduce ethnopharmacology in educational institutions through specific projects leading students to collect local remedies of popular medicine starting from a conceptual framework proposed by the teacher (Vallejo *et al.*, 2006). With such an approach, starting from objectives and ethnobiological methods, students can interview their families and people in their social environment as part of an investigation involving different areas. From the educational point of view, the process should be inspired by scientific models that focus on the following points: defining and enclosing a problem, designing a research project, bibliographical documentation and analysis, field work and elaboration of conclusions (Vallejo, 2004). Ethnopharmacological topics are a resource for learning scientific methods, including problem solving, and developing values around the ethnobiological knowledge. They are also an excellent tool in large cross-curricular subjects such as environmental education, health education, consumer education and moral and civic education.

Teachers may consider methodological aspects, such as using taxonomy of skills to organize the goals of ethnopharmacology, a strategy for properly structuring the contents and putting special emphasis on students' existing ideas about cultural biodiversity (Figure 10.1). An example of these ideas might be 'all natural things are good and safe'. Teachers should encourage cognitive conflict so that the student critically appraises this belief. This would help to build coherent knowledge schemes, integrating health, environment and tradition, from the experience of the student. Thus, it will lead to an appropriate behavioural change. The students' ideas come from their interaction with the social and natural environment, and academia. The main characteristics of students' preconceptions are their stability over time, their relative internal consistency and their generalization in the student group, hence they have great influence on the teaching and learning process. The students' psycho-evolutionary period following taxonomies and some models of Piaget and Ausubel, such as Bloom's taxonomy for the cognitive domain (Carr *et al.*, 1994), should be taken into account.

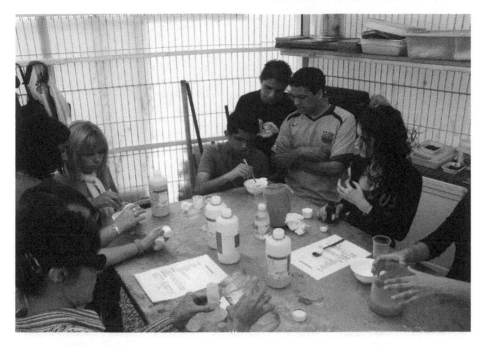

**Figure 10.1** Secondary education students developing skills using traditional methods in the greenhouse at Los Olmos High School, Albacete, Spain (image: A. Verde).

Another more ambitious and effective way to introduce ethnopharmacology is through specific school cross-curricular projects (PCC, proyecto curricular de centro). In Spain the PCC is the annual programme for every school where each centre can incorporate specific contents in the curriculum in an autonomous way, as a core idea (ITE, 2104). As ethnopharmacology covers contents ranging from chemistry to the history of medicinal animals and plants, and is based on tradition and cultural heritage, it lends itself to cross-curricular teaching (Verde *et al.*, 2010; González, 2014). Thus subjects as different as science, social science, biology, physics, chemistry, history, language and literature, and even others could be involved in a common project. The consensus of the whole educational community (teachers, parents, students and educational authorities) is fundamental in this issue, as it involves not only teaching staff and students, but also families. This consensus is largely dependent on the existence of a good leadership and the cooperation of all those involved. The curriculum needs to be organized from a philosophical and educational point of view that analyses local knowledge as a joint platform for teaching and learning scientific and humanistic education. The difficulties for implementing this proposal reside in the leadership of more motivated staff, their training and research capacity, as well as the development of curricular materials that enable the integration of the contents (Verde and Fajardo, 2003b; Verde *et al.*, 2004b). An easier alternative to this proposal is the organization of cultural weeks or specific science fair days focusing on ethnopharmacology, which could include different activities and could spread outside the school (Figure 10.2).

Secondary vocational education and training offer opportunities for ethnopharmacology-related activities. Work-based learning, notably apprenticeship and other models, helps to facilitate the transition from learning to work. This requires a clear regulatory framework defined by the educational authorities at the different levels (local, national and European), which

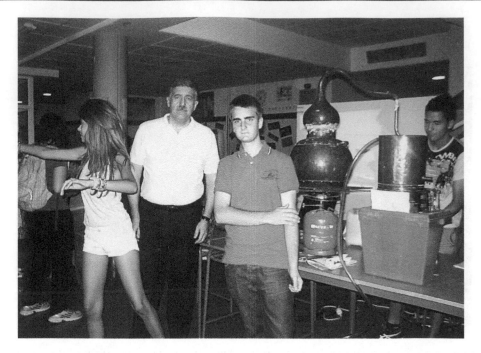

**Figure 10.2**   Secondary education students using traditional essential oil distillation facilities at the science fair at Los Olmos High School, Albacete, Spain (image: A. Verde).

clarify the roles for the different players and must be an integral part of the entire education system, focusing here on health and health-science related vocations (European Commission, 2012).

## 10.4   Conclusions

Currently there is a lack of space for the development of ethnopharmacology in pre-primary, primary or secondary education as a specific subject. However, it is possible to find options for learning ethnopharmacological knowledge, competences and skills using different interdisciplinary and transversal approaches, as is demonstrated by numerous experiences in this field. This chapter highlights the importance of working from the context of the student and, more ambitiously, through school cross-curricular projects, a unique Spanish legal framework.

The benefits of such an interdisciplinary ethnopharmacological approach in the various curricula of pre-primary, primary and secondary education include:

- *social benefits* like the active promotion of the link between generations, the reduction of excess local demand for health services, adding value to local products (e.g. the Mediterranean diet), promoting healthy life styles and promoting responsible medication use
- *cultural benefits*, including the maintenance and promotion of traditions and the local knowledge system, improved knowledge about local biodiversity, knowledge and appreciation of local natural resources
- *educational benefits* like learning about interdisciplinary cooperation of the various stakeholders (teachers, students, families) and facilitating the learning of other subjects.

Local communities could appreciate and add value to their TK as an essential part of their identities. In addition, teachers will have a great tool available that will facilitate interdisciplinary work and, finally, health authorities could promote the rational use of traditional herbal medicines as a less expensive way to assist health care in developing and developed societies.

# References

Ahmed, A.T., Oshiro, C.E., Loharuka, S. and Novotny, R. (2011) Perceptions of middle school educators in Hawai'I about school-based gardening and child health. *Hawaii Medical Journal*, **70**, 11–15.

Allen, D. and Hatfield, G. (2012) *Medicinal Plants in Folk Tradition: An ethnobotany of Britain and Ireland*. Timber Press.

Bennett, B.C. (2005) Ethnobotany Education, Opportunities, and Needs in the US. *Ethnobotanical Research Applications*, **3**, 113–121.

Blair, D. (2009) The child in the garden: An evaluative review of the benefits of school gardening. *Journal of Environmental Education*, **40**, 15–38.

Briody, M. (2007) *Irish Folklore Commission 1935–1970: History, Ideology, Methodology*. Gazelle Book Services.

Carr, M., Barker, M., Bell, B., *et al.* (1994) The Constructivist Paradigm and Some Implications for Science Content and Pedagogy, in *The Content of Science* (eds P. Fensham, R. Gunstone and R. White), The Farmer Press, London, pp. 147–159.

Coll, C. (2007) Una encrucijada para la educación escolar. *Cuadernos de Pedagogía*, **370**, 19–23.

Duschl, R.A. and Hamilton, R.J. (eds) (1992) *Philosophy of Science, Cognitive Psychology and Educational Theory and Practice*, State University of New York Press, Albany, NY.

EMA (2013) *Uptake of the traditional use registration scheme and implementation of the provisions of Directive 2004/24/EC in EU Member States*, available at www.ema.europa.eu/docs /en_GB/document_library/Report/2011/05/WC500106706.pdf, accessed 19 May 2014.

Etkin, N. (2001) Perspectives in ethnopharmacology: forging a closer link between bioscience and traditional empirical knowledge. *Journal of Ethnopharmacology*, **76**, 177–182.

European Commission (2012) Rethinking Education: Investing in skills for better socio-economic outcomes, COM/212/0669 final, 52012DC0669, Communication from the Commission to the European Parliament, The Council, The European Economic and Social Committee and the Committee of the Regions, available from http://eur-lex.europa.eu/LexUriServ/LexUriServ.do?uri=COM:2012: 0669:FIN:EN:PDF, accessed 25 June 2014.

Eurostat (2014a) *Glossary: International standard classification of education (ISCED)*, epp.eurostat.ec .europa.eu/statistics_explained/index.php/Glossary:Tertiary_education, accessed 1 September 2014.

Eurostat (2014b) Europe 2020 indicators – education, epp.eurostat.ec.europa.eu/statistics_explained /index.php/Europe_2020_indicators_-_education, accessed 1 September 2014.

Fajardo, J., Verde, A., Rivera, D., *et al.* (2008) Investigación y divulgación del conocimiento etnobiológico en Castilla-La Mancha. *Sabuco*, **6**, 137–156.

Gillespie, S.G. (1995) Ethnopharmacology: Design of an undergraduate course. *American Journal of Pharmacological Education*, **59**, 34–37.

Giovannini, P., Reyes-García V., Waldstein, A. and Heinrich, M. (2011) Do pharmaceuticals displace local knowledge and use of medicinal plants? Estimates from a cross-sectional study in a rural indigenous community, Mexico. *Social Science and Medicine*, **72**, 928–936.

González, L.C. (2014) Teaching plant science in school and community settings, in (ed. C.L. Quave), *Innovative Strategies for Teaching in the Plant Sciences*, Springer Publishing, pp. 161–185.

Heinrich, M., Kufer, J., Leonti, M. and Pardo-de-Santayana, M. (2006) Ethnobotany and ethnopharmacology: Interdisciplinary links with the historical sciences. *Journal of Ethnopharmacology*, **107**, 57–160.

ITE (2014) El proyecto curricular de centro (PCC), http://www.ite.educacion.es/formacion/materiales/72 /cd/curso/unidad2/u2.I.2.htm, accessed 2 September 2014.

Laaksoharju, T., Rappe, E. and Kaivola, T. (2012) Garden affordances for social learning, play, and for building nature-child relationship. *Urban Forestry & Urban Greening*, **11**, 195–203.

Leonti, M. and Casu, L. (2013) Traditional medicines and globalization: current and future perspectives in ethnopharmacology. *Frontiers in Pharmacology*, **4**, 1–13.

LOCE (2002) *Law/Organic Law, Spain*, Ley Orgánica 10/2002, de 23 de diciembre, de Calidad de la Educación, BOE, 24 de diciembre de 2002, available at http://www.boe.es/buscar/doc.php?id=BOE-A-2002-25037.

LOE (2006) *Law/Organic Law, Spain*. Ley Orgánica 2/2006, de 3 de mayo, de Educación, BOE, 4 de mayo de 2006, available at http://www.boe.es/buscar/doc.php?id=BOE-A-2006-7899.

LOGSE (1990) *Law/Organic Law, Spain*. Ley Orgánica 1/1990, de 3 de octubre de 1990, de Ordenación General del Sistema Educativo, BOE, 4 de octubre de 1990, available at http://www.boe.es/buscar/doc.php?id=BOE-A-1990-24172.

LOMCE (2014) *Law/Organic Law, Spain*. Ley Orgánica 8/2013, de 9 de diciembre, para la mejora de la calidad educativa, BOE, 10 de diciembre de 2013, available at http://www.boe.es/diario_boe/txt.php?id=BOE-A-2013-12886.

McClatchey, W. Bridges, W. (2014) Lesson learned in development of an interdisciplinary science curriculum support organization, in *Innovative Strategies for Teaching in the Plant Sciences* (ed. C.L. Quave), Springer Publishing, pp. 21–31.

Mignone, J., Bartlett, J., O'Neil, J. and Orchard, T. (2007) Best practices intercultural health: five case studies in Latin America. *Journal of Ethnobiology and Ethnomedicine*, **3**, 31.

Morales, R., Tardío, J., Aceituno, L., *et al.* (2011) Biodiversidad y etnobotánica en España, in *Biodiversidad. Aproximación a la diversidad botánica y zoológica de España* (ed. J.L. Viejo-Montesinos), Real Sociedad Española de Historia Natural, Madrid, pp 157–207.

OSN (2014) Open Science Network, available from http://www.opensciencenetwork.org/, accessed 25 June 2014.

Pardo de Santayana, M. and Gómez Peyón, E. (2003) Etnobotánica: aprovechamiento tradicional de plantas y patrimonio cultural. *Anales del Jardín Botánico de Madrid*, **60** (1), 171–182.

Pardo de Santayana, M., Morales, R., Aceituno, L., *et al.* (2012) Etnobiología y Biodiversidad. El Inventario español de los Conocimientos Tradicionales, Revista Ambienta 99, available from http://www.revistaambienta.es/WebAmbienta/marm/Dinamicas/secciones/articulos/Tradicional.htm, accessed 25 June 2014.

Pérez, F., Cabrero, J, Rey, A., *et al.* (2009) Innovación educativa sobre plantas medicinales en la educación secundaria, Proceedings 2° Congreso Iberoamericano de Fitoterapia, Lisboa.

Quave, C., Pardo-de Santayana, M. and Pieroni, A. (2012) Medical ethnobotany in Europe: From field ethnography to a more culturally sensitive evidence-based CAM? *Evidence -Based Complementary and Alternative Medicine*, available at 10.1155/2012/156846.

Reyes-García, V. (2010) The relevance of traditional knowledge systems for ethnopharmacological research: theoretical and methodological contributions. *Journal of Ethnobiology and Ethnomedicine*, **6**, 32.

Rivera, D. (2008) Etnobotánica OCW, http://ocw.um.es/ciencias/etnobotanica, accessed 25 June 2014.

Rivera, D. and Obón, C. (1998) *Manual de Etnobotánica*, Diego Marín, Murcia.

Ruíz-Gallardo, J.R., Verde, A. and Valdés, A. (2013) Garden-based learning: An experience with 'at risk' secondary education students. *Journal of Environmental Education*, **44**, 252–270.

UIO (2014) FRM5420 – Ethnopharmacology, www.uio.no/studier/emner/matnat/farmasi/FRM5420/index-eng.html, accessed 25 June 2014.

UNESCO (2014) *ISCED Fields of Education and Training 2013 (ISCED-F 2013)*, UNESCO, Paris, www.uis.unesco.org/Education/Documents/isced-fields-of-education-training-2013.pdf, accessed 1 September 2014.

Valdés, A., Verde, A., Benlloch, V., *et al.* (2008) The experience of integration of ethnobotany as cross-curricular material in secondary education (Instituto Los Olmos, Albacete, Spain), in 49th Annual Meeting of the Society for Economic Botany in Duke University, Durhnan (USA), p. 66.

Vallejo, J.R. (2004) Modelos y estrategias para la Educación ambiental en la Educación formal, in *Teoría y Práctica de la Educación Ambiental* (ed. F. Velásquez de Castro), Grupo Editorial Universitario, Granada, pp. 91–96.

Vallejo, J.R., Peral, D., Vázquez, F.M. and Gordón, F. (2006) Etnobotánica: investigando en la escuela a través de la medicina popular. *Encuentros en la Biología*, **112**, 3–5.

Vallejo, J.R., Peral, D. and Figuero, Mª.J. (2007) Algunas experiencias cooperativas entorno a la ciencia entre un centro de secundaria y la universidad. *Campo Abierto*, **26** (1), 79–92.

Vandebroek, I. (2013) Intercultural health and ethnobotany: How to improve healthcare for underserved and minority communities? *Journal of Ethnopharmacology*, **148**, 746–754.

Verde, A. and Fajardo, J. (2002) La Etnobotánica como recurso didáctico. *El huerto escolar. CREA. Revista del Centro de Recursos de Educación Ambiental*, **7**, 22–24.

Verde, A. and Fajardo, J. (2003a) La Etnobotánica en el currículo de Secundaria. *Educar en el* **2000**, 7, 52–55.

Verde, A. and Fajardo, J. (2003b) *Las plantas en la cultura popular de Castilla La Mancha Junta de Comunidades de Castilla La Mancha*, Consejería de Educación, Albacete, p. 102.

Verde, A. and Fajardo, J. (2014) La importancia de enseñar Etnobiología, in *Etnobiologia na educação ibero-americana: compreensão holística e pluricultural da Biologia* (eds G. Costa Santos, M. Vargas-Clavijo and E. Medeiros), UEFS, Feira de Santana, pp. 387–409.

Verde, A., Campos, A., Fernández, A., *et al.* (2004a) El jardín escolar como recurso didáctico para atender a la diversidad. *Educar en Castilla-La Mancha*, **25**, 20–21.

Verde, A., Fajardo, J., Rivera, D., *et al.* (2004b) *La alimentación en Castilla-La Mancha: de la escasez al desperdicio (el valor de los alimentos locales y su utilización sostenible)*, Editorial Azarbe, Murcia.

Verde, A., Benlloch, V. and Fajardo, J. (2005) La Etnobotánica como recurso didáctico en educación ambiental. *Idea La Mancha*, **2**, 240–245.

Verde, A., Valdés, A., Rivera, D., *et al.* (2009) La Etnobiología como materia transversal en el currículo de educación secundaria, Una experiencia en Castilla-La Mancha (España). *ENSAYOS, Revista de la Facultad de Educación de Albacete*, **24**, 149–162.

Verde, A., Rivera, D., Fajardo, J., *et al.* (2010) Folk medicine and health as cross-curricular material in secondary education in Castilla-La Mancha (Spain), in *Proceedings V Congreso Internacional de Etnobotánica ICEB 2009, Bariloche (Argentina)* (eds M. Pochetino, A. Ladio and P. Arenas), pp. 250–255.

Vilá, B. (2014) La Etnobiología y la Educación Ambiental en escuelas andinas del Altiplano: reflexiones y experiencias, in *Etnobiologia na educação ibero-americana: compreensão holística e pluricultural da Biologia* (eds G. Costa Santos, M. Vargas-Clavijo and E. Medeiros), UEFS, Feira de Santana, pp. 315–344.

# The Pharmacological Angle

# 11

# Anti-infective Agents: The Example of Antibacterial Drug Leads

Maíra Bidart de Macedo[1], Sofie Clais[1], Ellen Lanckacker[1], Louis Maes[1], Emerson Silva Lima[2] and Paul Cos[1]

[1] Laboratory of Microbiology, Parasitology and Hygiene, Faculty of Pharmaceutical, Biomedical and Veterinary Sciences, University of Antwerp, Belgium
[2] Faculdade de Ciências Farmacêuticas, Universidade Federal do Amazonas, Rua Alexandre Amorin, Manaus - AM, Brasil

## 11.1   Introduction

Infectious diseases are still a major threat to public health despite tremendous progress in human medicine (Cos *et al.*, 2006). Their impact is particularly large in developing countries due to the relative unavailability of medicines and the emergence of widespread drug resistance. Research on new anti-infective agents must therefore be continued and all possible strategies should be explored. Besides small molecules from medicinal chemistry, natural products are still major sources of innovative therapeutic agents for various conditions, including infectious diseases (Clardy and Walsh, 2004). Numerous natural products have been isolated and identified, with almost 50% of the new drugs introduced to the market from 1981 to 2010, and approximately 75% of anti-infective agents coming from natural products or natural product derivatives (Cragg and Newman, 2013). From all possible sources of natural products, plants have been viewed as one of the most promising, since they can be sourced more easily and be selected on the basis of their ethnopharmacological use, which is one attractive way to reduce arbitrariness and to enhance the probability of success in new drug-finding efforts (Cordell and Colvard, 2005; Patwardhan, 2005). This chapter evaluates different strategies for discovering novel plant-derived agents with antibacterial potential.

*Ethnopharmacology*, First Edition. Edited by Michael Heinrich and Anna K. Jäger.
© 2015 John Wiley & Sons, Ltd. Published 2015 by John Wiley & Sons, Ltd.

## 11.2    Bacterial resistance

Existing antibiotics all act similarly by disrupting the bacterial metabolism in order to inhibit growth (bacteriostatic) or kill the bacteria (bactericidal). This mode of action exerts a considerable selective pressure on the bacteria and induces bacterial resistance. Some bacteria that gained these resistance mechanisms are now of great medical importance, for example *Staphylococcus aureus* is resistant to β-lactam antibacterial drugs and *Klebsiella pneumoniae* shows resistance to third-generation cephalosporins and carbapenems. An important reason for the current resistance problem is the worldwide misuse of antibiotics. Moreover, the spread of resistant microorganisms occurs very quickly within communities, hospitals and even by travel. A perfect example of so-called 'resistance globalization' is the dispersal of New Delhi metallo-β-lactamase-1 (NDM-1) (Carlet *et al.*, 2012). NDM-1 is an enzyme (carbapenemase) that makes bacteria resistant against almost all antibiotics except tigecycline and colistin. It originated in India but has now been detected worldwide, spread by patients travelling to India to undergo medical treatments (So *et al.*, 2010).

Besides infection prevention and the rational use of antibiotics, a third measure for combating resistance is the continuous development of new antibiotics. A crucial concern is that since the late 1980s only a few novel antibacterial drugs have been discovered (Carlet *et al.*, 2012) and brought to the market. This is a result of the complex and time-consuming process of antibiotic development as well as the small return on investment in research and development compared to other drug classes. Moreover, there is a lack of compounds targeting multidrug resistant Gram-negative bacteria. The outer membrane of Gram-negatives renders them more resistant to antibiotics and they are often able to pump antibiotics out of the bacterial cell or produce enzymes that deactivate antibiotics, such as NDM-1. The formation and spread of resistant microorganisms is a complex phenomenon for which no simple approach will ever suffice. It is therefore indispensable that alternative measures are explored to avoid the post-antibiotic era, not only by looking for new antibiotics but also by focusing on alternative therapies for infectious diseases. As discussed in the following sections, ethnopharmacology can be an excellent source for the latter.

## 11.3    Plant-derived antibacterial agents

### 11.3.1    Direct antibacterial agents

The currently used antibiotics act as inhibitors of peptidoglycan synthesis (e.g. β-lactams, glycopeptides), protein synthesis (e.g. tetracyclines, chloramphenicol, macrolides, aminoglycosides) and nucleic acid synthesis by interrupting nucleotide metabolism (e.g. sulphonamides, diaminopyrimidines), inhibiting RNA polymerase (e.g. rifamycins) or DNA gyrase (e.g. quinolones). Other antibiotics interfere with membrane integrity (e.g. polymyxins). In contrast to antiparasitic drugs, no plant-derived antibiotics have reached the market. This is remarkable since a large number of plant extracts have been evaluated for antibacterial potential. Most of the extracts and isolated compounds show relatively high MIC values against Gram-positive bacteria and a lack of activity against Gram-negative bacteria. Examples are tannins, lignans, steroidal saponins and xanthones, which show weak-to-moderate antibacterial activities (Cowan, 1999). Flavonoids do not exhibit a significant direct antibacterial activity, but some of these compounds can have an indirect antibacterial effect (see below). Taking into account the sometimes high cytotoxicity and the non-specific mechanism of action, the most important application of these extracts and isolated compounds is as disinfectants. One example is the membrane-disrupting activities at high MIC values for ferulic acid and gallic acid (Borges *et al.*, 2013). It therefore appears that plants do not produce highly potent and specific inhibitors of bacterial targets (Lewis, 2013). Until now, the only exception was the coumarins, which inhibit bacterial DNA gyrase. Coumarins show good activity against Gram-positive bacteria, but their activity is still much lower than novobiocin, which is an aminocoumarin antibiotic produced by streptomycetes.

## 11.3.2   Antivirulence agents

A promising strategy currently gaining considerable attention is the inhibition of virulence factors. These are structural or physiological characteristics that help microorganisms to cause infection and disease (Figure 11.1) (Rasko and Sperandio, 2010). Virulence factors include structures such as pili for adhesion to cells and tissues, enzymes to evade host defences and toxins that can provoke deleterious effects on the host. Hence, inhibition of virulence factors is an interesting approach as it disarms pathogenic organisms. This could prevent further colonization and block the detrimental effects to the host in such a way that the host immune system is able to eliminate the pathogen more efficiently.

As antivirulence strategies do not directly kill a bacterium, they may exert less evolutionary pressure than standard antibiotics, whereby resistance development could be delayed. However, this remains a hypothesis that can only be proven once antivirulence compounds are used in clinical practice (Baron, 2013). Another possible advantage is the decreased impact on the normal bacterial flora since virulence inhibitors are pathogen-specific. This may also reduce drug-related side effects, such as diarrhoea, as well as the risk of secondary infections and colonization with drug-resistant organisms (Barczak and Hung, 2009). Nevertheless, the practical applicability of virulence inhibitors remains unknown. They could be used as prophylactic agents, as monotherapy or in combination with conventional antibiotic therapy. In the last few years, many compounds targeting different types of virulence factors have been evaluated *in vitro* and *in vivo*, but further research is definitely required (Baron, 2013). The following paragraphs discuss the main bacterial virulence factors and list some examples of putative plant-derived antivirulence compounds.

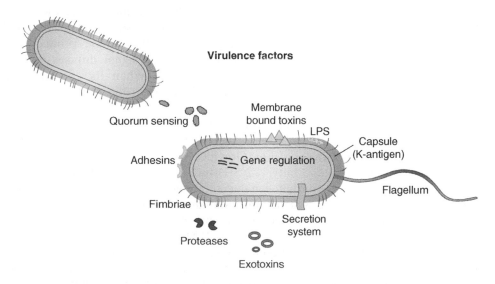

**Figure 11.1**   Overview of the most important virulence factors in bacteria.

### 11.3.2.1  Anti-adhesion agents

The first step in bacterial colonization consists of attachment to the host. Many types of bacterial appendages, including pili or fimbriae, contribute to this process by binding to cell-surface receptors on the host cell. Consequently, there are various possibilities for interfering with bacterial attachment mechanisms to prevent infection.

Cranberry juice (*Vaccinium macrocarpon* Aiton) has been used for decades to prevent urinary tract infections, which are among the most common bacterial infections in women. Although the mechanism of action is not completely elucidated, it has been shown that type A proanthocyanidins prevent the adherence of *P fimbriae* of *E. coli* to uroepithelial cell receptors. Moreover, cranberries can also reduce inflammatory cascades and immunological responses to bacterial evasion (Vasileiou *et al.*, 2013). The greatest challenge is to determine the optimal dose of proanthocyanidins required for *in vivo* activity (Beerepoot *et al.*, 2013). Berberine is an alkaloid known from plants used, for example, in traditional Chinese and Native American medicine, possessing significant antimicrobial activity. It causes *Streptococcus pyogenes* to release its lipoteichoic acids, thereby reducing its ability to bind to fibronectin. It also disrupts *E. coli* fimbriae through a still unknown mechanism of action (Cushnie *et al.*, 2015).

### 11.3.2.2  Quorum sensing inhibitors

Quorum sensing (QS) is a density-dependent bacterial cell-to-cell communication system. Bacterial synthases produce QS signals, which are called autoinducers (AI). When these molecules accumulate in the environment and reach a critical concentration (quorum), they flow back into the bacterial cell, bind to their receptor and trigger the expression of virulence genes and biofilm formation. In this way, QS inhibition allows a delay of virulence factor synthesis. Because of the apparent role of QS in biofilm formation, QS inhibitors are proposed as promising antibiofilm agents (Cos *et al.*, 2010). Disruption of the QS systems can generally be accomplished in three ways: quorum synthesis inhibitors, quorum quenching enzymes (which neutralize the quorum signal) and quorum receptor antagonists. The fact that plants survive in an environment with a high bacterial density may suggest that they possess active defence mechanisms against bacterial pathogens, like, for example, QS inhibitors.

The cell-to-cell signalling systems can be divided into four main categories (Parker and Sperandio, 2009). The most common is the LuxI/LuxR system, which is found in Gram-negative bacteria (Figure 11.2A). Homologues of LuxI synthase produce N-acyl homoserine lactones (AHLs), also called AI-1. This quorum signal diffuses across the bacterial membrane and accumulates in the environment. When its concentration is high enough, AI-1 diffuses back into the cell, where it binds to the transcription activator LuxR (Parker and Sperandio, 2009). Several extracts from honey, fruits, plants and secondary metabolites from fungi, nematodes and marine sponges block different AHL-type QS systems. De Nys *et al.* (1993) isolated some naturally occurring furanone compounds from the red alga *Delisea pulchra* (Greville) Montage. One of these compounds, (5Z)-4-bromo-5-(bromomethylene)-3-butyryl-2(5H)-furanone, inhibits AHL-based QS in several Gram-negative bacteria. The halogenated furanones bind to AHL receptors since its five-membered lactone scaffold is structurally similar to AHLs. To date, many furanone analogues capable of blocking AHL QS have been synthesized.

From horseradish (*Armoracia rusticana* P.Gaertn., B.Mey. & Scherb.), 1-isothiocyanato-3-(methylsulfinyl)propane, also known as iberin, was isolated and specifically targets two of the major QS networks in *P. aeruginosa*, the LasIR and RhlIR systems. It also down-regulates QS-controlled rhamnolipid production in *P. aeruginosa*. Propolis or bee hive glue disrupts

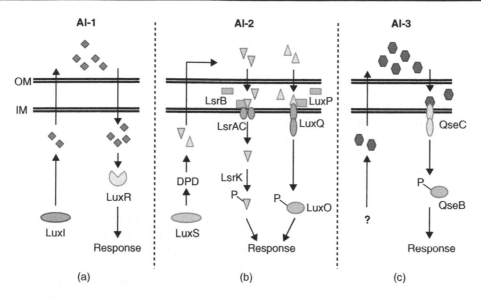

**Figure 11.2** Three QS systems in Gram-negative bacteria. A, AI-1-based strategy using AHL molecules. B, AI-2-based strategy using quorum sensing signals derived from the precursor DPD. C, AI-3-based strategy using an AI of unknown structure. Inner membrane (IM), outer membrane (OM). Adapted from Parker and Sperandio (2009).

AHL QS-controlled systems in bacteria (Bulman *et al.*, 2011). Swarming motility in *P. aeruginosa* PAO1 and its AHL-dependent LasR and RhlR-based QS behaviours are also inhibited.

A second QS pathway is the AI-2/LuxS-based system, which is found in Gram-positive and Gram-negative cells (Figure 11.2). It has been suggested that the AI-2 system serves for inter-species signalling. AI-2 is derived from the precursor 4,5-dihydroxy-2,3-pentadione (DPD), which is synthetized by LuxS. Cinnamaldehyde is known to affect AI-2 QS in *Vibrio* spp. by decreasing the DNA-binding activity of the response regulator LuxR (Brackman *et al.*, 2008). Another example is pyrogallol, isolated, for example, from *Emblica officinalis* Gaertn., which exhibits antagonism against AI-2 (Kalia, 2013). Recent studies claim that its activity is independent of QS because the addition of catalase is sufficient to abolish any pyrogallol-related effect (Defoirdt *et al.*, 2013). Furthermore, 7-hydroxyindole, isatin and several fatty acids block AI-2 regulated virulence factors.

A third cell-signalling system of Gram-negative microbes is the AI-3/QseC system (Figure 11.2). The sensor histidine kinase QseC detects AI-3 and undergoes autophosphory-lation. Subsequently, QseC transfers this phosphate to the response regulator QseB, which activates gene expression. The QseC pathway forms an attractive target for developing novel inhibitors as it possesses the potential to have a broad-spectrum activity. The citrus isolimonic acid is a potent inhibitor of *E. coli* O157:H7 biofilm formation by interfering with the AI-3 QS system (Vikram *et al.*, 2012).

The remaining QS system is the AIP/Agr system, which uses autoinducing peptides (AIPs) as signal molecules and is exclusively found in Gram-positive organisms. Hamamelitannin, i.e. a non-peptide analogue of the RNAIII inhibiting peptide, inhibits QS-regulated virulence in staphylococci (Brackman *et al.*, 2011).

Plants species used in local and traditional medical systems are still underexplored for their QS inhibitory activities. Most of the studied plant-derived QS inhibitors were only evaluated *in vitro*, but recent *in vivo* studies also show that QS inhibitors, for example baicalin and hamamelitannin, can increase the susceptibility of bacterial biofilms to antibiotics (Brackman *et al.*, 2011). Despite the promising findings *in vitro* and *in vivo*, no compound has yet reached clinical development.

### 11.3.2.3  Antibiofilm agents

Bacteria can grow as single cells (planktonic mode of growth) or as a sessile community, also known as a biofilm. According to the National Institutes of Health (NIH), biofilms are involved in over 80% of all bacterial infectious diseases. Biofilms consist of multiple bacteria attached to an inert or living surface and embedded by a self-produced extracellular matrix (Figure 11.3). This matrix consists of polysaccharides, proteins and extracellular DNA, and is often regarded as a slime layer (Cos *et al.*, 2010). It intercepts nutrients from the environment and protects the residing bacteria from environmental stress such as an attack by antimicrobials or the host immune system. A mature biofilm obtains a mushroom-shaped structure due to the formation of different microcolonies and the presence of typical water channels within the matrix, allowing the exchange of nutrients and waste products.

Biofilm formation can only start after a successful initial adhesion step and when the population is dense enough. Subsequently, the increase in QS signals triggers the bacteria to switch to the biofilm mode of growth. Hence, it is not surprising that molecules targeting adhesins or QS mechanisms also impact on biofilm formation, as previously discussed for the furanones. These QS inhibitors hinder biofilm formation in *E. coli* and *P. aeruginosa*. Other possibilities for interference with biofilm formation are the development of enzymes that degrade the biofilm matrix or inhibition of the synthesis of matrix components. A wide variety of natural products show antibiofilm activity, but in most cases the mechanism of action is still unknown. Epigallocatechin-3-gallate, an antimicrobial catechin found in green tea (*Camellia sinensis* (L.) Kuntze) extracts, inhibits slime production and biofilm formation in staphylococci and is also able to induce biofilm destruction (Cos *et al.*, 2010). Ursolic acid isolated from *Diospyros dendo* Welw. Ex Hiern also disrupts biofilms without QS inhibition, but the actual mechanism of action remains to be elucidated (Ren *et al.*, 2005).

### 11.3.2.4  Agents targeting secretion systems

Bacteria use secretion systems to inject toxins into the host cell. Seven distinct secretion systems have been described (Baron, 2013). A large majority of the studies have focused on

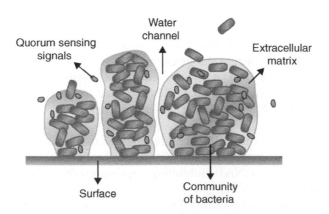

**Figure 11.3**  Overview of a biofilm. A biofilm is composed of multiple bacteria, which are attached to a surface and surrounded by an extracellular matrix.

the type III secretion system (TTSS), which is present in several Gram-negative pathogens including *Chlamydia*, *E. coli*, *Pseudomonas*, *Salmonella*, *Shigella* and *Yersinia*. TTSS consists of several proteins forming a needle-type structure that translocates effectors directly from the bacterial cytoplasm into the host cell cytoplasm.

From the leaf extracts of two Papua New Guinean rainforest plants, *Anisoptera thurifera* (Blanco) Blume and *Anisoptera thurifera* subsp. *polyandra* (Blume) P.S.Ashton. (syn. *A. polyandra* Blume), a complex tetrameric stilbenoid called (–)-hopeaphenol was identified. This compound inhibits TTSS in *Yersinia pseudotuberculosis* and *P. aeruginosa* (Zetterström *et al.*, 2013). Isolomonic acid is a potent inhibitor of TTSS in *E. coli* O157:H7 (Vikram *et al.*, 2012).

### 11.3.2.5  Agents targeting host immunity

Pathogenic microorganisms may possess factors that allow them to overcome host immune defences. For example, *S. aureus* produces a carotenoid pigment, staphyloxanthin, that protects it from reactive oxygen species produced by host neutrophils. In a recent study with 12 plant flavonoids, flavone reduced significantly the production of staphyloxanthin and α-hemolysin without inhibiting the planktonic growth of *S. aureus* (Lee *et al.*, 2012). The staphyloxanthin reduction rendered the *S. aureus* cells 100 times more vulnerable to hydrogen peroxide in the presence of flavone. This finding supports the usefulness of flavone as a potential antivirulence agent against antibiotic-resistant *S. aureus*.

## 11.3.3  Resistance-modifying agents

As their name suggests, resistance-modifying agents (RMAs) extend the lifespan of existing antibiotics by targeting bacterial resistance mechanisms (Abreu *et al.*, 2012). Four major mechanisms of resistance have been identified, each of which involves the alteration of a different bacterial structure: (i) targets of antibacterial action, (ii) membrane permeability, (iii) production of enzymes that inactivate antibiotics and (iv) antibiotic efflux pumps (Figure 11.4). The resistance mechanisms will be explained more in detail and some examples of plant-derived RMAs will be highlighted.

(i)  Alteration of the antibacterial target

Alteration of the target of an antibiotic is a widely used mechanism of drug resistance. A well-known example is quinolone resistance due to alterations in DNA gyrase and topoisomerase IV involved in DNA synthesis. At this moment, there are no plant-derived compounds exhibiting this mechanism of action.

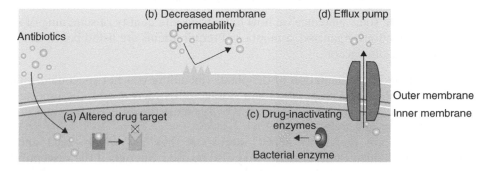

**Figure 11.4**  Four major antibiotic resistance mechanisms.

(ii)   Alteration of membrane permeability

To exert their antibacterial activities, antibiotics must access intracellular targets. The presence of two membranes in Gram-negative bacteria partially explains the enhanced resistance of Gram-negatives compared to Gram-positives. Thymol and carvacrol, isolated from the essential oil of *Thymus vulgaris* L., disintegrate the outer membrane and thus increase the permeability of antibiotics in Gram-negative bacteria (Abreu *et al.*, 2012). An ethanolic extract from *Holarrhena antidysenterica* Wall. acts as an RMA against *Acinetobacter baumannii* by weakening the outer membrane of the pathogen (Chusri *et al.*, 2014).

(iii)  Production of enzymes that inactivate antibiotics

β-lactam antibiotics act by inhibiting the transpeptidase or penicillin-binding proteins (PBPs) and are among the most commonly prescribed drugs. Resistance to many β-lactam antibiotics are most often caused by β-lactamases or by mutation in the PBPs resulting in reduced affinity. β-lactamases are bacterial enzymes that hydrolyze the β-lactam ring of the antibiotic and render the antibiotic inactive before it reaches the PBP target. In turn, clavulanic acid inhibits the β-lactamase and restores the antibiotic susceptibility when it is co-administered. A well-known example on the drug market is Augmentin®, which is the combination of the antibiotic amoxicillin with clavulanic acid. Altered PBPs are responsible for reduced sensitivity to β-lactam antibiotics, as shown for PBP2a in methicillin-resistant *S. aureus* (MRSA). The tea (*Camellia sinensis* (L.) Kuntze) catechins catechin gallate, epicatechin gallate and epigallocatechin gallate are able to reverse methicillin resistance in MRSA and penicillin resistance in β-lactamase-producing *S. aureus* (Abreu *et al.*, 2012). The mechanism of action is the prevention of PBP2a synthesis and the inhibition of β-lactamase secretion, respectively.

(iv)   Antibiotic efflux pumps

Another way to target resistance is by inhibiting the antibiotic efflux pumps of bacteria, which could restore susceptibility to multiple antibiotics simultaneously. From *Berberis* species the alkaloid,berberine was isolated and it increases the membrane permeability. However, berberine is rapidly pumped out of the bacteria through multidrug resistance pumps (MDRs). *Berberis* species also produce 5′-methoxy-hydnocarpin D and pheophorbide, which are inhibitors of the NorA MDR efflux pump in *S. aureus*. This clearly supports the idea that plant antibacterials are individually relatively weak but act in synergy (Lewis and Ausubel, 2006).

## 11.4   Basic requirements for successful antimicrobial drug discovery (Cos *et al.*, 2006)

In an effort to provide some guidance on how to improve the quality of screening of natural products against infectious organisms, a number of requirements are listed below in order to attain a robust 'proof-of-concept'.

1.   Identification and documentation of the plants (including voucher specimen, collection details and number) and preparation and storage of extracts need to be reported. In a bioassay-guided fractionation, a scattered activity across the different fractions is mostly indicative for non-selectivity.

2.   Test organisms are preferably ATCC strains as they are widely used and well-characterized. Defined clinical isolates may also be used, but only if the susceptibility to relevant reference compounds is reported.

3. *In vitro* models using the whole organism are the 'gold' standard and should be used whenever possible. If microorganisms can be cultivated either in cell-free medium ('axenic') or in cell cultures, the latter is preferred since it resembles more closely the *in vivo* situation.

4. Antimicrobial activity must be discriminated from non-specific toxicity by inclusion of a parallel cytotoxicity evaluation on mammalian cell lines or integration into a panel of unrelated microbial screens (bacteria, fungi, parasites, viruses).

5. Total extracts and derived primary fractions exhibiting strong non-selective action in the panel of *in vitro* screens can only be properly evaluated in animal models.

6. Extended dose ranges with at least three doses are needed for establishing representative dose-response curves. Descriptive values are IC50 and IC90. MIC and MBC values are also common end-points in antibacterial and antifungal screening.

7. To correct for too many false-positives, stringent end-point criteria must be adopted. For all anti-infective bioassays, IC50 values should be below 100 µg/ml for mixtures and below 25 µM for pure compounds. Some microorganisms even require more severe end-point criteria.

8. A universal panel of test organisms does not exist and is largely determined by the specific drug-finding objectives and the adopted plant selection criteria. Taking into account the sometimes broad traditional ethnobotanical use, a minimum panel of test organisms is recommended.

9. Inclusion of appropriate controls in each test replicate (blank-, infected- and reference controls) is necessary. For each test organism, one or more commercially available reference compounds can be considered.

10. Differences in composition of the growth medium can greatly affect the potency of a compound. Mueller–Hinton medium is recommended for antibacterial and Sabouraud for antifungal testing in agar and/or broth dilution tests. For fastidious bacteria, supplementation with growth factors or other media are allowed.

11. The infective dose can have a profound impact on the test results. For most bacteria, $10^5$ CFU/ml is adequate, while for yeasts and fungi about $10^3$ and $10^4$ CFU/ml is satisfactory, respectively. For viruses and parasites, optimal infective doses are species-specific.

12. For antibacterial and antifungal activities, follow-up of bioassay-guided fractionation can be performed with an assay of choice. Whenever possible, final reporting of active extracts or pure compounds should be done by applying the broth-dilution method. For essential oils, addition of solvents or emulsifiers may be necessary, but their final concentrations should be limited and reported.

13. The phenomenon of 'synergistic' effects in mixtures or extracts frequently causes loss of activity during bioassay-guided fractionation efforts and hence precludes the identification or characterization of the relevant fraction that could be retained for further evaluation. Synergistic vs additive effects need to be evaluated by the checkerboard method or time-kill curves.

# 11.5  Conclusion

There is still a great interest in plant-derived compounds as potential antibacterial agents. The compounds can act in three different ways, i.e. direct antibacterial activity, antivirulence activity or resistance-modifying activity. During the last few decades most research efforts have focused on finding novel antibiotics from plants. Here the outcome was very disappointing. One could even question whether plants synthesize target-specific compounds with a low MIC value against human pathogenic bacteria. Until now, the answer was negative, especially for compounds with an activity against Gram-negative bacteria. The more promising strategies for plant-derived compounds are those that study their antivirulence and resistance-modifying activities. This paradigm shift is now ongoing, but several hurdles may hamper its success. First, more complex and expensive bioassays are required for this type of research. Second, the correct interpretation of the results is difficult and prone to artefacts. Third, one should look for combination therapies with existing antibiotics, again complicating the set-up and interpretation of experiments. Nevertheless, recent publications are very promising and should encourage more researchers to join this exciting and novel field of ethno-antibacterial pharmacology.

# References

Abreu, A.C., McBain, A.J. and Simões, M. (2012) Plants as sources of new antimicrobials and resistance-modifying agents. *Natural Product Reports*, **29**, 1007–1021.

Barczak, A.K. and Hung, D.T. (2009) Productive steps toward an antimicrobial targeting virulence. *Current Opinion in Microbiology*, **12**, 490–496.

Baron, C. (2013) A novel strategy to target bacterial virulence. *Future Microbiology*, **8**, 1–3.

Beerepoot, M.A.J., Geerlings, S.E., van Haarst, E.P. and Mensing van Charante, N. (2013) Nonantibiotic prophylaxis for recurrent urinary tract infections: a systematic review and meta-analysis of randomized controlled trials. *Journal of Urology*, **190**, 1981–1989.

Borges, A., Ferreira, C., Saavedra, M.J. and Simoes, M. (2013) Antibacterial activity and mode of action of ferulic and gallic acids against pathogenic bacteria. *Microbial Drug Resistance*, **19**, 256–265.

Brackman, G., Defoirdt, T., Miyamoto, C., *et al.* (2008) Cinnamaldehyde and cinnamaldehyde analogs reduce virulence in *Vibrio* spp. by decreasing the DNA-binding activity of the quorum sensing response regulator LuXR. *BMC Microbiology*, **8**, 149.

Brackman, G., Cos, P., Maes, L., *et al.* (2011) Quorum sensing inhibitors increase the susceptibility of bacterial biofilms to antibiotics *in vitro* and *in vivo*. *Antimicrobial Agents and Chemotherapy*, **55**, 2655-2661.

Bulman, Z., Le, P., Hudson, P.L. and Savka, M.A. (2011) A novel property of propolis (bee glue): Anti-pathogenic activity by inhibition of N-acyl-homoserine lactone mediated signaling in bacteria. *Journal of Ethnopharmacology*, **138**, 788–797.

Carlet, J., Jarlier, V., Harbarth, S., *et al.* (2012) Ready for a world without antibiotics? The pensieres antibiotic resistance call to action. *Antimicrobial Resistance and Infection Control*, **1**, 11.

Chusri, S., Na-Phatthalung, P., Siriyong, T., *et al.* (2014) *Holarrhena antidysenterica* as a resistance modifying agent against *Acinetobacter baumannii*: its effect on bacterial outer membrane permeability and efflux pumps. *Microbiological Research*, **169**, 417–424.

Clardy, J. and Walsh, C. (2004) Lessons from natural molecules. *Nature*, **432**, 829–837.

Cordell G.A. and Colvard M.D. (2005) Some thoughts on the future of ethnopharmacology. *Journal of Ethnopharmacology*, **100**, 5–14.

Cos, P., Vlietinck, A.J., Vanden Berghe, D. and Maes, L. (2006) Anti-infective potential of natural products: how to develop a stronger in vitro 'proof-of-concept'. *Journal of Ethnopharmacology*, **106**, 290–302.

Cos, P., Toté, K., Horemans, T. and Maes, L. (2010). Biofilms: an extra hurdle for effective antimicrobial therapy. *Current Pharmaceutical Design*, **16**, 2279–2295.

Cowan, M.C. (1999) Plant products as antimicrobial agents. *Clinical Microbiology Reviews*, **12**, 564–582.

Cragg, G.M. and Newman, D.J. (2013) Natural products: a continuing source of novel drug leads. *Biochimica et Biophysica Acta*, **1830**, 3670–3695.

Cushnie, T.P.T., Cushnie, B. and Lamb, A.J. (2014) Alkaloids: an overview of their antibacterial, antibiotic-enhancing and antivirulence activities. *International Journal of Antimicrobial Agents*, **44**, 377–386.

Defoirdt, T., Brackman, G. and Coenye, T. (2013) Quorum sensing inhibitors: how strong is the evidence? *Trends in Microbiology*, **21**, 619–624.

De Nys, R., Wright, A.D., Konig, G.M. and Sticher, O. (1993) New halogenated furanones from the marine alga *Delisea pulchra*. *Tetrahedron*, **49**, 11213–11220.

Kalia, V.P. (2013) Quorum sensing inhibitors: an overview. *Biotechnology Letters*, **31**, 224–245.

Lee, J.H., Park, J.H., Cho, M.H. and Lee, J. (2012) Flavone reduces the production of virulence factors, staphyloxanthin and alpha-hemolysin, in *Staphylococcus aureus*. *Current Microbiology*, **65**, 726–732.

Lewis, K. (2013) Platforms for antibiotic discovery. *Nature Reviews Drug Discovery*, **12**, 371–387.

Lewis, K. and Ausubel, F.M. (2006) Prospects for plant-derived antibacterials. *Nature Biotechnology*, **24**, 1504–1507.

Parker, C.T. and Sperandio, V. (2009) Cell-to-cell signalling during pathogenesis. *Cellular Microbiology*, **11**, 363–369.

Patwardhan, B. (2005) Ethnopharmacology and drug discovery. *Journal of Ethnopharmacology*, **100**, 50–52.

Rasko, D.A. and Sperandio, V. (2010) Anti-virulence strategies to combat bacteria-mediated disease. *Nature Reviews Drug Discovery*, **9**, 117–128.

Ren, D.C., Zuo, R.J., Barrios, A.F.G., *et al.* (2005) Differential gene expression for investigation of *Escherichia coli* biofilm inhibition by plant extract ursolic acid. *Applied and Environmental Microbiology*, **71**, 4022–4034.

So, A., Furlong, M. and Heddini, A. (2010) Globalisation and antibiotic resistance. *British Medical Journal*, **341**, c5116.

Vasileiou, I., Katsargyris, A. and Theocharis, S. (2013) Current clinical status on the preventive effects of cranberry consumption against urinary tract infections. *Nutrition Research*, **33**, 595–607.

Vikram, A., Jesudhasan, P.R., Pillai, S.D. and Patil, B.S. (2012) Isolimonic acid interferes with *Escherichia coli* O157:H7 biofilm and TTSS in QseBC and QseA dependent fashion. *BMC Microbiology*, **12**, 261.

Zetterström, C.E., Hasselgren, J., Salin, O., *et al.* (2013) The resveratrol tetramer (–)-hopeaphenol inhibits type III secretion in the Gram-negative pathogens *Yersinia pseudotuberculosis* and *Pseudomonas aeruginosa*. *PloS One*, **8**, e81969.

# 12
# Searching for New Treatments of Malaria

Colin W. Wright

*Bradford School of Pharmacy, University of Bradford, West Yorkshire, UK*

## 12.1  Introduction

Globally, diseases caused by species of protozoa such as malaria, trypanosomiasis (African sleeping sickness, Chagas' disease) and leishmaniasis (cutaneous and visceral forms) are major causes of mortality and morbidity. To a large extent this is because many of the people affected do not have access to effective treatment but, in addition, new drugs are urgently needed as existing agents have important limitations of toxicity and/or reduced efficacy due to increasing parasite resistance. The most important of the protozoal diseases, malaria, is responsible for an estimated 627 million deaths each year, mostly among young children in Africa (World Malaria Report, 2013), and as space is restricted this will be the focus of this chapter. With reference to selected recent studies, the potential of natural products to contribute to the development of novel, effective and more affordable treatments for malaria will be explored, although several other protozoal diseases will be mentioned.

## 12.2  Traditional herbal remedies as a source of antimalarial lead compounds

Studies reporting the evaluation of plant species, especially those used traditionally for the treatment of malaria, have resulted in the isolation of many compounds with antiplasmodial activity, but only in relatively few cases have compounds been evaluated for *in vivo* antimalarial activity. (For recent reviews see Wright, 2010; Bero and Quetin-Leclercq, 2011; Pohlit *et al.*, 2013; Xu and Pieters, 2013). A selection of compounds is discussed below with a view to illustrating a variety of structural types possessing activity (**1–28**), as well highlighting some studies in which more extensive evaluations have been carried out, such as *in vivo* antimalarial

*Ethnopharmacology*, First Edition. Edited by Michael Heinrich and Anna K. Jäger.

tests, toxicity studies and pharmacokinetics. In addition, studies have been selected to illustrate some recent strategies that have been employed in the search for new antimalarial agents.

The Apocynaceae continues to be a rich source of indole alkaloids and several have been shown to have good selectivity against *Plasmodia* (as compared with their cytotoxic activities) (Xu and Pieters, 2013). The rationale for the investigation of the species mentioned below was on the basis of their alkaloidal constituents, i.e. they were not selected on the basis of any traditional use as antimalarials. For example, nicalaterine (**1**) and bisnicalaterine C (**2**), isolated from the bark of *Hunteria zeylanica* (Retz.) Gardner ex Thwaites, were found to be highly active against chloroquine-sensitive *P. falciparum* 3D7 ($IC_{50}$ = 0.11 and 0.05 μM and selectivity indices (SI) >450 and >1000, respectively); leuconicine B (**3**), a constituent of *Leuconotis griffithii* Hook.f., showed similar selectivity ($IC_{50}$ = 0.007 μM and SI = 543). Among several alkaloids reported from the stem bark of *Muntafara sessilifolia* (Baker) Pichon, 3′-oxotabernaelegantine (**4**), was less potent than the above alkaloids ($IC_{50}$ = 4.4 μM) but actually more selective as it did not exhibit significant cytotoxicity (SI > 31,412). Unfortunately, no *in vivo* antimalarial data has yet been reported for the above alkaloids.

One reason for the lack of published *in vivo* studies is the low abundance and difficulty of isolation of many phytochemicals, but in the case of Brazilian *Piper peltatum* L. (Piperaceae) multigram quantities of 4-nerolidylcatechol (**5**) have been obtained by means of standard extraction and chromatographic methods (Pohlit *et al.*, 2013). The latter compound was found to be active against both chloroquine-sensitive (3D7) and chloroquine-resistant (K1) strains of *P. falciparum* ($IC_{50}$ = 6.7 and 1.9 μM, respectively), and also suppressed parasitaemia in mice infected with *P. berghei* by 60% when given orally or subcutaneously in doses of 600 mg/kg/day. This relatively weak *in vivo* activity was markedly improved by *O,O*-diacetylation of **5** (up to 70% suppression at oral doses of 10–25 mg/kg/day). However, to show the viability of this compound as a lead antimalarial, derivatives with further improvements in activity (i.e. 100% suppression with no toxicity) will be required. Nevertheless, 4-nerolidylcatechol is interesting as it is believed to act by inhibiting the synthesis of terpenoid metabolites in *P. falciparum*.

The steroidal alkaloid conessine (**6**) is the major constituent of *Holarrhena pubescens* Wall. (Dua *et al.*, 2013; published as *Holarrhena antidysenterica*, an invalid taxon) (Apocynaceae) and is active against *Entamoeba histolytica*, the protozoan responsible for amoebic dysentery. This plant is used in India for the treatment of amoebic dysentery as well as for malaria and conessine has been shown to have potent activities against *P. falciparum in vitro* and against *P. berghei* in mice (89% suppression of parasitaemia at 10 mg/kg orally for 4 days), (Dua *et al.*, 2013). Although the *in vitro* selectivity index was low (<10) the authors suggest that chemical modification may improve its potential as an antimalarial. However, previous clinical studies have shown that conessine is neurotoxic (Steck, 1971).

Nitidine (**7**), a benzophenanthridine alkaloid found in *Zanthoxylum* sp. (Rutaceae), has been suggested to be a possible lead antimalarial compound as it is thought to be the main active constituent in several traditional antimalarial remedies (Bouquet *et al.*, 2012). It was found to have potent antiplasmodial activity against three strains of *P. falciparum* ($IC_{50}$ = 0.5–0.8 μM) with SIs of >10 compared with cytotoxic effects and was shown to have modest *in vivo* antimalarial activity (59% suppression of parasitaemia at 20 mg/kg/day) with no apparent toxicity. Confocal microscopy showed that the alkaloid localized in the parasite's cytoplasm rather than the nucleus and it was also found to inhibit β-haematin formation (i.e. suggesting that it has a chloroquine-like mode of action).

The seeds of *Garcinia kola* Heckel (Sterculiaceae) may be a potential lead to new antimalarial compounds since it was shown that kolaviron, a biflavanoid fraction from this species, suppressed parasitaemia by 90% in mice infected with *P. berghei* when given at a

**1 nicalaterine**

**2 bisnicalaterine C**

**3 leuconicine B**

**4 3'-oxotabernaelegantine**

**5 4-nerolidylcatechol**

**6 conessine**

**7 nitidine**

**8 ergosterol-5, 8-endoperoxide**

dose of 200 mg/kg (Oluwatosin *et al.*, 2014). The treated mice were also protected from the decrease in antioxidant status and packed cell volume seen in untreated infected mice. In another study, an alcoholic extract of the leaves of *Conyza sumatrensis* (Retz.) E.H. Walker (Asteraceae) was shown to have a modest effect on parasitaemia in *P. berghei* infected mice (62% suppression at 1 g/kg orally for 7 days), thus lending some support to its use as an antimalarial Cameroon folk medicine (Boniface and Pal, 2013). However, toxic deaths were observed with doses of 1.6 g/kg and this serves as a reminder that traditional medicines may not necessarily be safe.

Species of *Ajuga* (Lamiaceae) are used traditionally as antimalarials in Africa and *A. braceosa* Wall ex Benth. (now regarded as a synonym of *A. integrifolia* Buch.-Ham) has been investigated in some detail (reviewed in Cocquyt *et al.*, 2011). An ethanolic extract of the leaves presented modest *in vitro* antiplasmodial activities against chloroquine-sensitive and chloroquine-resistant *P. falciparum* (IC$_{50}$ = 55 and 57 μg/ml, respectively), and several compounds were isolated and tested, the most potent being ergosterol-5,8-endoperoxide (**8**) ($IC_{50}$ = 8.2 μM). The occurrence of this endoperoxide in *Ajuga* sp. is of interest since artemisinin is also an endoperoxide, but the antiplasmodial activity of ergosterol-5,8-endoperoxide is very weak compared to that of artemisinin. In mice infected with *P. berghei* strain NK65, the leaf ethanolic extract of *A. integrifolia* exhibited dose-dependent suppression of parasitaemia, but high doses were required to give suppression comparable to chloroquine (86% suppression at 1 g/kg/day) and on day 7 of the test 60% mortality of the mice was observed, suggesting a toxic effect. However, the authors of this study (Chandel and Bagai, 2010) reported that the $LD_{50}$ of the extract was >5 g/kg bodyweight in naïve mice and on this basis was considered to be safe. It is possible that mice with malaria are more sensitive to the extract, but the result may also suggest that while the extract has little acute toxicity it may exhibit toxicity when given in repeated doses and it should be noted that one of the isolated constituents, 8-*O*-acetylharpagide, has been reported to be cytotoxic. In contrast, a methanolic extract of the whole plant of *A. remota* Benth. (now also synonymous with *A. integrifolia* Buch.-Ham) was found to be inactive in mice infected with *P. berghei* strain NK65 when given orally at 1 g/kg/day. The lack of activity may be due to the use of the whole plant rather than the leaves as in the above study, or to variations in the plant constituents due to different growing conditions (Muregi *et al.*, 2007). Overall, the studies to date lend some support to the use of *A. integrifolia* as a traditional antimalarial but it may be potentially toxic. In addition to its direct antiplasmodial action, it has been postulated that this species could have immunomodulatory properties. This is based on the hypothesis that the constituent ergosterol-5,8-endoperoxide might mimic the action of dehydroepiandrosterone sulphate; the latter hormone has been shown to increase during puberty and correlates with resistance to malaria. In addition, phytoecdysones have been isolated from *A. integrifolia* and these could contribute to immunomodulatory/adaptogenic effects (Cocquyt *et al.*, 2011 and references therein).

## 12.3   Developments from established antimalarials

While novel antimalarial compounds are much needed, there is still scope for the continued development of established natural antimalarials. Recent progress with artemisinin (**9**) derivatives has been reviewed (Biamonte *et al.*, 2013), highlighting new methods of artemisinin production. The biosynthetic artemisinin precursor artemisinic acid may now be produced by a yeast fermentation process and then oxidized to yield artemisinin. Alternatively, a new synthesis from cyclohexenone requiring only five 'pots' has brought the prospect of industrial production closer. Newer derivatives of artemisinin include artemisone (**10**), which is up to 10-fold more potent than artesunate and, in combination with mefloquine, has been shown to cure *Aotus* monkeys with *P. falciparum* malaria with a single dose (10 mg and 5 mg/kg, respectively). Another approach has been the synthesis of peroxides known as ozonides based on the trioxane ring of artemisinin since the endoperoxide group is crucial for antimalarial activity. One of these, arterolane (**11**), is now available in combination with piperaquine as a three-day treatment of malaria in India, while a second-generation ozonide, OZ439 (**12**), has the advantage of a much longer half-life, which enables it to cure malaria in mice with a single dose of 10 mg/kg whereas this is only possible with other artemisinin derivatives in combination with a second drug (however, based on past experience it would be unwise to use OZ439 alone on account of the risk of parasite resistance development).

Febrifugine (**13**), a quinazolinone alkaloid from the Chinese herb *Dichroa febrifuga* Lour. (Hydrangeaceae) (Chang Shan), has long been known as a potentially effective antimalarial but it is metabolized in the liver to give a highly toxic epoxide derivative, precluding its clinical use. Derivatives of febrifugine designed so that epoxidation is blocked have been shown to be much less toxic, with high potency against malaria in monkeys (Zhu *et al.*, 2012).

The West African species *Cryptolepis sanguinolenta* (Lindl.) Schltr. (Asclepiadaceae) is used as a traditional antimalarial and contains the indoloquinoline alkaloids cryptolepine (**14**) and neocryptolepine (**16**). These alkaloids continue to be of interest as lead antimalarial compounds. Among synthetic cryptolepine analogues, 2,7-dibromocryptolepine (**15**) is of interest as it has encouraging *in vivo* activity in mice infected with *P. berghei* (90% suppression of parasitaemia when given intraperitoneally at 20 mg/kg/day) with no apparent toxicity to the mice (Onyeibor *et al.*, 2005). More recently, **15** given orally or parenterally has been shown to reduce parasitaemia and prolong survival time in mice infected with *Trypanosoma brucei*, the parasite responsible for African sleeping sickness (Oluwafemi *et al.*, 2009). Activity was also found against *Leishmania donovani* promastigotes and amastigotes although selectivity was relatively poor due to toxicity to the host macrophages (Hazra *et al.*, 2012). In another study, the mechanism(s) of action of cryptolepine were investigated in *L. donovani* promastigotes (Sengupta *et al.*, 2011). The results showed that cryptolepine induced apoptosis and oxidant stress in the parasites, but also that in *L. donovani* promastigotes cryptolepine toxicity is mitigated by autophagy, a parasite defence mechanism; when cryptolepine was given together with 3-methyladenine, an autophagy inhibitor, cryptolepine activity was enhanced and it is suggested that this finding could lead to new therapeutic strategies in the future.

Although **15** has potentially interesting antiprotozoal activities, with less toxicity compared to the parent compound, it has been shown to cause DNA damage in lymphocytes, but had no effect on human sperm DNA as assessed using the comet assay (Gopalan *et al.*, 2011). Regarding the metabolism of cryptolepine and its analogues, cryptolepine was shown to be a substrate for rabbit liver aldehyde oxidase but in contrast to cryptolepine, the metabolite cryptolepine-11-one was inactive against malaria parasites (Stell *et al.*, 2012). In contrast, **15** was not metabolized by aldehyde oxidase, a factor that may be important with respect to its *in vivo* antimalarial activity. In common with quinine, the antiplasmodial mode of action of **15** involves the inhibition of β-haematin formation, but it also has another, as yet unknown, mode of action. A dual mode of action may reduce the likelihood of parasite resistance development and this, coupled with the activity of **15** against three species of protozoa, provides impetus for further work on cryptolepine analogues in the future.

Neocryptolepine (**16**) and its analogues continue to be of interest; a number of analogues have been shown to have improved antiplasmodial activities and increased selectivity indices compared to neocryptolepine (Wang *et al.*, 2013). These compounds, in common with cryptolepine and its antiplasmodial analogues, were found to be inhibitors of β-haematin formation, but none has as yet been assessed for *in vivo* antimalarial activities.

## 12.4  Non-traditional medicine sources of potential antimalarials

Marine organisms continue to be an important source of novel antiplasmodial compounds (reviewed in Fattorusso and Taglialatela-Scafati, 2012). Bromphycolide A (**17**) is one of a novel class of meroditerpenes isolated from the marine red alga *Callophycus serratus* (Harvey ex Kützing) P.C. Silva and has been explored as an antimalarial lead compound (Teasdale *et al.*, 2013). This compound exhibits potent inhibition of both chloroquine-sensitive and chloroquine-resistant *P. falciparum* with low toxicity and good bioavailability, and despite liver metabolism and a short half-life it partially suppressed parasitaemia in mice infected

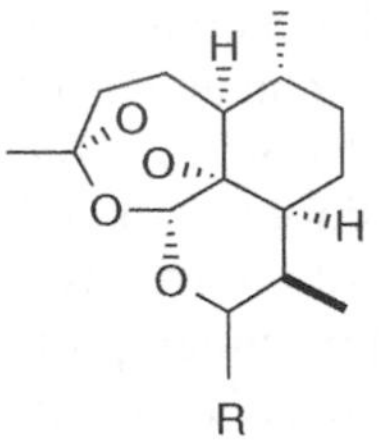

9  R = = O, artemisinin

10  R = —N (artemisone structure)          artemisone

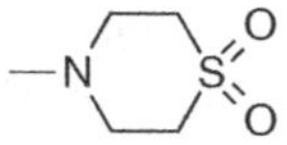

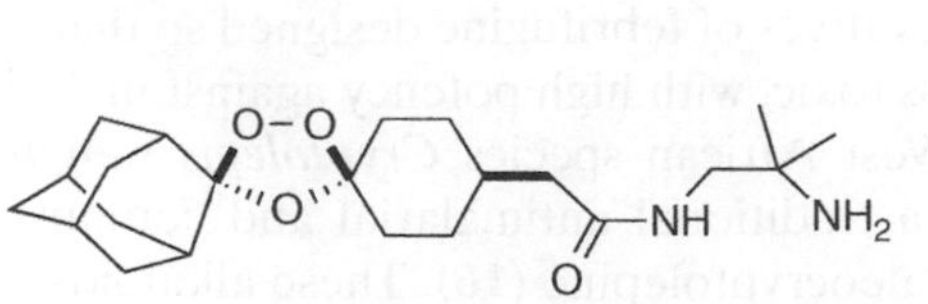

11  arterolane (OZ277)

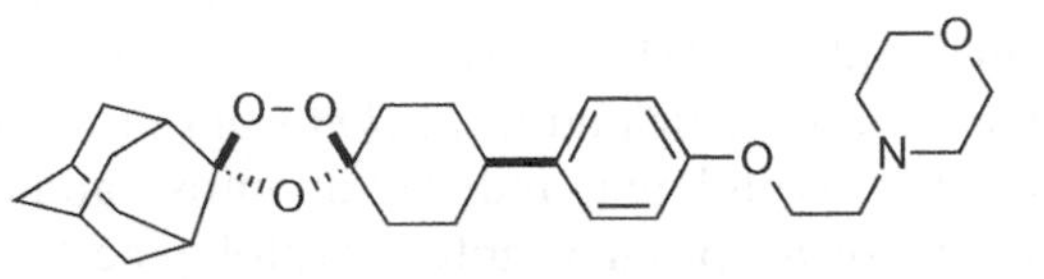

12  OZ439

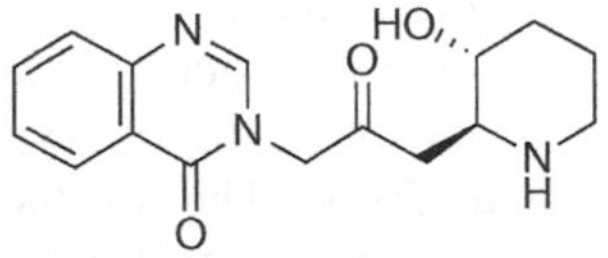

13  febrifugine

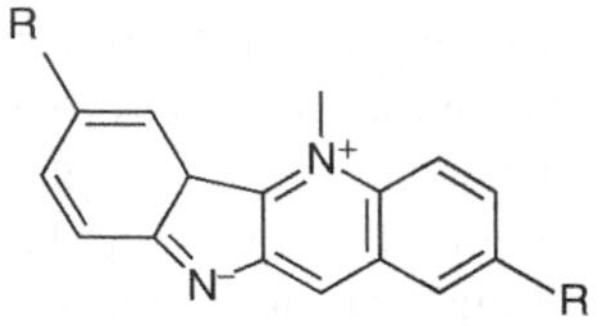

14  R = H, cryptolepine

15  R = Br, 2,7-dibromocryptolepine

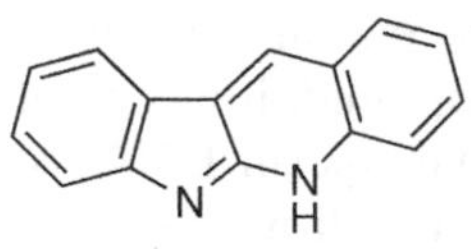

16  neocryptolepine

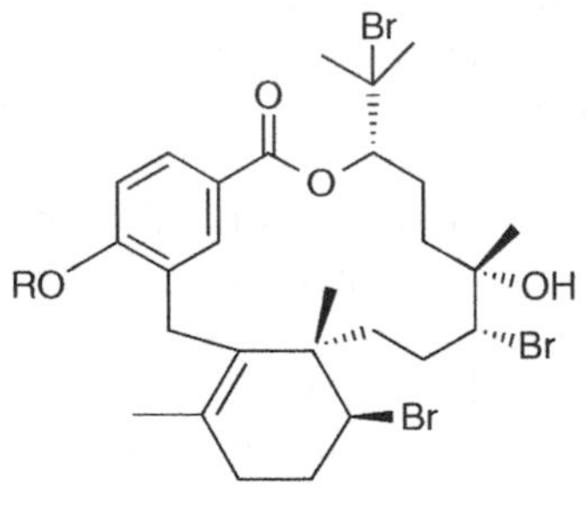

17  R = H, bromphycolide A

18  R = acetyl, 18-acetylbromphycolide A

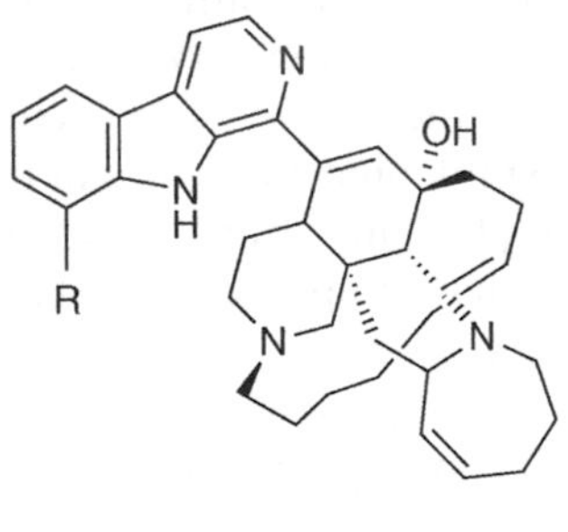

19  R = H, manzamine A

20  R = OH, 8-hydroxymanzamine A

with *P. yoelli* (47% suppression at 10mg/kg/day parenterally). Treatment of bromphycolide A with liver microsomal enzymes allowed the identification of possible phase I and II metabolites by LC-MS analysis and this knowledge has led to modifications of the molecule designed to prevent hydroxylation and/or glucuronidation. The semisynthetic analogue 18-acetylbromphycolide A (**18**) exhibits potent activity against *P. falciparum in vitro* but has yet to be assessed *in vivo*.

Marine sponges are of considerable interest as exemplified by compounds of the manzamine type, which are β-carboline alkaloids present in various sponge species found in the Indian and Pacific oceans (reviewed by Ashok *et al.*, 2014). Manzamine A (**19**), the first compound of this type, was isolated from Okinawa sponge (*Haliclona* sp. (Chalinidae)) in 1986 and in 2000 it was reported to have potent antiplasmodial activity ($IC_{50}$ = 4.5 and 8.0 ng/ml against *P. falciparum* strains D6 and W2, respectively) as well as >90% suppression of parasitaemia in malaria-infected mice with a single dose of 50 μM/kg given intraperitoneally while oral administration of two doses of 100 μM/kg suppressed parasitaemia by 90% for three days (Ang *et al.*, 2000). These promising results have prompted the investigation of natural and synthetic manzamine alkaloids as well as studies to determine their structure–activity relationships. The antimalarial mechanism of action of manzamines is uncertain but appears to involve the inhibition of DNA synthesis and this may explain the significant cytotoxicity observed with this class of compounds. Compared to manzamine A, some compounds, such as 8-hydroxymanzamine A (**20**), isolated from *Pachypellina* sp. (Phloeodictyidae), have better cytotoxic/antiplasmodial selectivity and potent *in vivo* antimalarial activity, but compounds with reduced *in vivo* toxicity need to be found/synthesized.

Another group of alkaloids with potential as antimalarials may be the pyrroloiminoquinones isolated from the Australian sponge *Zyzzya* sp. (Acarnidae) (Davis *et al.*, 2012). These compounds exhibited potent *in vitro* antiplasmodial activities ($IC_{50}$ < 100 nM) and makaluvamine G (**21**) was found to suppress parasitaemia in *P. berghei* infected mice by 48% when given subcutaneously at 8 mg/kg (higher doses could not be given due to limited compound availability). *In silico* physicochemical properties were calculated in order to determine the 'drug-likeness' of these alkaloids, while the potential for the metabolism of two compounds was tested using human and mouse hepatic microsomes *in vitro*. Makaluvamine G was found to be susceptible to metabolism and this is consistent with the low plasma levels observed following subcutaneous injection. In this study the authors carried out a more comprehensive evaluation of the compounds than is often the case and suggested that further work on one of the compounds, tsitsikammamine C (**22**), would be worthwhile.

## 12.5  Alternative strategies in the search for natural antimalarial compounds

With the development of molecular techniques and the 'omics' revolution, new strategies have become available for drug development and these are increasingly being employed in the search for new antiprotozoal agents (Becker, 2011). Many potential biochemical targets have been identified, such as *Plasmodium falciparum* thioredoxin reductase (*Pf*TrxR), so that compounds/extracts may be screened against specific parasite targets. An example of this approach is the use of mass spectrometry-based binding experiments, which led to the identification of oleamide (**23**) in an extract of *Guatteria recurvisepala* R.E.Fr. as a ligand to *Pf*TrxR (Munigunti *et al.*, 2011). Oleamide was found to exhibit modest activity against *P. falciparum in vitro* ($IC_{50}$ = 4.29 μg/ml). Cockburn *et al.* (2011) reported the screening of natural small molecules against *P. falciparum* heat shock protein (*Pf*Hsp70-1), which is believed to be essential for parasite survival and virulence in humans. Several compounds identified as modulators of *Pf*Hsp70-1 were found to have potent (low micromolar) activities against *P. falciparum*, including malonganenones A (**24**) and B (**25**), a new class of antiplasmodial compound. In another study, structure-based virtual screening was used to select potential falcipain-2 inhibitors from a natural products library (Wang *et al.*, 2014). Falcipain-2 is a malaria parasite cysteine protease enzyme that digests haemoglobin and is considered to be an attractive and promising target for antimalarials. The study identified 10 falcipain-2 inhibitors and one of these, the flavonoid glycoside quercetin-3-$O$-β-D-glucopyranoside (**26**), was found to have modest antiplasmodial activity ($IC_{50}$ = 5.54 and 4.05 µM, respectively, against chloroquine-sensitive (3D7) and chloroquine- resistant (Dd2) *P. falicaparum* strains). The activity of **26** against falcipain-2 was also relatively weak ($IC_{50}$ = 15.74 µM).

## 12.6   Herbal preparations for the treatment of malaria

Although most cases of malaria may be effectively treated with existing antimalarial drugs, these are not affordable and/or available to many of those who need them and this has led to a growing interest in the use of herbal medicines for malaria treatment (reviewed in Wright, 2010). In particular, a number of NGOs are promoting the local cultivation of *A. annua* L. in Africa and recommending the use of herbal teas made from the dried leaves. While clinical studies have shown that herbal teas prepared from high-artemisinin yielding cultivars of *A. annua* are effective in markedly reducing parasitaemia and symptoms in adult (semi-immune) malaria patients, recrudescent rates are high as not all parasites are killed. In addition, it cannot be assumed that the herbal teas will be similarly effective in young children, who have little immunity to malaria and are most at risk from severe disease and death from malaria. Furthermore, it is possible that the use of herbal preparations containing low levels of artemisinin may encourage the development of artemisinin-resistant parasites. Although it is argued that artemisinin may act synergistically with other constituents of *A. annua*, there is currently no evidence to show that herbal preparations are more effective than artemisinin alone in humans (especially with respect to recrudescence). However, in mice infected with *P. chabaudi* it was found that a single dose of dried *A. annua* reduced parasitaemia more effectively than an equivalent dose of artemisinin, possibly as a result of improved bioavailability of artemisinin, but the incidence of recrudescence in the two groups was not recorded (Elfawal *et al.*, 2012).

Interestingly, an examination of Chinese herbal texts has shown that in China *A. annua* (Qing Hao) was used as a fresh (rather than dried) herb and various methods of preparation are described, including pounding the herb to a pulp and then squeezing out the juice. The 'pounded juice' was found to have 20-fold higher artemisinin content than a herbal tea prepared from the same plant material (following drying) and was much more potent against malaria parasites *in vitro* and *in vivo* (Wright *et al.*, 2010). This study suggests that paying attention to the methods of preparation used by traditional healers may be worthwhile when evaluating traditional antimalarial remedies. In traditional Chinese medicine it is common for medicines to be prepared using a concoction of herbs and the investigation of combinations of herbs used with *A. annua* for malaria treatment may be worthwhile. A review of positive interactions between constituents of plant extracts of species used traditionally in the treatment of malaria has been published by Rasoanaivo *et al.* (2011). Curcumin (**27**), a phenolic compound found in the rhizomes of turmeric (*Curcuma longa* L., Zingiberaceae), has antiplasmodial activity and also has some effect in mice infected with malaria, but its effectiveness is compromised by glucuronidation in the small intestine. However, it has been proposed that as an adjunctive therapy, curcumin may act as an immunomodulator and have the potential to modulate or alleviate the effects of cerebral malaria (Jain *et al.*, 2013).

In the Democratic Republic of Congo an 80% ethanolic extract prepared from the stem bark of *Nauclea pobeguinii* (Pobég. ex Pellagr.) Merr. ex C.M.A. Petit (Rubiaceae) was evaluated in a Phase IIB clinical trial in adult patients with proven *P. falciparum* malaria (Mesla

21 makaluvamine G

22 tsitsikammamine C

23 oleamide

24 R = malonganenone A

25 R = malonganenone B

26 quercetin-3-O--D-glucopyranoside

27 curcumin

28 strictosamide

*et al.*, 2012). The extract contained 5.6% strictosamide (**28**), and patients received two 500 mg capsules three times a day for three days followed by one capsule three times a day for the next four days. A positive control group was treated with artesunate-amodiaquine. After 14 days, parasitological clearance rates were 87.9% in the extract-treated group compared to 96.9% in the artesunate-amodiaquine-treated group. No toxic effects were seen in the extract-treated group and side effects were reported to be less than in the positive control group. The authors concluded that the herbal extract is a promising candidate for the development of a herbal medicine for the treatment of uncomplicated malaria, but the medicine has not yet been evaluated in children.

## 12.7   Conclusion and future prospects

Although investigations into traditionally used antimalarials continue, an increasing range of natural product sources and drug-discovery strategies are being employed in the search for new treatments of malaria and this trend is expected to continue. In the coming decade it will be interesting to observe whether the new strategies are successful in delivering new antimalarials of similar calibre to artemisinin. Undoubtedly, many more natural products will be found that possess antiplasmodial properties and/or activity against a specific malaria parasite target, but the challenge will be to follow up on these compounds for *in vivo* antimalarial activity and for their potential as lead antimalarial compounds.

Encouragingly, morbidity rates due to malaria are falling, especially due to the wider availability of artemisinin combination therapy, and some authors suggest that malaria eradication may become possible. This would require effective antimalarial drugs acting not only against the trophic stages of malaria parasites infecting red blood cells (most current antimalarials) but also novel antimalarials targeting liver stage parasites in order to prevent the development of sporozoites inoculated by mosquitoes as well as drugs acting against gametocyte blood stages. Recently, an inexpensive and efficient assay for evaluating compounds for antigametocyte activity has been described (D'Alessandro *et al.*, 2013) that, with other developments such as a malaria vaccine, may one day make the prospect of a malaria-free world a closer reality.

## References

Ang, K.K.H., Holmes, M.J, Higa, T., *et al.* (2000) *In vivo* antimalarial activity of the beta-carboline alkaloid manzamine A. *Antimicrobial Agents and Chemotherapy*, **44**, 1645–1649.

Ashok, P., Ganguly, S. and Muruesan, S. (2014) Manzamine alkaloids: isolation, cytotoxicity, antimalarial activity and SAR studies. *Drug Discovery Today*, **19**, 1781–1791.

Becker, K. (2011) Apicomplexan parasites: molecular approaches toward targeted drug development, in *Drug Discovery in Infectious Diseases*, *Vol.* **2** (ed. P.M. Selzer), Taylor and Francis, Wiley-Blackwell.

Bero, J. and Quetin-Leclercq, J. (2011) Natural products published in 2009 from plants traditionally used to treat malaria. *Planta Medica*, **77**, 631–640.

Biamonte, M.A., Wanner, J. and Le Roch, K.G. (2013) Recent advances in malaria drug discovery. *Bioorganic & Medicinal Chemistry Letters*, **23**, 2829–2843.

Boniface, P.K. and Pal, A. (2013) Substantiation of the ethnopharmacological use of *Conyza sumatrensis* (Retz.) E.H. Walker in the treatment of malaria through *in vivo* evaluation in *Plasmodium berghei* infected mice. *Journal of Ethnopharmacology*, **145**, 373–377.

Bouquet, J., Rivaud, M., Chevalley, S., *et al.* (2012) Biological activities of nitidine, a potent anti-malarial lead compound. *Malaria Journal*, **11**, 67.

Chandel, S. and Bagai, U. (2010) Antiplasmodial activity of *Ajuga bracteosa* against *Plasmodium berghei* infected BALB/c mice. *Indian Journal of Medicial Research*, **131**, 440–444.

Cockburn, I.L., Pesce, E.-R., Pryzborski, J.M., *et al.* (2011) Screening for small molecule modulators of Hsp70 chaperone activity using protein aggregation suppression assays: inhibition of the plasmodial chaperone *Pf*Hsp70-1. *Biological Chemistry*, **392**, 431–438.

Cocquyt, K., Cos, P., Herewijn, P., *et al.* (2011) *Ajuga remota* Benth.: From ethnopharmacology to phytomedical perspective in the treatment of malaria. *Phytomedicine*, **18**, 1229–1237.

D'Alessandro, S., Silvestrini, F., Dechering, K., *et al.* (2013) A *Plasmodium falciparum* screening assay for anti-gametocyte drugs based on parasite lactate dehydrogenase detection. *Journal of Antimicrobial Chemotherapy*, **68**, 2048–2058.

Davis, R.A, Buchanan, M.S., Duffy, S., *et al.* (2012) Antimalarial activity of pyrroloiminoquinones from the Australian marine sponge *Zyzza* sp. *Journal of Medicinal Chemistry*, **55**, 5851–5858.

Dua, V.K., Verma, G., Singh, B., *et al.* (2013) Anti-malarial property of steroidal alkaloid conessine isolated from the bark of *Holarrhena antidysenterica*. *Malaria Journal*, **12**, 194.

Elfawal, M.A., Tolwer, M.J., Reich, N.G., *et al.* (2012) Dried whole plant *Artemisia annua* as an antimalarial therapy. *PLoS One*, **7**, e52746.

Fattorusso, E. and Taglialetela-Scafati, O. (2012) *The contribution of marine chemistry in the field of antimalarial research*, RSC Drug Discovery Series 25, *Drug Discovery from Natural Products*, Royal Society of Chemistry, Cambridge, pp. 374–390.

Gopalan, R.C., Emerce, E., Wright, C.W., *et al.* (2011) Effects of the antimalarial compound cryptolepine and its analogues in human lymphocytes and sperm in the Comet assay. *Toxicology Letters*, **207**, 322–325.

Hazra, S., Ghosh, S., Debnath, S., *et al.* (2012) Antileishmanial activity of cryptolepine analogues and apoptotic effects of 2,7-dibromocryptolepine against *Leishmania* donovani promastigotes. *Parasitology Research*, **111**, 195–203.

Jain, K., Sood, S. and Gowthamarajan, K. (2013) Modulation of cerebral malaria by curcumin as an adjunctive therapy. *Brazilian Journal of Infectious Diseases*, **17**, 579–591.

Mesia, K., Tona, L., Mampunza, N., *et al.* (2012) Antimalarial efficacy of a quantified extract of *Nauclea pobeguinii* stem bark in human adult volunteers with diagnosed uncomplicated *falciparum* malaria. Pat 2: A clinical phase IIB trial. *Planta Medica*, **78**, 853–860.

Munigunti, R., Nelson, N., Mulabagal, V., *et al.* (2011) Identification of oleamide in *Guatteria recurvisepala* by LC/MS-based *Plasmodium falciparum* thioredoxin reductase ligand binding method. *Planta Medica*, **15**, 1749–1753.

Muregi, F.W., Ishih, A., Miyase, T., *et al.* (2007) Antimalarial activity of methanolic extracts from plants used in Kenyan ethnomedicine and their interactions with chloroquine (CQ) against a CQ-tolerant rodent parasite, in mice. *Journal of Ethnopharmacology*, **111**, 190–195.

Oluwafemi, A.J., Okanla, O., Camps, P., *et al.* (2009) Evaluation of cryptolepine and huperzine derivatives as lead compounds towards new agents for the treatment of human African Trypanosomiasis. *Natural Product Communications*, **4**, 193–198.

Oluwatosin, A., Tolulope, A., Ayokulehin, K., *et al.* (2014) Antimalarial potential of kolaviron, a biflavonoid from *Garcinia kola* seeds against *Plasmodium berghei* infection in Swiss albino mice. *Asian Pacific Journal of Tropical Medicine*, **7**, 97–104.

Onyeibor, O., Croft, S.L., Dodson, H.I., *et al.* (2005) Synthesis of some cryptolepine analogues, assessment of their antimalarial and cytotoxic activities, and consideration of their antimalarial mode of action. *Journal of Medicinal Chemistry*, **48**, 2701–2709.

Pohlit, A.M., Lima, R.B.S., Frausin, G., *et al.* (2013) Amazonian plant natural products: Perspectives for discovery of new antimalarial drug leads. *Molecules*, **18**, 9219–9240.

Rasoanaivo, P., Wright, C.W., Willcox, M.L. and Giblert, B. (2011) Whole plant extracts versus single compounds for the treatment of malaria: synergy and positive interactions. *Malarial Journal*, **10** (Suppl 1), 54.

Sengupta, S., Chowdhury, S., Bose-Dasgupta, S., *et al.* (2011) Cryptolepine-induced cell death of *Leishmania donovani* promastigotes is augmented by inhibition of autophagy. *Molecular Biology International*, Article ID 187850.

Steck, E.A. (1971) *The Chemotherapy of Protozoan Diseases*, Walter Reed Army Institute of Research, Volume 3, pp. 138–142.

Stell, J.P., Wheelhouse, R.T. and Wright, C.W. (2012) Metabolism of cryptolepine and 2-fluorocryptolepine by aldehyde oxidase. *Journal of Pharmacy and Pharmacology*, **64**, 237–243.

Teasdale, M.E., Prudhomme, J., Torres, M., *et al.* (2013) Pharmacokinetics, metabolism and *in vitro* efficacy of the antimalarial natural product bromphycolide A. *ACS Medicinal Chemistry Letters*, **4**, 989–993.

Wang, N., Wicht, K.J., Wang, L., *et al.* (2013) Synthesis and *in vitro* testing of antimalarial activity of non-natural-type neocryptolepines: structure–activity relationship study of 2,11- and 9-11-disubstituted 6 methylindolo[2,3-*b*]quinolines. *Chemical and Pharmaceutical Bulletin*, **61**, 1282–1290.

Wang, L., Zhang, S., Zhu, J., *et al.* (2014) Identification of diverse natural products as falcipain-2-inhibitors through structure-based virtual screening virtual screening. *Bioorganic & Medicinal Chemistry Letters*, **24**, 1261–1264.

World Malaria Report (2013) http://w.w.w.who.int/malaria/media/world_malaria_report.2013/en/.

Wright, C.W. (2010) Recent developments in research on terrestrial plants used for the treatment of malaria. *Natural Product Reports*, **27**, 961–968.

Wright, C.W., Linley, P.A., Brun, R., *et al.* (2010) Ancient Chinese methods are remarkably effective for the preparation of artemisinin-rich extracts of Qing Hao with potent antimalarial activity. *Molecules*, **15**, 804–812.

Xu, Y-J. and Pieters, L. (2013) Recent developments in antimalarial natural products isolated from medicinal plants. *Mini-reviews in Medicinal Chemistry*, **13**, 1056–1072.

Zhu, S., Chandrashekar, G., Meng, L., *et al.* (2012) Febrifugine analogues: synthesis and antimalarial evaluation. *Bioorganic & Medicinal Chemistry*, **20**, 927–932.

# 13
# CNS Disorders

Anna K Jäger

*Department of Drug Design and Pharmacology, Faculty of Health and Medicinal Sciences, University of Copenhagen, Denmark*

## 13.1   Introduction

In many cultures there is a stigma attached to mental health problems. In some countries this stigma leads families to keep sick relatives out of sight, resulting in no medical care for them. Maybe there is no care available from the official healthcare system. Mental health care is under-prioritized in most healthcare systems, including in the western world.

Traditional healers generally use treatments that include the psychological, spiritual and socio-cultural aspects of mental health problems, as well as medicines. Activation of the patient, getting the patient to take responsibility for part of the process of healing, is often part of the treatment. Including 'mind aspects' might work especially well for mental health problems; similarly, the western approach might include both a psychiatrist and a psychologist.

The new WHO strategy for 2014–2023 on traditional medicine emphasises the important role for traditional medicine in healthcare, including mental health (WHO, 2013).

## 13.2   Epilepsy

Epilepsy is one of the most common diseases of the brain, affecting 50 million people world-wide (Quintans *et al.*, 2008). Globally, many patients with epilepsy are not under treatment with antiepileptic medicines, largely because of their lack of access to physicians and the cost of such medicines (Schachter, 2009). Of the patients receiving antiepileptic drugs, a third find that their seizures are resistant to treatment.

Cultures all over the world have used plants for centuries for treating epilepsy. Quintans *et al.* (2008) reviewed 355 plant species from different parts of the world that showed *in vivo* anticonvulsant activity. Likewise, a large number of purified compounds have been tested for various types of *in vitro* and *in vivo* antiepileptic and anticonvulsant activities (excellently reviewed by Zhu *et al.*, 2014).

*Ethnopharmacology*, First Edition. Edited by Michael Heinrich and Anna K. Jäger.
© 2015 John Wiley & Sons, Ltd. Published 2015 by John Wiley & Sons, Ltd.

Despite the widespread use of herbal therapies by patients with epilepsy, there is a striking lack of controlled evidence to support their use, and anecdotal reports suggest that some herbal therapies may pose a safety risk (Schachter, 2009). Of the ten best-selling medicinal plants for the treatment of epilepsy in the USA, there is no clinical data to support their use, only a case report on the use of Kava (*Piper methysticum* G.Forst – Piperaceae) in epilepsy (Pearl *et al.*, 2011). Despite promising results from preclinical *in vitro* and *in vivo* studies, the complete lack of clinical data to support efficacy highlights the need for well-conducted clinical trials. Lack of evidence is not evidence of lack of efficacy.

In our work on plants from Southern Africa used in the treatment of mental health problems we screened aqueous and ethanol extracts of 43 medicinal plants traditionally used to treat epilepsy and convulsions in the $GABA_A$-benzodiazepine receptor-binding assay (Risa *et al.*, 2004). These investigations led to the identification of the flavonoids apigenin, agathisflavone and amentoflavone as the active compounds from *Searsia* species (basionym: *Rhus* – Anacardiaceae) (Svenningsen *et al.*, 2006). Apigenin had previously not showed anticonvulsant activity *in vivo* (Viola *et al.*, 1995). Amentoflavone was reported to be a relatively weak negative allosteric modulator of GABA action, acting independently of the flumazenil binding site (Hanrahan *et al.*, 2003), thus the use of these plants as anticonvulsive agents suggested involvement of a different neurotransmitter system. Further functional characterization of the *Searsia* extracts showed inhibitory effects on spontaneous epileptiform discharges in mouse cortical slices (Pedersen *et al.*, 2008). Interestingly, the effect was not caused by the previous isolated flavonoids. The extracts contained N-methyl-D-aspartate (NMDA) receptor antagonists, which might explain the effect of the plants reported by traditional healers.

The example above illustrates the situation where an *in vitro* test shows a positive result, the active compounds are isolated, but there is no *in vivo* activity. In this case the expanded functional testing showed that the extracts worked via another mechanism than originally tested for, but that also resulted in anti-convulsive activity. This highlights the question of bioavailability, especially the passage through the blood–brain barrier for CNS-active plant extracts. It has been questioned whether flavonoids would reach the CNS. In recent years a number of studies have investigated this, showing that certain flavonoids are able to be absorbed after oral administration, pass through the blood–brain barrier and have various effects on the CNS (Jäger and Saaby, 2011).

In Africa the prevalence of epilepsy is more than double that in developed economies. This was thought to be due to birth defects caused by a lack of proper obstetrician facilities during delivery. However, when MRI scanners became available in Africa it quickly became clear that a high percentage of epilepsy patients had cysts in their brains from the eggs of the pork tapeworm *Taenia solium* (van As and Joubert, 1991; Garcia *et al.*, 2003; DeGiorgio *et al.*, 2005). These eggs cause small areas of the brain to die; in scans it looks like the brain is full of holes. Currently, clinical trials are being carried out to establish the effect of antiparasitic medicines in the treatment of neurocysticercosis-induced epilepsy.

Some years ago we tested a mixture of South African plants used to treat epilepsy (Jäger *et al.*, 2005). The healer claimed that this mixture had been used by healers in his family back to the 17th century, and that one treatment was sufficient to cure the patient of epilepsy. I was always very sceptical of this claim of a single treatment cure, but in light of the new insight, the healer might have been right, if the treatment killed the tapeworm larvae. It might have been the scientists that did not understand, or even know about, the underlying disease mechanism, and tested for the wrong activity.

Another thought-provoking consequence of neurocystosis-induced epilepsy is that it is contagious. Western medicine has for generations taught that you cannot be infected with epilepsy. Better sanitation and avoidance of 'crunchy meat' (pork meat with visible lumps of tapeworms, which give the meat a delicate crunch) might bring down the incidence rate of epilepsy.

## 13.3 Depression and anxiety

Depression and anxiety disorders are a major health burden in both developed and developing countries. One in three people in economically developed countries will during their lifetime experience episodes of depression. In areas stricken by war and natural disasters, the incidences are even higher. WHO estimates that by 2020 depression will be the second most prevalent disease in the world. Patients on extended sick leave due to depression are a huge socioeconomic burden for society.

### 13.3.1 Selective serotonin reuptake inhibitors

Selective serotonin reuptake inhibitors (SSRIs) block the reuptake of serotonin released into the postsynaptic gap back into the nerve cell, thus increasing the level of active serotonin in the postsynaptic gap. This increased serotonin level leads to a less depressed state of mind, and so these compounds have been the first choice treatment for depression for well over a decade. The serotonin transporter is the target for SSRIs.

*Sceletium tortuosum* (L.) N.E. Br (Aizoaceae), a succulent from South Africa used in traditional medicine, was one of the first plant species that attracted attention as an SSRI. In 2001 a patent was issued on mesembrine, a constituent of *S. tortuosum*, as an inhibitor of the serotonin transporter (US Patent, 2001). Further studies revealed that the extract also inhibits phosphodiesterase 4, suggesting that the effect of the extract is enhanced by dual action on the serotonin transporter and phosphdiesterase 4 (Harvey *et al.*, 2011). Smaller clinical studies indicate anxiolytic activity, and a recent functional magnetic resonance imaging study showed the attenuating effects of *S. tortuosum* on the threat circuitry of the human brain, providing supporting evidence that the dual serotonin reuptake inhibition and phosphodiesterase 4 inhibition of the extract might have anxiolytic potential by attenuating subcortical threat responsivity (Terburg *et al.*, 2013).

Depression might not be a diagnosis known by traditional healers. In our work in Southern Africa we included conditions like 'being put down by the spirits' within the indication category 'depression', as it had elements with similarities to the western diagnosis of depression. We screened 75 aqueous and ethanolic extracts from 34 plant species used in Southern Africa for depression for affinity to the serotonin transporter. Extracts of five species (*Agapanthus campanulatus* F.M.Leight. (Amaryllidaceae), *Boophane disticha* (L.f.) Herb. (Amaryllidaceae), *Datura ferox* L. (Solanaceae), *Mondia whitei* (Hook.f.) Skeels (Apocynaceae) and *Xysmalobium undulatum* (L.) W.T.Aiton (Apocynaceae)) had high affinity to the serotonin transporter.

As SSRIs are given as long-term treatment, we excluded *D. ferox* as a potentially useful ethnopharmacological medicine because of the well-known (side) effects of tropane alkaloids. During chemical characterization of *X. undulatum*, we discovered that what we had expected from TLC–Dragendorff analysis to be an alkaloid was in fact a cardiac glycoside. A medicinal plant containing cardiac glycosides should not be encouraged for long-time use for a non-heart-related condition, so we discontinued the work on *X. undulatum*.

The three remaining species were tested in three animal models for depression, the forced swim test (both mice and rats) and the tail suspension test on mice. *B. disticha* showed activity in all three assays, whereas the other Amarylidaceae species, *A. campanulatus*, only had activity in the mice forced swim test. *M. whitei* had an effect in the rat forced swim test, but not in any of the mice assays. The extracts were also characterized for activity on other transporters in COS-7 cells transfected with human serotonin, noradrenaline and dopamine transporters. The two Amaryllidaceous species affected all three transporters, whereas *M. whitei* showed selectivity for the serotonin transporter.

Bioassay-guided isolation from *B. disticha* led to the isolation of a series of buphanamine-type Amaryllidaceae alkaloids with affinity to the serotonin transporter (Neergaard *et al.*, 2009). *B. disticha* is a well-known, much-used medicinal plant, but also one that needs to be used with care due to its potential for toxic overdoses. The toxicology of *B. disticha* was recently reviewed by Nair and van Staden (2014), who concluded that the toxicity might mainly be due to lycorine, which is not one of the alkaloids with affinity to the serotonin transporter.

Bioassay-guided isolation from *M. whitey* led to the isolation of the monoterpene lactone (–)-loliolide as an SSRI (Neergaard *et al.*, 2010). It is unusual in that it is not an alkaloid, as CNS-active compounds normally are. *M. whitey* is distributed throughout sub-Saharan Africa, and is a valued medicine for depression and as an aphrodisiac (Oketch-Rabah, 2012), although no clinical data exist.

## 13.3.2 MAO-A inhibitors

Monoamine oxidases (MAOs) are mitochondria-bound enzymes that catalyse the oxidative deamination of primary, secondary and tertiary amines. They play an important role in controlling the concentration of monoamine neurotransmitters such as serotonin, dopamine, noradrenaline and adrenaline in the synapse.

There are two isoforms of MAOs in the brain, MAO-A and MAO-B. These are distinguished by different but overlapping substrate specificities. MAO-B is dealt with in the section on dementia.

MAO-A inhibitors have been shown to be effective antidepressants, but their severe side effects, such as hypertensive crisis and interaction with serotonergic drugs, limit their use so they are prescribed only to patients who fail to respond to other antidepressant medicines.

A large number of plants have been shown to possess MAO-A inhibitory activity and these have been recently reviewed by Vina *et al.* (2012). Certain plant-derived compounds have potent MAO-A inhibition. The widely distributed flavonoid quercetin has shown MAO-A inhibition in the nanomolar range (Chimenti *et al.*, 2006).

## 13.3.3 Clinical evidence

A recent review analysed all published studies on clinical trials on medicinal plants used for depression and anxiety (Sarris *et al.*, 2013). Currently, only one plant species has sufficient clinical data to support its use for depression: *Hypericum perforatum* L., St John's Wort (Hypericaceae). There exists partial evidence for the use of *Crocus sativus* L. (Iridaceae), *Rhodiola rosea* L. (Crassulaceae) and *Echium amoenum* Fisch. & C.A.Mey. (Boraginaceae) for depression. For generalized anxiety disorder there is evidentiary support from multiple trials for the use of *Piper methysticum* and *Galphimia glauca* Cav. (Malpighiaceae). For treatment of acute anxiolytic activity there is some evidence for the use of *Centella asiatica* (L.) Urb. (Apiaceae), *Salvia* spp. (Lamiaceae), *Melissa officinalis* L. (Lamiaceae), *Passiflora incarnate* L. (Passifloraceae) and *Citrus × aurantium* L. (Rutaceae), whereas for treatment of chronic anxiety *Piper methysticum*, *Matricaria chamomilla* L. (Asteraceae), *Ginkgo biloba* L. (Ginkgoaceae), *Scutellaria lateriflora* L. (Lamiaceae), *Silybum marianum* (L.) Gaertn. (Asteraceae), *Passiflora incarnata Withania somnifera* (L.) Dunal (Solanaceae), *Galphimia glauca, Centella asiatica, Rhodiola rosea, Echinacea* spp. (Asteraceae), *Melissa officinalis* and *Echium amoenum* have shown some evidence. For treatment of anxiolytic effects in people with cognitive decline there is some evidence for the use of *Bacopa monnieri* (L.) Wettst. (Plantaginaceae).

## 13.4 Insomnia

Both acute and chronic insomnia are major health burdens. People who do not get a good night's sleep do not function well. The prevalence of insomnia is relatively high, with 17.4% of adults self-reporting insomnia or having trouble sleeping during a 12-month period (Pearson *et al.*, 2002). A systematic review of insomnia identified ten randomized clinical trials of a sufficient quality studying the hypnotic effect of *Valeriana officinalis* L. (Caprifoliaceae), *Humulus lupulus* L. (Cannabaceae) and *Piper methysticum* and combinations thereof (Sarris and Byrne, 2011). The studies on *V. officinalis*, which were conducted over 2–6 weeks, were inconclusive, with three positive and three negative results. Two studies on a combination of *V. officinalis* and *H. lupulus* indicated an effect on sleep latency and reduced severity of insomnia. For *P. methysticum*, one study showed improved quality of sleep, whereas another study did not find any kind of effect.

As pointed out in the review by Wheatley (2005), the positive effects of *V. officinalis* might be in chronic insomnia, although there is no clear evidence for this. Overall, there is only weak evidence for herbal extracts in treating insomnia.

## 13.5 Sedatives

Several species of the Lamiaceae, such as *Salvia* sp., *Melissa officinalis* and *Lavandula angustifolia* Mill., have long had a reputation in European popular medicine as having a sedative effect. An extract of *Salvia officinalis* L. has been shown to lower agitation in patients with Alzheimer's disease (Akhondzadeh *et al.*, 2003). Likewise, aromatherapy with essential oils from *L. angustifolia* and *M. officinalis* reduced agitation in patients suffering from Alzheimer's disease (Holmes *et al.*, 2002; Snow *et al.*, 2004; Lin *et al.*, 2007).

From our database on Southern African mental health plants we selected the species used for sedation. We screened extracts for binding to the benzodiazepine site of the GABA$_A$-receptor. One of the plants that stood out was *Piper capense*. From the roots of this plant we isolated by bioassay-guided fractionation two alkaloids, piperine and 4,5-dihydropiperine, the latter slightly more active than piperine (Pedersen *et al.*, 2009). We synthesised a small library of analogues and determined their affinity to the benzodiazepine site. Structure–activity relationship analysis showed that we could not make a compound more active than the one made by nature in *P. capense*, namely 4,5-dihydropiperine (Pedersen *et al.*, 2009). No further work has been published on 4,5-dihydropiperine, but there a lot of research activity around piperine. Piperine is a well-known constituent of *Piper* species.

## 13.6 Dementia

An ageing population is a reality in many western countries, but simple demographic projections show that within a few decades developing countries will also have massive elderly populations. With age comes dementia: 5% of people over 65 and about half of those over 85 suffer from dementia (Evans *et al.*, 1989). Dementia is thus a major public health concern.

Aging in humans is generally associated with deterioration of cognitive performance, especially learning and memory. Dementia is not a disease, but a number of symptoms stemming from other disease or conditions. Alzheimer's disease accounts for about 60% of dementia cases, with vascular dementia the second most prevalent form of dementia, with 20% of cases, and Parkinson's disease and vascular dementia with Lewy bodies each accounting for 5% of cases (Kalaria *et al.*, 2008).

## 13.6.1   Countering neurotransmitter abnormalities: acetylcholinesterase inhibitors

A deficiency in cholinergic neurotransmission is a cause of dementia. In order to increase the level of choline available for neurotransmission, inhibitors of cholinesterase were developed. The development of medicines based on the alkaloid galanthamine from snowdrops (Galanthus sp. – Amaryllidaceae) is described in Chapter 8. Rivastigmine, a semi-synthetic derivative of the alkaloid physostigmine (from *Physostigma venenosum* Balf. – Fabaceae), has also been approved in many countries as an acetylcholinesterase inhibitor. The acetyl-cholinesterase inhibitor huperzine A, a sesquiterpene alkaloid from *Huperzia serrata* (Thunb.) Trevis. (Lycopodiaceae) used traditional Chinese medicine for dementia, is also sold in parts of the world as a (generally unlicensed) supplement. A recent meta-analysis of randomized clinical trials showed beneficial effects of huperzine A on cognitive functions, but also stated that the findings should be interpreted with caution due to the poor methodological quality of the included trials (Yang *et al.*, 2013).

The success of galanthamine inspired a search for other acetylcholinesterase inhibitors. The relative ease of the assay technique made it accessible for researchers in less affluent universities to conduct these studies. Today, we know of hundreds of plants and compounds with acetyl/butyrylesterase inhibitory activity (for recent reviews see Howes and Perry, 2011; Kumar *et al.*, 2012; Natarajan *et al.*, 2013; Konrath *et al.*, 2013). However, despite several of these compounds showing higher *in vitro* activity that the current registered medicines, there is probably no scope for further cholinesterase inhibitors on the market. The challenge now is therefore to identify the species with the best potential as phytomedicines for use in traditional and complementary treatment.

## 13.6.2   Countering neurotransmitter abnormalities: MAO-B inhibitors

MAO-B plays a role in controlling the level of monoamine neurotransmitters. As part of the normal ageing process in humans the level of MAO-B increases in the brain, and it is generally higher in patients with neurodegenerative diseases as Alzheimer's and Parkinson's. Inhibition of MAO-B confers neuroprotection through anti-apoptotic mechanisms, stabilization of the mitochondrial membrane and a reduction of reactive oxygen species.

A high number of plant compounds and extracts have shown MAO-B inhibition, these have been reviewed recently (Carradori *et al.*, 2014). The authors of this review point out that it is very difficult to compare results from different studies as the methodology varies widely. Nevertheless, there is consensus that flavonoids are a promising source of MAO-B inhibitors. The flavonoids tend to inhibit both the MAO-A and MAO-B isoform, so to avoid unintended effects it is necessary to select the flavonoids which have high selectivity towards MAO-B. Gancaonin A (5,7-dihydroxy-4'-methoxy-6-prenylisoflavone) from the fruits of *Cudrania tricuspidata* (unresolved name, probably a Moraceae) had an $IC_{50}$ value of 0.8 µM and a

MAO-B SI ($IC_{50}$ MAO-A/$IC_{50}$ MAO-B) of 1000 (Han *et al.*, 2005). 5-Hydroxyflavanone from *Sinofranchetia chinensis* (Franch.) Hemsl. (Lardizabalaceae) had an $IC_{50}$ of 3.8 µM and an SI of 10 (Haraguchi *et al.*, 2004). Formononetin and kushenol F, both isolated from *Sophora flavescens* Aiton (Fabaceae), were active in the lower micromolar range, with SI of 2 for MAO-B (Hwang *et al.*, 2005).

The alkaloid methylpiperate, isolated from *Piper longum* L. (Piperaceae), inhibited MAO-B with an $IC_{50}$ of 1.6 µM and SI of 17 (Lee *et al.*, 2008). Chemical modification of coumarin has produced a brominated coumarin with an extreme SI of 135870 (Penin *et al.*, 2010), but as such compounds are not found in nature, it has little relevance in traditional medicine.

## 13.6.3 Reducing the formation and fibrillation of amyloid β peptides

Another target for the treatment of dementia is reduction of the production of amyloid β peptides (Aβ) by inhibition of β-secretase (BACE1), which is the rate-limiting enzyme involved in the formation of Aβ. Soluble Aβ can fibrillate to form the main component of intracellular neurofibrillary tangles and extracellular senile plaques in synaptic terminals.

A number of plant-derived compounds have shown inhibition of BACE1. Among the most active compounds *in vitro* are ellagic acid and punicalagin, both isolated from husk of *Punica granatum* L. (Lythraceae), which have *Ki* values below the micromolar range (Kwak *et al.*, 2005). Compounds with *Ki* values in the low micromolar range include catechins from green tea (*Camellia sinensis* (L.) Kuntze (Theaceae), *trans/cis*-resveratrol, oxyresveratrol, veraphenol and *cis*-scirpusin A from *Smilax china* L. (Smilacaceae), tellimagradin II and a pentagalloyl-glucopyranoside from Sanguisorbae radix (likely *Sanquisorba officinalis* L. – Rosaceae), and epiberberine and groenlandicine from the rhizome of *Coptis chinensis* Franch. (Ranunculaceae) (Jeon *et al.*, 2003, 2007; Lee *et al.*, 2005; Jung *et al.*, 2009). Slightly lower activity was observed with rosmarinic acid, known from several Lamiaceaous species, and the ubiquitous flavone luteolin (Choi *et al.*, 2008).

Several compounds and plant extracts possess the ability to prevent fibrillation of Aβ or even defibrillate the already formed tangles and plaques.

Quercetin, gossypetin and myricetin from green tea, rutin, rosmarinic acid, curcumin, salvianolic acid B from *Salvia miltiorrhiza* Bunge (Lamiaceae) and a penta-galloyl-glucopyranose from *Paeonia* × *suffriticosa* Andrews (Paeoniaceae) all prevented fibrillation of Aβ (Natarajan *et al.*, 2013).

Extracts of *Ginkgo biloba*, *Withania somnifera*, walnut (likely *Juglans regia* L. – Juglandaceae) and *Uncaria rhynchophylla* (Miq.) Miq. ex Havil. (Rubiaceae) reduced the formation of fibrils of Aβ (Natarajan *et al.*, 2013).

Perhaps most interestingly, resveratrol from red wine deaggregated Aβ-fibrils, and aqueous extract from *Caesalpinia crista* L. (Fabaceae) both inhibited and disaggretated the preformed fibrils (Natarajan *et al.*, 2013). Curcumin has been shown to disrupt existing plaques *in vivo*. It has even been suggested that the lower rate of dementia in India could be due the high consumption of curry dishes rich in turmeric (*Curcuma longa* L. – Zingiberaceae), the source of curcumin (Ng *et al.*, 2006).

## 13.6.4 Anti-inflammatory and antioxidant activity

Inflammation is often associated with neurodegeneration and might worsen the situation. Inhibition of cyclooxygenase or NF-κB transactivation could reduce the damaging inflammatory condition. A long list of plants have shown potential as anti-inflammatory agents *in vitro* (Natarajan *et al.*, 2013).

The inflammatory condition might lead to production of reactive oxygen species. The elevated levels of reactive oxygen species and reactive nitrogen species might cause oxidative stress and are potential causes of neurodegeneration. A high number of plants have demonstrated antioxidant activity in chemical tests. Some of these results must be viewed critically as such tests might not reflect a real clinical effect.

The best preventative treatment for dementia might be a combination of anti-inflammatory and antioxidant activities. A number of plant species possess this dual activity. An example is green tea, where the catechins act as reactive oxygen species scavangers and the flavonoids have antioxidant activity (Rice-Evans *et al.*, 1996). However, it could of course also be a treatment combining two plant species with anti-inflammatory and antioxidant activity, respectively.

Overall, looking at the plants used in the treatment of dementia, cholinesterase inhibitors have a lower therapeutic index and the source plants are classified as medicinal plants. For the treatment of senile plaques and tangles, and reduction of inflammation and lowering of oxidative reactants, many of the compounds are found in dietary plants. As has been argued convincingly by ethnopharmacologists in most traditional medicine systems, diet is also part of the treatment.

## 13.7   Conclusion

One common feature of mental diseases is that they are a huge burden for the society. Diseases in the CNS present in many ways and have a number of underlying causes, which we do not always fully understand. We need better treatment, and we need accessible, reliable treatment. To provide this, we need to identify the plant species with proven activity. There is a wealth of pre-clinical work, a lot of it scattered, so there need to be a focused effort to get the work to the stage that justifies going on to clinical trials. Most importantly, there is a serious lack of clinical trials.

A question that needs some thought is whether we need a battery of mental health plants for each climatic zone/continent/traditional medicine system? Are healers and patients prepared to use 'foreign' plants, and will they be available at a financially accessible price?

This chapter shows that there are plants out there to treat the major CNS diseases.

## References

Akhondzadeh, S., Noroozian, J., Mohammadi, M., *et al.* (2003) *Saliva officinalis* extract in the treatment of patients with mild to moderate Alzheimer's disease: a double blind, randomized and placebo-controlled trial. *Journal of Clinical Pharmacology and Therapeutics*, **28**, 53–59.

Carradori, S., D'Ascenzio, M., Chimenti, P., *et al.* (2014) Selective MAO-B inhibitors: a lesson from natural products. *Molecular Diversity*, **18**, 219–243.

Chimenti, F., Cottiglia, F., Bonsignore, L., *et al.* (2006) Quercetin as the active principle of *Hypericum hircinum* exerts a selective inhibitory activity against MAO-A: Extraction, biological analysis, and computational study. *Journal of Natural Products*, **69**, 945–949.

Choi, S.H., Hur, J.M., Yang, E.J., *et al.* (2008) Beta-secretase (BACE1) inhibitors from *Perilla fructescens* var. *Acuta*. *Archives of Pharmacal Research*, **31**, 183–187.

DeGiorgio, C., Pietsch-Escueta, S., Tsang, V., *et al.* (2005) Sero-prevalence of *Taenia solium* cysticercosis and *Taenia solium* taeniasis in California, USA. *Acta Neurologica Scandinavica*, **111**, 84–88.

Evans, D.A., Funkenstein, H.H., Albert, M.S., *et al.* (1989) Prevalence of Alzheimer's disease in a community population of older persons. Higher than previously reported. *Journal of the American Medical Association*, **262**, 2551–2556.

Garcia, H.H., Gonzalez, A.E., Evans, C.A. and Gilman, R.H. (2003) Cysticercosis Working Group in Peru. *Taenia solium cysticercosis. Lancet*, **362**, 547–556.

Han, X.H., Hong, S.S., Hwang, J.S., *et al.* (2005) Monoamine oxidase inhibitory constituents from the fruits of *Cundrania tricuspidata. Archives of Pharmacal Research*, **28**, 1324–1327.

Hanrahan, J.R., Chebib, M., Davucheron, N.M., *et al.* (2003) Semisynthetic preparation of amentoflavone: a negative modulator at GABAA receptors. *Bioorganic and Medicinal Chemistry Letters*, **13**, 2281–2284.

Haraguchi, H., Tanaka, Y., Kabbash, A., *et al.* (2004) Monoamine oxidase inhibitors from *Gentiana lutea. Phytochemistry*, **65**, 2255–2260.

Harvey, A.L., Young, L.C., Viljoen, A.M. and Gericke, N.P. (2011) Pharmacological actions of the South African medicinal and functional food plant *Sceletium tortuosum* and its principal alkaloids. *Journal of Ethnopharmacology*, **137**, 1124–1129.

Holmes, C., Hopkins, V., Hensford, C., *et al.* (2002) Lavender oil as a treatment for agitated behaviour in severe dementia: a placebo controlled study. *International Journal of Geriatric Psychiatry*, **17**, 305–308.

Howes, M.J.R. and Perry, E. (2011) The role of phytochemicals in the treatment and prevention of dementia. *Drugs Aging*, **28**, 439–468.

Hwang, J.S., Lee, S.A., Hong, S.S., *et al.* (2005) Monoamine oxidase inhibitory components from the roots of *Sophora flavescens. Archives of Pharmacal Research*, **28**, 190–194.

Jäger, A.K. and Saaby, L. (2011) Flavonoids and the CNS. *Molecules*, **16**, 1471–1485.

Jäger, A.K., Mohoto, S.P., van Heerden, F.R. and Viljoen, A.M. (2005) Activity of a traditional South African epilepsy remedy in the GABA-benzodiazepine receptor assay. *Journal of Ethnopharmacology*, **96**, 603–606.

Jeon, S.Y., Seong, Y.H. and Song, K.S. (2003) Green tea catechins as a BACE1 (beta-secretase) inhibitor. *Bioorganic & Medicinal Chemistry Letters*, **13**, 3905–3908.

Jeon, S.Y., Kwon, S.H., Seong, Y.H., *et al.* (2007) Beta-secretase (BACE1)-inhibiting stilbenoids from *Smilax rhizome. Phytomedicine*, **14**, 403–408.

Jung, A.Y.H., Byung-Sun, M.I.N., Yokozawa, T., *et al.* (2009) Anti-Alzheimer and antioxidant activities of coptidis rhizome alkaloids. *Biological and Pharmaceutical Bulletin*, **32**, 1433–1438.

Kalaria, R.N., Maestre, G.E., Arizaga, R., *et al.* (2008) Alzheimer's disease and vascular dementia in developing countries: prevalence, management, and risk factors. *Lancet Neurology*, **7**, 812–826.

Konrath, E.L., Passos, C.D.S., Klein-Junior, L.C. and Henriques, A.T. (2013) Alkaloids as a source of potential anticholinesterase inhibitors for the treatment of Alzheimer's disease. *Journal of Pharmacy and Pharmacology*, **65**, 1701–1725.

Kumar, H., More, S.V., Han, S.D., *et al.* (2012) Promising therapeutics with natural bioactive compounds for improving learning and memory – A review of randomized trials. *Molecules*, **202**, 10503–10539.

Kwak, H.M., Jeon, S.Y., Sohng, B.H., *et al.* (2005) Beta-secretase (BACE1) inhibitors from pomegranate (*Punica granantum*) husk. *Archives of Pharmacal Research*, **28**, 1328–1332.

Lee, H.J., Seong, Y.H., Bae, K.H., *et al.* (2005) Beta-secretase (BACE1) inhibitors from sanguisorbae radix. *Archives of Pharmacal Research*, **28**, 799–803.

Lee, S.A., Hwang, J.S., Han, X.H., *et al.* (2008) Methylpiperate derivatives from *Piper longum* and their inhibition of monoamine oxidase. *Archives of Pharmacal Research*, **31**, 679–683.

Lin, P.W., Chan, W.C., Ng, B.F. and Lam, L.C. (2007) Efficacy of aromatherapy (*Lavandula angustifolia*) as an intervention for agitated behaviours in Chinese older persons with dementia: a cross-over randomized trial. *International Journal of Geriatric Psychiatry*, **22**, 405–410.

Nair, J.J. and van Staden, J. (2014) Traditional usage, phytochemistry and pharmacology of the South African medicinal plant Boophone disticha (L.f.) Herb. (Amaryllidaceae). *Journal of Ethnopharmacology*, **151**, 12–26.

Natarajan, S., Shunmugiah, K.P. and Kasi, P.D. (2013) Plants traditionally used in age-related brain disorders (dementia): an ethnopharmacological survey. *Pharmaceutical Biology*, **51**, 492–523.

Neergaard, J.S., Andersen, J., Pedersen, M.E., *et al.* (2009) Alkaloids from *Boophone disticha* with affinity to the serotonin transporter. *South African Journal of Botany*, **75**, 371–374.

Neergaard, J.S., Rasmussen, H.B., Stafford, G.I., *et al.* (2010) Serotonin transporter affinity of (–)-loliolide, a monoterpene lactone from Mondia whitei. *South African Journal of Botany*, **76**, 593–596.

Ng, T.P., Chiam, P.C. and Lee, T. (2006) Curry consumption and cognitive function in the elderly. *American Journal of Epidemiology*, **164**, 898–906.

Oketch-Rabah, H.A. (2012) *Mondia whitei*, a medicinal plant from Africa with aphrodisiac and antidepressant properties: a review. *Journal of Dietary Supplements*, **9**, 272–284.

Pearl, P.L., Drillings, I.M. and Conry, J.A. (2011) Herbs in epilepsy: evidence for efficacy, toxicity, and interactions. *Seminars in Pediatric Neurology*, **18**, 203–208.

Pearson, N.J., Johnson, L.L. and Nahin, R.L. (2006) Insomnia, trouble sleeping, and complementary and alternative medicine: analysis of the 2002 national health inverview survey data. *Archives of Internal Medicine*, **166**, 1775–1782.

Pedersen, M.E., Vestergaard, H.T., Stafford, G.I., *et al.* (2008) The effect of extracts of *Searsia* species on epileptiform activity in slices of the mouse cerebral cortex. *Journal of Ethnopharmacology*, **119**, 538–541.

Pedersen, M.E., Metzler, B., Stafford, G.I., *et al.* (2009) Amides from *Piper capense* with CNS activity – A preliminary SAR analysis. *Molecules*, **14**, 3833–3843.

Penin, L.S., Cambiero, F.O., Castelao D.V., *et al.* (2010). Uso de derivados de 3-fenilcumarinas 6-sustituidas y preparacion de vuevos derivados. Universidade de Santiago de Compostela. Patent No. WO2010086484 A1.

Quintans, L.J.J., Almeida, J.R.G.S., Lima, J.T., *et al.* (2008) Plants with anticonvulsant properties – a review. *Brazilian Journal of Pharmacognosy*, **18**, 798–819.

Rice-Evans, C.A., Miller, N.J. and Paganga, G., 1995. Structure-antioxidant activity relationships of flavonoids and phenolic acids. *Free Radical and Biology and Medicine*, **20**, 933–956.

Risa, J., Risa, A., Adsersen, A., *et al.* (2004) Screening of plants used in southern Africa for epilepsy and convulsions in the GABA$_A$-benzodiazepine receptor assay. *Journal of Ethnopharmacology*, **93**, 177–182.

Sarris, J. and Byrne, G.J. (2011) A systematic review of insomnia and complementary medicine. *Sleep Medicine Reviews*, **15**, 99–106.

Sarris, J., McIntyre, E. and Camfield, D.A. (2013) Plant-based medicines for anxiety disorders, Part 2: A review of clinical studies with supporting preclinical evidence. *CNS Drugs*, **27**, 301–319.

Schachter, S.C. (2009) Botanicals and herbs: a traditional approach to treating epilepsy. *Neurotherapeutics*, **6**, 415–420.

Snow, A.L., Hovanec, L. and Brandt, J. (2004) A controlled trial of aromatherapy for agitation in nursing home patients with dementia. *Journal of Alternative and Complementary Medicine*, **10**, 431–437.

Svenningsen, A.B., Madsen, K.D., Liljefors, T., *et al.* (2006) Biflavones from *Rhus* species with affinity for the GABA$_A$-benzodiazepine receptor. *Journal of Ethnopharmacology*, **103**, 276–280.

Terburg, D., Syal, S., Rosenberger, L.A., *et al.* (2013) Acute effects of *Sceletium tortuosum* (Zembrin), a dual 5-HT reuptake and PDE4 inhibitor, in the human amygdala and its connection to the hypothalamus. *Neuropsychopharmacology*, **38**, 2708–2716.

US Patent (2001) Pharmaceutical compositions containing mesembrine and related compounds. *United States Patent* **6**, 288, 104.

van As, A.D. and Joubert, J. (1991) Neurocysticercosis in 578 black epileptic patients. *South African Medical Journal*, **80**, 327–328.

Vina, D., Serra, S., Lamela, M. and Delogu, G. (2012) Herbal natural products as a source of monoamine oxidase inhibitors: A review. *Current Topics in Medicinal Chemistry*, **12**, 2131–2144.

Viola, H., Wasowski, C., Levi de Stein, M., *et al.* (1995) Apigenin, a component of *Matricaria recutita* flowers, is a central benzodiazepine receptors-ligand with anxiolytic effects. *Plant Medica*, **61**, 213–216.

Wheatley, D. (2005) Medicinal plants for insomnia: a review of their pharmacology, efficacy and tolerability. *Journal of Paychopharmacology*, **19**, 414–421.

WHO (2013) WHO traditional medicine strategy 2014–2023, WHO Press, Geneva, http://apps.who.int/iris/bitstream/10665/92455/1/9789241506090_eng.pdf?ua=1.

Yang, G., Wang, Y., Tian, J. and Liu, J. (2013) Huperzine a for Alzheimer's disease: A systematic review and meta-analysis of randomized clinical trials. *PLoS ONE*, **8** (9), e74916. doi:10.1371/journal.pone.0074916.

Zhu, H.L., Wan, J.B., Wang, Y.T., *et al.* (2014) Medicinal compounds with antiepileptic/anticonvulsant activities. *Epilepsia*, **55**, 3–16.

# 14
# Respiratory Conditions

Adolfo Andrade-Cetto[1] and Jorge García-Alvarez[2]

*Department of Cell Biology, School of Sciences, National Autonomous University of Mexico, Mexico*

## 14.1 Introduction

### 14.1.1 The respiratory system

Breathing is one of the essential functions of living beings, in which gas exchange is necessary to obtain energy and maintain active metabolism in all tissues. The respiratory system consists of very specialized structures, including the nasal cavity, pharynx, larynx, trachea, bronchi, bronchioles and lungs, and facilitates the passage of oxygen from the air into the body, where it is then captured by the bloodstream. Erythrocytes are essential components of the blood that capture, transport and distribute oxygen from the lungs to the body's cells. Subsequently, these cells capture carbon dioxide to remove it from the body via a process that is essentially the reverse of oxygen uptake.

In the lung, the alveolar epithelium is the respiratory unit and is characterized by two types of cell: type I pneumocytes and type II pneumocytes. Type I pneumocytes are flat cells with a nucleus protruding into the alveolar surface, whereas type II pneumocytes have rounded edges and surface microvilli and secrete surfactant liquid, a phospholipid layer that coats the alveoli. The alveolar epithelium represents the interphase between the oxygen introduced from outside and the blood capillaries. This respiration unit is therefore a very thin, rapidly permeable and widely vascularized diffusion barrier, and this structural organization allows gas exchange through diffusion between the blood and air containing oxygen (Petechuk, 2004).

### 14.1.2 Respiratory diseases

Similar to other systems, the respiratory system requires a delicate balance to maintain homeostasis, and the environment largely determines the proper functioning of such systems. When maintenance functions are carried to the limit, control mechanisms are overwhelmed and disease ensues, which can adversely affect an individual's quality of life and ultimately a nation's economy. The World Health Organization (WHO, 2014) has classified respiratory diseases into groups. This classification is the international standard used to classify mortality and morbidity, and the impact on the public health and social security strategies of most countries. The groups are:

A.  Diseases affecting the upper respiratory tract (nasal cavity, pharynx, larynx, etc.) due to microorganisms.
B.  Diseases affecting the lower respiratory tract (bronchi, bronchioles), further divided into those that are caused by microorganisms and caused by external agents (e.g. cigarette smoke).
C.  Conditions in the alveoli caused by chronic particles that may be present on a daily basis or acute inhalation of a toxin/irritating substance.
D.  Diseases that alter the structure of the alveoli, preventing gas exchange.

The diseases include the following:

A.  Acute upper respiratory tract infections: colds, sinusitis, pharyngitis, tonsillitis, tracheitis and epiglotitis.
    Influenzas and pneumonia: H1N1 influenza, viral pneumonia and pneumonia caused by bacteria such as *Haemophilus influenzae*.
    Other diseases of the upper respiratory tract: allergic rhinitis, chronic rhinitis, chronic sinusitis and chronic laryngitis tonsillitis.
    Infections of the upper respiratory tract: acute bacterial rhino sinusitis.
B.  Acute lower respiratory infections: acute bronchitis and acute bronchiolitis.
    Lower respiratory tract chronic diseases: bronchitis, emphysema, chronic obstructive pulmonary disease (COPD) and asthma.
C.  Lung diseases caused by external agents: pneumoconiosis caused by inhalation of organic and inorganic particles such as silica, asbestos, actinomycetes and fungal spores.
D.  Other respiratory diseases principally affecting the interstitium: pulmonary edema, pulmonary eosinophilia and idiopathic pulmonary fibrosis.
    Suppurative and necrotic conditions of the lower respiratory tract: gangrene and necrosis of lung abscesses with and without pneumonia.
    Other pleural diseases: pleural plaque pneumothorax.
    Other diseases of the respiratory system: acute and chronic respiratory failure, apnea and lung collapse.

## 14.1.3   Common cold

The common cold is an infectious disease caused by rhinovirus and adenovirus, which causes an inflammatory reaction in the nasal passage. It mainly affects the nose and throat, causing discomfort. The most common feature is the persistent nasal discharge with sneezing, which can last for several days; infection usually resolves without treatment. In children it is more common and increases in periods of cold, cough and nasal congestion gets worse at night and nasal discharge may last for more than three days. It is very difficult to differentiate bacterial infections. The most notable difference is that viral infection improves spontaneously in 7 to 12 days, and nasal discharge is watery and clear (although it may change over time). For bacterial infections, nasal discharge is usually thicker, purulent and mucoid (Grief, 2013).

### 14.1.4   Influenza

Influenza is a debilitating disease caused by viruses that infect the upper respiratory tract (nose, throat, bronchi and lungs). The infection is often accompanied by fever, headache, runny nose, nasal congestion, joint pain and muscular pain, although these symptoms may vary according to age. Influenza viruses are spherical, with a coat consisting mainly of hemagglutinin, and have a diameter of 80–120 nm. The main types of influenza viruses are influenza A, B and C. Influenza A viruses are usually transmitted between birds and mammals, and can cause death. Influenza B viruses are found only in humans, while the C viruses are not very common, but can also cause disease. Type A viruses are classified depending on two coat proteins, hemagglutinin and neuraminidase, which are present in varying amounts (Gopinath *et al.*, 2014).

### 14.1.5   Acute lower respiratory tract infections: acute bronchitis

Acute bronchitis is caused by inflammation of the bronchial tree and affects both adults and children without chronic lung disease. These infections are caused by agents that circulate in the environment on a seasonal basis and are also responsible for causing respiratory infections of the upper airway, including rhinovirus, coronavirus and adenovirus. Acute bronchitis is characterized by the presence of acute cough, which worsens as the disease progresses. The pulmonary secretions (sputum) in bronchitis cases are purulent but do not necessarily indicate bacterial infection. Fever may also be present (Wenzel and Fowler, 2006).

### 14.1.6   Other diseases of the upper respiratory tract: allergic rhinitis and rhinitis

Allergic rhinitis is an inflammatory disorder of the nasal mucosa induced by a reaction mediated by immunoglobulin E (IgE) in subjects sensitized by an allergen. This condition is characterized by sneezing, runny nose, nasal congestion and nasal itching, and is usually accompanied by redness, watering and itchy eyes. These symptoms can lead to physical and mental complications, including sleep disorders and bad breath, in children and adolescents, which may result in inefficient performance in daily activities. In some cases, allergic rhinitis is associated with asthma (Schatz, 2007).

Rhinitis mainly affects the nose and throat, although it can spread to the larynx. The most common feature of rhinitis is a persistent nasal discharge or cough (or both), which lasts more than 10 days. In children, nasal congestion and cough worsen at night, and nasal discharge may last for more than 3 days. It is very difficult to distinguish bacterial from viral rhinitis, although the most notable difference is that viral rhinitis improves spontaneously within 7 to 12 days, and the nasal discharge is watery and clear (but may change over time). In contrast, bacterial rhinitis is associated with nasal discharge that is usually thicker, purulent and mucoid (Wald *et al.*, 1981; Meltzer *et al.*, 2006).

### 14.1.7   Chronic lower respiratory tract diseases: COPD

COPD is a preventable and treatable disease with significant extrapulmonary effects. This disease is characterized by a typically progressive chronic airflow limitation associated with an abnormal inflammatory response to the inhalation of toxic particles or gases. Patients with COPD may develop emphysema, chronic bronchitis, bronchiolitis and cardiovascular disorders with hypertension. COPD is associated with high morbidity and mortality rates, and the main risk factor for this disease is inhaling cigarette smoke as a result of tobacco addiction (smoking). The pathologic progress of COPD is mainly measured by airflow obstruction, showing a decreased expiratory volume. The damage is progressive and irreversible, and is associated with an abnormal inflammatory response followed by destruction of the lung parenchyma (Markewitz *et al.*, 1999; Thorley and Tetley, 2007).

### 14.1.8   Lung diseases caused by external agents: hypersensitivity pneumonitis

Hypersensitivity pneumonitis, also known as extrinsic allergic alveolitis, is a disease caused by an exaggerated inflammatory immune response in the bronchioles and lung alveoli to inhaled antigen particles present in the environment. A wide variety of antigens have been described, but the most common are organic particles such as fungi, bacteria, animal proteins and chemical compounds of lower molecular weight that function as haptens and bind to albumin to create an antigenic particle. Hypersensitivity pneumonitis is subdivided into acute and chronic hypersensitivity pneumonitis. The acute phase is characterized by fever, chills, sweating, headache and nausea. These symptoms last for a few hours and may be accompanied by coughing and dyspnea (shortness of breath when performing daily activities). If these problems persist, cough and dyspnea become more severe over the course of days or weeks after exposure. When the disease becomes chronic, the symptoms described above are accompanied by fatigue and weight loss (Selman, 2004).

### 14.1.9   Other respiratory diseases principally affecting the interstitium: idiopathic pulmonary fibrosis

Idiopathic pulmonary fibrosis is a chronic and lethal disease. As its name suggests, this disease is of unknown etiology and primarily affects older adults between 50 and 70 years of age. In most patients, disease progression is slow and the median survival is estimated at 2 to 5 years after diagnosis. In addition, this disease currently has no cure. Clinical manifestations are often characterized by progressive dyspnea, accompanied by cough and lung volume reduction with subsequent deterioration of gas exchange. These alterations are due to damage to the alveolar epithelium and lead to abnormal connective tissue remodelling. This phenomenon is the result of fibroblast proliferation, which leads to the loss of gas exchange between the alveolar epithelium and blood capillaries (Selman *et al.*, 2001).

### 14.1.10   Suppurative and necrotic lower respiratory tract conditions: pneumonia with necrosis

Pneumonia with necrosis is a rare complication of lung infections caused by bacterial agents, such as *Staphylococcus aureus*, *Streptococcus pyogenes*, *Streptococcus pneumoniae* and *Klebsiella pneumoniae*, or fungi such as *Aspergillus*. In these infections, necrotic foci form in localized areas and may be accompanied by other complications such as pulmonary abscess and gangrene, in which the lung tissue is destroyed. During this disease, thrombosis occurs in larger blood vessels and plays a role in pathogenesis. Patients with these complications show symptoms that often accompany infection, such as dyspnea, cough commonly accompanied with fluids, fever, chest pain and loss of consciousness. Risk factors include advanced age with habits of alcoholism, smoking, diabetes mellitus, chronic lung disease or liver disease. However, appropriate use of broad-spectrum antibiotics can result in successful treatment. In more severe cases with gangrene, surgical procedures may be required (Penner *et al.*, 1994; Norte *et al.*, 2012).

### 14.1.11    Other pleural diseases: pleural plaque

Pleural plaques are dense and fibrotic lesions that occur in the parietal pleura, which is the tissue lining the lungs that enables their extension. These lesions are detected by thorax X-ray or computed tomography (CT) scan, and their size varies from a few millimetres to a centimetre. These plaques are very common in people who were exposed to asbestos or silica but have also been observed in unexposed individuals. Pathologically, the lesions are mainly composed of avascular and acellular collagen fibres, with only a few fibroblasts present between the fibres. These lesions limit the extension of the lung during the breathing process, and this disease is therefore characterized by breathlessness. This symptom may also be accompanied by coughing and tightness in the chest (Clarke *et al.*, 2006).

### 14.1.12    Other diseases of the respiratory system: acute respiratory failure

Acute respiratory failure can develop rapidly, within minutes to hours, and is more common in infants than adults. Respiratory failure can have various causes, and most of the fatalities are observed in developing countries. Malnutrition in children under 5 years of age is a major risk factor for this condition, as these children are likely to develop chronic fatigue and subsequent respiratory failure. Another risk factor is severe chronic anemia, which prevents the efficient transport of oxygen (Balfour-Lynn *et al.*, 2014).

Traditional plant-based medicines have long been used to treat respiratory conditions, mainly for the relief of associated symptoms such as cough, sneezing or rhinitis. They have a number of pharmacological actions relevant to treat diseases of both the upper and lower respiratory tract, including asthma, sinusitis, rhinitis and others. In addition to their traditional use, phytomedicines and even isolated compounds from plants play an important role in treating respiratory conditions and as supportive measures in more serious diseases such as: bronchitis, emphysema and pneumonia (Heinrich *et al.*, 2012). They are now sold in many pharmacies worldwide.

Ethnopharmacological research in countries where people mainly depend on traditional medicine for the treatment of respiratory diseases provides an excellent strategy to discover new plant species or new compounds to treat respiratory conditions, as exemplified by the species discussed in the following sections.

## 14.2    Case studies

Medicinal plants are used worldwide to treat respiratory conditions, and some useful natural products used to treat respiratory problems, such as codeine or ephedrine, are now included in manufactured products. Indeed, the modern literature provides several examples of how plants serve both as important components of traditional medicines and new phytotherapeutic agents found in over-the-counter medications.

Many plant preparations have been studied clinically but have not been developed as phytomedicines. In a review of clinical trials of phytomedicines used in otorhinolaryngology and pulmonology, currently under development as potential novel medications, Ghazi-Moghadam *et al.* (2012) reported that species such as *Lycopersicon esculentum* Miller yielded a bioactive naringenin chalcone shown to inhibit the release of histamine from mast cells during the initial phase of inflammation. In addition, this plant compound decreased the level of eosinophils and eosinophil cationic proteins in patients with mild to moderate perennial allergic rhinitis. A herbal tablet formulated with *Cinnamomum zeylanicum* Nees, *Malpighia glabra* L. and *Bidens pilosa* L. was shown to significantly reduce nasal symptoms and inhibit the release of prostaglandin D2 in patients with allergic rhinitis. In Japan, *Rubus chingii* var. suavissimus (S. K. Lee) L. T. Lu is used for the treatment of allergic rhinitis, and a randomized, double-blind, placebo-controlled study reported that this plant improved patients' nasal symptoms. *Nigella sativa* L., a plant used in Middle Eastern and Mediterranean regions, has been reported to have anti-inflammatory and anti-allergic effects, which are mediated by changes in the phagocytosis and killing activity of polymorphonuclear leucocytes, leukotriene synthesis and inhibition of histamine release. In particular, patients treated with its fatty oil for 30 days showed significant improvements of nasal signs and symptoms. Furthermore, this plant was shown to function as a histamine antagonist and inhibitor of the histamine receptor; a placebo-controlled trial reported that treatment of asthmatic patients with an extract of this plant for 3 months improved symptoms and pulmonary function tests. The extracts of *Pelargonium sidoides* DC from Southern Africa also are used widely in the treatment of respiratory tract infections, acute rhino sinusitis and bronchitis, and are now a well-established element in European phytotherapy with licensed products widely available. The antimicrobial and anti-inflammatory activity of this botanical drug is based on inducing the release of tumor necrosis factor (TNF)-α and increased activity of natural killer (NK) cells. Following a therapeutic dose of 30 drops three times per day for at least 7 days, patients show significant improvements in the symptoms of common cold and acute bronchitis. The leaves of *Eucalyptus globulus* Labill are reported to possess antibacterial activity against oral bacteria, and extracts in chewing gum have been shown to significantly inhibit plaque formation, inflammation and bleeding of the gingiva. The main active principle is the monoterpene cineol. *Andrographis paniculata* (Burm. f.) Ness. (Acanthaceae) is an important medicinal plant widely used in Chinese traditional medicines and mentioned in ancient scriptures of Ayurveda. The prevention and treatment of uncomplicated upper respiratory tract infections in adults and children stand out because there is considerable clinical evidence to back up such uses (Joseph, 2014), extracts of the plant present a consistent inhibitory effect on the secretion of influenza virus, regulated on expressed and secreted activation of normal T cells (Wang and Liu, 2014).

The following section covers brief but more detailed examples of species that have already been developed into phytomedicines.

## 14.2.1 *Althaea officinalis* L. Malvaceae

Medicinal plants with antitussive effects and a broad-spectrum effect function to reduce coughing through demulcent action, by removing the irritation (expectorant) or by depressing the cough reflex.

The medicinal use of *Althaea officinalis* (marshmallow root) has been documented in Europe since Roman times. It is traditionally used as a demulcent and emollient to treat irritation of the oral and pharyngeal mucosa and associated dry cough (European Medicines Agency, 2009). In the Middle Ages the species was prescribed by Lonicerus and Matthiolus as an expectorant and diuretic. Today the roots are collected in the autumn from plants not less than 2 years old.

The demulcent effects of *A. officinalis* are due to its high content of polysaccharide hydrocolloids, which form a protective coating on the oral and pharyngeal mucosa to soothe local irritation and inflammation (Shah *et al.*, 2011). This botanical drug is also indicated for the treatment of acute or chronic bronchitis and dry cough. Specifically, a formulation is used as a gargle to treat inflammation of the mucous membranes of the mouth and throat. Ten to 15 g of the root are mixed with 150 ml of cold water and stirred for 90 minutes prior to application.

The root extract and the isolated polysaccharide were tested at oral doses of 50–100 mg/kg body weight for treatment of cough induced by mechanical stimulation, and the results were compared with those obtained for *Althaea* syrup (1000 mg/kg), prenoxdiazine (30 mg/kg), dropropizine (100 mg/kg) and codeine (10 mg/kg). Both the extract and isolated polysaccharide significantly reduced the intensity and the number of cough efforts from the laryngopharyngeal and tracheobronchial areas. Polysaccharides from this plant also exhibited statistically significant cough-suppressing activity, which was noticeably higher than that of the control drug. In particular, the greatest antitussive activity was observed with the polysaccharide containing the highest proportion of the uronic acid constituent (Al-Snafi, 2013).

Mucilage polysaccharides contain 5–11% mucilage and consist of a mixture of colloidally soluble polysaccharides, particularly acid arabinogalactans, rhamnans, arabans, glucans and acidic heteropolysaccharides, including D-galactose, L-rhamnose, D-glucuronic acid and D-galacturonic acid (European Medicines Agency, 2009).

## 14.2.2 Codeine and noscapine

These compounds occur naturally in opium (*Papaver somniferum* L.) and are clearly derived from local and traditional knowledge but are currently produced using a semi-synthetic process. In particular, 3-methylmorphine is used for its antitussive properties. This drug is on the WHO's list of essential medicines. Codeine sulfate causes respiratory depression, in part by a direct effect on the brainstem respiratory centres. It depress the cough reflex through direct effects on the cough centre in the medulla. Noscapine is a benzyl isoquinoline alkaloid also isolated from opium. It is used for its cough-suppressing effects, and the agonist is the σ- receptor (Kamei, 1996).

## 14.2.3 *Echinacea purpurea* (L.) Moench and *Ecinacea angustifolia* DC.

These species are mentioned in the European Pharmacopoeia as a support treatment for flu-like infections and recurrent infections of the upper respiratory tract. It is known that these plant extracts activate the immune system and anti-inflammatory reactions through the up-regulation of TNF-α. In one double-blind study that included 100 patients with acute flu-like infections, patients received 30 ml of an *Echinacea* preparation or placebo and after 2 days the dose was reduced to 15 ml/day. Eight cold symptoms (lethargy, limb, pain, headache, rhinitis, cough, sore throat and pharyngeal redness) were rated for severity using a semi-quantitative scoring system (WHO, 1999c).

In a double-dummy controlled trial, the effects of a combined *Echinacea* and sage spray were compared to a chlorhexidine/lidocaine combination for the treatment of sore throat, and 60%

of patients in each group became symptom-free after 3 days with no significant difference between these two combinations (Ghazi-Moghadam *et al.*, 2012). The main compounds present in *E. purpurea* are chicoric acid, caffeic acid and two immuno-stimulatory polysaccharides (PSI and PSII). PSI was identified as 4-O-methyl glucurono-arabinoxylan (composed mainly of glucuronic acid and the sugars arabinose and xylose), while PSII was shown to be an acidic arabino rhamnogalactan (mainly composed of the sugars arabinose, rhamnose and galactose). In a meta-analysis from 2006 the authors concluded that the standardized extracts of Echinaceae were effective in the prevention of the symptoms of the common cold after clinical inoculation (Rhinovirus). In a review of randomized controlled trials Linde *et al.* (2009) found that the available Echinacea products differ greatly in terms of chemical composition and plant part used, and that the majority of these products have not been tested in clinical trials. They therefore suggested that alcoholic and pressed juice preparations that are based primarily on the aerial parts of *E. purpurea* might have the best evidence base and have beneficial effects on cold symptoms in adults if treatment is started early.

## 14.2.4  *Ephedra sinica* Stapf. (Ephedraceae)

Medicinal plants with anticatarrhal effects are used to reduce excessive discharge from mucous membranes. These plant medicines are particularly useful for nasal and sinus congestion and mucosal edema, and they can also reduce airway hypersensitivity.

For over 5000 years the Chinese have used ephedra medicinally. It is listed as one of the original 365 medicinal plants from the classical 1st century AD text on Chinese herbalism by Shen Nong. Chinese traditional medicinal uses include the alleviation of sweating, lung and bronchial constriction, water retention, coughing, shortness of breath, common cold and fevers without sweat (WHO, 1999a). ESCOP recommend the plant to treat nasal congestion due to hay fever, allergic rhinitis, acute coryza, common cold and sinusitis.

The main active constituents of ephedra, including ephedrine and pseudoephedrine, are potent bronchodilators and sympathomimetic drugs that stimulate α-, β1- and β2- adrenoceptors to relax the bronchial muscles. Ephedrine, like other sympathomimetics with α-receptor activity, causes vasoconstriction and blanching when applied topically to nasal and pharyngeal mucosal surfaces. In addition, the continued prolonged use of these preparations (3 days) may cause rebound congestion and chronic rhinitis. Part of ephedrine's peripheral mechanism of action is related to the release of norepinephrine, with rapidly repeated doses being less effective owing to the depletion of norepinephrine stores. Ephedrine is also a potent stimulator of the CNS, and the effects of this drug may last for several hours after oral administration. Furthermore, the use of this botanical drug can produce side effects such as nervousness, tremor, sleeplessness, loss of appetite and nausea. The plant has a risk of abuse, and for this reason products sold as over-the-counter herbal medicines or dietary supplements are now banned in most countries (WHO, 1999a).

A recent study (Yen *et al.*, 2014) evaluated the traditional medicine Yakammaoto, which for more than 2000 years has been used to treat flu-like symptoms in China and Japan. This preparation containing nine ingredients, including *Ephedra sinica*, was evaluated for its effects on coxsackie virus B4 (CVB4), which causes flu-like symptoms and life-threatening diseases such as pneumonia. These authors concluded that Yakammaoto showed antiviral activity against CVB4-induced cellular injuries in the airway mucosa, preventing viral attachment, internalization and replication.

## 14.2.5  *Thymus vulgaris L.* (Lamiaceae)

Antitussive drugs are used to control coughing, particularly in patients with a dry, nagging, unproductive cough.

*Thymus vulgaris* is indigenous to southern and Central Europe, although it is currently a pan-European species that is cultivated in Europe, America and other parts of the world. The plant has been used traditionally to treat coughs due to colds, bronchitis, laryngitis and tonsillitis. The leaves and flowers are indicated for the treatment of irritable and whooping cough, catarrh of the upper respiratory tract, bronchial catarrh, the supportive treatment for tussis, and for mouthwashes and gargles used to lessen inflammation of the mouth (WHO, 1999b).

The principal components of this plant (including chemo varieties) are thymol and carvacrol (up to 64% of the oil), along with linalool, p-cymol, cymene, thymene, α-pinene, apigenin, luteolin, 6-hydroxyluteolin glycosides and di-, tri- and tetra-methoxylated flavones (WHO, 1999b). Its expectorant properties, which function via a bronchospasmolytic effect, have been demonstrated in animal and *in vitro* experiments and were attributed to the compounds thymonin, cirsilineol and 8-methoxycirsilineol. An extract containing 0.072% thymol was also shown to antagonize contractions of isolated guinea pig trachea. Furthermore, extracts of this plant showed activity against *Mycobacterium tuberculosis* strain H37Rv, *Klebsiella pneumoniae* and *Diplococcus pneumoniae*. In clinical studies, *T. vulgaris* also showed activity against non-productive cough resulting from uncomplicated respiratory infections. In particular, 93.5% of 154 children treated with 15–30 ml of syrup containing 97.6 mg of thyme fluid extract showed improved cough intensity in cases presenting bronchial catarrh (ESCOP, 2003).

# 14.3  Conclusions

Respiratory conditions have been treated with medicinal plants since ancient times and there are many examples of plants that are effective in treating the main symptoms of catarrh, cough, sneezing, etc. Since these conditions can be recognized easily by traditional healers, medicinal plants have been commonly used for their treatment. For cases in which the origin of the disease cannot be recognized (by healers), as in a respiratory viral infection, the traditional medicine seldom targets the virus itself but rather treats the symptoms, which is often sufficient to achieve patient recovery. In more serious diseases, such as pulmonary fibrosis, emphysema or influenza, traditional medicine has a more limited action, but it can still play an important role as supportive treatment.

A variety of natural products are used to treat respiratory ailments, including saponins, chalcones, monoterpenes, phenolic compounds and alkaloids. In particular, the alkaloids codeine, noscapine and ephedrine are used in many prescriptions, although a specific pharmacological action has not yet been correlated to a certain class of compound.

It is important to note how traditional medicines used for centuries in Europe are currently being developed as phytomedicines. Moreover, traditional preparations that are still used in the Americas (Mesoamerica and Brazil as examples), China, India and Africa can provide new medicinal plants for the treatment of respiratory conditions. As an example; in many lesser developed countries a major concern is tuberculosis, and there are quite a few R&D activities focusing on medicinal plants for such conditions. Thus new ethnopharmacological studies can lead us to find new species to target this bacterial infection.

Traditional medicines have provided us with phytomedicines and natural products for the treatment of respiratory ailments. For this reason ethnopharmacological field studies in countries where traditional medicine still plays an important role could lead us to discover new therapeutic agents that can be developed in a more global way as new phyto-medicines or isolated compounds.

# Acknowledgments

Thanks to Dr Prof. Michael Heinrich for his help in editing the manuscript. This work was partially supported by grants from DGAPA, PAPIIT (project IN214413) and CONACyT CB-0151264.

# References

Al-Snafi, A. E. (2013) The pharmaceutical importance of *Althaea officinalis* and *Althaea rosea*: A review. *International Journal of PharmTech Research*, **5**, 1378–1385.

Balfour-Lynn, R.E., Marsh, G., Gorayi, D., *et al.* (2014) Non-invasive ventilation for children with acute respiratory failure in the developing world: literature review and an implementation example. *Pediatric Respiratory Reviews*, **15**, 181–187.

Clarke, C.C., Mowat, F.S., Kelsh, M.A. and Roberts, M.A. (2006) Pleural plaques: a review of diagnostic issues and possible non asbestos factors. *Archives of Environmental and Occupational Health*, **61**, 183–192.

ESCOP (2003) *Monographs*. Thieme, Norfolk, 556 pp.

European Medicines Agency (2009) *Evaluation of Medicines for Human Use. Assessment report on* Althaea officinalis L. Radix, document reference MEA/HMPC/98718/2008, London.

Ghazi-Moghadam, K., Inançli, H.M., Bazazy, N., *et al.* (2012) Phytomedicine in otorhinolaryngology and pulmonology: Clinical trials with herbal remedies. *Pharmaceuticals*, **5**, 853–874.

Gopinath, S.C., Tang, T.H., Chen, Y., *et al.* (2014) Sensing strategies for influenza surveillance. *Biosensors and Bioelectronics*, **61C**, 357–369.

Grief, S.N. (2013) Upper respiratory infections. *Primary Care Clinics in Office Practice*, **40**, 757–770.

Heinrich, M., Barnes, J., Gibbons, S. and Williamson, E. (2012) *Fundamentals of Pharmacognosy and Phytotherapy, Elsevier-Churchill Livingstone,* p. **336**.

Joseph, S.M. (2014). Scientific aspects of the therapeutic use of *Andrographis paniculata* (Kalmegh): A review. *International Journal of Pharmaceutical Sciences Review and Research*, **27**, 10–16.

Kamei, J. (1996) Role of opioidergic and serotonergic mechanisms in cough and antitussives. *Pulmonary Pharmacology*, **9**, 349–356.

Linde, K., Barrett, B., Bauer, R., *et al.* (2009) *Echinacea for preventing and treating the common cold (Review)*, The Cochrane Collaboration, Wiley & Sons, p. 104.

Markewitz, B.A., Owens, M.W. and Payne, D.K. (1999) The pathogenesis of chronic obstructive pulmonary disease. *American Journal of the Medical Sciences*, **318**, 74–78.

Meltzer, E.O., Hamilos, D.L., Hadley, J.A., *et al.* (2006) Rhinosinusitis: developing guidance for clinical trials. *Otolaryngology Head and Neck Surgery*, **135**, S31–S80.

Norte, A., Santos, A., Gamboa, F., *et al.* (2012) Necrotizing pneumonia: a rare complication. *Acta Medica Portuguesa*, **25**, 51–55.

Penner, C., Maycher, B. and Long, R. (1994) Pulmonary gangrene, a complication of bacterial pneumonia. *Chest*, **105**, 567–573.

Petechuk, D. (2004) *The Respiratory System*, Greenwood Press, Westport, p. 240.

Schatz, M.A. (2007) A survey of the burden of allergic rhinitis in the USA. *Allergy*, **62** (Suppl. 85), 9–16.

Selman, M. (2004) Hypersensitivity pneumonitis: a multifaceted deceiving disorder. *Clinical Chest Medicine*, **25**, 531–547.

Selman, M., King, T.E. and Pardo, A. (2001) Idiopathic pulmonary fibrosis: prevailing and evolving hypotheses about its pathogenesis and implications for therapy. *Annals of Internal Medicine*, **134**, 136–151.

Shah, S.M., Akhtar, N., Akram, M., *et al.* (2011) Pharmacological activity of *Althaea officinalis* L. *Journal of Medicinal Plant Research*, **5**, 5662–5666.

Thorley, A.J. and Tetley, T.D. (2007) Pulmonary epithelium, cigarette smoke and chronic obstructive pulmonary disease. *International Journal of Chronic Obstructive Pulmonary Disease*, **2**, 409–428.

Wald, E.R., Milmoe, G.J., Bowen, A.D., *et al.* (1981) Acute maxillary sinusitis in children. *New England Journal of Medicine*, **304**, 749–754.

Wang, X.G. and Liu, Z.J. (2014) Prevention and treatment of viral respiratory infections by traditional Chinese herbs (Review). *Chinese Medical Journal*, **127**, 344–1350.

Wenzel, R.P. and Fowler, A.A. (2006) Clinical practice. *Acute bronchitis. New England Journal of Medicine*, **355**, 2125–2130.

WHO (1999a) *Monographs on Selected Medicinal Plants. Herba Ephedrae*, World Health Organization, Geneva/Malta, pp. 145–153.

WHO (1999b) *Monographs on Selected Medicinal Plants. Herba Thymi*, World Health Organization, Geneva/Malta, 259–266.

WHO (1999c) *Monographs on Selected Medicinal Plants. Herba Echinaceae purpurae*, World Health Organization, Geneva/Malta, 136–144.

WHO (2014) *International Classification of Diseases (ICD-10)*, available from http://www.who .int/classifications/icd/en/.

Yen, M.H., Lee, J.J., Yeh, C.F. *et al.* (2014) Yakammaoto inhibited human coxsackievirus B4 (CVB4)-induced airway and renal tubular injuries by preventing viral attachment, internalization, and replication. *Journal of Ethnopharmacology*, **151**, 1056–1063.

# 15

# Can there be an Ethnopharmacology of Inflammation?

Michael Heinrich and Anthony Booker

*Research Cluster 'Biodiversity and Medicines'/Centre for Pharmacognosy and Phytotherapy, UCL School of Pharmacy, London, UK*

## 15.1  Introduction

The body's inflammatory response is a localized pathophysiological condition forming part of the body's response to (often xenobiotic) stimuli. The classical signs based on European traditions are *calor* (heat), *dolor* (pain), *rubor* (redness) and *tumor* (swelling). These cardinal signs can be traced back to Celsus (c. 25 BCE to c. 50 CE), a Roman encyclopedist. The four classical signs of inflammation very often are a reaction to injury, infection or disease. Our modern understanding of proinflammatory processes is based on detailed mechanistic biochemical studies identifying the signalling networks involved in such processes.

While most notably some upstream targets are disease and/or organ specific, there are many effector proteins that are common to different disease states. Numerous signalling cascades have been identified, involving as one of the last steps the activation of inducible transcription factors that bind to the promoter regions of pro-inflammatory genes. Such targets include the genes for adhesion molecules (chemokines) and cytokines (TNF-a, interleukins). Famously, the nuclear factor of kappa-light-chain-enhancer B cells (NF-kB) is one of the principle inducible transcription factors in mammals and has been shown to play a pivotal role in the mammalian innate immune response of chronic inflammatory conditions such as rheumatoid arthritis. Mediators of inflammation that are under the influence of activated NF-kB include inducible nitric oxide synthase (iNOS), the subsequent production of NO and prostaglandin (PG) synthase (cyclo-oxygenase), especially COX-2. PGs have also been shown to inhibit NF-kB activation. Consequently, a compound shown to interfere with NO/iNOS and/or

*Ethnopharmacology*, First Edition. Edited by Michael Heinrich and Anna K. Jäger.
© 2015 John Wiley & Sons, Ltd. Published 2015 by John Wiley & Sons, Ltd.

COX-2 may well act via inhibiting NF-kB. Toll-like receptors (TLRs) are, on the other hand, an example of upstream mediators that recognize molecules that share characteristics with pathogens, but are distinguishable from such molecules, collectively referred to as pathogen-associated molecular patterns. They again link into a range of pro-inflammatory pathways, including NF-kappaB-mediated signalling systems. Numerous upstream mediators have now been identified and a large diversity of disease conditions are linked to an orchestrated change of these signalling systems. Thus, the broad concept of inflammation (and consequently anti-inflammatory effects) is now generally broken down into understanding disease-specific signalling cascades.

This biomedical concept of 'inflammation' has provided a unified concept that helps to understand processes that in essence are protective tissue responses to injury, infection or destruction of tissue, and this topic has been reviewed widely (cf. the numerous textbooks on the topic, such as Rang *et al.*, 2011, Mutschler *et al.*, 2013). In the broadest sense Celsus' initial observation was transformed into a mechanistic and descriptive interpretation covering the entire range of the body's responses to such challenges. However, in local and indigenous systems the starting point is generally a specific bodily condition, e.g. an inflamed part of the skin, that resulted from an infection or an injury or some chronic pain condition (e.g. lower back pain) and which requires treatment. In these systems, and again in general terms, the therapeutic strategy starts with some organ-specific symptoms and defines a treatment to overcome it. In essence in biomedical practice a practitioner may prescribe a non-steroidal anti-inflammatory drug (NSAID) like aspirin or ibuprofen, which has both anti-inflammatory and pain-reducing effects, with the understanding that it acts on the basis of specific effects on pharmacological targets in these signalling networks. If this does not work the practitioner may shift to a combination of an antibiotic and an opioid, with the understanding that both the infection and the associated pain are treated. In this case an antibiotic is given to reduce the inflammation.

Chronic inflammation has also been linked to the development of cancers by potentially promoting and initiating carcinogenesis(Hanahan and Weinberg, 2011; Candido and Hagemann, 2013; Elinav *et al.*, 2013) by modulating the relevant signalling pathways relevant in the development of cancers (including, importantly, the NF-kappaB pathway).

In traditional medicine the treatment would generally start from the perspective that there is a need to treat a certain part of the body (like an infected wound on the hand or heat and pain in a part of the body) based on what has been observed to be therapeutically useful for this condition or by providing a holistic treatment of an abnormal bodily state. In this regard this chapter is different to others in the book as it does not deal with an illness caused by a specific pathogen (like a bacterium or a parasite) nor is it restricted to a specific organ system (like the respiratory system). Instead a plethora of diseases are associated with acute and chronic forms of inflammation.

In particular, the concept of inflammation in traditional Chinese medicine (TCM) is rather complex and it is not always possible to make a meaningful connection to biomedical theory. For example, in the treatment of arthritis the TCM diagnosis for this condition begins with the precept that all pain is caused by the poor or obstructed flow of qi through the meridians (channels). This obstruction to the qi flow may be caused by different pathogenic factors, i.e. wind, cold, damp, heat and combinations of these factors. A patient presenting with a painful hot, red and swollen joint may be diagnosed with an invasion of damp and heat, whereas a patient presenting with pain that affects different joints and is worse in cold weather would more likely be diagnosed with an invasion of wind and cold. In each case a different treatment strategy would be employed (including a different herbal formula). Moreover a condition that began as an acute cold invasion may over time become a chronic heat condition, necessitating a moving treatment strategy as the disease progresses. Whereas it is reasonably straightforward to equate heat and damp-heat with inflammation, it needs more of an epistemological jump to appreciate how wind and cold might also be causative factors.

A classical ethnopharmacological approach linking a specific use with an *in vitro* pharmacological study therefore may not be as straightforward as it would be with, for example, an antibacterial screening approach. In other cultures (as exemplified in Celsus' work) a relatively well-defined concept of acute inflammatory diseases, most importantly on the skin and the mucosa, would enable a direct link between local and indigenous use and the bioscientific evaluation. Inflammatory processes have also been implicated in a plethora of conditions, including chronic pain and degenerative CNS disorders, therefore in pharmacological terms a much wider range of diseases and conditions could form a basis for assessing, for example, a plant in a range of anti-inflammatory assays.

As a general note of caution, there is never a direct and unilateral correlation between a local/traditional use and some biomedical or bioscientific parameters, but in the context of inflammatory conditions it is essential to appreciate the breadths of the conditions potentially associated with a specific bioscientific pro-inflammatory parameter.

In this chapter we will use a few examples of important herbal medicines for which some evidence for clinical effectiveness exists and which are derived from diverse medical traditions. Of course, the most famous anti-inflammatory medicine – aspirin – is a semi-synthetic derivative of a natural product derived from plants with a long tradition of use as a medicine. In 1828 the German pharmacist Johannes Andreas Buchner (1783–1852) first isolated salicin from Salix spp. (willow bark, Salicaceae). It was derivatized first to yield salicylic acid (1838, Rafaele Pirea, 1814–1865, Italy) and later, by the company Bayer in 1899, to yield acetyl salicylic acid, or aspirin – a compound previously known but which had not been studied pharmaceutically. This latter discovery is often associated with the German chemist Felix Hoffmann (1868–1946), who worked for Bayer. Controversially, the German Jewish chemist Arthur Eichengrün (1867–1949) late in his life claimed to have planned and directed the compound's synthesis and the early clinical testing. Only at the turn of the millennium did these claims receive some attention (Sneader, 2000) and the controversy about the two versions of the drug discovery process continues (Sneader, 2000; Heinrich, 2013). From an ethnopharmacological perspective, there can be no doubt that these discoveries are based on European local uses of species containing salicin and related glycosides, and while the later part of the discovery and development has received considerable scrutiny, much less attention has been paid to the specific basis for the early developments of this anti-inflammatory drug. A more detailed assessment of the local uses which formed the basis of J.A. Buchner's discovery would be of great interest.

In the context of this chapter we will focus less on new drugs, but – using several examples from medical traditions around the world – will look at bioscientific studies of plants with a wider importance as local medicines with uses that are associated with anti-inflammatory effects in the broadest sense.

## 15.2 Ethnopharmacology of inflammation: some examples

Plants have yielded a large number of species with acclaimed anti-inflammatory effects. From an ethnopharmaoclogical perspective a key challenge remains to define how 'inflammatory' conditions are described and defined in indigenous and local cultures. Contrary to other chapters, this chapter is not dealing with a single disease or a group of clearly differentiated diseases but with a wide range of pathophysiological responses that all show the hallmarks of chronic or acute inflammatory conditions.

## 15.2.1   The arnica complex

The most iconic of all medicinal plants that is used to treat acute inflammatory conditions may well be *Arnica montana* L. (Asteraceae). Today, arnica is an important medicinal plant with pharmaceutical uses exclusively for treating bruises, sprains and as a counter-irritant in the form of creams and gels. Uses of arnica in the Middle Ages and the Renaissance were seemingly very limited and it was hardly known in Greek, Roman and Arabic medicine. The first reliable evidence dates back to the 14th (Matthaeus Silvaticus) and 15th centuries (Mayer and Czygan, 2000), so the documented use of this species as a medicine is relatively recent. The situation is even more complicated since *A. montana* was associated or confused with water plantain (*Alisma plantago-aquatica* L.). In Jacobus Theodorus Tabernomontanus' *New vollkommentlich Kreuterbuch* (1588), a picture of *A. montana* is included, with a text referring to *A. plantago-aquatica* (Obón *et al.*, 2012). As shown later in the text this could be an intentional use as part of a plant complex or it may simply be an error in the text. In the 16th century the species became a very important remedy in treating wounds (Mayer and Czygan, 2000; Heinrich *et al.*, 2005). Today it is a pan-European licensed or registered herbal medical product, but also an important element of popular medicine.

There is some clinical evidence to support the use of arnica for reducing bruising, but not for other indications. Its use is plausible based on known biologically active sesquiterpene lactones, which are known to be absorbed through the skin, inhibit the transcription factor NF-κB and act as anti-inflammatory agents (Bremner and Heinrich, 2002; Merfort, 2003).

What makes this example particularly fascinating is the widespread use of species labelled as 'arnica', but which very often are not *A. montana*. The concept of a plant complex was initially proposed by Linares and Bye (1987) for a group of different species sharing common names, morphological and aromatic characteristics, and which have similar uses. In essence these are a group of species, which are culturally linked together because of common (often morphological) characteristics. These characteristics may well be very different from those used, for example, in botany. In the original case study by Linares and Bye (1987) a key characteristic of the cachani complex was the secondary underground storage organs. This complex is composed of four species (*Iostephune madrensis* (S.Watson) Strother, *Liatris punctatu* Hook, *Psacalium* sp. and *Senecio sessilifolius* (Hook. & Arn.) Hemsl. [listed as *Rolduna sessilifolia* (Hook. & Arn.) H.Rob. & Brettell] and one species of the Rosaceae *(Potentilla* sp.). In the context of the arnica complex there seems to be a dissemination based on topical uses for acute inflammatory skin conditions. Obón de Castro *et al.* (2012) investigated the distribution and dissemination of the árnica complex on the Iberian Peninsula and showed that it included 32 different plant species belonging to six Angiosperm families (including 24 species of Asteraceae, as well as one or two species each of Hypericaceae, Lamiaceae, Liliaceae, s.str., Plantaginaceae and Rosaceae) which also partially share therapeutic uses and morphological characteristics. *Chiliadenus glutinosus* (L.) Fourr., *Inula montana* L. and *Dittrichia viscosa* (L.) Greuter are the most widely reported species, all more important than *Arnica montana* L. Many of the other 32 taxa are very popular in Spain and Portugal, and are mainly used to treat inflammation, wounds, hematomas and contusions. The term 'árnica' thus served as a label helping in the dissemination of the use of this plant complex on the Peninsula. The use of species labelled 'árnica' has also spread to South and Central America, as well as to Mexico. For example, in Mexico *Heterotheca inuloides* is labelled 'árnica' and is used widely in the treatment of bruises, contusions and swellings. Other common árnica species include Asteraceae like *Tithonia diversifolia* (Hemsl.) A. Gray and *Neurolaena lobata* (L.) R.Br. ex Cass. These are species that are all larger yellow flowering subshrubs or shrubs, but also other morphologically distinct species may be labelled 'arnica' (Heinrich *et al.*, 1998, 2014).

In conclusion, the example of árnica illustrates that the use of a species may have resulted from therapeutic experiences in treating inflammatory conditions and that this use together with morphology classifies these species into popular plant complexes. Today we have many arnicas and their popularity is linked to a widespread experience with these botanical drugs as therapeutic agents for inflammatory conditions.

## 15.2.2 *Harpagophytum procumbens* (Burch.) DC. ex Meisn. (Pedaliaceae)

The Devil's claw or grapple plant is aptly named for its formidable 'claws' – the dried hooked thorns of the fruit used in seed dispersal – which are a hazard to any passing clove-footed animal or careless human. The plant is native to south-western Africa and it is collected in regions bordering the Kalahari Desert. It thrives in clay or sandy soils and is often found in the South African veldt of the west/north of Northern Province and the southern regions of South West Province. (Volk, 1964)

The species is used traditionally as a tonic for 'illnesses of the blood', fever, problems during pregnancy, and kidney and bladder problems. An ointment made from the fresh root is applied topically for sores, ulcers, boils and other skin lesions, including external 'cancerous growths'. The link between local and traditional use and the development of a product used in 'rational phytotherapy' seems to be based on the use being adopted by European farmers in south-west Africa. The first uses of the drug were as a tea for inflammatory conditions (painful rheumatic conditions) and for gastrointestinal problems (Wegener, 2005). While interned by the British in south-west Africa (now Namibia) in the late 1930s the German farmer and former soldier G.H. Mehnert experimented with a devil's claw preparation and used it clinically in a wide range of diseases that the inmates were suffering from (Mehnert, 2007; Wichtl, 2009). Subsequent studies were carried out at the University of Jena (German Democratic Republic) on the anti-inflammatory effects of extracts from this drug (Zorn, 1958). However, the history of its introduction into European phytotherapy is only partially understood.

In a critical appraisal of local and traditional uses Mncwangi *et al.* (2012) showed that the species in fact has a very wide range of uses, some of which are linked to the bitterness of a key class of secondary metabolites – the iridoids, which would explain the species' use in treating gastrointestinal complaints and as a 'tonic' (Wichtl, 2009). Starting in the mid 1980s and with considerable research effort (African) devil's claw has been developed into a very successful and relatively well-characterized phytomedicine (Mncwangi *et al.* 2012).

There is good clinical evidence for some of the chemically well-defined commercial Devil's claw products available, especially on the European market, in terms of their clinical effectiveness for treating pain, especially lower back pain. Most pharmacological and clinical research has been conducted on standardized extracts used in the treatment of rheumatic conditions and lower back pain as well as other degenerative conditions of the musculo-skeletal system. There is also pre-clinical evidence for anti-inflammatory effects (Edwards *et al.*, 2015), especially based on inhibitory effects on TNF-$\alpha$ and on arachidonic acid metabolism by acting on the COX-2 mRNA expression (Fiebich *et al.*, 2001, 2012).

The secondary storage roots are collected and while they are still fresh they are cut into small pieces and dried. The main exporters are South Africa and Namibia. Attempts are currently underway to cultivate the species. The dried and powdered root of the plant is now included in the *European Pharmacopeia* (2002). Several constituents, including iridoids and phenylethanoids, are known, but the active constituents have not been identified with certainty.

## 15.2.3   *Scutellaria baicalensis* Georgi (Huang Qin, Baical skullcap; Lamiaceae)

This native to southern China has been considered to be one of the fundamental 50 herbs of TCM. It has a long tradition of uses for removing heat, particularly in the lung, alleviating pain and for a range of urological and gynaecological problems (difficult micturition and menstrual problems). Considerable research has gone into understanding its chemistry and pharmacological mechanism of action (Shang *et al.*, 2010).

Famously, *S. baicalensis* is a part of PHY906, a decoction which also contains *Glycyrrhiza uralensis* Fisch., *Paeonia lactiflora* Pall. and *Ziziphus jujuba* Mill. used in the adjuvant treatment of cancer for reducing chemotherapy-induced toxicities and/or increasing chemotherapeutic efficacy (Chen *et al.*, 2008; Liu and Cheng, 2012). In China this tetraherbal combination has a long tradition of use for common gastrointestinal distress, including diarrhoea, abdominal spasms, fever, headache, vomiting, nausea, extreme thirst and subcardiac distention. Beneficial effects on the outcomes of advanced colorectal, liver and pancreatic cancers, and increased survival if given as a co-adjuvant treatment with conventional chemotherapy are well established (Liu and Cheng, 2012). However, most of the uses of this complex preparation seem to only have limited direct links with inflammatory processes.

## 15.2.4   *Curcuma longa* L. (Zingiberaceae)

The ancient peoples of India called turmeric, which is probably native to south-east Asia, the Oushadhi – the medicinal herb. It is not known to occur in the wild and is only cultivated. The name 'turmeric' may originate from the old English word *tamaret*, possibly coming from the Latin name *terra merita*, becoming *terre merite* in French – deserving earth. Contrary to other examples in this chapter, over centuries it has been traded intercontinentally. It is traditionally indicated as an anti-inflammatory and for the treatment of flatulence, jaundice, menstrual difficulties, haematuria, haemorrhage and colic. As an external treatment it is used in poultices to relieve pain and inflammation. In China, different parts of the root and rhizome are accorded different medicinal properties (Anonymous, 2002; Booker, 2014; Booker *et al.*, 2015). The di-phenylheptanoid curcumin is often regarded as being responsible for the therapeutic effect of turmeric. In the context of inflammatory conditions it modulates the inflammatory response by down-regulating the activity of cyclooxygenase-2 (COX-2), lipoxygenase-5, (LOX-5) and iNOS by inhibiting the production of the inflammatory cytokines, TNF-α, interleukin 1, 2, 6, 8, and 12, monocyte chemo-attractant protein (MCP) and migration inhibitory protein (MIP), and by down-regulating mitogen-activated and Janus kinases (Abe *et al.*, 1999; Kim *et al.*, 2012). However, this does not explain the use of turmeric in TCM, where aqueous decoctions are the main phytopharmaceutical preparations used. As curcumin is poorly soluble in aqueous solution, any therapeutic effect must be due to other more polar compounds found within turmeric which are more readily soluble in water, e.g. polysaccharides.

Despite several thousand research studies on the plant or its main active compounds, good clinical evidence for the effectiveness of turmeric in humans is lacking. Only a few small clinical trials showing robust evidence are available, but in the context of inflammatory conditions the promising effects of curcumin in patients with diseases like arthritis, Crohn's disease, ulcerative colitis, peptic ulcer, gastric ulcer, irritable bowel disease, gastric inflammation, vitiligo, psoriasis and atherosclerosis provide some evidence (Edwards *et al.*, 2015).

Its wide use as a spice has guaranteed a long-standing interest in this plant and contrary to other examples it seems that research on this species' pharmacological effects is not driven by specific health claims. Instead, research on a plethora of conditions has been conducted, but there is a strong focus on antioxidant, hepato-protective and anti-inflammatory effects. Current research has also focused on turmeric's anti-carcinogenic and antimicrobial properties, in addition to its use in cardiovascular disease and gastrointestinal disorders (Thorne, 2002). Importantly, good evidence points to turmeric effectively blocking the proliferation of tumour cells through the suppression of NF-kB and STAT3 pathways, which also provides evidence for potential anti-inflammatory effects. Another mechanism for chemoprevention has been linked to NRF2 and its ability to regulate reactive oxygen species and reactive nitrogen species (Shureiqi and Baron, 2011), although some caution is needed as NRF2 has also been linked to oncogenesis because of its ability to create a more favourable intracellular environment for the survival of tumour cells (Sporn and Liby, 2012).

All this points to prominent anti-inflammatory effects and to the species' therapeutic potential.

## 15.2.5 *Capsicum frutescens* L.

Archaeological records of *Capsicum annuum*'s use (Long-Solis, 1986), presumably as a food and medicine in the Teohucán Valley, in Puebla, and in Tamaulipas, Mexico includes coprolites and carbonized seeds. These may have been the first cultivated chilies (7000 BCE–5000 BCE), but, of course, there is no information on the species' uses.

Originally, *C. frutescens* had a more southerly Southern American distribution (presumably originating in the western Amazonian region or Bolivia). The species commonly known as chili (English)/chile (Spanish) has been used widely in Mesoamerican Indian cultures and was discovered by the Spanish conquistadores. Pungent varieties are known both from *Capsicum annuum* L. and *C. frutescens*. Multiple medical uses were recorded during the Aztec period, including as a remedy for dental problems, infections of the ear and various types of wounds as well as digestive problems. Consequently, chillies were also an important element of tribute requested by the Aztec rulers. Soon after the conquest the Aztec term *chilli* was adopted into Spanish and the fruit was introduced in many warmer regions of the world. Most notably as early as 1542 *C. frutescens* cultivars were introduced into India by the Portuguese and *C. annuum*, for example, into the Eastern Mediterranean, the Near East and south-central Europe (Hungary). In 1543 Leonhard Fuchs described *Indianischer Pfeffer* in his *New Kreüterbuch*. Subsequently, the plant was incorporated into numerous cultures and today is widely cultivated, therefore it also has a large number of popular and local uses. For example, it is a typical Balkan (Hungarian) spice. In 1846 L. Thresh isolated *capsaicin* from *Capsicum frutescens* L., s.l. In 1919 the structure was partly elucidated by E.K. Nelson. *C. frutescens* has been used as a rubefacient to locally stimulate blood circulation.

Importantly, during the 20th century pungent fruits were used topically for rheumatism in Europe. Anti-inflammatory plasters were common going back to antiquity (Heinrich, 2013 and references cited). The irritation causing increased blood flow to the area was considered to help with relieving the inflammation. For example, in 2009 a plaster with capsaicin came onto the market in many European countries. There is evidence for efficacy for the use of externally applied capsaicin products in treating pain (Edwards *et al.*, 2015).

Research in recent decades is an exciting example of research driven by traditional knowledge and which resulted in the discovery of the transient receptor potential vanilloid type 1 protein (TRPV1). These channels were originally cloned while researchers were looking for a molecular target of this highly pungent natural product and the phorboid resiniferatoxin from species of the genus *Euphorbia*.

In this case the link between local and traditional use and recent biomedical discoveries is somewhat more indirect. While there is a large body of evidence pointing to anti-inflammatory effects, this can only partially be linked to such uses.

## 15.3 Conclusions

This chapter's title raises a question that is difficult to answer. Taking, for example, respiratory conditions (see Chapter 14), local and traditional uses may give rise to a wide range of possible groups of activities like antiviral, antibacterial, spasmolytic, cough-suppressant or immunomodulatory effects. One group of uses (in essence defined on the basis of a classical pharmacological definition of diseases of the respiratory system) therefore gives rise to a wide group of targets. Clearly, for inflammatory conditions there is a unified biomedical concept linking the various diseases to one specific concept, which helps to explain the disease mechanisms and to develop new treatment strategies and medicines. However, since many different types of local/traditional therapeutic claims can be linked to inflammatory processes, there can therefore be no unified ethnopharmacology of inflammation. Instead it is a broad concept that enables a wide range of therapeutic targets to be explored. Acute forms of inflammation especially of the skin, conversely, have been an essential element in helping the dissemination of the medicinal use of some plants, as exemplified for the arnica complex. Consequently, the ethnopharmacologies of inflammation will offer numerous research challenges and opportunities for developing better herbal medicinal products or medicines.

## References

Abe, Y., Hashimoto, S. and Horie, T. (1999) Curcumin inhibition of inflammatory cytokine production by human peripheral blood monocytes and alveolar macrophages. *Pharmacology Research*, **39** (1), 41–47.

Anonymous (2002) *Curcuma longa*. Alternative Medicine Review Monographs, Thorne Research Inc.

Booker, A. (2014) *The Transformation of Traditional Asian Medical Knowledge into International Commodities – the Link between Traditional Medicines and the International Market*, PhD dissertation, UCL, London.

Booker, A., Johnston, D. and Heinrich, M. (2015) Value Chains of Herbal Medicines, in *Ethnopharmacological and Analytical Challenges in a Globalizing World Evidence-Based Validation of Herbal Medicine* (ed. P. Mukherjee), Elsevier, Chennai.

Bremner, P. and Heinrich, M. (2002) Natural products as modulators of the NF-κB-pathway. *Journal of Pharmacy and Pharmacology*, **54**, 453–472.

Candido, J. and Hagemann, T. (2013) Cancer-related inflammation. *Journal of Clinical Immunology*, **33** (Suppl. 1), S79–S84.

Chen, S.T., Dou, J., Temple, R., *et al.* (2008) New therapies from old medicines. *Nature Biotechnology*, **26**, 1077–1083.

Edwards, S., da Costa Rocha, I., Williamson, E.M. and Heinrich, M. (2015) *Phytopharmacy – an Evidence-based Guide to Herbal Medicines*. Wiley, Chichester.

Elinav, E., Noworski, R., Thaiss, C.A., *et al.* (2013) Inflammation-induced cancer: crosstalk between tumours, immune cells and microorganisms. *National Review of Cancer*, **13**, 759–771.

European Pharmacopoeia (2002) *Council of Europe (Directorate for the Quality of Medicines). European Pharmacopoeia*, 4th edn. Strasbourg

Fiebich, B.L., Heinrich, M., Hiller, K.O. and Kammerer, N. (2001) Inhibition of TNF-alpha synthesis in LPS-stimulated primary human monocytes by *Harpagophytum* extract STEIHAP 69. *Phytomedicine*, **8** (1), 28–30.

Fiebich, B.L., Muñoz, E., Rose, T., *et al.* (2012) Molecular targets of the antiinflammatory *Harpagophytum procumbens* (Devil's claw): Inhibition of TNFα and COX-2 gene expression by preventing activation of AP-1. *Phytotherapy Research*, **26** (6), 806–811.

Hanahan, D. and Weinberg, R.A. (2011) Hallmarks of cancer: the next generation. *Cell*, **144**, 646–674.

Heinrich, M. (2013) Ethnopharmacology and drug discovery, in *Elsevier Reference Module in Chemistry, Molecular Sciences and Chemical Engineering* (ed. J. Reedijk), Elsevier, Waltham, MA. doi: 10.1016/B978-0-12-409547-2.02773-6

Heinrich, M., Robles, M., West, J.E., *et al.* (1998) Ethnopharmacology of Mexican Asteraceae (Compositae). *Annual Review of Pharmacology and Toxicology*, **38** (1), 539–565.

Heinrich, M., Pieroni, A. and Bremner, P. (2005) *Medicinal plants and phytomedicines*, in The Cultural History of Plants (consulting ed. Prance, G., scientific ed. Nesbitt, M.), Routledge (Taylor and Francis), New York, pp. 205–238.

Heinrich, M., Leonti, M. and Frei Haller, B. (2014) A perspective on natural products research and ethnopharmacology in México. The eagle and the serpent on the prickly pear cactus. *Journal of Natural Products*, **77**, 678–689.

Kim, J.H., Gupta, S.C., Park, B., *et al.* (2012) Turmeric (*Curcuma longa*) inhibits inflammatory nuclear factor (NF)-kappaB and NF-kB-regulated gene products and induces death receptors leading to suppressed proliferation, induced chemosensitization, and suppressed osteoclastogenesis. *Molecular Nutrition and Food Research*, **56**, 454–465.

Linares, E. and Bye, R. (1987) A study of four medicinal plants complexes of Mexico and adjacent United States. *Journal of Ethnopharmacology*, **19**, 153–183.

Liu, S.H. and Cheng, Y.C. (2012) Old formula, new Rx: the journey of PHY906 as cancer adjuvant therapy. *Journal of Ethnopharmacology*, **140** (3), 614–623.

Long-Solis, J. (1986) *Capsicum y cultura. La historia del Chilli*, Fondo de Cultura Económica, México.

Mayer, J.G. and Czygan, F.-Ch. (2000) *Arnica montana* L., oder Bergwohlverleih. *Zeitschrift für Phytotherapie*, **21**, 30–36.

Mehnert, G.M. (2007) Mit Schwert und Pflugschar in Sachsen und Südwestafrika. Anekdoten und Geschichten eines Südwester Pioniers. Überrarbeitet von Bernd Kroemer. Glanz & Gloria Verlag. Windhook Namibia

Merfort, I. (2003) Arnica: new insights on the molecular mode of action of a traditional medicinal plant. *Forschende Komplementärmedizin und klassische Naturheilkunde*, **10** (Suppl 1), 45–48.

Mncwangi, N., Chen, W., Vermaak, I., *et al.* (2012) Devil's Claw – a review of the ethnobotany, phytochemistry and biological activity of *Harpagophytum procumbens*. *Journal of Ethnopharmacology*, **143** (3),755–771

Mutschler, E.G., Geisslinger, H.K. Kroemer, S., *et al.* (2013) *Pharmakologie, Klinische Pharmakologie, Toxikologie*, 10th edn, Govi Verlag, Eschborn.

Obón, C. Rivera, D. Verde, A., *et al.* (2012) Árnica: a multivariate analysis of the botany and ethnopharmacology of a medicinal plant complex in the Iberian Peninsula and the Balearic Islands. *Journal of Ethnopharmacology*, **144**(1), 44–56.

Rang, H.P., Ritter, J.M. Flower, R. and Henderson, G. (2011) *Rang and Dales Pharmacology*, 7th edn, Churchill Livingstone, New York/London.

Shang, X., He, X., He, X., *et al.* (2010) The genus *Scutellaria* – an ethnopharmacological and phytochemical review. *Journal of Ethnopharmacology*, **128** (2), 279–313.

Shureiqi, I. and Baron, J.A. (2011) Curcumin chemoprevention: the long road to clinical translation. *Cancer Prevention Research*, **4**, 296–298.

Sneader, W. (2000) The discovery of aspirin: a reappraisal. *British Medical Journal*, **321** (7276), 1591–1594.

Sporn, M.B. and Liby, K.T. (2012) NRF2 and cancer: the good, the bad and the importance of context. *Nature Reviews. Cancer*, **12** (8), 564–571.

Volk, O.H. (1964) Zur Kenntnis von *Harpagophytum procumbens* DC. Botanik und Verbreitung. *Deutsche Apotheker Zeitung*, **104**, 573–576.

Watt, J.M. and Breyer-Brandwick, M.G. (1962) *Medicinal and Poisonous Plants of Southern and Eastern Africa*, 2nd edn, E & S. Livingstone Ltd, Edinburgh.

Wegener, T. (2005) *Zur klinischen Wirksamkeit der südafrikanischen Teufelskrallenwurzel (Harpagophyti radix) bei Patienten mit Cox- und Gonarthrose*, PhD dissertation, Universität Osnabrück, Germany

Wichtl, M. (ed.) (2009) *Teedrogen & Phytopharmaka*, Wissenschaftliche Verlagsgesellschaft, Stuttgart.

Zorn, B. (1958) Über die antiarthritische Wirkung der Harpagophytum-Wurzel. *Deutsche Rheumaforschung*, **17**, 134.

# 16

# Epidermal Growth Factor Receptors and Downstream Signalling Pathways as Cancer Treatment Targets for Medicinal Plants

Ean Jeong Seo[1], Ching-Fen Wu[1], Henny J. Greten[2] and Thomas Efferth[1]

[1]*Department of Pharmaceutical Biology, Institute of Pharmacy and Biochemistry, Johannes Gutenberg University, Mainz, Germany*
[2]*Abel Salazar Biomedical Sciences Institute, University of Porto, Portugal, and Heidelberg School of Chinese Medicine, Heidelberg, Germany*

## 16.1 Role of epidermal growth factor receptors for cancer biology

The gene family of human epidermal growth factor receptors consists of four members (HER1–HER4), which of HER1 (EGFR, erbB1) and HER2 (erbB2, c-neu) are best characterized. On binding to their respective ligands, they activate the signal transduction pathways involved in basic biological processes such as cell proliferation, differentiation, apoptosis, metastasis and angiogenesis. HER1 and HER2 are frequently over-expressed in tumours and are associated with an unfavourable prognosis of patients (Scagliotti *et al.*, 2004).

The receptors are inactive monomers, which are activated by binding of specific ligands. As of yet, 10 ligands belonging to two families are known, i.e. the epidermal growth factor family (EGF, transforming growth factor-α, β-cellulin, epiregulin, HB-EGF and AR) and the neuregulin family (heregulin and neuregulins) (Riese *et al.*, 1995; Beerli and Hynes, 1996). Activation is associated with either homo-dimerization with a second EFGR molecule or with another

*Ethnopharmacology*, First Edition. Edited by Michael Heinrich and Anna K. Jäger.

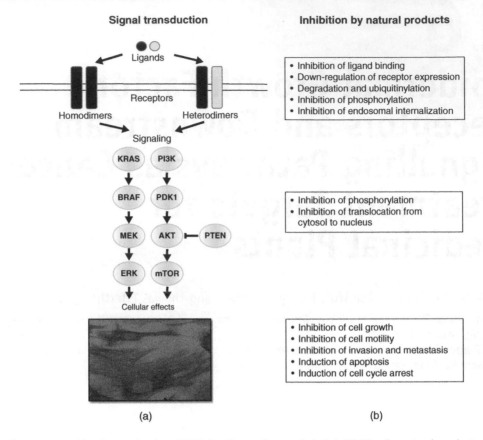

**Figure 16.1**    Signal transduction of HER family members and their inhibition by natural products.

HER member. Similarly, HER2 can dimerize with HER3 or HER4 and HER3 with HER4. Interestingly, HER3 lacks an intracellular kinase domain. Hence, it can bind ligands, but the enzymatic activity of the heterodimers depends on the binding partner, i.e. EGFR, HER2 or HER4 (Olayioye *et al.*, 2000). Dimers are only formed if one receptor molecule of the pair binds to a ligand. The flexibility in heterodimerization and binding of 10 different ligands results in a large complexity and variability in mediating signal transduction (Riese *et al.*, 1995; Beerli and Hynes, 1996). Heterodimers expand substrate selection and signalling pathway activation. Furthermore, the duration and strength of receptor signalling affect altered receptor internalization and recycling as well as rates of phosphorylation and dephosphorylation (Earp *et al.*, 1995).

Dimerization stimulates the intrinsic tyrosine kinase activity of EGFR, which regulates specific signal transduction cascades, e.g. Raf/Mek/Erk, PI3K/PDK1/Akt, PLCγ/PKC, MAPK and JNK-signalling routes (Figure 16.1). Constitutive EGFR activation as consequence of point mutations or gene amplification causes deregulated cellular processes such as proliferation, invasion, angiogenesis, cell motility, cell adhesion, inhibition of apoptosis and DNA synthesis. The kinase activity is also associated with auto-phosphorylation of five tyrosine residues in the C-terminal EGFR domain. Mutations affecting EGFR expression foster carcinogenesis.

The extraordinary relevance of EGFR in tumour biology makes it an exquisite molecular target for tumour therapy. Apart from therapeutic antibodies, several small molecules have been developed as EGFR inhibitors (Oliveira *et al.*, 2006). For example, gefitinib (Iressa®, Astra Zeneca, DE, USA) and erlotinib (Tarceva®, OSI-774, Genentech Inc., CA, USA) are first-generation inhibitors used for the treatment of non-small cell lung cancer and other tumour types (Astsaturov *et al.*, 2006). Both quinazolinamines exhibit their inhibitory activity by competing with ATP for the ATP binding pocket of EGFR.

Despite considerable successes with EGFR tyrosine kinase inhibitors in cancer therapy, resistance against these chemical compounds has developed due to the selection of point-mutated EGFR variants (Perea and Hidalgo, 2004). There is therefore an urgent need for the identification of novel EGFR tyrosine kinase inhibitors. In recent years, medicinal plants became the centre of interest as resources for novel treatment strategies to target EGFR family members.

Since the development of monoclonal antibody C225 to treat EGFR-positive cancers (Mendelsohn, 1997), many other therapeutic antibodies and small molecule tyrosine kinase inhibitors against EGFR and HER2 have been developed (Roskoski, 2014). In contrast, HER4 does not serve as target for drug development because of its positive prognostic significance. While EGFR- or HER2-overexpressing cancers are adverse prognostic factors for standard cytotoxic chemotherapy, the contrary occurs on application of EGFR- or HER2-targeting drugs. Tumours with high EGFR or HER expression are preferentially killed by such targeted antibodies and small molecule inhibitors (Figueroa-Magalhaes *et al.*, 2014). This is an instructive example of how the specific therapeutic targeting of proteins with worse prognosis can be exploited to improve treatment success rates. Unfortunately, tumours can also develop resistance against EGFR- or HER2-directed antibodies, and small molecules and the search for novel drugs to fight cancer continues. In this context, the tremendous chemodiversity of phytochemicals comes into play. Novel compounds from natural sources may serve as lead compounds for a new generation of drugs eradicating resistant tumours.

## 16.2   Inhibition of epidermal growth factor signalling by phytochemicals and medicinal plants

### 16.2.1   Natural products as a resource for cancer treatment

As pointed out by a survey of the National Cancer Institute, USA, the majority of established cancer drugs are natural products, derivatives of natural products or drugs mimicking the mode of action of natural products (Newman and Cragg, 2007). Searching in nature for novel scaffolds is a promising way to find new chemical tools to bypass and overcome such drug resistance. Novel natural product inhibitors may serve as lead compounds for drug development. A plethora of data in the literature shows that natural products can serve as inhibitors for EGFR-associated signalling molecules such as the RAS/RAF/MEK/ERK and PI3K/AKT/mTOR pathways. This indicates that the identification of novel inhibitors from natural resources is not beyond the scope of expectations.

### 16.2.2   Inhibitors of EGFR signalling

Phytochemicals from different chemical classes such as flavonoids, terpenoids and alkaloids have been shown to exert their cytotoxic activity towards cancer cells by affecting EGFR signalling. Some specific compounds were intensively investigated, such as genistein, curcumin and resveratrol (Park *et al.*, 2010; Wang *et al.*, 2010; Lee *et al.*, 2011). The frequent observation that natural products act in a multifactorial manner (Efferth and Koch, 2011) applies here as well.

Furthermore, natural compounds inhibited the phosphorylation of downstream kinases either as consequence of EGFR inhibition or by binding of compounds to corresponding kinase domains of signal transducers. In addition, translocation of kinases (e.g. ERK, MAPK) from the cytosol to the nucleus can be blocked by some compounds. As consequence of silencing EGFR signalling routes, various effects were observed in cancer cells, e.g. induction of cell cycle arrest and apoptosis, inhibition of cell mobility and inhibition of invasion of metastasis. It is important to note that several compounds have been shown to exert their effects not only *in vitro* but also *in vivo* (Park *et al.*, 2010; Lee *et al.*, 2011).

Furthermore, natural products can reduce the side effects of standard anticancer therapy on normal organs as shown by the combination of curcumin and gefitinib, which led to reduced gastrointestinal side effects compared to gefitinib alone in xenograft tumour-bearing mice (Lee *et al.*, 2011).

In addition to isolated phytochemicals, there are also a number of investigations reporting on the inhibition of EGFR by single plant extracts or extracts from complex herbal mixtures used in TCM to treat cancer (Table 16.1). The use of these plants and mixtures in TCM has been previously reported (Cai, 1998; Guo and Wei 2007; Hsu *et al.*, 2008; Shen *et al.*, 2008; Hao *et al.*, 2009; Lu *et al.*, 2009; Xiong *et al.*, 2010; Way *et al.*, 2010; Zhou *et al.*, 2010; Hou *et al.*, 2011; Liu and Cheng, 2012). The majority of these studies described the down-regulated EGFR expression rather than inhibition of phosphorylation. This might indicate that inhibition of EGFR mRNA or protein expression results from the multifactorial action of complex compound mixtures in the extracts, while the inhibition of EGFR phosphorylation necessitates the binding of a specific compound to the tyrosine kinase domain of the receptor. The molecular mechanisms causing down-regulation of EGFR expression remain, however, unknown. A few studies report on the inhibition of kinases downstream of EGFR, e.g. AKT and STAT3 as well as the down-regulation of expression, e.g. ERK1/2 (Table 16.1). A synopsis of the published literature indicates that Chinese medicinal plants affect EGFR signalling by multiple modes – an observation that supports the more general view that medicinal plants exert multifactorial activities (Efferth and Koch, 2011). It is important to point out that several investigations reported on the *in vivo* activity of medicinal plants and herbal preparations in rats and mice (Table 16.1). Hence, it can be speculated that these medicinal plants might also be active in cancer patients.

## 16.2.3   Inhibitors of HER2/HER3 signalling

Although the inhibition of other EGFR family members was much less investigated, several studies provided results for the inhibition of HER2 and HER3, and their related downstream signalling routes. Evidence has been gathered for (–)-epigallocatechin-3-gallate, genistein and curcumin (Masuda *et al.*, 2003; Li *et al.*, 2004; Shimizu *et al.*, 2005; Hou *et al.*, 2011; Sun *et al.*, 2012). The mechanisms of actions how these phytochemicals affect HER2 and HER3 are comparable with those observed for EGFR. They include inhibition of HER2/HER3 phosphorylation and expression as well as inhibition of downstream signal transducers, e.g. ERK1/2, AKT and STAT3.

Several studies also described anticancer active medicinal plants from Chinese medicine inhibiting HER2, HER2-downstream signal routes, leading to inhibition of cell proliferation induction of apoptosis, postponing and reducing both carcinogenesis and tumour recurrence (Table 16.2). Here again, it is important to note that the activity of Chinese medicinal plants

**Table 16.1** Plants and mixtures from traditional Chinese medicine with activity against EGFR.

| Plant/mixture | Tumour type | Effect | Reference |
| --- | --- | --- | --- |
| Hechanpian | A549 lung cancer | Down-regulation of EGFR mRNA Growth inhibition Induction of apoptosis | Xiong *et al.* (2010) |
| *Saussurea involucrata* Kar. et Kir. | PC3 prostate cancer | Inhibition of EGFR phosphorylation and activation of AKT and STAT3 | Way *et al.* (2010) |
| Maimendong and qianjin weijing decoction | A549 lung cancer | Down-regulation of EGFR and ERK Growth inhibition and apoptosis induction | Zhou *et al.* (2010) |
| *Scutellaria baicalensis* Huds. | HepG2 liver cancer | Down-regulation of EGFR and ERK1/2 protein expression | Ye *et al.* (2009) |
| Mixture of Radix Astragali and Radix Rehmanniae | Normal keraqtinoxytes | Up-regulation of EGFR expression | Ren *et al.* (2012) |
| *Ganoderma tsugae* Murrill | A431 epidermoid cancer | Inhibition of EGFR expression | Hsu *et al.* (2009) |
| Jinguo Weikang | Gastric precancerous lesions | Down-regulation of EGFR protein expression *in vivo* (rats) | Shen *et al.* (2008) |
| Astragalus injection | MDA-MB-468 breast cancer | Down-regulation of EGFR protein expression *in vivo* | Ye and Chen (2008) |
| Xiaotan Sanjie | MKN-45 gastric cancer | Down-regulation of EGFR protein expression *in vivo* | Guo and Wei (2007) |
| Kanglaite | Lewis lung cancer | Down-regulation of EGFR | Pan *et al.* (2012) |
| Mixture of *Sophora tonkinensis* Gagnep, *Polygonum bistorta* L., *Prunella vulgaris* L., *Sonchus arvensis* L., *Dictamnus dasycarpous* Turcz., *Dioscorea* bulbifera L. | 4NQO-induced oral squamous cell carcinomas | Down-regulation of EGFR | Wang *et al.* (2013) |
| Radix Caulophylli | A431 epidermoid cancer | | Hou *et al.* (2011) |

have not only been demonstrated *in vitro*, but also *in vivo*. Among other diseases, the plants and herbal recipes listed in Table 16.2 have been used in traditional Chinese medicine to treat cancer (Chen *et al.*, 2001; Liu *et al.*, 2001, 2008; Ko *et al.*, 2004; Hwang *et al.*, 2012; Zhang *et al.*, 2012).

## 16.3 Conclusions and perspectives

The identification of tumour target molecules with prognostic relevance for patients has opened avenues for the development of more specific treatment options. Important examples in current cancer biology and pharmacology are EGFRs and specific small molecules inhibiting their signalling in tumours. Nevertheless, resistance can also occur towards targeted therapies and novel drugs attacking these receptors are needed. Natural products have been

**Table 16.2**   Plants and mixtures from traditional Chinese medicine with activity against HER2.

| Plant | Tumour type | Effect | Reference |
| --- | --- | --- | --- |
| *Pharbitis (Ipomoea) nil* L. | MCF7 breast cancer | Inhibition of phosphorylation of HER2, AKT and ERK Inhibition of proliferation and induction of apoptosis | Ju *et al.* (2011) |
| Rupifang | Mammary hyperplasia in rats | Down-regulation of EGFR protein expression | Zhang *et al.* (2012) |
| Ru'ai Shuhou | Spontaneous breast cancer | Postponing and reducing the carcinogenesis of primary breast tumours in HER2-transgenic mice | Wu *et al.* (2010) |
| Ru'ai Shuhou | Spontaneous breast cancer | Inhibition of tumour recurrence | Wu *et al.* (2012) |
| Si-Wu-Tang | BT-474 and SK-BR-3 breast cancer | Reversion of trastuzumab-induced antiproliferative effects | Chen *et al.* (2013) |
| *Salvia milthiorrhiza* Bunge | MCF-7 and MCF-7 HER2 breast cancer | Down-regulation of AKT and G1 cell cycle arrest MCF-7 HER2 cells were more resistant to danshen than MCF-7 cells | Yang *et al.* (2010) |
| Actaea (Cimicifuga) racemosa (L.) Nutt. | Spontaneous breast cancer | No effect on primary breast cancer development in MMTV-neu mouse model Increased incidence of lung metastasis | Davis *et al.* (2008) |

identified as possible novel drug candidates specifically inhibiting EGFR in tumour cells. An important perspective for EGFR/HER2/HER3 inhibiting natural products is their use for personalized treatment options. The individual testing of the mutational status would allow the right EGFR/HER2/HER3 inhibitor to be selected for each patient. In this respect, natural products may represent valuable tools for the development of personalized therapy in the years to come.

# References

Astsaturov, I., Cohen, R.B. and Harari, P. (2006) Targeting epidermal growth factor receptor signaling in the treatment of head and neck cancer. *Expert Reviews in Anticancer Therapy*, **6**, 1179–1193.

Beerli, R.R. and Hynes, N.E. (1996) Epidermal growth factor-related peptides activate distinct subsets of ErbB receptors and differ in their biological activities. *Journal of Biological Chemistry*, **271**, 6071–6076.

Cai, S. (1998) Chemical constituents and pharmcological activity of eight species herb Xuelianhua. *Chinese Pharmaceutical Journal*, **33**, 449–452.

Chen, X.G., Li, Y., Yan, C.H., *et al.* (2001) Cancer chemopreventive activities of S-3-1, a synthetic derivative of danshinone. *Journal of Asian Natural Product Research*, **3**, 63–75.

Chen, J.L., Wang, J.Y., Tsai, Y.F., *et al.* (2013) In vivo and in vitro demonstration of herb-drug interference in human breast cancer cells treated with tamoxifen and trastuzumab. *Menopause*, **20**, 646–654.

Davis, V.L., Jayo, M.J., Ho, A., *et al.* (2008) Black cohosh increases metastatic mammary cancer in transgenic mice expressing c-erbB2. *Cancer Research*, **68**, 8377–8383.

Earp, H.S., Dawson, T.L., Li, X. and Yu, H. (1995) Heterodimerization and functional interaction between EGF receptor family members: a new signaling paradigm with implications for breast cancer research. *Breast Cancer Research Treatment*, **35**, 115–132.

Efferth, T. and Koch, E. (2011) Complex interactions between phytochemicals. The multi-target therapeutic concept of phytotherapy. *Current Drug Targets*, **12**, 122–132.

Figueroa-Magalhaes, M.C., Jelovac, D., Connolly, R.M. and Wolff, A.C. (2014) Treatment of HER2-positive breast cancer. *Breast*, **23**, 128–136.

Guo, X.D. and Wei, P.K. (2007) Effect of Xiaotan Sanjie Recipe on growth of transplanted tumor and expressions of proliferating cell nuclear antigen and epidermal growth factor receptor in tissue of gastric carcinoma of nude mice. *Journal of Chinese Integrative Medicine*, **5**, 432–436.

Hao, Q., Wang, J., Niu, J., *et al.* [Study on phytoestrogenic-like effects of four kinds of Chinese medicine including Radix Rehmanniae Preparata, Radix Paeoniae Alba, Radix Angelicae Sinensis, Rhizoma Chuanxiong]. *Zhongguo Zhong Yao Za Zhi*, **34**, 620–624.

Hou, X., Wang, S., Hou, J. and He, L. (2011) Establishment of A431 cell membrane chromatography-RPLC method for screening target components from Radix Caulophylli. *Journal of Separation Science*, **34**, 508–513.

Hsu, S.C., Ou, C.C., Li, J.W., *et al.* (2008) Ganoderma tsugae extracts inhibit colorectal cancer cell growth via G(2)/M cell cycle arrest. *Journal of Ethnopharmacology*, **120**, 394–401.

Hsu, S.C., Ou, C.C., Chuang, T.C., *et al.* (2009) Ganoderma tsugae extract inhibits expression of epidermal growth factor receptor and angiogenesis in human epidermoid carcinoma cells: In vitro and in vivo. *Cancer Letters*, **281**, 108–116.

Hwang, Y.H., Kim, T., Cho, W.K., *et al.* (2012) Food- and gender-dependent pharmacokinetics of paeoniflorin after oral administration with Samul-tang in rats. *Journal of Ethnopharmacology*, **142**, 161–167.

Ju, J.H., Jeon, M.J., Yang, W., *et al.* (2011) Induction of apoptotic cell death by Pharbitis nil extract in HER2-overexpressing MCF-7 cells. *Journal of Ethnopharmacology*, **133**, 126–131.

Ko, S.G., Koh, S.H., Jun, C.Y., *et al.* (2004) Induction of apoptosis by Saussurea lappa and Pharbitis nil on AGS gastric cancer cells. *Biological and Pharmaceutical Bulletin*, **27**, 1604–1610.

Lee, J.Y., Lee, Y.M., Chang, G.C., *et al.* (2011) Curcumin induces EGFR degradation in lung adenocarcinoma and modulates p38 activation in intestine: the versatile adjuvant for gefitinib therapy. *PLoS One*, **6**, e23756.

Li, Y., Mi, C., Wu, Y.Z., *et al.* (2004) [The effects of genistein on epidermal growth factor receptor mediated signal transduction pathway in human ovarian carcinoma cells lines SKOV3 and its xenograft in nude mice]. *Zhonghua Bing Li Xue Za Zhi*, **33**, 546–549.

Liu, S.H. and Cheng, Y.C. (2012) Old formula, new Rx: the journey of PHY906 as cancer adjuvant therapy. *Journal of Ethnopharmacology*, **140**, 614–623.

Liu, Z., Yang, Z., Zhu, M. and Huo, J. (2001) Estrogenicity of black cohosh (Cimicifuga racemosa) and its effect on estrogen receptor level in human breast cancer MCF-7 cells. *Journal of Medicinal Food*, **30**, 77–80.

Liu, S., Zhao, J., Liu, J., *et al.* (2008) Effects of Ru'ai Shuhou Recipe on 5-year recurrence rate after mastectomy in breast cancer. *Journal of Chinese Integrative Medicine*, **6**, 1000–1004.

Lu, Y., Wu, L.Q., Dong, Q. and Li, C.S. (2009) Experimental study on the effect of Kang-Lai-Te induced apoptosis of human hepatoma carcinoma cell HepG2. *Hepatobiliary Pancreatic Disease International*, **8**, 267–272.

Masuda, M., Suzui, M., Lim, J.T. and Weinstein, I.B. (2003) Epigallocatechin-3-gallate inhibits activation of HER-2/neu and downstream signaling pathways in human head and neck and breast carcinoma cells. *Clinical Cancer Research*, **9**, 3486–3491.

Mendelsohn, J. (1997) Epidermal growth factor receptor inhibition by a monoclonal antibody as anticancer therapy. *Clinical Cancer Research*, **3**, 2703–2707.

Newman, D.J. and Cragg, G.M. (2007) Natural products as sources of new drugs over the last 25 years. *Journal of Natural Products*, **70**, 461–477.

Olayioye, M.A., Neve, R.M., Lane, H.A. and Hynes, N.E. (2000) The ErbB signaling network: receptor heterodimerization in development and cancer. *EMBO Journal*, **19**, 3159–3167.

Oliveira, S., van Bergen en Henegouwen, P.M., Storm, G. and Schiffelers, R.M. (2006) Molecular biology of epidermal growth factor receptor inhibition for cancer therapy. *Expert Opinion in Biological Therapy*, **6**, 605–617.

Pan, P., Wu, Y., Guo, Z.Y., *et al.* (2012) Antitumor activity and immunomodulatory effects of the intraperitoneal administration of Kanglaite in vivo in Lewis lung carcinoma. *Journal of Ethnopharmacology*, **143**, 680–685.

Park, S.J., Kim, M.J., Kim, Y.K., *et al.* (2010) Combined cetuximab and genistein treatment shows additive anti-cancer effect on oral squamous cell carcinoma. *Cancer Letters*, **292**, 54–63.

Perea, S. and Hidalgo, M. (2004) Predictors of sensitivity and resistance to epidermal growth factor receptor inhibitors. *Clinical Lung Cancer*, **6** (Suppl. 1), S30–S34.

Ren, J.W., Chan, K.M., Lai, P.K., *et al.* (2012) Extracts from Radix Astragali and Radix Rehmanniae promote keratinocyte proliferation by regulating expression of growth factor receptors. *Phytotherapy Research*, **26**, 1547–1554.

Riese, D.J., 2nd,, van Raaij, T.M., Plowman, G.D., *et al.* (1995) The cellular response to neuregulins is governed by complex interactions of the erbB receptor family. *Molecular Cellular Biology*, **15**, 5770–5776.

Roskoski, R., Jr., (20140 ErbB/HER protein-tyrosine kinases: Structures and small molecule inhibitors. *Pharmacology Research*, **87C**, 42–59.

Scagliotti, G.V., Selvaggi, G., Novello, S. and Hirsch, F.R. (2004) The biology of epidermal growth factor receptor in lung cancer. *Clinical Cancer Research*, **10**, 4227s–4232s.

Shen, S.W., Yuwen, Y., Zhang, Z.L., *et al.* (2008) Effect of Jinguo Weikang Capsule on proto-oncogene expression of gastric mucosa in rats with gastric precancerous lesions. *Chinese Journal of Integral Medicine*, **14**, 212–216.

Shimizu, M., Deguchi, A., Joe, A.K., *et al.* (2005) EGCG inhibits activation of HER3 and expression of cyclooxygenase-2 in human colon cancer cells. *Journal of Experimental Therapy in Oncology*, **5**, 69–78.

Sun, S.H., Huang, H.C., Huang, C. and Lin, J.K. (2012) Cycle arrest and apoptosis in MDA-MB-231/Her2 cells induced by curcumin. *European Journal of Pharmacology*, **690**, 22–30.

Wang, Y., Romigh, T., He, X., *et al.* (2010) Resveratrol regulates the PTEN/AKT pathway through androgen receptor-dependent and -independent mechanisms in prostate cancer cell lines. *Human Molecular Genetics*, **19**, 4319–4329.

Wang, Y., Yao, R., Gao, S., *et al.* (2013) Chemopreventive effect of a mixture of Chinese Herbs (antitumor B) on chemically induced oral carcinogenesis. *Molecular Carcinogens*, **52**, 49–56.

Way, T.D., Lee, J.C., Kuo, D.H., *et al.* (2010) Inhibition of epidermal growth factor receptor signaling by Saussurea involucrata, a rare traditional Chinese medicinal herb, in human hormone-resistant prostate cancer PC-3 cells. *Journal of Agricultural and Food Chemistry*, 2010, **58**, 3356–3365.

Wu, X.Q., Wan, H. and Li, X.R. (2010) [Effect of ru'ai shuhou recipe on immune response in HER2/neu tranagenic mice undergoing breast cancer carcinogenesis process]. *Zhongguo Zhong Xi Yi Jie He Za Zhi*, **30**, 717–719.

Wu, X.Q., Shao, S.J. and Qu, W.C. (2012) [Effects of ru'ai shuhou recipe on the matrix metalloproteinases and the inhibitive factors in the recurrence and metastasis of HER2 positive breast cancer]. *Zhongguo Zhong Xi Yi Jie He Za Zhi*, **32**, 1526–1530.

Xiong, S.Q., Zhou, D.H. and Lin, L.Z. (2010) [Apoptosis inducing effect of Hechanpian on human lung adenocarcinoma A549 cells]. *Zhongguo Zhong Xi Yi Jie He Za Zhi*, **30**, 607–610.

Yang, W., Ju, J.H., Jeon, M.J., *et al.* (2010) Danshen (Salvia miltiorrhiza) extract inhibits proliferation of breast cancer cells via modulation of Akt activity and p27 level. *Phytotherapy Research*, **24**, 198–204.

Ye, M.N. and Chen, H.F. (2008) Effects of Astragalus injection on proliferation of basal-like breast cancer cell line MDA-MB-468. *Journal of Chinese Integrative Medicine*, **6**, 399–404.

Ye, F., Che, Y., McMillen, E., *et al.* (2009) The effect of Scutellaria baicalensis on the signaling network in hepatocellular carcinoma cells. *Nutrition and Cancer*, **61**, 530–537.

Zhang, G., Li, D., Guo, H., *et al.* (2012) Modulation of expression of p16 and her2 in rat breast tissues of mammary hyperplasia model by external use of rupifang extract. *Journal of Traditional Chinese Medicine*, **32**, 651–656.

Zhou, Y., Zhan, Z., Tang, Y., *et al.* (2010) [Mechanisms of proliferative inhibition by maimendong & qianjinweijing decoction in A549 cells]. *Zhongguo Fei Ai Za Zhi*, **13**, 477–482.

# 17

# From Ethnopharmacological Field Study to Phytochemistry and Preclinical Research: The Example of Ghanaian Medicinal Plants for Improved Wound Healing

Andreas Hensel[1], Emelia Kisseih[1], Matthias Lechtenberg[1], Frank Petereit[1], Christian Agyare[2] and Alex Asase[3]

[1]*Institute of Pharmaceutical Biology and Phytochemistry, University of Münster, Corrensstraße, Germany*
[2]*Department of Pharmaceutics, Faculty of Pharmacy and Pharmaceutical Sciences, College of Health Sciences, Kwame Nkrumah University of Science and Technology, Kumasi, Ghana*
[3]*Department of Botany, University of Ghana, Legon, Ghana*

## 17.1 Introduction

Ethnopharmacological knowledge is widespread and important among local and indigenous people around the world but much of the information is empirical at best, lacking scientific validation. Despite widespread use of plant resources in traditional medicines, bioassay analysis of few plant species have been conducted to investigate their pharmacological properties and to ascertain safety and efficacy of herbal remedies (Kunwar *et al.*, 2009). An enormous amount of knowledge on how to use the plants against different diseases may be expected to have accumulated in communities where the use of plants is still relevant (Farnsworth, 1998).

*Ethnopharmacology*, First Edition. Edited by Michael Heinrich and Anna K. Jäger.
© 2015 John Wiley & Sons, Ltd. Published 2015 by John Wiley & Sons, Ltd.

Traditional medicine uses knowledge, skills and practices for the well-being of the local people and is based on the expertise gained by herbalists over a long period of time (WHO, 2000; Ved and Goraya, 2008).

The present study in a defined geographical and cultural area in Ghana on plants used for wound healing highlights the importance of plants used for wound healing. Our aim is both to provide an example of an ethnopharmacological research strategy and to demonstrate how this can be used in the analysis of plants used locally in the treatment and management of wounds. The latter provides a scientific basis for the traditional use of these plants, and provides an example highlighting that certain species can be used for the strategic development of high-quality galenical preparations for topical wound healing in African (and also western) countries.

## 17.2  Results

### 17.2.1  The start of a research project: validated field study on wound-healing plants

A validated survey was carried out in the Bosomtwi-Atwima-Kwanwoma district, Ashanti region, Ghana and could only be performed thanks to an extensive collaboration between scientists from Kwame Nkrumah University (Kumasi, Ghana), Münster University (Germany), a botanist from the University of Ghana, Accra, executives and members of the district branch of the Ghana Association of Traditional Medicine (GHAFTRAM) and 76 healers from the rural community. It was essential for the research team to build up a climate of trust and honour for the healers, and to show them very clearly that the study was science-driven and not aiming to 'steal' knowledge from them. The relevant permits were obtained prior to the start of the interviews.

One year after the field study was completed German scientists visited some selected healers of the community to communicate the outcome of the study and to express their gratitude. In this context, despite the very basic conditions under which the healers perform their role, all German scientists were deeply impressed by the personality and the knowledge of these people.

### 17.2.2  Before starting laboratory work: who the healers are and some socioeconomic aspects

Evaluation of the status of the interview partners revealed that professional healers were mainly older than 40 years (86%), with 14% older than 80 years. About two-thirds of the healers were men. The level of education of the healers does not increase their potential qualification to practice as a traditional healer. Only one healer had a university degree, while 40% had no formal education, 50% has at most middle school/junior secondary school (elementary) education and 8% had high school education. Younger healers had comparably higher levels of education than the old practitioners. The only practitioner with a university education fell within the 21–30 age group. The level of education could determine the level of readiness to apply scientifically validated methods of preparation of their medicines and treatment of the ailment. The practical work of healers depended mostly on their intuition and experience achieved during practical work over the years. Herbal practitioners constituted the majority (58%) of the healers. Fetish priests and traditional healers constituted 36% and 6% of the group, respectively. It is important to note, however, that there was no clear distinction of practice between the three kinds of healers. Each could play the role of the other, and this is common in traditional medical practice.

A significant proportion of the healers have been in practice for long periods of time. Moreover, the profession requires long experience to be able to identify plants for effective management and treatment of diseases.

## 17.2.3   Evaluation of the data collection and cross-referencing to published literature

Overall, 104 plant species from 89 genera (47 families) were recorded (Table 17.1). In order to investigate whether these species are already known plants for wound healing, cross-referencing was made to standard literature (Neuwinger, 1989; Burkill, 2000) (Table 17.1). Of the 104 plants from the survey only 26 are listed for wound-healing by Burkill, nine by Neuwinger and nine in both references.

## 17.2.4   The next step: selection of plants for *in vitro* investigations

Based on the frequency of use, species were clustered into three groups (Table 17.1):

- group I – very frequently used species
- group II – frequently used species
- group III – species used fewer than 7 times.

Overall, 18 medicinal plants comprise 57% of all records from the healers.

The top 18 plants were subjected to an intense review concerning the details of use given by the healers. Eleven plant species were selected (Table 17.2) for further *in vitro* investigation for their influence on the cell physiology of human skin cells. One of the most cited species, *Chromolaena odorata*, was excluded from this screening because its activity on the human skin is well documented and the evidence for such effects has been well documented (Phan *et al.*, 1998, 2001). *Colocasia esculentus* was also excluded since it remained unclear from the survey which part of the plant is used.

## 17.2.5   Screening of selected plant extracts: influence on skin cells under *in vitro* conditions

Extracts were prepared from the selected species (Table 17.2) and investigated at 10 and 100 µg/ml, focusing on a potential influence on mitochondrial activity on human keratinocytes. Aqueous extracts from *Combretum mucronatum*, *Phyllanthus muellerianus* and *Pycnanthus angolensis* turned out to significantly increase viability (MTT assay).

Aqueous extracts from these three species were subjected to a more detailed investigation using human keratinocytes and primary dermal fibroblasts by using standard methods of cell biology (Deters *et al.*, 2004, 2005, 2008; Zippel *et al.*, 2009; Table 17.3). The stimulating effects of *P. muellerianus* on keratinocytes were dose dependent (10–100 µg/ml) and the increased cellular energy status was accompanied by an increased cellular proliferation. Aqueous extracts from *P. angolensis* (50–100 µg/ml) stimulated keratinocytes in MTT and BrdU assay.

**Table 17.1**   Medicinal plants used for the management of various wounds in Bosomtwi-Atwima-Kwanwonwa district, Ghana, according ethnopharmacological survey.

| Plan species/scientific name/ local name (Asante-Twi) | Type of wound | Formulation | Part of plant used |
|---|---|---|---|
| **Acanthaceae** | | | |
| *Justicia flava* Vahl. Afema This species had a frequency of use of 11 hits and was sorted into group I (very frequent use, recorded more than 10 times by the 78 healers) for intensified experimental investigation. | New, old, deep, chronic wounds, boils, burns, stomach ulcer Also described in 2 | Poultice, decoction | Fresh leaves |
| **Amaranthaceae** | | | |
| *Althernanthera pungens* (L.) Link. Abirimmuro | New wounds, boils | Decoction | Leaves |
| *Pupalia lappacea* (L.) A Juss. Aposompo This species had a frequency of use of 11 hits and was sorted into group I (very frequent use, recorded more than 10 times by the 78 healers) for intensified experimental investigation. | New wounds, boils Also described in 2 | Poultice | Leaves |
| **Anacardiaceae** | | | |
| *Lannea welwitschii* (Hiern) Engl. Kumnini | Chronic wounds, stomach ulcer/sores | Decoction | Leaves, stem bark |
| *Mangifera indica* L. Mango | Chronic and new wounds Also described in 2 | Poultice | Leaves, stem bark |
| **Annonaceae** | | | |
| *Annona squamosa* L. Apre | Burns | Poultice | Leaves |
| *Pachypodanthium staudtii* Engl. et Diels Duawusa | Measles, skin rashes Also described in 1 | Cream with shear butter | Leaves |
| *Uvaria mocoli* De Wild & T. Durand. Apraduro | Shingles | Poultice | Leaves |
| *Xylopia aethiopica* A.Rich. Hwentia | Chronic wounds Also described in 1 | Powder, poultice | Fruits |
| **Apocynaceae** | | | |
| *Alstonia boonei* De Wild. Nyamedua This species had a frequency of use of seven hits and was sorted into group II (frequent use, recorded seven to nine times by the 78 healers) for intensified experimental investigation. | Chronic, new wounds, boils Also described in 2 | Poultice | Stem bark, root |
| *Funtumia elastica* (Preuss) Stapf. Funtum | Stomach ulcer/sores | Decoction | Stem bark |
| *Hunteria ghanensis* J. B. Hall & Leeuwenb. Akuama | Stomach ulcer/sores | Enema | Seeds |

**Table 17.1** *(Continued)*

| Plan species/scientific name/ local name (Asante-Twi) | Type of wound | Formulation | Part of plant used |
|---|---|---|---|
| *Rauwolfia vomitoria* Afzel. Kakapenpen | Haemorrhoids Also described in 1 | Root | Decoction |
| *Strophanthus hispidus* DC. Omaatwa | Chronic wounds, stomach ulcer Also described in 1 | Leaves, root | Poultice, decoction |
| *Voacanga africana* Stapf ex Scott-Eliot Paaku | New, old wounds | Decoction | Stem bark |
| **Araceae** | | | |
| *Anchomanes difformis* Engl. Opɛ This species had a frequency of use of seven hits and was sorted into group II (frequent use, recorded seven to nine times by the 78 healers) for intensified experimental investigation. | Snake bites, burns Also described in 1 | Decoction poultice | Leaves, stem bark |
| *Colocasia esculentus* (L.) Schott Kooko This species had a frequency of use of 10 hits and was sorted into group I (very frequent use, recorded more than 10 times by the 78 healers) for intensified experimental investigation. | Stings/bites, chronic wounds, deep wounds Also described in 2 | Poultice, decoction | Leaves, stem bark |
| **Arecaceae** | | | |
| *Elaeis guineensis* Jacq. Abe | Chronic wounds | Powder | Leaves |
| **Asclepiadaceae** | | | |
| *Parquetina nigrescens* (Afzel). Bullock. Abakamo This species had a frequency of use of seven hits and was sorted into group II (frequent use, recorded seven to nine times by the 78 healers) for intensified experimental investigation. | Boils, carbuncles, snake bites, new, old wounds Also described in 1 | Poultice | Leaves, root |
| *Secamone afzelii* (Roem. & Shult.) K. Schum Kwantemaa | Chronic wounds, skin tumour, bites | Poultice | Aerial parts |
| **Asteraceae** | | | |
| *Ageratum conyzoides* L. Guakro | New, old wounds, burns Also described in 2 | Poultice | Leaves |
| *Blumea aurita* DC. Plaaduru | New, old wounds Also described in 2 | Poultice | Leaves |
| *Chromolaena odorata* (L.) R.M King & H. Rob. Mfofo (Acheampong) This species had a frequency of use of 11 hits and was sorted into group I (very frequent use, recorded more than 10 times by the 78 healers). | New, old wounds | Poultice | Leaves |

*(Continued overleaf)*

**Table 17.1**   (*Continued*)

| Plan species/scientific name/ local name (Asante-Twi) | Type of wound | Formulation | Part of plant used |
|---|---|---|---|
| *Eclipta alba* Hassk. Ntum | Deep wounds Also described in 2 | Poultice | Leaves |
| *Melanthera scandens* Schu, Nach. & Thonn. Mfofo | Stomach ulcer/sores Also described in 2 | Decoction | Leaves |
| *Vernonia amygdalina* Delile. Odwono | Stomach sores/ulcer | Decoction (enema) | Leaves |
| **Bignoniaceae** | | | |
| *Kigelia africana* (Lam.) Benth. Nufuhene | Stomach ulcer/sores Also described in 1 and 2 | Decoction | Stem bark |
| *Nerbouldia laevis* Seem. Sesemasa/Sasanemasa | Stomach ulcer Also described in 2 | Decoction, enema | Leaves, stem bark |
| *Spathodea campanulata* P. Beauv. Kuokuonesuo This species had a frequency of use of eight hits and was sorted into group II (frequent use, recorded seven to nine times by the 78 healers) for intensified experimental investigation. | Skin rashes, haemorrhoids, stomach ulcer Also described in 1 and 2 | Decoction | Leaves, stem bark |
| **Bombacaceae** | | | |
| *Bombax buonopozense* P. Beauv. Akata | Stomach ulcer, burns | Decoction | Leaves |
| *Ceiba pentandra* (L.) Gaetn. Onyina | Stomach ulcer/sores Also described in 2 | Decoction | Stem bark |
| **Capparidaceae** | | | |
| *Euadenia trifoliolata* Oliv. Densinkro | Chronic wounds | Poultice | Leaves |
| **Caricaceae** | | | |
| *Carica papaya* L. Bofere | New, old, stomach ulcer/sores Also described in 2 | Poultice, decoction | Leaves |
| **Caesalpiniaceae** | | | |
| *Cassia alata* L. Osempe | Chronic wounds, shingles, burns | Poultice | Leaves |
| *Cassia occidentalis* L. Mmofraborodee | Stomach ulcer/sores | Decoction | Leaves |
| *Erythrophleum ivorensis* A. Chev. Pɔtrɔdom | Old wounds | Decoction | Leaves |
| **Cecropiaceae** | | | |
| *Myrianthus arboreus* P. Beauv. Nyankama | Stomach ulcer/sores | Decoction | Leaves |
| **Chrysobalanceae** | | | |
| *Acioa dinklagei* Engl. Atwere | Old and new wounds | Poultice | Leaves |

**Table 17.1** (*Continued*)

| Plan species/scientific name/ local name (Asante-Twi) | Type of wound | Formulation | Part of plant used |
|---|---|---|---|
| **Combretaceae** | | | |
| *Combretum mucronatum* G. Don. Hwiremoo This species had a frequency of use of seven hits and was sorted into group II (frequent use, recorded seven to nine times by the 78 healers) for intensified experimental investigation. | New, old wound, boils, burns Also described in 2 | Poultice | Leaves |
| *Terminalia ivorensis* A. Chev. Emire | Haemorrhoids, stomach ulcer, burns | Decoction | Stem bark |
| **Crassulaceae** | | | |
| *Kalanchoe integra* Kuntze. Egorɔ | Boils | Poultice | Leaves |
| **Cucurbitaceae** | | | |
| *Momordia charantia* L. Nyanya | Mouth sores, chronic wounds, stomach ulcer Also described in 1 and 2 | Poultice, decoction | Leaves, stem bark |
| **Dioscoreaceae** | | | |
| *Dioscorea cayensis* Lam. Bayere | Stomach ulcer/sores | Decoction | Leaves |
| **Euphorbiaceae** | | | |
| *Acalypha ciliata* Forssk. Mofoa | Chronic wounds, stomach ulcer Also described in 2 | Decoction | Leaves |
| *Alchornea cordifolia* Muell. Arg. Gyama This species had a frequency of use of 13 hits and was sorted into group I (very frequent use, recorded more than 10 times by the 78 healers). | Deep wounds, fractures, haemorrhoids, stomach ulcer Also described in 2 | Decoction poultice | Leaves, stem bark |
| *Euphorbia hirta* L. Kakaweadwe | Deep wounds, carbuncles Also described in 1 and 2 | Poultice | Leaves |
| *Jatropha curcas* L. Nkrangyedua | Chronic and old wounds, boils, stomach sores Also described in 1 and 2 | Poultice, decoction | Leaves |
| *Mallotus oppositifolius* Muel. Arg. Nyanyafurowa (Pimpim) This species had a frequency of use of eight hits and was sorted into group II (frequent use, recorded seven to nine times by the 78 healers). | New, old, chronic wounds, fractures, burns Also described in 2 | Poultice | Leaves |

*(Continued overleaf)*

**Table 17.1**    (*Continued*)

| Plan species/scientific name/ local name (Asante-Twi) | Type of wound | Formulation | Part of plant used |
|---|---|---|---|
| *Manihot esculentus* L. Bankye | New wounds, stomach ulcer/sores Also described in 2 | Poultice, decoction | Leaves |
| *Phyllanthus muellerianus* (Kuntze.) Exell. Awobɛ This species had a frequency of use of nine hits and was sorted into group II (frequent use, recorded seven to nine times by the 78 healers) for intensified experimental investigation. | New, old, deep and chronic wounds Also described in 2 | Poultice | Leaves |
| *Phyllanthus urinaria* L. Bowomaguwokyi | Chronic wounds | Poultice | Leaves |
| *Ricinodendron heudelotii* (Baill.) Pierre ex Heckel Nwama | Stomach ulcer/sores | Decoction | Stem bark |
| **Fabaceae** | | | |
| *Acacia pennata* Willd. Nwere | Burns, new and old wounds | Poultice | Leaves, stem bark |
| *Albizia ferruginea* Benth. Awiemfoɔsamena | Measles | Poultice | Leaves |
| *Albizia zygia* J.F. Macbr. ɔkoro | Chronic wounds, swellings, carbuncles | Powder | Seeds, bark |
| *Baphia nitida* Lodd. Odwono | New, old and deep wounds, stomach ulcer | Poultice | Leaves, root |
| *Milletia zechiana* Harm. Frafraha | New, old wounds | Decoction | Root, stem bark |
| **Lamiaceae** | | | |
| *Hoslundia opposita* Vahl. Nunum nini This species had a frequency of use of 16 hits and was sorted into group I (very frequent use, recorded more than 10 times by the 78 healers) for intensified experimental investigation. | Chronic and deep wounds, stomach ulcer | Poultice, decoction | Leaves, root |
| *Ocimum gratissimum* L. Nunum | Burns, boils, stomach ulcer | Poultice, decoction | Leaves |
| **Lecythidaceae** | | | |
| *Petersianthus macrocarpus* (P. Beauv.) Liben. Asia | Boils | Poultice, decoction | Leaves |
| **Loranthaceae** | | | |
| *Tapinanthus bangwenis* Engl. & K. Krause Nkranpan | New and chronic wounds | Poultice | Leaves, stem bark |

**Table 17.1** (*Continued*)

| Plan species/scientific name/ local name (Asante-Twi) | Type of wound | Formulation | Part of plant used |
|---|---|---|---|
| **Malvaceae** | | | |
| *Abelmoschus esculentus* Moench. Nkuruma | Chronic wounds | Powder | Seeds |
| *Gossypium hirsutum* L. Asaawa | Boils, skin rashes | Poultice | Leaves |
| *Sida acuta* Burm. f. Tweta | New and old wounds Also described in 2 | Poultice | Leaves |
| *Theobroma cacao* L. Kokoo | Deep wounds | Poultice | Leaves |
| **Meliaceae** | | | |
| *Khaya ivorensis* A. Chev. Dubini | Boils, haemorrhoids, swellings, fractures | Poultice | Stem bark, leaves |
| *Khaya senegalensis* A. Juss. Kuntunkuri | Snake bites, chronic wounds | Powder, decoction | Stem bark |
| **Mimosaceae** | | | |
| *Caepsalpinia bunduc* (L.) Roxb. Abubuo | Haemorrhoids Also described in 1 | Decoction | Stem bark |
| **Moraceae** | | | |
| *Ficus capensis* Thunb. Doma | New and old wounds | Poultice | Leaves |
| *Ficus elastica* Roxb. Amanyedua | Boils, new and old wounds | Poultice | Leaves, stem bark |
| *Ficus exasperata* Vahl Nyankyerenee This species had a frequency of use of 15 hits and was sorted into group I (very frequent use, recorded more than 10 times by the 78 healers) for intensified experimental investigation. | New, old, deep wounds, boils, burns Also described in 1 | Poultice | Leaves, stem bark |
| *Ficus leprieurii* Miq. Amasusuwa | Boils | Decoction | Stem bark |
| *Ficus sur* Forskal Doma | Stomach ulcer Also described in 1 | Decoction | Stem bark |
| **Musaceae** | | | |
| *Musa paradisiaca* L. Bɔɔdee This species had a frequency of use of seven hits and was sorted into group II (frequent use, recorded seven to nine times by the 78 healers). | New wounds Also described in 2 | Poultice | Stem, leaves |
| **Myristicaceae** | | | |
| *Pycnanthus angolensis* (Welw.) Warb. Otie This species had a frequency of use of eight hits and was sorted into group II (frequent use, recorded seven to nine times by the 78 healers) for intensified experimental investigation. | Haemorrhoids, stomach ulcer, chronic wounds Also described in 2 | Decoction | Stem bark, leaves |

(*Continued overleaf*)

**Table 17.1**   (*Continued*)

| Plan species/scientific name/ local name (Asante-Twi) | Type of wound | Formulation | Part of plant used |
|---|---|---|---|
| **Myrtaceae** | | | |
| *Psidium guajava* L. Gua (Guava) | Chronic wounds | Decoction | Leaves |
| **Passifloraceae** | | | |
| *Adenia cissampeloides* (Planch.ex Benth.) Harms. Homakyem | Stings/bites | Decoction | Whole plant |
| **Piperaceae** | | | |
| *Piper guineense* Schumach. & Thonn. Sorowisa | Stomach ulcer/sores | Enema | Dried fruits |
| *Piper umbellatum* L. Mumuaha | Burns Also described in 1 and 2 | Poultice | Leaves |
| **Phytolaccaceae** | | | |
| *Hilteria latifolia* (Lam.) H. Wall. Anafranaku | Chronic and deep wounds | Poultice | Leaves |
| **Poaceae** | | | |
| *Brachyachne obtusiflora* (Benth.) C.E. Hubb. Aberekyere abodwesɛ | Boils | Poultice | Roots, leaves |
| *Cymbopogon citratus* (DC) Stapf. Akutukankan | Boils, swellings | Poultice | Leaves |
| *Eleusine indica* (L.) Gaetn Nsensan | New and old wounds Also described in 2 | Poultice | Aerial parts |
| *Zea mays* L. Aburo | Boils, carbuncles | Poultice, powder | Fruits, leaves |
| **Portulaceae** | | | |
| *Portulaca oleracea* L Adwera | Boils Also described in 2 | Poultice | Leaves |
| **Rubiaceae** | | | |
| *Morinda lucida* Benth. Konkroma | Haemorrhoids, stomach ulcer | Decoction | Stem bark |
| *Psydrax subcordata* (DC.) Bridson Ntatiadupon | Haemorrhoids, stomach ulcer | Decoction | Stem bark |
| **Rutaceae** | | | |
| *Zanthoxylum gilletii* (De Wild.) Waterman Okuo | Stomach ulcer/sores Also described in 2 | Decoction | Stem bark |
| *Zanthoxylum leprieurii* (Guil. & Perr.) Engl. Oyaa | Stomach ulcer/sores Also described in 2 | Decoction | Stem bark |
| **Sapindaceae** | | | |
| *Blighia sapida* Kon. Akyee | Snake bites, stings | Poultice | Stem bark |
| *Paullinia pinnata* L. Toa-ntini This species had a frequency of use of eight hits and was sorted into group II (frequent use, recorded seven to nine times by the 78 healers). | New, old and chronic wounds, haemorrhoids, stomach ulcer Also described in 1 and 2 | Poultice, decoction | Roots, leaves |

**Table 17.1** (*Continued*)

| Plan species/scientific name/ local name (Asante-Twi) | Type of wound | Formulation | Part of plant used |
|---|---|---|---|
| **Solanaceae** | | | |
| *Datura metel L.* Pepediewuo | Chronic, old and new wounds, stomach ulcer, haemorrhoids | Decoction, poultice | Leaves |
| *Lycopersicum esculentum* Mill. Tomato | Chronic wounds, burns | Poultice | Fruits |
| *Nicotiana tabacum L.* Ataa/taa | Stomach ulcer/sores Also described in 1 and 2 | Decoction | Leaves |
| *Physalis angulata L* Totɔtotɔ | Chronic wounds | Poultice | Leaves |
| *Schwenchia americana L.* Agyennyensu | Snake bites, chronic and new wounds | Powder, poultice | Leaves |
| *Solanum torvum Sw.* Kwaonsusua | New wounds, boils Also described in 1 and 2 | Poultice | Leaves |
| **Sterculiaceae** | | | |
| *Cola nitida* (Vent.) Schott & Endl. Bese (Kola) | Boils | Poultice | Leaves |
| *Triplochiton scleroxylon* K. Schum. Wawa | Burns, stomach ulcer, haemorrhoids | Decoction, powder | Stem bark |
| **Tiliaceae** | | | |
| *Duboscia viridiflora* Mildbr. Akokoragyehin | New wounds | Poultice, powder | Stem bark, leaves |
| **Urticaceae** | | | |
| *Laportea ovalifolia* (Schumach.) Chew. Akyekyenswonsa | Boils, swellings | Poultice | Leaves |
| **Vitaceae** | | | |
| *Ampelocissus multistriata* (Bak.) Planch. Anunum | New and old wounds | Poultice | Leaves |
| **Zingiberaceae** | | | |
| *Aframomum melegueta* K. Schum. Famwisa This species had a frequency of use of nine hits and was sorted into group II (frequent use, recorded seven to nine times by the 78 healers). | Mouth sores, boils, skin rashes, fractures Also described in 2 | Decoction (gargle), powder | Dried seeds |
| *Zingiber officinale* Roscoe. Akakaduro | Chronic wounds, boils | Poultice | Rhizome |

Wound healing activity cross-referenced in published literature: 1, Neuwinger (1989); 2, Burkill (2000).

**Table 17.2** Influence of aqueous extracts and ethanolic extracts at 10 and 100 μg/ml for 72 h on mitochondrial activity of HaCaT keratinocytes (MTT test).

| Plant and extracts | 10 μg/ml | 100 μg/ml | Plant and extracts | 10 μg/ml | 100 μg/ml |
|---|---|---|---|---|---|
| *Anchomames difformis* | | | *Astonia boonei* | | |
| $H_2O$ extract | 97 ± 7% | 94 ± 8% | $H_2O$ extract | 101 ± 5% | 103 ± 9% |
| EtOH/$H_2O$ extract | 95 ± 7% | 98 ± 7% | EtOH/$H_2O$ extract | 101 ± 8% | 103 ± 8% |
| *Combretum mucronatum* | | | *Ficus exasperata* | | |
| $H_2O$ extract | 112 ± 7% * | 100 ± 5% | $H_2O$ extract | 97 ± 6% | 98 ± 6% |
| EtOH/$H_2O$ extract | 100 ± 6% | 98 ± 8% | EtOH/$H_2O$ extract | 97 ± 6% | 102 ± 8% |
| *Hoslundia opposita* | | | *Justicia flava* | | |
| $H_2O$ extract | 100 ± 8% | 102 ± 8% | $H_2O$ extract | 95 ± 9% | 97 ± 9% |
| EtOH/$H_2O$ extract | 96 ± 8% | 97 ± 9% | EtOH/$H_2O$ extract | 95 ± 7% | 89 ± 5% |
| *Parquetina nigrescens* | | | *Phyllanthus muellerianus* | | |
| $H_2O$ extract | 84 ± 9%* | 84 ± 6%* | $H_2O$ extract | 107 ± 6%* | 116 ± 7%* |
| EtOH/$H_2O$ extract | 91 ± 4%* | 94 ± 7%* | EtOH/$H_2O$ extract | 105 ± 5% | 99 ± 7% |
| *Pycnanthus angolensis* | | | *Pupalia lappacea* | | |
| $H_2O$ extract | 104 ± 6% | 115 ± 7%* | $H_2O$ extract | 102 ± 8% | 100 ± 5% |
| EtOH/$H_2O$ extract | 99 ± 9% | 104 ± 8% | EtOH/$H_2O$ extract | 99 ± 9% | 98 ± 7% |
| *Spathodea campanulata* | | | **Positive control:** | | |
| $H_2O$ extract | 102 ± 6% | 113 ± 8%* | 123 ± 6%* | | |
| EtOH/$H_2O$ extract | 98 ± 8% | 103 ± 8% | | | |

Data with standard deviation SD are from three independent experiments each with $n = 6$ replicates. Negative control: untreated cells; positive control: FCS 1%. *$p < 0.05$, **$p < 0.01$ compared to the untreated control group (ANOVA). For experimental details see Agyare *et al.* (2009).

MTT activity in dermal fibroblasts was also increased, while the cell proliferation decreased. *C. mucronatum* extract raised keratinocyte and fibroblast mitochondrial activity at 10 μg/ml significantly, while higher concentrations turned out to have an inhibitory effect.

Based on these data it was decided to focus further phytochemical research on *P. muellerianus* and *C. mucronatum*.

## 17.2.6 Phytochemical aspects of *P. muellerianus* and the ICH-validated HPLC method for quality control (ICH, 2014)

The total tannin content of an aqueous extract from the dried leaves of *P. muellerianus* was 14%. From a methanol-water (7:3) extract (Bicker *et al.*, 2009) the ellagitannin geraniin (**1**; 2.9% w/w) with two isomers (**1a, 1b**) was identified as a major constituent (Foo, 1993) along with furosin (**2**, 0.03%) and corilagin (**3**, 0.004%) (Figure 17.1). Quercetin-3-O-β-D-glucoside, kaempferol-3-O-β-D-glucoside, quercetin-3-O-D-β-rutinosid, caffeoyl-malic acid, gallic acid, methyl gallate, caffeic acid, 5-O-caffeoylquinic acid and 3,5-O-dicaffeoylquinic acid were also identified.

An HPLC method for standard quality control was developed for the identification and quantitation of geraniin and rutin as lead compounds of the extract. A typical chromatogram

**Table 17.3** Influence of aqueous extracts at 10, 50 and 100 μg/ml for 72 h on mitochondrial activity (MTT test) and mitogenic proliferation (BrdU incorporation ELISA) of HaCaT keratinocytes and primary skin fibroblasts.

| Extract (μg/ml) | Keratinocytes | | | | | | Primary fibroblasts | | | | | | | | | | | |
|---|---|---|---|---|---|---|---|---|---|---|---|---|---|---|---|---|---|---|
| | MTT assay (%) | | | BrdU-ELISA (%) | | | MTT assay (%) | | | | | | BrdU-ELISA (%) | | | | | |
| | 10 | 50 | 100 | 10 | 50 | 100 | 1 | 5 | 10 | 20 | 50 | 100 | 1 | 5 | 10 | 20 | 50 | 100 |
| *P. muellerianus* | 107 ±6 | 112* ±7 | 116* ±7 | 106 ±7 | 123* ±7 | 126* ±8 | 103 ±6 | 109 ±5 | 114* ±5 | 119* ±5 | 74 ±10 | 68 ±9 | 102 ±12 | 100 ±8 | 116 ±15 | 121* ±13 | 62** ±8 | 54** ± |
| *P. angolensis* | 102 ±6 | 108 ±5 | 115* ±7 | 105 ±7 | 122* ±11 | 115 ±8 | | | 106 ±9 | | 122 ±7 | 131* ±15 | | | 116 ±5 | 90 ±10 | | 78* ± 13 |
| *C. mucronatum* | 112* ±7 | 105 ±5 | 96 ±8 | 106 ±10 | 131** ±12 | 169 ±10 | | | 116* ±9 | | 108 ±8 | 82 ±8 | | | 88 ±9 | | 76 ±11 | 64** ±12 |
| Positive control | | 123* ±6 | | | 118* ±9 | | | | 121* ±6 | | | 115* ±8 | | | 115* ±10 | | 119* ±7 | |

Data and SD values are from three independent experiments each with *n* = 6 replicates. Negative control: untreated cells; positive control: FCS 1%. *p < 0.05, **p < 0.01 compared to the untreated control group (ANOVA). For experimental details see Agyare *et al.* (2009).

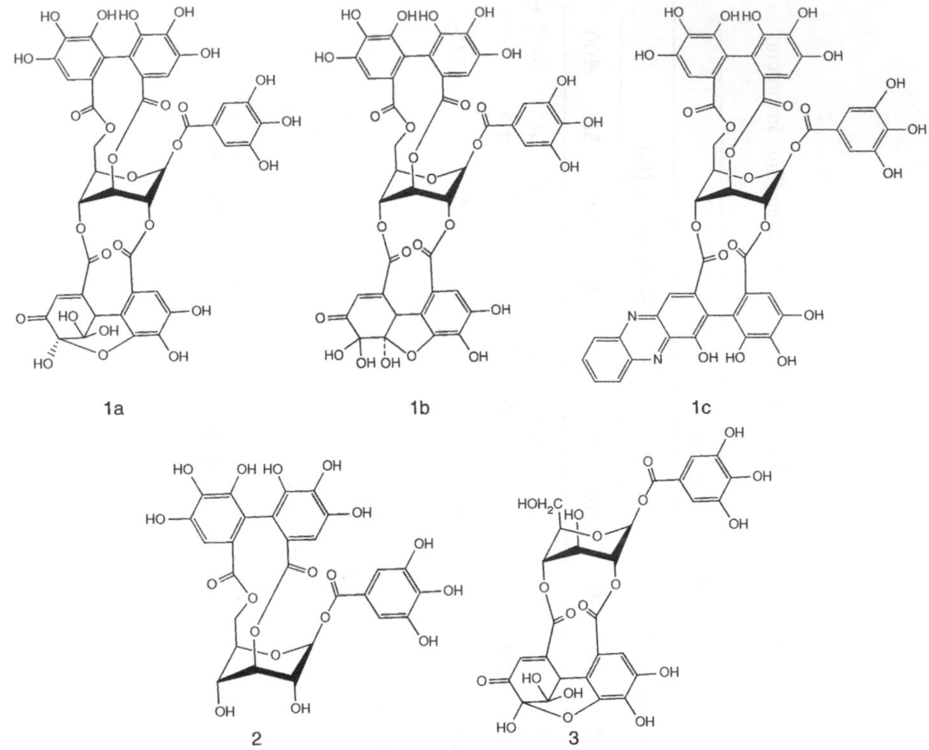

**Figure 17.1** Structural features of hydrolysable ellagitannins from *P. muellerianus:* **1a** and **1b** equilibrium geraniin, **1c** phenazine derivative of geraniin, **2** corilagin, **3** furosin.

of a representative batch is shown in Figure 17.2. Using a validated method the contents of the marker compound geraniin were determined with 4.3% (w/w, related to the dried leaves).

## 17.2.7 Influence of *P. muellerianus* on the cell physiology of human skin cells

In the next step the influence of geraniin and furosin on skin cells was investigated using primary dermal fibroblasts and HaCaT keratinocytes. Geraniin exhibited strong stimulating effects on both cell types.

During the development of human skin towards an intact barrier system keratinocytes undergo cellular proliferation followed by a switch to cellular differentiation. The potential differentiation behaviour of keratinocytes in the presence of geraniin and furosin was investigated using differentiation-specific protein expression of cytokeratins CK1,10 and involucrin. Geraniin and furosin had a positive influence on cellular differentiation. The differentiation-inducing effect on keratinocytes is in the same concentration range (50–100 µM) as the stimulation of cell vitality and proliferation.

Besides the stimulation of the epidermal keratinocytes barrier function, the formation of extracellular matrix markers from the fibroblasts as typical dermis cells was also investigated. The influence of the aqueous extract, geraniin and furosin on the induction of collagen

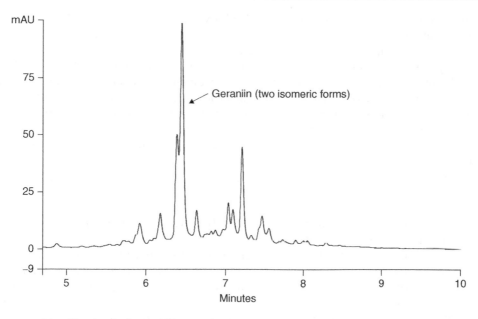

**Figure 17.2** Identification and quantification of geraniin in a methanol/water (7:3) extract from *P. muelleri-anus* by HPLC. For experimental details see Agyare *et al.* (2011).

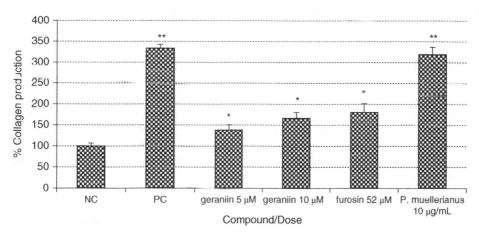

**Figure 17.3** Influence of aqueous extract from *P. muellerianus,* geraniin and furosin on collagen production in NHDF as determined by ELISA. PC, positive control (1% ascorbic acid); NC, negative control (untreated cells).

synthesis, an important texture marker protein for extracellular matrix, was investigated (Figure 17.3). The aqueous extract was found to increase the synthesis of collagen highly significantly, almost the same as the positive control. Furosin and geraniin also had a significant influence on collagen formation and this may be attributed to the strong redox properties of the ellagitannins (Murad *et al.*, 1981; Chojkier *et al.*, 1989; Agyare *et al.*, 2009).

The extract obtained from *P. muellerianus* was screened for antiviral activity and was shown to be active against *Herpes simplex* virus 1 (HSV-1) at 10 μg/ml. Using geraniin gave a remarkably low $IC_{50}$ of $1.4\,\mu M$, with a selectivity index of 15 compared to cell toxicity, indicating that this polyphenol might be a very interesting compound for further antiviral investigations (A. Hensel, unpublished results).

Other reports on the antiviral activity of geraniin have been published (Notka *et al.*, 2004; Yang *et al.*, 2007), indicating that this compound is an efficient blocker of viral cell entry. Additionally, geraniin increases the functionality of macrophages towards an increased phagocytosis (Ushio *et al.*, 1991) and is described as an anti-inflammatory compound by inhibition of TNF-α release (Okabe *et al.*, 2001; for a review see Fujiki *et al.*, 2003) and NO formation (Kumaran and Karunakaran, 2006). Additionally the inflammatory response provoked by bacterial infection can effectively be diminished by geraniin.

Using these data the effect of the aqueous extract of *P. muellerianus* and geraniin during wound healing can be assessed as follows:

(i)   Stimulation of keratinocyte and dermal fibroblast viability, energy production and proliferation for tissue regeneration.

(ii)  Induction of keratinocyte terminal differentiation for initiation of barrier formation.

(iii) Induction of collagen for remodelling of tissue and regeneration of extracellular matrix.

(iv)  Reduction of cellular damages due to oxidative stressors by radical-scavenging effects.

(v)   Prevention of bacterial or viral infection.

(vi)  Inhibition of inflammation processes during the healing process.


## 17.2.8   Phytochemistry of *C. mucronatum*

Using an EtOH 50% extract a variety of polyphenols were isolated, dominated by epicatechin, a series of unsubstituted procyanidins and isovitexin.

For analytical quality control an HPLC method was developed and validated according to ICH protocol, using epicatechin, isovitexin and procyanidin B2 as lead compounds. This method should enable the African partners to easily establish rationalized specifications and a validated production chain. The authors have the strong feeling that the development of a stable and robust analytical method is a prerequisite for the transfer of such methods to West Africa. This should also encourage the scientists and mercantilists in Africa to start product development, drug registration and build up their own high-quality business for the optimized therapy of patients.


## 17.2.9   Influence of *C. mucronatum* on the cell physiology of human skin cells

Earlier investigations shown the activity of the extract against skin cells (Agyare *et al.*, 2009). Detailed *in vitro* investigations using human primary keratinocytes and dermal fibroblast indicated that viability was significantly increased by EtOH 50% extract. Interestingly, the extract had no activity on the cellular proliferation at low concentrations, while higher doses inhibited proliferation. Cytototoxic effects could be excluded. Additionally, the differentiation of specific markers in primary keratinocytes were investigated using confocal laser scanning microscopy and immunostaining against differentiation-specific proteins CK1/CK10 and involucrin (Figures 17.4 and 17.5). Both differentiation markers were obviously upregulated. Treatment of the keratinocytes with the extract and Western-blot analysis again showed a significant increase in both differentiation-specific proteins, therefore the *C. smeathmanii* extract

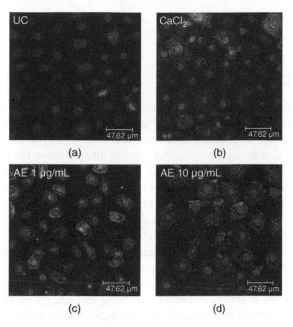

(a)                                    (b)

(c)                                    (d)

**Figure 17.4** Influence of 1 and 10 μg/ml of *C. mucronatum* aqueous extract on expression of differentiation-specific involucrin in pNHEK after 7 days treatment as determined by mmunofluorescence assay using a confocal laser scanning microscope. A, untreated cells, negative control; B, CaCl$_2$ (2 mM), positive control; C, 1 μg/ml; D, 10 μg/ml. Magnification ×88.

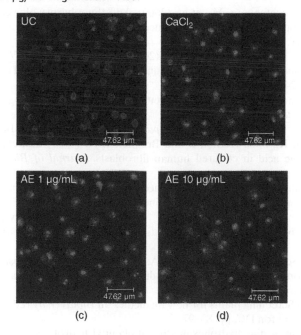

(a)                                    (b)

(c)                                    (d)

**Figure 17.5** Influence of 1 and 10 μg/ml of *C. mucronatum* aqueous extract on expression of differentiation-specific cytokeratin CK1 in pNHEK after 7 days of treatment as determined by immunofluorescence assay using a confocal laser scanning microscope. A, untreated cells, negative control; B, CaCl$_2$ (2 mM), positive control; C, 1 μg/ml; D, 10 μg/ml. Magnification ×88.

is assessed to be an inductor of keratinocyte differentiation. Bioassay-guided fractionation led to the finding that the oligomeric procyanidins are the active compounds.

## 17.3 Conclusion

Ethnopharmacological field studies provide an excellent tool for collecting information on traditionally used plants if they are performed under validated and structured scientific conditions. *In vitro* screening to evaluate the data from the field study can pinpoint very interesting plants for further detailed investigations, but also is an indicator for the knowledge of the healers interviewed. During our investigations in Ghana a very high degree of concordance between traditional use and *in vitro* laboratory data was found. In contrast to that, similar studies with plant selection from other continents (e.g. wound-healing plants from TCM; Wang *et al.*, 2013) showed very inconsistent data. On the other hand, Ghana's healers definitely represent an important element of the Ghanian health system. Wound healing and other medicinal plants can provide valuable data on highly interesting plants with good potential for preclinical and clinical research towards product development. Intense networking between European and West African economies should build up a system for the structured development of galenical formulations for markets, especially in West Africa, by using local raw materials, cheap and easy manufacturing, high-quality standards according to the regulations of international pharmacopoeias and defined marketing strategies.

## References

Agyare, C., Asase, A., Lechtenberg, M., *et al.* (2009) An ethnopharmacological survey and *in vitro* confirmation of ethnopharmacological use of medicinal plants used for wound healing. *Journal of Ethnopharmacolology*, **125**, 393–403.

Agyare, C., Deters, A., Lechtenberg, M., *et al.* (2011) Ellagitannis from *Phyllanthus muellerianus* (Kuntze) Exell: influence on cell physiology of human skin keratinocytes and dermal fibroblasts. *Phytomedicine*, **18**, 617–624.

Bicker, A., Petereit, F. and Hensel, A. (2009) Proanthocyanidins and a phloroglucinol derivative from *Rumex acetosa* L. *Fitoterapia*, **80**, 483–495.

Burkill, H.M. (2000) *The Useful Plants of West Tropical Africa*, 3rd edn, Royal Botanic Gardens, Kew.

Chojkier, M., Houglum, K., Solis-Herrzo, J. and Brenner, D.A. (1989) Stimulation of collagen gene expression by ascorbic acid in cultured human fibroblasts. *Journal of Biological Chemistry*, **264**, 16957–16962.

Deters, A., Brunold, C. and Hensel, A. (2004) Polysaccharides from *Hibiscus sabdariffa* flowers stimulate proliferation and differentiation of human keratinocyte. *Planta Medica*, **70**, 370–373.

Deters, A.M., Lengsfeld, C. and Hensel, A. (2005) Oligo- and polysaccharides exhibit a structure-dependent bioactivity on human keratinocytes in vitro. *Journal of Ethnopharmacology*, **102**, 191–199.

Deters, A., Petereit, F., Schmidgall, J. and Hensel, A. (2008) N-Acetyl-D-glucosamine oligosaccharides induce mucin secretion from colonic tissue and induce differentiation of human keratinocytes. *Journal of Pharmacy and Pharmacology*, **60**, 197–204.

Farnsworth, N.R. (1998) Screening plants for new medicines, in *Biodiversity* (ed. E.O. Wilson), National Academy Press, Washington DC, pp. 83–97.

Foo, L.Y. (1993) Amariin, a di-dehydrohexahydroxydiphenoyl hydrolysable tannin from *Phyllanthus amarus*. *Phytochemistry*, **33**, 487–491.

Fujiki, H., Suganuma, M., Kurusu, M., *et al.* (2003) New TNF-alpha releasing inhibitors as cancer preventive agents from traditional herbal medicine and combination cancer prevention study with EGCG and sulindac or tamoxifen. *Mutation Research*, **523**, 119–124.

ICH (2014) *Validation of Analytical Procedures: Methodology*, ICH Harmonized Tripartite Guideline, ICH, ICH-Q2(R1), http://www.ICH.org/products/guidelines/quality/article/quality-guidelines.htm, accessed 20 March 2014.

Kumaran, A. and Karunakuran, R.J. (2006) Nitric oxide radical scavenging active components from *Phyllanthus emblica* L. *Plant Foods for Human Nutrition*, **61**, 1–5.

Kunwar, R.M., Uprety, Y., Burlakoti, C., *et al.* (2009) Indigenous use and ethnopharmacology of medicinal plants in far-west Nepal. *Ethnobotany Research and Applications*, **7**, 5–28.

Murad, S., Grove, D., Lindberg, K.A., *et al.* (1981) Regulation of collagen synthesis by ascorbic acid. *Proceedings of the National Academy of Sciences*, **78**, 2879–2882.

Neuwinger, H.D. (1989) *Afrikanische Heilpflanzen und Jagdgifte*, 2nd edn, Wissenschaftliche Verlagsgesellschaft, Stuttgart.

Notka, F., Meier, G. and Wagner, R. (2004) Concerted inhibitory activities of *Phyllanthus amarus* on HIV replication in vitro and ex vivo. *Antiviral Research*, **64**, 93–102.

Okabe, S., Suganuma, M., Imayoshi, Y., *et al.* (2001) New TNF-alpha releasing inhibitors, geraniin and corilagin, in leaves of *Acer nikoense*, Megusurino-ki. *Biological Pharmaceutical Bulletin*, **10**, 1145–1148.

Phan, T.T., Hughes, M.A. and Cherry, G.W. (1998) Enhanced proliferation of fibroblast and endothelial cells treated with an extract of leaves of *Chromolaena odorata* (Eupolin) an herbal remedy for treating wounds. *Plastical Reconstruction Surgery*, **101**, 76–65.

Phan, T.T., Hughes, M.A. and Cherry, G.W. (2001) Effect of an aqueous extract from the leaves of *Chromolaena odorata* (Eupolin) on the proliferation of human keratinocytes and on the migration in an *in vitro* model of reepithclialization. *Wound Repair Regeneration*, **9**, 301–313.

Ushio, Y., Fang, T., Okuda, T. and Abe, H. (1991) Modificational changes in function and morphology of cultured macrophages by geraniin. *Japanese Journal of Pharmacology*, **57**, 187–196.

Ved, D.K. and Goraya, G.S. (2008) *Demand and Supply of Medicinal Plants in India*, Bishen Singh, Mahendra Pal Singh, Dehra Dun and FRLHT, Bangalore.

Wang, R., Lechtenberg, M., Sendker, J., *et al.* (2013) Wound-healing plants from TCM: in vitro investigations on selected TCM plants and their influence on human dermal fibroblasts and keratinocytes. *Fitoterapia*, 308–317.

WHO (2000) *General Guidelines for Methodologies on Research and Evaluation of Traditional Medicine*, Geneva, pp. 1–80.

Yang, C.M., Cheng, H.Y., Lin, T.C., *et al.* (2007) The in vitro activity of geraniin and 1,3,4,6-tetra-O-galloyl-beta-D-glucose isolated from *Phyllanthus urinaria* against herpes simplex virus type 1 and type 2 infection. *Journal of Ethnopharmacology*, **110**, 555–558.

Zippel, J., Deters, A., Pappai, D. and Hensel, A. (2009) A high molecular arabinogalactan from *Ribes nigrum* L.: influence on cell physiology of human skin fibroblasts and keratinocytes and internalization into cells via endosomal transport. *Carbohydrate Research*, **344**, 1001–1008.

# 18

# Gynaecological, Andrological and Urological Problems: An Ethnopharmacological Perspective

Tinde van Andel, Hugo de Boer and Alexandra Towns

*Naturalis Biodiversity Center, Leiden University, Leiden, the Netherlands*

## 18.1   Introduction

Herbal medicine is used widely in the context of reproductive health, including gynaecological, andrological and urological ailments. In this chapter we will focus on medicinal plants used for salient reproductive health issues in Latin America, the Caribbean, Sub-Sahara Africa and South and South-East Asia. These populations have limited access to biomedical health care, frequently use medicinal plants and maintain the largest body of knowledge on plant-based medicine (Beal, 1998; WHO, 2008). Moreover, the high levels of biodiversity in the tropics represent a wealth of pharmacological properties, many of which are as yet unknown to science. The greatest challenge for ethnopharmacologists, however, is not only to discover new phytochemical properties of tropical plants, but also to study the potential risks and benefits of herbal medicine use by those whose health largely depends upon it. We describe several reproductive health issues for which medicinal plants are used, discuss the prevalence and medical causes of these ailments and, in the case of cultural-bound health concepts, explain underlying belief systems motivating medicinal plant use. We conclude each section by highlighting several frequently used plants, identifying their pharmacological properties that justify traditional usage and suggesting directions for future research.

*Ethnopharmacology*, First Edition. Edited by Michael Heinrich and Anna K. Jäger.
© 2015 John Wiley & Sons, Ltd. Published 2015 by John Wiley & Sons, Ltd.

## 18.2    Menstrual disorders

Although not always life-threatening, menstrual disorders can be particularly disruptive to daily activity patterns, particularly in the absence of appropriate sanitary facilities or analgesics for cases of painful menstruation (Tjon A Ten, 2007). Moreover, menstrual disorders may be risk markers for other reproductive morbidities (Harlow and Campbell, 2000). Some scholars argue that in countries where access to modern healthcare facilities is limited and traditional medicine is considered more culturally appropriate, research on the efficacy and safety of indigenous therapies for menstrual disorders should be encouraged to promote their use as an acceptable alternative to synthetic pharmaceuticals (Lindsey *et al.*, 1998; Michel *et al.*, 2007; Monera and Gwekwe, 2012). Other researchers advocate culturally sensitive integration of traditional and modern practices to reduce maternal mortality without replacing significant cultural heritage (de Boer *et al.*, 2011).

Recent review papers on medicinal plants for women's health show that more than 2000 plant species are used in Latin America, the Caribbean, sub-Saharan Africa and South and South-East Asia to treat menstrual disorders, reflecting the importance of menstruation as a major reproductive health issue among women in those regions (de Boer and Cotingting, 2014; van Andel *et al.*, 2014). Most species were used to treat painful menstruation, to induce or regulate menses and/or to provoke an abortion. The most widely used genera were *Citrus*, *Senna*, *Phyllanthus* and *Gossypium*. Less than half of the 59 predominant species used in the tropics have been tested for their pharmacological properties and/or mechanisms of action. From the tested species, 48% work as uterine spasmolytics and may ease uterine cramps and contractions, while 31% act as uterine spasmogenics and probably ease menstrual pains by inducing the menses.

### 18.2.1    Dysmenorrhea and uterine spasmolytics

Painful menstruation results partly from an excess production of prostaglandins that stimulate or intensify uterine contractions. These compounds are used clinically to induce labour and as abortifacients (Lange, 1986). Biomedical treatment prescribes inhibitors of the biosynthesis of prostaglandins (Ortiz de Montellano and Browner, 1985). Essential oils (e.g. estragole, bisabolol, limonene, eugenol) often contain compounds that inhibit prostaglandin biosynthesis and therefore could be effective as smooth muscle relaxants in the treatment of dysmenorrhea (Achterrath Tuckermann *et al.*, 1980; Ortiz de Montellano and Browner, 1985). Frequently used species for dysmennorhea that contain such oils are *Citrus aurantiifolia* (Christm.) Swingle, *Ocimum gratissimum* L., *Zingiber officinale* L., *Matricaria recutita* L., *Rosmarinus officinalis* L. and *Psidium guajava* L. (van Andel *et al.*, 2014). Except for *M. recutita*, all of these species have shown smooth muscle relaxant properties under laboratory conditions. Some species with spasmolytic effects (e.g. *Z. officinale*, *Citrus* spp.) are also used to induce abortion or for uterine cleansing, which could imply a dose-dependent reversal of effect. Women in Bénin used complicated herbal mixtures containing up to 31 species to treat several gynaecological disorders simultaneously, varying from painful, irregular or complicated menstruation to uterine fibroids and cysts (Towns and van Andel, 2014). Such practices complicate the study of the effect and safety of herbal medicines, as compounds from different species may have synergistic or mutually counteracting effects.

## 18.2.2   Uterine spasmogenics

Plants that have the ability to increase the strength or frequency of the contraction of the uterus can increase menstrual flow and could also act as abortifacient by causing the expulsion of the implanted embryo. Laboratory tests have shown smooth muscle contracting properties for a number of commonly used plant species for painful menstruation (e.g. *Leonurus japonicus* Houtt., *Ricinus communis* L., *Scoparia dulcis* L., *Senna alexandrina* Mill., *Xylopia aethiopica* (Dunal) A.Rich.; see van Andel *et al.*, 2014, for an overview). However, the mechanisms of action remain mostly unclear. Results from clinical trials on humans were published only for *L. japonicus* (Zhou, 2010). This medicinal plant stimulated uterine contractions and reduced postpartum hemorrhage, corroborating its traditional use to induce menstruation and to expel the placenta after childbirth. Strong laxatives, such as the oil of *R. communis* seeds and leaves of *Senna alata* (L.) Roxb., may stimulate not only peristaltic action, but also the smooth muscles of the uterus (Belew, 1999). Menstrual complaints and research into the risks and benefits of medicinal plants used to treat these ailments should be given a higher priority in reproductive health programmes that respect traditional knowledge and local perceptions and preferences.

# 18.3   Postpartum use

## 18.3.1   Puerperal infections

In developing countries, maternal death from sepsis following puerperal infections is one of the leading causes of maternal mortality (Ronsmans *et al.*, 2006). A meta-analysis of maternal mortality found that deaths due to sepsis were higher in Africa (odds ratio 2.71), Asia (1.91), and Latin America and the Caribbean (2.06) than in developed countries (Khan *et al.*, 2006). After parturition the pH of the vagina becomes more basic because of the neutralizing effect of the alkaline amniotic fluid, blood and lochia, as well as a decrease in lactic acid-producing lactobacilli. The more alkaline vagina is a suitable environment for aerobic bacteria. Moreover, 48 hours postpartum, the intrauterine environment becomes favourable for growth of anaerobic bacteria because of progressive necrosis of endometrial and placental remnants. Vaginal microorganisms invade the uterine cavity and anaerobic organisms account for 70% of puerperal infections, with *Peptostreptococcus*, *Peptococcus*, *Streptococcus* and *Bacteroides fragilis* most common. Subsequent invasion of the lymphatic system, causing a more widespread infection and sepsis, is also possible. Symptoms of puerperal infection are a rising fever and increasing uterine tenderness on postpartum days 2 or 3 (Kim *et al.*, 2009).

Many medicinal plants have well-documented *in vitro* and *in vivo* antimicrobial properties, but none have been tested for the treatment of systemic bacterial infections, such as those found in puerperal fever. Plant species with antimicrobial properties could be efficacious if used to prevent puerperal fever through perineal cleansing, washes, steam baths and poultices. Plant species that are commonly used by South-East Asian women in postpartum remedies such as *Blumea balsamifera* (L.) DC., *Amomum villosum* Lour. and *Amomum microcarpum* C.F.Liang & D.Fang all are rich in essential oil constituents with antimicrobial properties (de Boer *et al.*, 2011).

### 18.3.2    Postpartum haemorrhage

Postpartum menstrual flow and expulsion of the lochia during the postpartum period are natural processes that cease without intervention, but these are nevertheless salient health issues frequently treated with traditional herbal remedies. A possible complication after giving birth is postpartum haemorrhage, defined as blood loss in excess of 500 ml within the first 24 hours after a vaginal delivery. Normally, uterine musculature contracts around the blood vessels that supplied the placenta and acts as a physiologic-anatomic ligature. However, excessive placental bleeding can occur if the uterus fails to contract or if placental tissue is retained. In the latter case, the uterus is unable to maintain contraction and involutes around the retained tissues (Kim *et al.*, 2009). Atonic uterus and placental remnants account for 80% of primary postpartum haemorrhage cases (Oats and Abraham, 2010). Control of the bleeding can be achieved by increasing uterine contraction with uterotonic or spasmogenic plants, such as L. *japonicus* (van Andel *et al.*, 2014).

### 18.3.3    Perineal healing

Plants that enhance wound healing can also be beneficial during postpartum recovery. Trauma to the perineal area resulting from childbirth can be a cause of postpartum haemorrhage, increases susceptibility to microbial infections and can cause acute discomfort (de Boer and Cotingting, 2014). Direct application of these plants to the affected areas would confer the greatest benefit, and ethnobotanical research in Laos confirms that such remedies are mainly used in cleansing baths and steam saunas (de Boer and Lamxay, 2009; de Boer *et al.*, 2012, 2011). Several plant species commonly used in the postpartum context have promising wound healing properties, as was shown in studies of the leaves (Barua *et al.*, 2010; Ghosh and Gupta, 2011) and whole plant (Edwin *et al.*, 2008) of *Achyranthes aspera* L. Research into pure curcumin from *Curcuma longa* L. showed that it enhanced wound healing in animals (Panchatcharam and Miriyala, 2006; López-Jornet, 2011). Furthermore, in a human clinical study, the rhizome extract improved wound healing after episiotomy (Golmakani *et al.*, 2009). Future research into some of these compounds will hopefully see the complementation of current pharmaceuticals with novel remedies based on plant-derived metabolites. Continuing research in ethnopharmacology focusing on species with high consensus in traditional postpartum care could yield novel lead compounds for *in vivo* assays and clinical trials.

## 18.4    Vaginal applications

Large numbers of women use medicinal plants to clean, tighten, warm or dry their vagina. These practices, commonly referred to as 'dry sex', encompass washing, douching or steaming with herbal decoctions and the insertion of medicinal plants directly into the vagina (Brown *et al.*, 1993; Hilber *et al.*, 2007). These practices have commonly been documented in sub-Saharan Africa (Civic and Wilson, 1996; Beksinska *et al.*, 1999; Low *et al.*, 2011; Towns and van Andel, 2014) and also in the Caribbean (Halperin, 1999; van Andel *et al.*, 2008) and South-East Asia (Joesoef *et al.*, 1996). Women's motivations to engage in such practices vary from maintaining personal hygiene, preventing sexually-transmitted and post-partum infections, disguising undesirable odours, limiting vaginal secretions and obtaining a dry, contracted vagina to enhance male sexual arousal and maintain partner fidelity (Runganga *et al.*, 1992; van Andel *et al.*, 2008; Hilber *et al.*, 2010).

Dry sex practices have been suggested as a risk factor that may increase women's susceptibility to HIV infection and cervical cancer (Brown *et al.*, 1993; Beksinska *et al.*, 1999). Several attempts have been made to clarify the link between intravaginal herbal insertions and the occurrence of physical abrasions in the vaginal epithelium (Shattock and Moore, 2003), bacterial vaginosis, the disturbance of vaginal flora and an increased risk of HIV infection (Myer *et al.*, 2005; McClelland *et al.*, 2006; Hilber *et al.*, 2007). The results of these review papers, however, are inconclusive, as differences in definitions of intravaginal practices make it difficult to compare findings directly. There is a need to identify harmful vaginal practices so that their effects on the vaginal flora and susceptibly to sexually transmitted infections (STIs) and HIV can be better studied (Hilber *et al.*, 2007; Low *et al.*, 2011). Most medical authors do not specify the different plants used, but categorize them instead simply as 'herbs' (Hilber *et al.*, 2007), 'leaves' (Brown *et al.*, 1993), 'traditional products' (Low *et al.*, 2011) or publish lists of herbal ingredients with vernacular names only (Irwin *et al.*, 1991; Runganga *et al.*, 1992) and appear to assume they all have a similar effect.

The few ethnobotanical studies on vaginal practices report a wide variety of medicinal plants used in Suriname (177 species), Ghana (22 spp.), Uganda (c. 39 spp.), Benin (23 spp.) and Gabon (41 spp.) (Kamatenesi-Mugisha *et al.*, 2008; van Andel *et al.*, 2008; van Onselen, 2011; Towns and van Andel, 2014). While Surinamese women mostly use genital steam baths, Beninese wash with cooled plant decoctions, Ghanaians insert cotton wool soaked in plant extracts and Ugandans insert plants directly into the vagina or smear macerated medicinal plants on the areas affected by AIDS and *Herpes zoster*. In Gabon, women roll fresh leaves into egg-shaped balls (known as 'ovules') and insert these vaginally. Ethnobotanists seldom subject their respondents to medical research and pharmacologists hardly ever test plants on properties that may affect the vaginal flora or tissue. The challenge for ethnopharmacologists is to bridge this gap between medical and ethnobotanical research by studying the pharmacological effects of vaginally applied medicinal plants and making a distinction between harmless, beneficial or possibly dangerous practices.

Aromatic plants play a key role in intravaginal practises: Piperaceae, Lamiaceae, Verbenaceae and Myrtaceae are used both in Suriname and Africa. When heated by steam or body temperature, essential oils spread a pleasant odour, which might explain the traditional use of genital baths for refreshment. Essential oils are also known to have antibacterial properties (Burt, 2004). *Ocimum gratissimum* L., a frequently used species for intravaginal practises, is known to contain eugenol, a volatile compound with antiseptic properties (Nakamura *et al.*, 1999). Other common ingredients in vaginal cleansers are barks from Anacardiaceae (e.g. *Spondias mombin* L., *Anacardium occidentale* L., *Mangifera indica* L.). These are known to be rich in tannins (Mole, 1993) and are probably responsible for the astringent (drying and tightening) effect on the vaginal tissue. Leaves of *Vismia guianensis* (Aubl.) Pers., a popular steam bath ingredient in Suriname, proved to be effective against *Candida albicans*, the main fungus that causes vaginal yeast infection (Camelo *et al.*, 2011). The leaves of *Alchornea cordifolia* (Schumach. & Thonn.) Müll.Arg., commonly used in Ghana and Gabon for direct vaginal insertion, demonstrated a very broad spectrum of antimicrobial activity (Okeke *et al.*, 1999). Guava leaves (*Psidium guajava*), another frequent ingredient in vaginal applications, possess analgesic and anti-inflammatory properties (Ojewole, 2006). Plants with astringent, antimicrobial or anti-inflammatory assets may be helpful in treating bacterial and fungal infections (Kamatenesi-Mugisha *et al.*, 2008), but they are also likely to affect the vaginal flora itself. Future ethnopharmacologcial research should focus on frequently used plants and their antimicrobial effects in vaginal applications on both harmful and benevolent bacteria. Results should be incorporated in rural education programmes, which should be sensitive to the personal and cultural significances of intravaginal practices and offer alternative suggestions that meet the beliefs and local knowledge associated with these traditions (Runganga *et al.*, 1992).

## 18.5   Female infertility

Recent studies have estimated that infertility affects 48.5 million couples worldwide (Boivin *et al.*, 2007; Mascarenhas *et al.*, 2012). Sub-Saharan Africa has the highest rates of secondary infertility, up to 30% of couples, compared to 23% in South-East Asia, 20% in Central America and the Caribbean, 14% in South America, and 10% or less in developed countries (Rutstein and Shah, 2004; Mascarenhas *et al.*, 2012). Infertility is considered a major reproductive health issue in Africa (Larsen, 2000), with serious psychological and social consequences (Naab *et al.*, 2013). The ability of a woman to have children is closely linked to a female identity and social status in most African societies (Caldwell and Caldwell, 1987). High infertility rates have been linked to elevated rates of sexually transmitted and upper genital tract infections (Collet *et al.*, 1988), eliciting calls for more accessible fertility treatments in this region, known as the 'infertility belt' of Central Africa (Cui, 2010).

In Africa, infertility is often linked with concepts of blockages in the womb, resulting in the use of plants that contract the uterus (van Andel *et al.*, 2014). From a Western biomedical perspective, however, promising plant species for infertility are those that address ovulation disorders or stimulate hormone production. Many of the plants used in Africa for infertility, therefore, have local applicability but are unlikely to be of major pharmacological interest outside of the continent. Plant species for treating infertility were documented in South Africa (90 species), Bénin (58 spp.), Cameroon (46 spp.), Ghana (42 spp.) and Gabon (13 spp.) (Steenkamp, 2003; Telefo *et al.*, 2011; van Onselen, 2011; Abdillahi and Staden, 2013; Towns and van Andel, 2014). Species such as *Solanecio biafrae* (Oliv. & Hiern) C. Jeffrey, *Eremomastax speciosa* (Hochst.) Cufod., *Aloe buettneri* A.Berger and *Justicia insularis* T. Anderson have shown estrogenic and ovulatory effects in a range of clinical and pharmacological studies (Telefo *et al.*, 2011). Medicinal plant use for infertility has also been documented to a lesser extent in South-East Asia (de Boer and Cotingting, 2014) and in the Caribbean (Ososki *et al.*, 2002; Lans, 2007).

Although modern fertility treatments are available in developing countries (van Balen and Gerrits, 2001), the high costs of these procedures together with the social stigma against infertility will likely result in most African women continuing to use medicinal plants as an affordable and private form of treatment (Telefo *et al.*, 2011). In spite of the large number of plants used for women's infertility, few pharmacological studies are available on their effects. More research is needed to ensure the safe and effective use of medicinal plants for treating infertility.

## 18.6   Andrology

### 18.6.1   Aphrodisiacs and male sterility

Medicinal plant use in the tropics for andrology is generally limited to sexual stimulants, erectile dysfunction, urological infections (including STIs) and prostrate problems. Given the general interest in virility and sexual satisfaction, the claimed increase of erectile dysfunction, the commercial value of synthetic treatments (e.g. Viagra, Cialis) and the intensified search for natural alternatives with fewer side effects and lower costs (Sandroni, 2001; Patel *et al.*, 2011), medicinal plants with aphrodisiac properties and their mechanisms of action are generally well documented. Ethnobotanists have published extensively on plants used in the field of andrology in Africa (Noumi *et al.*, 1998, 2011; Kamatenesi-Mugisha and Oryem-Origa, 2005; van Wyk, 2008), Latin America (Duke, 2008), the Caribbean (Lans, 2007; Mitchell, 2011), and Asia (Hopkins, 2006; Melnyk and Marcone, 2011; Thakur *et al.*, 2011). Most of these traditional remedies are drunk as slightly fermented or strongly alcoholic plant mixtures, which are claimed to work as aphrodisiacs, but also double as general strengtheners, tonics, blood purifiers, diuretics, laxatives and remedies for impotence, infertility, urinary tract infections (including STIs) and kidney problems (Volpato and Godínez, 2004; Vandebroek *et al.*, 2010; van Andel *et al.*, 2012). Apart from erectile dysfunction, male infertility can also be due to malfunctioning sperm motility (oligozoospermia) and low or absent sperm production (oligospermia). The latter two ailments are harder to diagnose in traditional medicine and treatments that specify these complaints are rarer.

From an ethnopharmacological perspective, the popularity of these bitter tonics is related to the widespread belief that the presence of 'dirt' or 'cold' inside a man's blood, veins or other hollow organs will reduce his strength and his capacity to have intercourse and reproduce. A free flow of bodily fluids, enhanced by diuretics, laxatives and aphrodisiacs, will therefore guarantee a healthy and reproductive life (Laguerre, 1987; van Andel *et al.*, 2012).

Aphrodisiacs can be categorized according to their mode of action into three groups: substances that (i) increase libido (arousal), (ii) intensify sexual potency (effectiveness of erection) and (iii) increase sexual pleasure (Malviya *et al.*, 2011). The causes of erectile dysfunction may be physiological (e.g. cardiovascular leakage and diabetes) or psychological (Bosch *et al.*, 1991). The psychological effects of aphrodisiacs increase sexual desire and pleasure through hallucinogenic properties or other mood-stimulating properties. Aphrodisiacs can also act physiologically, enhancing erection through hormonal changes, increased blood flow and smooth muscle-relaxing properties (Sandroni, 2001). Research on medicinal plants used as aphrodisiacs and to treat both erectile dysfunction and male infertility has been done mostly on rodents in laboratory settings. Several species have been shown to enhance sexual behaviour, testosterone levels and/or erection functionality, such as *Mondia whitei* (Hook.f.) Skeels, *Aframomum melegueta* K.Schum., *Piper guineense* Schumach. & Thonn., *Curculigo orchioides* Gaertn., *Vangueria agrestis* (Schweinf. ex Hiern.) Lantz, *Eurycoma longifolia* Jack and *Microdesmis keayana* J.Léonard (Kamtchouing *et al.*, 2002; Chauhan *et al.*, 2007; Zamblé *et al.*, 2009). Others appeared to relax corpus cavernosum smooth muscle tissue and thus facilitate erection due to increased blood flow in the penis, including *Securidaca longipedunculata* Fresen. and *Eriosema kraussianum* Meissner (Drewes *et al.*, 2002; Marion Meyer *et al.*, 2008).

Very few aphrodisiac plants have been tested on humans in randomized, placebo-controlled, double-blind trials. The intake of yohimbine (an alkaloid extracted from *Pausinystalia johimbe* (K.Schum.) Pierre ex Beille) increased erectile function, ejaculation, interest in sex and sexual thoughts among patients with psychogenic erectile dysfunction (Montorsi *et al.*, 1994). Men who consumed 1500 or 3000 mg of *Lepidium meyenii* Walp. reported significantly improved sexual desire relative to a placebo (Gonzales *et al.*, 2002). *P. johimbe* and *L. meyenii* extracts are also commonly used in western countries to treat oligospermia and oligozoospermia (Rowland and Tai, 2003). More clinical studies are needed to understand mechanisms and drug interactions, and to establish safe doses (Melnyk and Marcone, 2011).

Another complicating factor is that traditionally these plants are mostly ingested as mixtures, and not always solely to enhance sexual activities. Chemical processes related to synergism and additive or reduced therapeutic effects are likely to occur in mixtures, in particular when they are boiled or soaked in alcohol for a prolonged period (Wang *et al.*, 2005). Studying the botanical contents of traditional mixtures is further complicated by the difficulty of identifying small plant fragments, especially when they consist of wood, bark or roots, organs not often present on herbarium sheets (Veldman *et al.*, 2014). The challenge for ethnobotanists is to match the fragmented, woody ingredients sold on local markets, often under popular 'commercial' names, with fertile herbarium vouchers collected in their natural environment to guarantee their scientific identification. Popular aphrodisiac ingredients sold under the name 'sarsaparilla' could refer to many different species of *Smilax* (Ferrufino-Acosta, 2010) and no fewer than ten different species were being commercialized under the name 'bois bandé' in the French Caribbean and the Guianas (van Andel *et al.*, 2012). Moreover, since the introduction of Viagra and sildenafil citrate-based generics in 1998, adulteration of traditional remedies with sildenafil has also become extensive (Reepmeyer *et al.*, 2007; Wollein *et al.*, 2011).

## 18.7  Urology

Common urological health issues in the tropics include urinary tract infections (UTIs), STIs, general urinary and bladder infections, and, in the case of sub-Saharan Africa, urinary schistosomiasis. Worldwide, an estimated 150 million cases of UTIs occur annually and are a particularly severe problem for women and malnourished children (Reed and Wegerhoff, 1994; Maclennan *et al.*, 2005). Urinary schistosomiasis is caused by the parasite *Schistosoma haematobium*; together with the intestinal form of the disease, it causes more than 200,000 deaths annually in Africa (USAID, 2014).

From an ethnopharmacological perspective, plants used against urological complications have antibacterial, antifungal and antiviral properties or function as diuretics, diluting the infection or removing it from the body through urination. Recent research from Bangladesh has documented the use of 31 plants species to treat UTIs and other sexual and urinary complications (Hossan *et al.*, 2010). The leaves and bark of *Garcinia mangostana* L., used to treat urinary disorders in South-East Asia, have shown strong antibacterial activity (Obolskiy and Pischel, 2009). The stem bark of *Ocotea bullata* (Burch.) E. Meyer in Drege, commonly used to treat urinary disorders in South Africa, has demonstrated prostaglandin synthesis inhibitory activity in pharmacological studies (Fennell *et al.*, 2004). Medicinal plant remedies for urinary schistosomiasis have been documented across the African continent, with extracts of *Berkheya speciosa* (DC.) O.Hoffm., *Trichilia emetica* Vahl and *Euclea natalensis* A.DC. demonstrating efficacy against the parasite in laboratory studies (Ndamba *et al.*, 1994; Sparg *et al.*, 2000; Mølgaard *et al.*, 2001; Fennell *et al.*, 2004; Bah *et al.*, 2006). Hundreds of medicinal plants are used worldwide against STIs with documented antibacterial, antifungal and antiviral properties (Vermani and Garg, 2002).

One of the great challenges of ethnopharmacological research on urology is to focus on the use of medicinal plants for urinary schistosomiasis. Currently *praziquantel* is the only medicine approved by the WHO for its treatment, raising concerns that the parasite may develop resistance (Wang *et al.*, 2012). The use of medicinal plants to treat vaginal infections is another area for future research, as their use may interact with biomedical treatments for STIs (Allen *et al.*, 2010). This example highlights the need for improved communication between ethnobotanists, pharmacologists and local biomedical health providers in order to avoid the adverse effects of combining medical systems.

# References

Abdillahi, H. and van Staden, J. (2013) Application of medicinal plants in maternal healthcare and infertility: a South African perspective. *Planta Medica*, **230**, 591–599.

Achterrath Tuckermann, U., Kunde, R., Flaskamp, E., *et al.* (1980) Pharmacological investigations with compounds of chamomile. V. Investigations on the spasmolytic effect of compounds of chamomile and Kamillosan on the isolated guinea pig ileum. *Planta Medica*, **39**, 38–50.

Allen, C.F., Desmond, N., Chiduo, B., *et al.* (2010) Intravaginal and menstrual practices among women working in food and recreational facilities in Mwanza, Tanzania: implications for microbicide trials. *AIDS Behaviour*, **14**, 1169–1181.

Bah, S., Diallo, D., Dembélé, S. and Paulsen, B.S. (2006) Ethnopharmacological survey of plants used for the treatment of schistosomiasis in Niono District, Mali. *Journal of Ethnopharmacology*, **105**, 387–399.

Barua, C.C., Begum, S.A. and Talukdar, A. (2010) Wound healing activity of methanolic extract of leaves of *Achyranthes aspera* Linn using in vivo and in vitro model: a preliminary study. *Indian Journal of Animal Science*, **80**, 969–972.

Beal, M.W. (1998) Women's use of complementary and alternative therapies in reproductive health care. *Journal of Nurse-Midwifery*, **43**, 224–234.

Beksinska, M.E., Rees, H.V., Kleinschmidt, I. and McIntyre, J. (1999) The practice and prevalence of dry sex among men and women in South Africa: a risk factor for sexually transmitted infections? *Sexually Transmitted Infections*, **75**, 178–180.

Belew, C. (1999) Herbs and the childbearing woman: guidelines for midwives. *Journal of Nurse-Midwifery*, **44**, 231–252.

Boivin, J., Bunting, L., Collins, J.A. and Nygren, K.G. (2007) International estimates of infertility prevalence and treatment-seeking: potential need and demand for infertility medical care. *Human Reproduction*, **22**, 1506–1512.

Bosch, R.J., Benard, F., Aboseif, S.R., *et al.* (1991) Penile detumescence: characterization of three phases. *Journal of Urology*, **146**, 867–871.

Brown, J.E., Ayowa, O.B. and Brown, R.C. (1993) Dry and tight: Sexual practices and potential (AIDS) risk in Zaire. *Social Science and Medicine*, **37**, 989–994.

Burt, S. (2004) Essential oils: their antibacterial properties and potential applications in foods: a review. *International Journal of Food Microbiology*, **94**, 223–253.

Caldwell, J.C. and Caldwell, P. (1987) The cultural context of high fertility in sub-Saharan Africa. *Popul Developmental Review*, **13**, 409–437.

Camelo, S.R.P., Costa, R.S., Ribeiro-Costa, R.M., *et al.* (2011) Phytochemical evaluation and antimicrobial activity of ethanolic extract of *Vismia guianensis* (Aubl.) Choisy. *International Journal of Pharmaceutical Science Review Research*, **2**, 3224–3229.

Chauhan, N.S., Rao, C. V. and Dixit, V.K. (2007) Effect of Curculigo orchioides rhizomes on sexual behaviour of male rats. *Fitoterapia*, **78**, 530–534.

Civic, D. and Wilson, D. (1996) Dry sex in Zimbabwe and implications for condom use. *Social Science Medicine*, **42**, 91–98.

Collet, M., Reniers, J., Frost, E., *et al.* (1988) Infertility in Central Africa: infection is the cause. *International Journal of Gynaecology and Obstetrics*, **26**, 423–428.

Cui, W. (2010) Mother or nothing: the agony of infertility. *Bulletin of the World Health Organization*, **88**, 881–882.

de Boer, H.J. and Cotingting, C. (2014) Medicinal plants for women's healthcare in Southeast Asia: a meta-analysis of their traditional use, chemical constituents, and pharmacology. *Journal of Ethnopharmacology*, **151**, 747–767.

de Boer, H.J. and Lamxay, V. (2009) Plants used during pregnancy, childbirth and postpartum healthcare in Lao PDR: a comparative study of the Brou, Saek and Kry ethnic groups. *Journal of Ethnobiology and Ethnomedicine*, **5**, 25.

de Boer, H.J., Lamxay, V. and Björk, L. (2011) Steam sauna and mother roasting in Lao PDR: practices and chemical constituents of essential oils of plant species used in postpartum recovery. *BMC Complementary and Alternative Medicine*, **11**, 128.

de Boer, H.J., Lamxay, V. and Björk, L. (2012) Comparing medicinal plant knowledge using similarity indices: a case of the Brou, Saek and Kry in Lao PDR. *Journal of Ethnopharmacology*, **141**, 481–500.

Drewes, S.E., Horn, M.M., Munro, O.Q., *et al.* (2002) Pyrano-isoflavones with erectile-dysfunction activity from *Eriosema kraussianum*. *Phytochemistry*, **59**, 739–747.

Duke, J.A. (2008) *Duke's Handbook of Medicinal Plants of Latin America*, CRC Press, Boca Raton.

Edwin, S., Jarald, E.E. and Deb, L. (2008) Wound healing and antioxidant activity of *Achyranthes aspera*. *Pharmaceutical Biology*, **46**, 824–828.

Fennell, C.W., Lindsey, K.L., McGaw, L.J., *et al.* (2004) Assessing African medicinal plants for efficacy and safety: pharmacological screening and toxicology. *Journal of Ethnopharmacology*, **94**, 205–217.

Ferrufino-Acosta, L. (2010) Taxonomic revision of the genus Smilax (Smilacaceae) in Central America and the Caribbean Islands. *Willdenowia*, **40**, 227–280.

Ghosh, P. and Gupta, V. (2011) Wound-healing potential of aqueous and ethanolic extracts of apamarga leaves. *International Journal of Green Pharmacy*, **5**, 12–15.

Golmakani, N., Motlagh, E.R. and Tara, F. (2009) The effects of turmeric (*Curcuma longa* L.) ointment on healing of episiotomy site in primiparous women. *Iranian Journal of Obstetrics, Gynecology and Infertility*, **11**, 29–38.

Gonzales, G.F., Córdova, A., Vega, K., *et al.* (2002) Effect of *Lepidium meyenii* (Maca) on sexual desire and its absent relationship with serum testosterone levels in adult healthy men. *Andrologia*, **34**, 367–372.

Halperin, D.T. (1999) Dry sex practices and HIV infection in the Dominican Republic and Haiti. *Sexually Transmitted Infectections*, **75**, 445–446.

Harlow, S.D. and Campbell, O.M.R. (2000) Menstrual dysfunction: a missed opportunity for improving reproductive health in developing countries. *Reproductive Health Matters*, **8**, 142–147.

Hilber, A.M., Chersich, M.F., van de Wijgert, J.H.H.M., *et al.* (2007) Vaginal practices, microbicides and HIV: what do we need to know? *Sexually Transmitted Infections*, **83**, 505–508.

Hilber, A.M., Hull, T.H., Preston-Whyte, E., *et al.* (2010) A cross-cultural study of vaginal practices and sexuality: Implications for sexual health. *Social Science Medicine*, **70**, 392–400.

Hopkins, J. (2006) *Asian Aphrodisiacs: From Bangkok to Beijing – the search for the ultimate turn-on*, Tuttle Publishing, North Clarendon.

Hossan, S., Agarwala, B., Sarwar, S., *et al.* (2010) Traditional use of medicinal plants in Bangladesh to treat urinary tract infections and sexually transmitted diseases. *Ethnobotanical Research Applications*, **8**, 61–74.

Irwin, K., Bertrand, J., Mibandumba, N., *et al.* (1991) Knowledge, attitudes and beliefs about HIV infection and AIDS among healthy factory workers and their wives, Kinshasa, Zaire. *Social Science Medicine*, **32**, 917–930.

Joesoef, M.R., Sumampouw, H., Linnan, M., *et al.* (1996) Douching and sexually transmitted diseases in pregnant women in Surabaya, Indonesia. *American Journal of Obstetrics and Gynecology*, **174**, 115–119.

Kamatenesi-Mugisha, M. and Oryem-Origa, H. (2005) Traditional herbal remedies used in the management of sexual impotence and erectile dysfunction in western Uganda. *African Health Science*, **5**, 40–49.

Kamatenesi-Mugisha, M., Oryem-Origa, H., Odyek, O. and Makawiti, D.W. (2008) Medicinal plants used in the treatment of fungal and bacterial infections in and around Queen Elizabeth Biosphere Reserve, western Uganda. *African Journal of Ecology*, **46**, 90–97.

Kamtchouing, P., Mbongue, G.Y., Dimo, T., *et al.* (2002) Effects of *Aframomum melegueta* and *Piper guineense* on sexual behaviour of male rats. *Behavioural Pharmacology*, **13**, 243–247.

Khan, K.S., Wojdyla, D., Say, L., *et al.* (2006) WHO analysis of causes of maternal death: a systematic review. *Lancet*, **367**, 1066–1074.

Kim, M., Hayashi, R.H. and Gambone, J.C. (2009) Obstetric hemorrhage and puerperal sepsis, in *Hacker and Moore's Essentials of Obstetrics and Gynecology* (eds N. Hacker, J. Gambone and C. Hobel), Saunders Elsevier, Philadelphia, pp. 128–138.

Laguerre, M. (1987) *Afro-Caribbean Folk Medicine*, Bergin & Garvey Publishers, South Hadley.

Lange, A.P. (1986) Induction of labour, in *Prostaglandins and their Inhibitors in Clinical Obstetrics and Gynaecology* (eds M. Bygdeman, G.S. Berger and L.G. Keith), Springer, Amsterdam, pp. 165–202.

Lans, C. (2007) Ethnomedicines used in Trinidad and Tobago for reproductive problems. *Journal of Ethnobiology and Ethnomedicine*, **3**, 13.

Larsen, U. (2000) Primary and secondary infertility in sub-Saharan Africa. *International Journal of Epidemiology*, **29**, 285–291.

Lindsey, K., Jäger, A.K., Raidoo, D.M. and van Staden, J. (1998) Screening of plants used by Southern African traditional healers in the treatment of dysmenorrhoea for prostaglandin-synthesis inhibitors and uterine relaxing activity. *Journal of Ethnopharmacology*, **64**, 9–14.

López-Jornet, P. (2011) Topical curcumin for the healing of carbon dioxide laser skin wounds in mice. *Photomedicine and Laser Surgery*, **29**, 809–814.

Low, N., Chersich, M.F., Schmidlin, K., *et al.* (2011) Intravaginal practices, bacterial vaginosis, and HIV infection in women: individual participant data meta-analysis. *PLOS Med* **8**, e1000416.

Maclennan, C., Swingler, G. and Craig, J. (2005) *Urinary tract infections in infants and children in developing countries in the context of IMCI*, Discussion Papers on Child Health 05.11, World Health Organization, Geneva.

Malviya, N., Jain, S., Gupta, V.B. and Vyas, S. (2011) Recent studies on aphrodisiac herbs for the management of male sexual dysfunction – a review. *Acta Poloniae Pharmaceutica*, **68**, 3–8.

Marion Meyer, J.J., Rakuambo, N.C. and Hussein, A.A. (2008) Novel xanthones from *Securidaca longipedunculata* with activity against erectile dysfunction. *Journal of Ethnopharmacology*, **119**, 599–603.

Mascarenhas, M.N., Flaxman, S.R., Boerma, T., *et al.* (2012) National, regional, and global trends in infertility prevalence since 1990: a systematic analysis of 277 health surveys. *PLoS Med*, **9**, e1001356.

McClelland, R.S., Lavreys, L., Hassan, W.M., *et al.* (2006) Vaginal washing and increased risk of HIV-1 acquisition among African women: a 10-year prospective study. *AIDS*, **20**, 269–273.

Melnyk, J.P. and Marcone, M.F. (2011) Aphrodisiacs from plant and animal sources: a review of current scientific literature. *Food Research International*, **44**, 840–850.

Michel, J., Duarte, R.F., Bolton, J.L., *et al.* (2007) Medical potential of plants used by the Q'eqchi Maya of Livingston, Guatemala for the treatment of women's health complaints. *Journal of Ethnopharmacology*, **114**, 92–101.

Mitchell, S.A. (2011) The Jamaican root tonics: a botanical reference. *Focus on Alternative and Complementary Therapy*, **16**, 271–280.

Mole, S. (1993) The systematic distribution of tannins in the leaves of angiosperms: A tool for ecological studies. *Biochemical System Ecology*, **21**, 833–846.

Mølgaard, P., Nielsen, S.B., Rasmussen, D.E., *et al.* (2001) Anthelmintic screening of Zimbabwean plants traditionally used against schistosomiasis. *Journal of Ethnopharmacology*, **74**, 257–264.

Monera, T.G. and Gwekwe, N.S. (2012) *Herbal medicine use in dysmenorrhea: determining extent of use and commonly used herbs*, International Pharmaceutical Federation, Amsterdam.

Montorsi, F., Strambi, L.F., Guazzoni, G., *et al.* (1994) Effect of yohimbine-trazodone on psychogenic impotence: a randomized, double-blind, placebo-controlled study. *Urology*, **44**, 732–736.

Myer, L., Kuhn, L., Stein, Z.A., *et al.* (2005) Intravaginal practices, bacterial vaginosis, and women's susceptibility to HIV infection: epidemiological evidence and biological mechanisms. *Lancet Infectious Diseases*, **5**, 786–794.

Naab, F., Brown, R. and Heidrich, S. (2013) Psychosocial health of infertile Ghanaian women and their infertility beliefs. *Journal of Nursing Scholarship*, **45**, 1–9.

Nakamura, C.V., Ueda-Nakamura, T., Bando, E., *et al.* (1999) Antibacterial activity of *Ocimum gratissimum* L. essential oil. *Memórias do Instituto Oswaldo Cruz*, **94**, 675–678.

Ndamba, J., Nyazema, N., Makaza, N., *et al.* (1994) Traditional herbal remedies used for the treatment of urinary schistosomiasis in Zimbabwe. *Journal of Ethnopharmacology*, **42**, 125–132.

Noumi, E., Amvan Zollo, P.H. and Lontsi, D. (1998) Aphrodisiac plants used in Cameroon. *Fitoterapia*, **69**, 125–134.

Noumi, E., Eboule, A.F. and Nanfa, R. (2011) Traditional health care of male infertility in Bansoa, West Cameroon. *International Journal of Biomedical and Pharmaceutical Science*, **2**, 42–50.

Oats, J. and Abraham, S. (2010) *Llewellyn-Jones Fundamentals of Obstetrics and Gynaecology*, 9th edn, Mosby Elsevier, Edinburgh.

Obolskiy, D. and Pischel, I. (2009) *Garcinia mangostana* L.: a phytochemical and pharmacological review. *Phytotherapy Research*, **1065**, 1047–1065.

Ojewole, J.A.O. (2006) Anti-Inflammatory and analgesic effects of *Psidium guajava* Linn. (Myrtaceae) leaf aqueous extracts in rats and mice. *Methods and Findings in Experimental and Clinical Pharmacology*, **28**, 441–446.

Okeke, I.N., Ogundaini, A.O., Ogungbamila, F.O. and Lamikanra, A. (1999) Antimicrobial spectrum of *Alchornea cordifolia* leaf extract. *Phytotherapy Research*, **13**, 67–69.

Ortiz de Montellano, B.R. and Browner, C.H. (1985) Chemical bases for medicinal plant use in Oaxaca, Mexico. *Journal of Ethnopharmacology*, **13**, 57–88.

Ososki, A.L., Lohr, P., Reiff, M., *et al.* (2002) Ethnobotanical literature survey of medicinal plants in the Dominican Republic used for women's health conditions. *Journal of Ethnopharmacology*, **79**, 285–298.

Panchatcharam, M. and Miriyala, S. (2006) Curcumin improves wound healing by modulating collagen and decreasing reactive oxygen species. *Molecular Cell Biochemistry*, **290**, 87–96.

Patel, D.K., Kumar, R., Prasad, S.K. and Hemalatha, S. (2011) Pharmacologically screened aphrodisiac plants: a review of current scientific literature. *Asian Pacific Journal of Tropical Biomedicine*, **1**, S131–S138.

Reed, R.P. and Wegerhoff, F.O. (1994) Urinary tract infection in malnourished rural African children. *Annals of Tropical Paediatrics*, **15**, 21–26.

Reepmeyer, J.C., Woodruff, J.T. and d'Avignon, D.A. (2007) Structure elucidation of a novel analogue of sildenafil detected as an adulterant in an herbal dietary supplement. *Journal of Pharmaceutical and Biomedical Analysis*, **43**, 1615–1621.

Ronsmans, C., Graham, W.J. and the Lancet Maternal Survival Series steering group (2006) Maternal mortality: who, when, where, and why. *Lancet*, **368**, 1189–1200.

Rowland, D.L. and Tai, W. (2003) A review of plant-derived and herbal approaches to the treatment of sexual dysfunctions. *Journal of Sexual Marital Therapy*, **29**, 185–205.

Runganga, A., Pitts, M. and McMaster, J. (1992) The use of herbal and other agents to enhance sexual experience. *Social Science Medicine*, **35**, 1037–1042.

Rutstein, S. and Shah, I. (2004) Infecundity infertility and childlessness in developing countries, *DHS Comparative Reports 9*, USAID, Calverton.

Sandroni, P. (2001) Aphrodisiacs past and present: A historical review. *Clinical Autonomic Research*, **11**, 303–307.

Shattock, R.J. and Moore, J.P. (2003) Inhibiting sexual transmission of HIV-1 infection. *Natural Reviews in Microbiology*, **1**, 25–34.

Sparg, S.G., van Staden, J. and Jäger, A.K. (2000) Efficiency of traditionally used South African plants against schistosomiasis. *Journal of Ethnopharmacology*, **73**, 209–214.

Steenkamp, V. (2003) Traditional herbal remedies used by South African women for gynaecological complaints. *Journal of Ethnopharmacology*, **86**, 97–108.

Telefo, P.B., Lienou, L.L., Yemele, M.D., *et al.* (2011) Ethnopharmacological survey of plants used for the treatment of female infertility in Baham, Cameroon. *Journal of Ethnopharmacology*, **136**, 178–187.

Thakur, M., Thompson, D., Connellan, P., *et al.* (2011) Improvement of penile erection, sperm count and seminal fructose levels in vivo and nitric oxide release in vitro by ayurvedic herbs. *Andrologia*, **43**, 273–277.

Tjon A Ten, V. (2007) *Menstrual Hygiene: A neglected condition for the achievement of several Millennium Development Goals*, Europe External Policy Advisors, Zoetermeer.

Towns, A.M. and van Andel, T.R. (2014) Comparing local perspectives on women's health with statistics on maternal mortality: an ethnobotanical study in Bénin and Gabon. *BMC Complementary and Alternative Medicine*, **14**, 113.

USAID (2014) *Schistosomiasis*, USAID Neglected Tropical Diseases Program, http://www.neglecteddiseases.gov/target_diseases/schistosomiasis/index.html, assessed 20 June 2014.

van Andel, T.R., de Korte, S., Koopmans, D., *et al.* (2008) Dry sex in Suriname. *Journal of Ethnopharmacology*, **116**, 84–88.

van Andel, T.R., Mitchell, S., Volpato, G., *et al.* (2012) In search of the perfect aphrodisiac: Parallel use of bitter tonics in West Africa and the Caribbean. *Journal of Ethnopharmacology*, **143**, 840–850.

van Andel, T.R. van, de Boer, H.J., Barnes, J. and Vandebroek, I. (2014) Medicinal plants used for menstrual disorders in Latin America, the Caribbean, sub-Saharan Africa, South and Southeast Asia and their uterine properties: a review. *Journal of Ethnopharmacology*, **155**, 992–1000.

van Balen, F. and Gerrits, T. (2001) Quality of infertility care in poor-resource areas and the introduction of new reproductive technologies. *Human Reproduction*, **16**, 215–219.

van Onselen, S. (2011) *The knowledge of midwives, priestesses and market sellers about medicinal plants for women's reproductive health matters in five Southern regions in Ghana*, MSc thesis, Department of Cultural Anthropology, Leiden University.

van Wyk, B.E. (2008) A broad review of commercially important southern African medicinal plants. *Journal of Ethnopharmacology*, **119**, 342–355.

Vandebroek, I., Balick, M.J., Ososki, A., *et al.* (2010) The importance of botellas and other plant mixtures in Dominican traditional medicine. *Journal of Ethnopharmacology*, **128**, 20–41.

Veldman, S., Otieno, J., Gravendeel, B., *et al.* (2014) Conservation of endangered wild harvested medicinal plants: use of DNA barcoding, in *Novel Plant Bioresources* (ed. A. Gurib-Fakim), John Wiley & Sons, Chichester, pp. 81–88.

Vermani, K. and Garg, S. (2002) Herbal medicines for sexually transmitted diseases and AIDS. *Journal of Ethnopharmacology*, **80**, 49–66.

Volpato, G. and Godínez, D. (2004) Ethnobotany of Pru, a traditional Cuban refreshment. *Economic Botany*, **58**, 381–395.

Wang, M., Lamers, R.J.A.N., Korthout, H.A.A.J., *et al.* (2005) Metabolomics in the context of systems biology: bridging traditional Chinese medicine and molecular pharmacology. *Phytotherapy Research*, **19**, 173–182.

Wang, W., Wang, L. and Liang, Y.S. (2012) Susceptibility or resistance of praziquantel in human schistosomiasis: a review. *Parasitology Research*, **111**, 1871–1877.

WHO (2008) Traditional medicine, *Factsheet 134*, World Health Organization, Geneva.

Wollein, U., Eisenreich, W. and Schramek, N. (2011) Identification of novel sildenafil-analogues in an adulterated herbal food supplement. *Journal of Pharmaceutical and Biomedical Analysis*, **56**, 705–712.

Zamblé, A., Martin-Nizard, F., Sahpaz, S., *et al.* (2009) Effects of Microdesmis keayAbdillahi, H., Staden, J. Van, 2013. Application of medicinal plants in maternal healthcare and infertility: a south African perspective. *Planta Medica*, **230**, 591–599.

Zhou, X. (2010) The clinical observation of reducing Cesarean section hemorrhage by using the motherwort injection. *Journal of Qiqihar Medical College*, **10**, 10.

# 19
# Ethnopharmacological Aspects of Bone and Joint Health

Elizabeth M. Williamson

*The School of Pharmacy, University of Reading, Whiteknights, Reading, Berkshire*

## 19.1   Introduction

Currently there are no drugs available for bone disorders developed from ethnobotanical leads, for many reasons, but mainly because the view of bone as a tissue has changed dramatically in recent decades. There is historical and cultural evidence of bone diseases throughout history, but a link with bone was not necessarily made, making an evaluation of medicinal plants traditionally used in this context difficult. For example, a basic understanding of osteoporosis did not arise until the last half of the 20th century, although its presence in older women is well documented in artworks and literature as 'dowager's hump'. The incidence of osteoporosis varies with ethnicity and race as well as gender, so references to this disease in traditional medicine will also depend on where the report originates from. In addition, osteoporosis is primarily a disease of ageing, so its occurrence is much more apparent in modern societies with larger ageing populations. The other main causes of osteoporosis relate to lifestyle (diet, exercise, lack of sunlight), other diseases (rheumatoid and other inflammatory conditions, obesity and anorexia) and drug treatment (such as with corticosteroids and aromatase inhibitors), which are more carefully scrutinized in modern societies compared to in previous centuries.

For all these reasons, ethnomedical records need to be interpreted very carefully, and few actually refer directly to treatments for loss of bone mass. It is much more common to find traditional remedies for bone fracture than for bone loss, but in more sophisticated forms of ethnomedicine such as TCM and Ayurveda, and their variants as practised in different Asian countries, bone tissue is considered to be part of a connecting system of organs, and medicinal plants which nourish bone and its linked organs are described. In many other cultures no reference is made to osteoporosis and the main use of medicinal plants which affect

*Ethnopharmacology*, First Edition. Edited by Michael Heinrich and Anna K. Jäger.
© 2015 John Wiley & Sons, Ltd. Published 2015 by John Wiley & Sons, Ltd.

bone is for the treatment of fractures. The other significant bone and joint disorders, which are indeed widely described in the ethnomedical literature, are osteoarthritis and gout. Gout has highly characteristic and painful symptoms and a well-documented history, and acute attacks of gout are still treated with colchicine, an alkaloid discovered from the ethnopharmacological use of the autumn crocus *Colchicum autumnale*. In this brief review, medicinal plants traditionally used to treat bone loss, bone fracture, osteoarthritis and gout will be considered; purely anti-inflammatory agents which would certainly be taken to relieve bone and joint pain are not included but covered elsewhere in this book.

## 19.2   Current views of bone and joint disorders

By far the most prevalent bone disease of modern times is osteoporosis, which is a huge and increasing health burden for most societies. The term was coined in the 1830s by a French pathologist, Jean Lobstein, but no significance was attached at the time to the fact that some patients' bones were riddled with larger than normal holes (Patlak, 2001). Even now, osteoporosis may not be diagnosed until either bone pain or fracture occurs, giving rise to its description as a 'silent disease', and then the only real treatment is to prevent further degeneration. Osteoporosis is most common in post-menopausal women, due to lack of oestrogen, and it also occurs in men as a result of androgen deficiency, and as life expectancy increases, its prevalence can only increase.

Bone fracture is a common consequence of osteoporosis but also occurs very widely in young and healthy patients who have met with some kind of injury. This type of breakage heals more easily than osteoporotic fracture and nowadays drugs are not given, only physical support and pain relief. There are reports of medicinal plants traditionally used to aid fracture healing, sometimes by application of a poultice, although it is more common simply to set the bone using bamboo or similar splints and give anti-inflammatory medicinal plants to reduce pain and swelling. Unfortunately traditional bone-setting, for example in Nigeria (where 85% of patients first consult a traditional bone-setter), can be a serious problem due to lack of regulation and poor training of bone-setters, and the complication rate including gangrene and eventual amputation is very high (Dada *et al.*, 2011).

It has long been known that calcium is necessary for bone health, as bone is composed of mainly calcium salts and before the metabolic aspects of osteoporosis became known the only treatment for bone mineral loss was calcium and, upon the discovery of vitamin D in 1922, a combination of both. Rickets, a softening of the bones which can cause deformities such as bow legs and pelvis abnormalities, is caused by a deficiency of vitamin D and was commonplace in societies where nutrition was poor (especially with a lack of dairy products) and there was restricted access to sunlight (Patlak, 2001). Ironically, the incidence of rickets is once again increasing as children are prevented from being in the sun for fear of skin cancer or as a result of restrictive dairy-free diets.

Joint disorders include osteoarthritis, an autoimmune inflammatory disease which causes injury bone tissue, and gout, an extremely painful swelling of the joint caused by deposition of crystals of sodium urate inside and around joints. Gout incidence varies also with race, gender and age. Damage to joints caused by gout and other diseases or injuries can also lead to osteoarthritis, and both conditions are exacerbated by modern lifestyles which encourage obesity, high meat and fructose intake, and reduced levels of exercise.

As the main bone disorders have only been really known as such from the 20th century, it is difficult to find many records of ethnobotanical treatment for them. The incidence of these disorders also differs according to race and ethnicity, which must be borne in mind when evaluating reports from different geographical regions and ethnic groups. Osteoporosis is more common in white and Hispanic women than in African and Asian women (Cauley, 2011), and gout is more common in Pacific Islanders, the Māori of New Zealand and African men compared to Europeans and Australian aborigines (Singh, 2013). Diet is also a significant factor in the development of osteoporosis (Putnam *et al.*, 2007) and weight-bearing exercise also enhances bone formation. In traditional societies most ordinary people probably ate more fruit and vegetables and walked much more than they do in modern western societies. Polyphenols are now known to have beneficial effects on bone production, soluble fibre enhances the absorption of calcium and magnesium, and monounsaturated fatty acids suppress the production of cytokines involved in bone resorption (Putnam *et al.*, 2007). A diet of unprocessed foods, as is more common in traditional societies, therefore contributes to bone health and may reduce the incidence of osteoporosis.

Although plant remedies specifically for bone disorders are not widely cited in the ethnopharmacological literature directly, it can be productive to consider the reputed role of bone and connective tissue in traditional medicine, with herbal treatments intended to nourish these and related tissues. Bone as a tissue is metabolically dynamic despite its static appearance and rigidity, and undergoes constant construction and deconstruction, involving the formation of matrix and mineralization, and resorption. These processes are known as bone remodelling and are necessary for preserving bone strength through repair and growth, and maintaining calcium homoeostasis throughout the whole body. Bone remodelling processes are controlled by a complex interaction between inhibitory and stimulatory factors for bone production and resorption, which include oestrogens, androgens, calcitonin, vitamin D, parathyroid hormone, cortisol, prostaglandins and tumour necrosis and growth factors. Some effects are dose dependent, for example parathyroid hormone in small doses increases bone formation but in large doses causes resorption, in order to replenish calcium in the bloodstream. The two opposing effects are controlled by each other, for example mediators produced by osteoblasts (cells which build bone), such as RANK-L and osteoprotegerin, influence the activity of osteoclasts (which resorb bone). The 'raw material' of bone is protein, mainly collagen, which forms the osteoid matrix in which the osteocytes (immobile cells derived from osteoblasts) are embedded and the minerals calcium and phosphorus, in the form of hydroxyapatite, are laid down to provide strength and hardness. An adequate supply of these from the diet is therefore essential for bone health.

Bone is also highly vascularized and for regeneration and maintenance angiogenesis is essential to develop the microvasculature and establish microcirculation. A close relationship has been observed between bone growth, fracture healing and angiogenesis, and the microvasculature is provided by endothelial cells during bone remodelling. This is mediated via vascular endothelial growth factor (VEGF) and the effects of VEGF on skeletal growth have been widely reported (see Yang *et al.*, 2014).

The complexity of bone metabolism and its influences from other bodily systems, together with the enormous differences in the incidence of bone disorders due to diet, lifestyle, race, ethnicity, age and gender, demonstrates how these disorders may not be recognized as such, and may also explain the paucity of traditional bone healing agents reported in ethnopharmacological texts. However, bone metabolism is part of general metabolism and 'nourishing bone' as a holistic concept is notable in TCM and Ayurveda. Inflammation and injury to the joints eventually destroys bone and connective tissue, and therefore medicinal plants used for 'swollen joints' and osteoarthritis in all societies are relevant in the context of bone health.

## 19.3    Traditional views of bone disorders

Bone and joint disorders have, arguably, become more prevalent in modern times and in western societies due to lifestyle factors and a greater ageing population. There is also a deeper understanding of them, leading to more diagnoses. However, osteoporosis has certainly been recorded throughout history and Egyptian mummies from 4000 years ago have been found with curvature of the spine. In 19th century England, in the novel *Great Expectations*, Charles Dickens described Miss Haversham in these terms: 'her chest had dropped, so that she stooped'. This description suggests that the condition 'dowager's hump' was not necessarily thought to be due to weakness of the bone but was certainly linked to old age, especially in women (Patlak, 2001).

Gout has also been known for centuries, especially in wealthy people who could afford to eat a high-protein diet with plenty of meat, sugar and alcohol, and as a result has been termed the 'King's disease'. Its first documentation is also from Egypt, in 2600 BC, in a description of 'arthritis of the big toe'. The overt manifestations of osteoporosis, gout and fracture are therefore well-documented throughout history, unlike the more subtle symptoms of bone and joint disorders.

The role of oestrogen in osteoporosis was proposed in 1940 by the clinical researcher Fuller Albright at Massachusetts General Hospital, who then began to treat post-menopausal patients with oestrogen injections (Patlak, 2001). It is now known from epidemiological studies, particularly in Asian women, that phytoestrogens in the diet can also prevent osteoporosis to some extent and some herbal drugs have a traditional use based on this mechanism of action, even though it was not known at the time. These include *Epimedium* species and others shown in Table 19.1, which covers a selection of medicinal plants from the European, North American, Chinese and Ayurvedic medical systems. There are of course similar records from cultures in South America, Africa, Australia, New Zealand and elsewhere, but for reasons of space these are not discussed here.

### 19.3.1    European traditional herbal medicine

Apart from a few specific medicinal plants used to treat bone disorders, for example the herb *Symphytum officinale* (knitbone or comfrey) which has a long history of use, most traditional European herbal medicine systems do not really deal with bone disorders. There are, however, numerous references to 'rheumatic disorders' and these have been well reviewed by Adams *et al.* (2009). The *British Herbal Pharmacopoeia*, first published in 1983, which summarizes the most important medicinal plants used by traditional medical herbalists in the UK but also reflects other European use, mentions only *Symphytum* and *Pilosella officinarum* in the context of bone fracture and no medicinal plants at all for osteoporosis (BHP, 1983). *Symphytum* contains allantoin (Staiger, 2012) and clinical studies have demonstrated relief of pain and swelling in joint trauma. *Pilosella* is rich in phenolic antioxidants (Stanojević *et al.*, 2009), but neither *Symphytum* nor *Pilosella* have been investigated for effects on bone metabolism to date.

Gout is mentioned much more frequently in European sources and is usually considered as a rheumatic disease. Plants used for treatment of gout include many medicinal plants from the Asteraceae, which have demonstrable antiinflammatory activity, but have not yet been investigated for effects on xanthine oxidase. Gout was considered to result from an accumulation of 'thick slime' in the body (Adams *et al.*, 2009) and to expel this slime drastic purgatives such as colocynth (*Citrullus colocynthus*) and white bryony (*Bryonia dioica*) were often used, although

**Table 19.1** A selection of medicinal plants traditionally used to treat bone and joint disorders, including gout.

| Species and family | Common name(s) | Tradition/ region/ people | Rationale for use in bone and/or joint health and mechanisms if known | Constituents (relating to bone/joint use if known) |
|---|---|---|---|---|
| *Aegopodium podagraria* L. (Apiaceae) | Goutwort, goutweed, ground elder | Europe | Herb used to treat gout (Williamson, 2003) Anti-inflammatory: falcarindiol is a COX-1 inhibitor | Polyacetylenes, e.g. falcarindiol |
| *Angelica atropurpurea* L. (Apiaceae) | Purple stem angelica | N. Am. Iroquois | Root applied as poultice and taken internally for fracture and rheumatism (Lewis and Elvin-Lewis, 2003). | Not known Most angenlicas contain phthalides and polyphenols |
| *Aralia racemosa* L. (Araliaceae) | American spikenard | N. Am. Chippewa | Root applied as poultice and taken internally for sprains and fractures (Lewis and Elvin-Lewis, 2003) | Not known Most aralias contain triterpene saponins |
| *Angelica sinensis* (Oliv.) Diels (Apiaceae) | Dang gui, Chinese angelica | TCM | Root used to replenish qi Increases proliferation of osteoblasts, promotes angiogenesis by various mechanisms, including oestrogenic (Yang *et al.*, 2014) | Phthalides (i.g. ligustilide); polyphenols (esp. ferulic acid) |
| *Apium graveolens* L. (Apiaceae) | Celery | Europe | Fruits ('seeds') used for gout and other inflammatory conditions (Williamson, 2003; Grieve, 1931) | Essential oil (limonene, selinene); phthalides (ligustilide etc); coumarins |
| *Araiostegia divaricata* var. *formosana* (Hayata) M. Kato (syn: *Davallia formosana* Hayata) (Davalliaceae) | Da ye gu sui bu (= 'mender of bones' from Da ye) | TCM Taiwan | Kidney yang tonic; root used for bone fractures, osteoporosis and gout Xanthine oxidase-inhibiting activity (Chen *et al.*, 2014) | Epicatechin, flavones and other polyphenolics |
| *Astragalus propinquus* Schischkin (syn. A. *membranaceus* (Fisch.) Bunge. (Leguminosae) | Huang qi, membraneous milk vetch | TCM | Tonifies qi Root promotes osteoblast differentiation and reduces bone loss by various mechanisms, including oestrogenic (Yang *et al.*, 2014) | Astragalosides and isoflavones, polysaccharides |
| *Boswellia serrata* Roxb. and other species (Burseraceae) | Salai guggul, sallaki, Indian olibanum/ frankincense | AYV | Resin reduces kapha (water) and vāta (air) doshas Nourishes asthi (bone) and dhātu (tissue) (Williamson, 2003; Pole, 2009) Used for osteoarthritis | Boswellic acids and related pentacyclic triterpenes, essential oil |

*(Continued overleaf)*

**Table 19.1** (Continued)

| Species and family | Common name(s) | Tradition/ region/ people | Rationale for use in bone and/or joint health and mechanisms if known | Constituents (relating to bone/joint use if known) |
|---|---|---|---|---|
| *Cicuta maculata* L. (Apiaceae) | Spotted water hemlock | N. Am. Iroquois | Decoction of plant taken for sprains and broken bones (Lewis and Elvin-Lewis, 2003) Sometimes described as North America's most toxic plant | Not known Contains cicutoxin, a potent neurotoxin that is unstable and *may be* denatured on boiling |
| *Cissus quadrangularis* L. (Vitaceae) | Bone setter Asthisanhari Hadjod | AYV | Stems used to nourish asthi dhātu, pacify vāta and pitta Used internally and as a poultice for fractures Stimulates osteogenesis (Williamson, 2002) | Quadrangularins, resveratrol and other stilbenoids |
| *Colchicum autumnale* L. (Colchicaceae) | Autumn crocus, meadow saffron | Europe, UK | Mitotic poison; also inhibits neutrophil motility, leading to anti-inflammatory effects Corms used to treat acute gout (BHP, 1983; Williamson, 2003) | Alkaloids, mainly colchicine (colchicine still used today) |
| *Commiphora mukul* Hook ex Stocks (Burseraceae) | Guggul Indian bdellidum | AYV | Resin sandhāñya (action) = 'bone mender' Also used for osteoarthritis Inhibits RANKL signalling (Williamson, 2003; Pole, 2009). | Guggulsterones, guggullignans, essential oil |
| *Curcuma longa* L. (syn *C. domestica* Val. (Zingiberaceae) | Haldi, haridara, turmeric | AYV, TCM | Balances all doshas Kidney yang tonic (TCM) and anti-inflammatory Rhizome used for osteoarthritis (Williamson, 2003; Pole, 2009) | Phenylpropanoids known as curcuminoids, glycans, essential oil |
| *Cullen corylifolium* (L.) Medik. (Syn *Psoralea corylifolia* L.) (Leguminosae) | Bhu gu zi, babchi, bakuchi | TCM, AYV, Siddha | Fruits used to tonify kidney yang (TCM; Leung and Siu, 2014) Alleviates kapha (water) and vāta (air) dosha (Pole, 2009) Oestrogenic effects | Coumarins; psoralen, isopsoralen and their glycosides, isoflavonoids |
| *Daucus carota* L. (Apiaceae) | Wild carrot; Queen Anne's lace | Europe | Herb and fruits used for kidney stones and gout (Williamson, 2003) Anti-inflammatory | Essential oil (asarone, carotol), phthalides, coumarins, flavonoids |
| *Dipsacus inermis* Wall. (= *Dipsacus asperoides* C. Y. Cheng et T. M. Ai; *D. asper* Wall) (Dipsacaceae) | Xu duan ('joiner of fractures'), Himalayan teasel | TCM | Root tonifies kidney yang, for strengthening bone and healing bone fractures Induces osteoblast differentiation through bone morphogenetic protein-2/p38 (Niu et al., 2011) | Dipsacus saponins, iridoid glycosides and other polyphenolics |

| Species (Family) | Common name | Tradition/Region | Uses | Active compounds |
|---|---|---|---|---|
| *Drynaria roosii* Nakaike (syn. *D. fortunei* (Kunze ex Mett.) J. Sm (Polypodiaceae) | Gu sui bu (= 'mender of shattered bones'), basket fern | TCM | Kidney yang tonic, rhizome traditionally used for bone fractures and osteoporosis (Putnam *et al.*, 2007) | Flavan-3-ols and propelargonidins |
| *Eleutherococcus senticosus* (Rupr. & Maxim) Maxim (= *Acanthopanax senticosus* (Rupr. & Maxim) Harms. (Araliaceae) | Wu jia pi, Eleuthero, Siberian ginseng | TCM Korea Russia | Root tonifies kidney qi and strengthens kidney yang (for osteoporosis) Mechanisms not yet fully known but may not include oestrogenic effects (Lim *et al.*, 2013) | Saponins, the eleutherosides and polyphenolic compounds |
| *Epimedium breviconu* Maxim. and other spp (Berberidaceae) | Yin yang huo, barrenwort, horny goat weed | TCM | Herb used to tonify yang Strengthens bones via oestrogenic properties (Leung and Siu, 2014) but more widely used for erectile dysfunction | Isoflavones, including icariin |
| *Eucommia ulmoides* Oliv. (Eucommiaceae) | Du zhong | TCM Korea, Malaysia | Bark tonifies kidney qi and strengthens kidney yang Increases osteoblast and inhibits osteoclast activity (Zhang *et al.*, 2014), increases longitudinal bone growth in rat (He *et al.* 2015). Oestrogenic | Lignans, iridoids, flavones, phenylpropanoids, mono- and tri-terpenes |
| *Eupatorium perfoliatum* L. (Asteraceae) | Boneset, feverwort, ague-weed | N. Am. | Herb originally used for 'break-bone' (Dengue) fever, now used for gout and other rheumatic disorders Anti-inflammatory and antiplasmodial (Millspaugh, 1974; Hensel *et al.*, 2011) | Sesquiterpene lactones, including eupafolin; caffeic acid derivatives |
| *Eurycoma longifolia* Jack. (Simaroubaceae) | Tongkat ali, long Jack | SE Asia Malaysia | Root used for bone pain and for androgenic effects (which are responsible for bone enhancing properties) (Shuid *et al.*, 2012) | Quassinoids: eurycomanone and derivatives |
| *Ficus religiosa* L. (Moraceae) | Pippala, pipal, sacred fig, bo-tree | AYV | Pacifies kapha and vata Aerial parts taken internally for bone fractures (Williamson, 2002) | Saponins and phytosterols (e.g. β-sitosterol) |
| *Harpagophytum procumbens* (Burch.) DC. ex Meisn (Pedaliaceae | Devil's claw | Southern and Eastern Africa | Extracts of tubers used for back pain Anti-inflammatory and immune modulatory Some clinical evidence to support use (Williamson, 2003) | Iridoids, e.g. harpagoside and procumbide |

*(Continued overleaf)*

**Table 19.1** (Continued)

| Species and family | Common name(s) | Tradition/region/people | Rationale for use in bone and/or joint health and mechanisms if known | Constituents (relating to bone/joint use if known) |
|---|---|---|---|---|
| Ligustrum lucidum Ait. (Oleaceae) | Nu zen zhi, glossy privet, Chinese wax tree | TCM | Fruits used as a yin tonic for age-related problems; effects on bone both oestrogen-dependent and independent (Putnam et al., 2007) | Phenolics, including nuzhenide, salidroside and tyrosol derivatives |
| Malva neglecta Wallr. (Malvaceae) | Common mallow | N. Am. Iroquois | Decoction of leaves applied as a poultice for broken bones and bruising in babies (Lewis and Elvin-Lewis, 2003) | Not known Many mallows contain sulphated flavonol glycosides |
| Pilosella officinarum Vaill (Hieracium pilosella L.) (Compositae) | Mouse ear; mouse ear hawkweed | Europe N Am. | Herb extracts applied externally as a lotion or compress to bone fractures (BHP, 1983; Stanojević et al., 2009) | Phenolics, e.g. chlorogenic acid, apigenin, umbelliferone |
| Pistacia chinensis subsp. integerrima (Stew. ex Brandis) Rech. f. (=P. integerrima Stew ex. Brandis (Anacardiaceae) | Mastic tree kakra, karkatshringi | AYV | Pacifies kapha and vata doshas, used for gout The whole plant is anti-inflammatory Xanthine oxidase-inhibiting activity shown (Ahmad et al., 2009) | Essential oil (pinenes, phellandrene etc.); triterpenes (e.g. pistagremic acid); flavonoids |
| Quercus bicolor Willd. (Fagaceae) | Swamp white oak | N. Am. Iroquois | Bark decoction taken to treat fracture (Lewis and Elvin-Lewis, 2003) | Not known, but most oaks contain tannins |
| Rhus spp., e.g. R. glabra L., R. aromatica Ait. (Anacardaceae) | Sumac; sumach | N. Am. Iroquois | Bark poultice applied to dislocated shoulders and elbows (Lewis and Elvin-Lewis, 2003) | Not known, but most species contain polyphenols based on gallic acid |
| Salvia miltiorrhiza Bunge (Lamiaceae) | Dan shen, red root sage | TCM | Root used to nourish kidney qi Blocks collagenase, stimulates osteogenesis and inhibits bone resorption (Guo et al., 2014) | Diterpenoids (e.g. tanshinones), phenolics (e.g. salvianolic acids) |
| Salix species (Salicaceae). | Willow species | Europe N. Am. | Bark used for bone and joint pain Anti-inflammatory and analgesic effects via various mechanisms (Williamson, 2003) | Phenolic glycosides, e.g. salicin |

| Plant | Common name | Region/tradition | Uses | Chemistry |
|---|---|---|---|---|
| *Sassafras albidum* (Nutt.) Nees. (Lauraceae) | Sassafras, ague tree | USA Europe | Bark formerly used for gout and other inflammatory conditions (BHP, 1983) No longer used as safrole is carcinogenic | Essential oil (mainly safrole), lignans, e.g. sesamin |
| *Sesamum indicum* L. (Pedaliaceae) | Tila, Zhi ma, sesame | AYV, TCM | Seeds nourish asthi dhātu and pacify vata (Pole, 2009) Kidney yang tonic (TCM) Stimulates osteoblast differentiation (Wanachewin et al., 2012) Oestrogenic, source of calcium | Fixed oil (oleic and linoleic acids); lignans (e.g. sesamol, sesamin) |
| *Senecio aureus* Georgi (Asteraceae/Compositae) | Life root, squaw weed | Europe, N. Am. Iroquois | Herb decoction ingested for bone fracture and menopausal symptoms (Lewis and Elvin-Lewis, 2003; Williamson, 2003) | Eremophilane diterpenes (also toxic pyrollizidine alkaloids) |
| *Silphium perfoliatum* L. (Asteraceae/Compositae) | Cup plant | N. Am. Chippewa Ojibwa | Root decoction ingested for lumbago and other back pain Root smoked by Ponca, Omaha and Winnebago for rheumatism (Lewis and Elvin-Lewis, 2003) | Labdane diterpenes, e.g. silphanepoxol, chlorosilphanol A |
| *Symphytum officinale* L. (Boraginaceae) | Comfrey, knitbone, consolida | Europe | Root and herb used for joint pain and bone fracture Anti-inflammatory activity Not for internal use (Williamson, 2003; Staiger, 2012) | Allantoin, triterpene saponins (and toxic pyrollizidine alkaloids) |
| *Tanacetum vulgare* L. (Asteraceae) | Tansy, buttons | Scotland | Herb used as a specific for gout in Scotland but no record elsewhere (Grieve, 1931) | Essential oil (mainly thujone and sesquiterpenes) |
| *Uvularia perfoliata* L. (= *Erythronium carolinianum* J.F. Gmel.) (Colchicaceae) | Perforate bellwort | N. Am. Iroquois | Herb seed internally and externally for bone fracture (Lewis and Elvin-Lewis, 2003) | Not known |

AYV, Ayurveda; TCM, traditional Chinese medicine; N. Am., North America, with nation if known.

This is a selection of some important herbal medicines used for bone and joint disorders from the best documented sources, mainly the Asian scientific literature, and classical North American and European herbals references. The references generally apply to the ethnomedical use but further chemical and pharmacological information may have been added from accepted standard sources (mainly general references, which are included in the reference list).

The list does not include purely anti-inflammatory medicinal plants unless bone and/or gout and/or swollen joints are mentioned specifically. These are dealt with elsewhere in this book.

Plant names have been checked with the most recent lists from Kew. Only common synonyms are given, for reasons of space and to avoid perpetuating obsolete or confusing names.

there is no scientific rationale for this practice. Most inflammatory diseases were thought to result from a build-up of 'toxins' and some form of cleansing was often recommended as part of the treatment. Some anthraquinone glycosides are also powerful laxatives and plants containing them were used traditionally to treat gout, for example rhubarb, *Rheum palmatum* (Adams *et al.*, 2009). In fact, anthraquinones often possess anti-inflammatory and immunological effects, which may have been helpful in treating inflammatory pain, despite the unpleasant purging the patient had to undergo.

## 19.3.2   North America

Medicinal plants from North and South America were brought back to Europe by colonialists and some plants used by North American and Canadian native peoples are now widely used in European herbal medicine. In North America, medicinal plants for treating fracture are commonplace and often used in the form of a poultice. Out of all the traditions covered in this chapter, the North American medicinal plants are the least well investigated both chemically and pharmacologically, as can be seen in Table 19.1, but an excellent account of how plants are used there for musculo-skeletal ailments is given by Lewis and Elvin-Lewis (2003), with further details of the plants themselves in Millspaugh (1974). An interesting note of caution is raised by the common names of the North American plants known as 'boneset', *Eupatorium perfoliatum* (boneset, ague weed, feverwort) and *E. purpureum* (purple boneset, gravel weed, Joe-pye weed): the name 'boneset' derives from their use in treating Dengue fever, which was common in the southern States and was also known as 'break-bone fever', rather than being an indication of usefulness in healing fractures. However, these plants are now used to treat gout and other rheumatic disorders (Millspaugh, 1974).

## 19.3.3   Traditional Chinese medicine

TCM principles are aimed at maintaining physiological harmony and specific changes in bone pathology were of course unknown in ancient times. Osteoporosis was not described as such in TCM, although Chinese medicinal plants are widely used in orthopaedics, but was considered to be closely related to kidney function. In western terms, this is not contradictory, since people suffering from kidney failure have lower bone density than healthy people of the same age. Osteoporosis in TCM is described as 'bone atrophy' or 'bone rheumatism', caused by weakness in the kidney, spleen and liver (Leung and Siu, 2014). This results in 'blood stasis' and can be thought of as a weakness in vascularization, which also explains the link between angiogenesis and osteogenesis in TCM theory. 'Kidney deficiency' (shēn xū) is considered to be the root of all bone and joint pathologies, including arthritis and osteoporosis, so medicinal plants which strengthen the kidney by tonifying kidney qi (vital energy) and increasing kidney yang (yang is the 'active' force of the universe) are the basis for treating bone and joint diseases. Examples of medicinal plants described as 'kidney tonifying' are *Ligustrum lucidum*, *Eucommia ulmoides*, *Dipsacus inermis*, *Cullen corylifolium* (syn *Psoralea corylifolia*) and *Drynaria roosii* (see Table 19.1). Medicinal plants described in these terms may provide useful leads for modern bone therapies, but it is of course crucial that the mechanism of action is known, since some also have phytoestrogenic effects and may be contraindicated in certain disorders. In TCM, medicinal plants are rarely used singly but as part of a formula that is intended to approach treatment from various aspects aimed at restoring balance to the system, in accordance with the principles of yin and yang (the opposing forces of the universe which must be in harmony for good health) and other TCM concepts. It may be challenging to identify a specifically 'bone active' herb from such a formula, and it may not be productive either since the components are expected to act together rather than individually. Chinese prescriptions are often named according to their intended organ targets and/or main herbal constituents, for example the formula Bu Pi Yen Shèn Xuè, meaning nourishing (bu) spleen (pi), kidney (shèn) and blood (xuè) circulation, and like many such formulae, contains Dan Shen (*Salvia miltiorrhiza*) to correct blood stasis. This formula has been clinically tested and found to be effective in relieving bone pain in osteoporosis patients. Other formulae containing Dan Shen, such as Jian Gu San and Kang Gu Song ('gu' is Chinese for bone) have also been demonstrated to be effective in clinical studies (Guo *et al.*, in press). Although identifying a specific herb or natural product as a therapy for bone disorders may not be possible from a formula, it may be possible to use the principles of TCM as a multi-factorial approach to treatment by nourishing related organs of the body, rather than simply viewing TCM as a source of lead molecules for drug development.

Gout in TCM is considered to be an obstructive disorder characterized by stagnation of qi and blood stasis, and therefore has elements in common with osteoporosis. In western terms, both are inflammatory disorders, so this link is not surprising. Some of the same medicinal plants used in TCM for osteoporosis are also used for gout, for example the rhizome of the fern *Davillia formosana* (now called *Araiostegia divaricata* var. *formosana*) is used particularly in Taiwan for both diseases. *In vivo* experiments in mice have confirmed both xanthine oxidase inhibitory activity and anti-osteoporotic activity for the extract (Chen *et al.*, 2014).

## 19.3.4 Ayurveda

In Ayurveda, bone (asthi) is one of the seven tissues (dhatus) and osteoporosis is known as asthi-sushirta (bone porousness). It is said to be due to two main causes, the first is poor metabolism or mand-asthiagni (agni = digestive fire) and the other is the result of an excess of the vata 'dosha'. The three doshas (tridosha), vata, pitta and kapha, are 'humours', subtle energies or functional principles used to describe the characteristics of all living things and the environment, including people, diseases, medicines and food. The doshas govern the function of the body on both the physical and emotional level. Bone is a container of vata dosha and Ayurvedically, osteoporosis is a vata disorder, caused by a disturbance of that dosha. A person described as a 'vata' type person would be more prone to disorders caused by disturbances of vata, including osteoporosis, by impairing the flow and assimilation of nutrients to the bones. The other doshas are involved in other ways, for example a pitta imbalance would result in poor digestion and metabolism, preventing the bones from receiving the nutrients, and a disruption of kapha could prevent bone growth even when the nutrients are available. For more detail on this complex subject, see Pole (2009). As with other holistic systems of medicine, in Ayurveda bone tissue is considered to be dynamic and linked to other bodily tissues, for example fat (medas dhātu), and bone marrow and nerve tissue (majja dhātu), via channels known as 'srotas'. In western medicine it is known that obesity is linked to osteoporosis, and that the bone marrow produces connective tissue cell types including osteoblasts, osteoclasts and chondrocytes, as well as endothelial cells required for vascularization, confirming once again the usefulness of the holistic approach of traditional medicine. The most important Ayurvedic medicinal plants for treating bone disorders are probably *Boswellia serrata*, *Cissus quadrangularis*, *Commiphora mukul*, *Sesamum indicum* and *Ficus religiosa* (see Table 19.1) and all are described in terms of their effect on vata dosha (mainly) and asthi dhātu (Williamson, 2003; Pole, 2006). Since Ayurveda is so complicated, an expert would be needed to interpret the descriptions, but in ethnopharmacological terms medicinal plants described as 'pacifying vata' or 'nourishing asthi dhātu' may have an application in the treatment of osteoporosis.

Gout in Ayurveda, as in TCM, is described in similar terms to osteoporosis in that is it caused by an imbalance, in this case a disturbance in vata dosha, and the herb *Pistacia integerrima* is used to treat both disorders. It has been shown to possess both anti-osteoporotic and xanthine oxidase inhibiting activity (Ahmad *et al.*, 2008).

## 19.4    Conclusions

Osteoporosis and other bone diseases are multifactorial in origin and their causes and treatments are only recently starting to be understood. To use the ethnopharmacological literature to identify useful agents for bone and joint disorders, it is necessary to understand how they are viewed in the context of traditional medicine. Clues to identifying bone active properties may be found by looking at medicinal plants described in the TCM literature as 'nourishing kidney' and in the Ayurvedic literature as 'pacifying the vata dosha'. At present, Asian systems of herbal medicine are more likely to document medicinal plants with anti-osteoporotic effects, but the western herbal literature contains many phytoestrogenic plants, used to treat menopausal symptoms, which may yield SERMs suitable for therapeutic use. Medicinal plants used to treat gout and related inflammatory conditions are much more commonly cited. It is notable that medicinal plants from all traditions used for the same indications contain similar or related components, which adds weight to the ethnobotanical evidence that they may be effective, and suggests that more specific tests could be employed to confirm the activity and elucidate the mechanism(s) of action.

## References

Adams, M., Berset, C., Kessler, M. and Hamburger, M. (2009) Medicinal herbs for the treatment of rheumatic disorders – a survey of European herbals from the 6th and 17th century. *Journal of Ethnopharmacology*, **121**, 343–359.

Ahmad, N.S., Farman, M., Najmi, M.H., *et al.* (2008) Pharmacological basis for use of *Pistacia integerrima* leaves in hyperuricemia and gout. *Journal of Ethnopharmacology*, **117**, 478–482.

BHP (1983) *The British Herbal Pharmacopoeia*, British Herbal Medicine Association, Keighley. W. Yorks, UK.

Cauley, J.A. (2011) Defining ethnic and racial differences in osteoporosis and fragility fractures. *Clinical Orthopedics and Related Research*, **469**,1891–1899.

Chen, C.Y., Huang, C.C., Tsai, K.C., *et al.* (2014) Evaluation of the antihyperuricemic activity of phytochemicals from *Davallia formosana* by enzyme assay and hyperuricemic mice model. *Evidence Based Complementary and Alternative Medicine*. doi: 10.1155/ 2014/ 873607.

Dada, A.A., Yinusa, W. and Giwa, S.O. (2011) Review of the practice of traditional bone setting in Nigeria. *African Health Sciences*, **11**, 262–265.

Grieve, M. (1931) *A Modern Herbal*, available at http://botanical.com/.

Guo, Y., Li, Y., Xue, L., *et al.* (in press) DanShen: an ancient Chinese herbal medicine and a new source of innovative anti-osteoporotic drugs. *Journal of Ethnopharmacology*,**155**,1401–1416.

Hensel, A., Maas, M., Sendker, J., *et al.* (2011) *Eupatorium perfoliatum* L.: phytochemistry, traditional use and current applications. *Journal of Ethnopharmacology*, **138**, 641–651.

Kim, J.Y., Lee, J.L., Song, J., *et al* (2015) Effects of *Eucommia ulmoides* extract on longitudinal bone growth rate in adolescent female rats. *Phytotherapy Research* **29**, 148–153

Leung, P.C. and Siu, W.S. (2014) Herbal treatment for osteoporosis: a current review. *Journal of Traditional and Complementary Medicine*, **3**, 82–87.

Lewis, W.H. and Elvin-Lewis, M.P.F. (2003) Musculo-skeletal system, in *Medical Botany. Plants Affecting Human Health*, 2nd edn, Wiley, New York.

Lim, D.W., Kim, J.G., Lee, Y., *et al.* (2013) Preventive effects of *Eleutherococcus senticosus* bark extract in OVX-induced osteoporosis in rats. *Molecules*, **18**, 7998–8008.

Millspaugh, C.F. (1974) *American Medicinal Plants*, Dover, New York. A republication of *Medicinal plants*, from 1892.

Niu, Y., Li, Y., Huang, H., *et al.* (2011) Asperosaponin VI, a saponin component from *Dipsacus asper* Wall, induces osteoblast differentiation through bone morphogenetic protein-2/p38 and extracellular signal-regulated kinase 1/2 pathway. *Phytotherapy Research*, **25** (11), 1700–1706.

Patlak, M. (2001) Bone builders: the discoveries behind preventing and treating osteoporosis. *FASEB Journal*, **15** (10), 1677E-E

Pole, S. (2006) *Ayurvedic Medicine. The Principles of Traditional Practice*, Churchill-Livingstone, London, UK.

Putnam, S.E., Scutt, A.M., Bicknell, K., *et al.* (2007) Natural products as alternative treatments for metabolic bone disorders and maintenance of bone health. *Phytotherapy Research*, **21**, 99–112.

Shuid, A.N., El-arabi, E., Effendy, N.M., *et al.* (2012) *Eurycoma longifolia* upregulates osteoprotegerin gene expression in androgen-deficient osteoporosis rat model. *BMC Complementary and Alternative Medicine*. doi: 10.1186/1472-6882-12-152.

Singh, J.A. (2013) Racial and gender disparities among patients with gout. *Current Rheumatology Reports*, **15** (2), 307. doi: 10.1007/s11926-012-0307-x.

Staiger, C. (2012) Comfrey: a clinical overview. *Phytotherapy Research*, **26**,1441–1448.

Stanojević, L., Stanković, M., Nikolić, V., *et al.* (2009) Antioxidant activity and total phenolic and flavonoid contents of *Hieracium pilosella* L. extracts. *Sensors*, **9**, 5702–5714.

Wanachewin, O., Boonmaleerat, K., Pothacharoen, P., *et al.* (2012) Sesamin stimulates osteoblast differentiation through p38 and ERK1/2 MAPK signaling pathways. *BMC Complementary and Alternative Medicine*. doi: 10.1186/1472-6882-12-71.

Williamson, E.M. (ed.) (2002) *Major Herbs of Ayurveda*, Churchill-Livingstone, London, UK.

Williamson, E.M. (2003) *Potter's Herbal Cyclopedia*, CW Daniels, Saffron Walden.

Yang, Y., Chin, A., Zhang, L., *et al.* (2014) The role of traditional Chinese medicine in osteogenesis and angiogenesis. *Phytotherapy Research*, **28**, 1–8.

Zhang, R., Pan, Y.L., Hu, S.J., *et al.* (2014) Effects of total lignans from *Eucommia ulmoides* bark prevent bone loss *in vivo* and *in vitro*. *Journal of Ethnopharmacology*, **141**, 78–92.

# 20
# Diabetes and Metabolic Disorders: An Ethnopharmacological Perspective

Adolfo Andrade Cetto

*Department of Cell Biology, School of Sciences, National Autonomous University of Mexico, Mexico*

## 20.1   Introduction

Metabolism is the process by which organisms acquire and distribute energy from food, which is composed of proteins, carbohydrates and fats. Chemicals in the digestive system break these components down into sugars and acids, the body's fuel. The body can use this fuel immediately or it can store the energy in body tissues, including the liver, muscles and body fat. A metabolic disorder occurs when abnormal chemical reactions in the body disrupt this process (National Library of Medicine, 2014).

Most metabolic diseases are rare (e.g. Gaucher's disease or hereditary hemochromatosis), but type-2 diabetes (T2D) and metabolic syndrome (MS) incidence is growing rapidly worldwide. All metabolic diseases are linked to genetic factors, but T2D and MS are also correlated with lifestyle, obesity and a lack of physical activity. The International Diabetes Federation (IDF) estimates that as of 2013, worldwide more than 382 million people have diabetes and that this number will increase to 592 million by 2035 (International Diabetes Federation, 2014). WHO estimates that 347 million people currently have diabetes and that by 2030 it will be the seventh leading cause of death (World Health Organization, 2014). The IDF also estimates that approximately one quarter of the world's adults have MS. The clustering of cardiovascular disease (CVD) risk factors that typify metabolic syndrome is now considered a driving force for a new CVD epidemic (International Diabetes Federation, 2014).

*Ethnopharmacology*, First Edition. Edited by Michael Heinrich and Anna K. Jäger.
© 2015 John Wiley & Sons, Ltd. Published 2015 by John Wiley & Sons, Ltd.

The use of medicinal plants to treat various diseases is common practice worldwide. In countries such as India, China and Mexico, traditional medicine plays an important role in official or unofficial healthcare systems. Such medicinal plants are used primarily in unprocessed forms. In developed countries such as Germany, the UK and France, traditional medicine now plays an important role as part of the official health system, primarily in the form of phytomedicines.

Ethnopharmacological research, in countries where traditional medicine plays an important role in the health system, can provide us with new compounds or new phytomedicines for the management of metabolic disorders.

In this chapter we present an ethnopharmacological perspective on the main metabolic disorders: T2D and MS.

## 20.2    Type-2 diabetes

Diabetes mellitus is defined as an elevated blood glucose level associated with absent or inadequate pancreatic insulin secretion, which may occur with or without the impairment of insulin signalling. T2D is characterized by tissue resistance to insulin combined with a relative deficiency in insulin secretion. A given individual may exhibit either increased insulin resistance or increased β-cell deficiency, and these abnormalities may be mild or severe. Although in these patients insulin is produced by β cells, their production is inadequate to overcome insulin resistance, and blood glucose therefore increases. Impaired insulin signalling also affects fat metabolism, resulting in increased free fatty acid flux, elevated triglyceride levels and reciprocally low levels of high-density lipoprotein (HDL) (Expert Committee, 2003).

T2D is a polygenic disorder; the additive effects of an as-yet unknown number of genetic polymorphisms (risk factors) are required for its development, and they may not be sufficient in the absence of environmental (acquired) risk factors. The most important risk factors are those that influence insulin sensitivity: obesity (visceral obesity), physical inactivity, high-fat/low-fibre diets, smoking, and low birth weight (Alsahli and Gerich, 2012).

The onset of T2D, then, depends on two types of factors: (i) genetic factors that affect obesity, β-cell potential or insulin resistance, and (ii) environmental factors such as inactivity and excess in food intake or in inadequate food. These two causes lead to insulin resistance, which is initially compensated by β cells. The β cells will then work too hard, which reduces their mass and creates glucose intolerance and glucotoxic effects on the cells. Further decreases in their mass create more severe glucotoxicity and decomposition with severe hyperglycemia.

The long-term complications of diabetes include retinopathy with a potential loss of vision, nephropathy leading to renal failure, peripheral neuropathy with risk of foot ulcers, amputations, and Charcot joints, autonomic neuropathy causing gastrointestinal, genitourinary, and cardiovascular symptoms, and sexual dysfunction (Expert Committee, 2003).

The pathophysiology of these diseases is complicated; many metabolic pathways and cell types are involved. Herein, we provide a short description of the main metabolic aspects.

### 20.2.1    Insulin

Insulin-like signalling integrates the storage and release of nutrients with somatic growth during development and in adulthood. It is a feature of all metazoans, revealing a common mechanism used by animals to integrate metabolism and growth with environmental signals (White, 2012).

Insulin exerts critical control over carbohydrate, fat and protein metabolism; β cells in the islets of Langerhans are the only cells in the body that produce a meaningful quantity of insulin to maintain glucose levels within a range from 70 to 150 mg/dl in normal individuals. The β cells release insulin in two phases. The first phase release is rapidly triggered in response to increased blood glucose levels, and the second phase is a sustained, slow release of newly formed vesicles triggered independently of sugar. Other substances known to stimulate insulin release include the amino acids arginine and leucine, the parasympathetic release of acetylcholine (via phospholipase C), sulfonylurea, cholecystokinin (CCK, via phospholipase C) and the gastrointestinally derived incretins glucagon-like peptide-1 (GLP-1) and glucose-dependent insulinotropic peptide.

## 20.2.2   Insulin effects in peripheral tissues

Insulin activity in the peripheral tissues is mediated via the insulin receptor, which on hormone binding initiates a cascade of intracellular protein phosphorylation. The intracellular subunit of the receptor is a tyrosine-specific kinase that auto-phosphorylates and catalyses the phosphorylation of several proteins that in turn promotes the multifaceted effects of the hormone. Different tissues are known to respond distinctly to insulin; tissue sensitivity correlates with the levels of insulin receptors expressed on the plasma membrane. Insulin stimulates glucose turnover, favouring its influx into cells, followed by oxidative metabolism to release energy, produce lipids or store glucose as glycogen via non-oxidative metabolism. Insulin-stimulated glucose transport is observed only in skeletal muscle, adipose cells and the heart because these tissues express the insulin-dependent glucose transporter, GLUT4. In the liver and kidney, insulin inhibits gluconeogenesis because of the tissue-specific expression of hormone-sensitive metabolic enzymes involved in this process. Insulin simultaneously stimulates lipid synthesis while preventing lipolysis in adipose cells, skeletal muscle and liver. Insulin promotes protein synthesis in almost all tissues. Insulin acts as a mitogen via increased DNA synthesis and the prevention of programmed cell death, or apoptosis. In addition, insulin stimulates ion transport across the plasma membrane of multiple tissues. There is increasing evidence for a direct role of insulin, acting through the insulin or insulin growth factor (IGF) receptors, in the regulation of pancreatic β-cell growth, survival and insulin release (White, 2012).

The most prominent abnormality in T2D is an impairment of glucose-induced insulin secretion, which is more severe in the first phase than in the longer second phase of secretion. In contrast, β-cell responses to non-glucose secretagogues, such as GLP-1 or sulfonylureas, remain intact; β cells exposed to abnormally high glucose concentrations lose the differentiation that normally equips them with the unique metabolic machinery needed for glucose-induced insulin secretion (Gordon *et al.*, 2012).

## 20.2.3   Insulin resistance (skeletal muscle and adipose tissue)

Insulin resistance occurs when cells in the body (liver, skeletal muscle and adipose tissue) become less sensitive and eventually resistant to insulin, and occurs when normal hormone concentrations produce a substandard biological response. T2D mellitus is characterized in almost all cases by insulin resistance. This has been clearly demonstrated by the glucose clamp technique, in which glucose clamps were performed in normal subjects, subjects with impaired glucose tolerance (IGT) and subjects with T2D. Despite similar steady-state insulin levels, the glucose disposal rate was decreased by 24% in the subjects with IGT and by 58% in those with T2D compared with normal controls. In the basal state, 30% of glucose uptake is insulin mediated, whereas in the post-prandial state insulin-mediated glucose disposal increases by 85%. Studies have shown that 80–90% of this increased insulin-mediated glucose disposal is into skeletal muscle. Consequently, in insulin-resistant states an inability to respond to insulin stimulation with an adequate increase in glucose disposal largely contributes to post-prandial hyperglycemia (Courtney and Olefsky, 2003).

### 20.2.4   Liver

Glucose metabolism in the liver is controlled by the pancreatic hormones insulin and glucagon. A high insulin:glucagon ratio in the post-prandial state favours glucose storage and disposal, glycogen synthesis and glycolysis, whereas a low ratio in the fasted state favours glucose production, glycogenolysis and gluconeogenesis. This tightly regulated control of hepatic glucose metabolism is disrupted in diabetes, leading to inappropriate increases in glucose production by the liver (Clark and Newgard, 2003).

The liver contributes to glucose homoeostasis through the rapid postprandial clearance of glucose from the portal vein in the absorptive state after a meal; when blood glucose falls below normal concentrations, glycogen is mobilized and glucose is produced via gluconeogenesis. When the blood glucose concentration increases, hepatic glucose uptake increases proportionally, stimulating glucokinase and glycogen synthesis. Elevated blood glucose concentrations normally increase insulin release and reduce glucagon release, thus increasing the insulin to glucagon ratio, which in turn inactivates glycogen phosphorylase (inhibiting glycogenolysis), activates glycogen synthase (stimulating glycogen synthesis) and increases the concentration of fructose-1,6-bisphosphate. These events reduce the hepatic production of glucose and increase the hepatic storage of glucose as glycogen. The main enzymatic targets for controlling the elevation of blood sugar levels are the inhibition of glucose-6-phosphatase, the inhibition of fructose-1, 6-bisphosphatase and the inhibition of glycogen phosphorylase (Andrade-Cetto, 2012).

### 20.2.5   Gut

Incretins are hormones released by the gut in response to food ingestion that augment insulin release by what is known as the incretin effect. Two primary incretins are GLP-1 and glucose-dependent insulinotropic polypeptide (GIP). Other gut hormones that influence glucose homeostasis include ghrelin and peptide YY. Ghrelin acts on the hypothalamus to stimulate appetite and also inhibits insulin secretion. The incretin effect can be measured because there is a greater insulin response after oral than intravenous glucose delivery despite comparable glycemia (Alsahli and Gerich, 2012).

The α-glucosidase enzyme is located in the brush border of the small intestine and is required for the breakdown of carbohydrates to absorbable monosaccharides. The α-glucosidase inhibitors (AGIs) delay but do not prevent the absorption of ingested carbohydrates, reducing the postprandial glucose and insulin peaks (Andrade-Cetto *et al.*, 2008).

## 20.3   Metabolic syndrome

MS is a cluster of conditions with the most dangerous effect being an increased risk of heart attack; the main risk factors are elevated fasting plasma glucose (>110 mg/dl but <126 mg/dl) and abdominal (or central) obesity, which is defined by having a waist circumference of at least 102 cm for men and 89 cm for women, although these values can vary by ethnicity.

The underlying cause of MS continues to challenge experts, but both insulin resistance and central obesity are considered significant factors. Genetics, physical inactivity, ageing, a pro-inflammatory state and hormonal changes may also be causative, but the role of these factors can vary depending on the ethnic group. Central obesity is associated with insulin resistance and MS; it contributes to hypertension, high serum cholesterol, low HDL-c and hyperglycemia, and it is independently associated with higher CVD risk.

According to the IDF, for a person to be defined as having MS, they must have central obesity (defined by waist circumference, with ethnicity-specific values) along with any two of the following four predispositions: elevated triglycerides (≥150 mg/dl), reduced HDL cholesterol (<40 mg/dl in males, <50 mg/dl in females), elevated systolic blood pressure (BP) (≥130) or diastolic BP (≥85 mm Hg) and elevated fasting plasma glucose (≥100 g/dl) (http://www.idf.org).

People with metabolic syndrome are at increased risk of

- atherosclerosis, peripheral vascular disease and other diseases related to fatty build-ups in artery walls (these blockages narrow the arteries and restrict blood circulation throughout the body but are especially dangerous when they affect the arteries leading to the brain, heart, kidneys and legs)
- coronary heart disease and heart attack
- stroke, which occurs when the blood supply to a part of the brain is interrupted by a blocked or burst blood vessel, depriving the brain of oxygen and nutrients
- T2D (American Heart Association, 2014).

In obesity, plasma free fatty acids (FFAs) are elevated, causing insulin resistance in muscle, liver and endothelial cells, and this contributes to the development of T2D, hypertension, dyslipidemia and non-alcoholic fatty liver disease. Elevated FFA levels cause insulin resistance in skeletal muscle and liver, which contributes to the development of T2D and MS (Boden, 2006).

## 20.4  Case studies

It is important to embed such an ethnopharmacological perspective in a discussion on the use of plants in traditional medicine to treat these diseases. As we can deduce from the background information presented here, the diagnosis of T2D and MS is quite difficult in a traditional medicine-based framework. For T2D, the blood glucose level is necessary to establish a diagnosis, and MS is not even considered among many of the traditional medicines worldwide. Central obesity can be easily observed, but insulin resistance, HDL-c and triglyceride levels are difficult to detect without laboratory testing. The plants that are primarily used to treat T2D are selected by diabetic patients once they have a diagnostic examination performed by a physician. For MS, the patients look for plants used to treat obesity, T2D or hypertension, and thus fewer plants with centuries of use and evaluation exist to treat these increasingly modern-day problems. In many parts of the world, diabetic patients or people with obesity are trying new plants at their own risk.

### 20.4.1  Liver targeting

In South and Central Mexico as well as Guatemala traditionally the dry leaves (15 g) of *Cecropia obtusifolia* Bertol. (Cecropiaceae) are boiled in water (c. 500 ml) and the resulting infusion is cooled and filtrated, with the cold infusion being consumed over the day or when people are thirsty (Andrade-Cetto and Heinrich, 2005). Studies have assessed its hypoglycemic effects in animal models and T2D patients.

An open, controlled clinical trial was conducted with 12 recently diagnosed ($2 \pm 0.8$ years) T2D patients, eight women and four men with an average age of $48 \pm 4$ years, who controlled their diabetes with diet and exercise. None of the patients had ever taken any hypoglycemic drug. Over a 34-week period the patients received daily an aqueous leaf extract. Glucose, cholesterol, triglycerides and insulin levels were determined every 15 days, and HbA1c was measured monthly. A significant reduction in the glucose levels was detected after 4 weeks of administration, and HbA1c was significantly reduced after 3 months of treatment. No significant effect on cholesterol, triglycerides or insulin could be observed (Revilla-Monsalve *et al.*, 2007).

*C. obtusifolia* contains chlorogenic acid (CA) and isoorientin. CA is an inhibitor of glucose-6-phosphate translocase (Figure 20.1) and thus the authors proposed that the hypoglycemic effects of the plant were due at least in part to this inhibition. They proposed that glucose-6-phosphate translocase inhibition would inhibit gluconeogenesis and reduce hepatic glucose production. To test this hypothesis, they measured the effects of plant extracts on gluconeogenesis (*in vivo*) and glucose-6-phosphate translocase enzyme activity (*in vitro*). A pyruvate tolerance test (2 g/kg) was performed in 18-h fasted n5-STZ rats to determine whether inhibition of gluconeogenesis occurred *in vivo*. The effect of the extracts on glucose-6-phosphatase translocase activity was assayed *in vitro* in intact rat liver microsomes. The diabetic rats treated with plant extracts had a lower glucose curve; the extracts reduced the elevation in glucose blood levels and inhibited glucose-6-phosphatase translocase activity with $IC_{50}$ values of 224 g/ml for *Cecropia obtusifolia* aqueous extract, 160 g/ml for *C.obtusifolia* butanolic extract and 254 g/ml for chlorogenic acid. The authors concluded that the administration of the plant could improve glycemic control by blocking hepatic glucose output, especially in the fasting state (Andrade-Cetto, 2012).

## 20.4.2   Gut targeting

An aqueous extract from the aerial parts of *Brickellia cavanillesii* (Cass.) A. Gray (Asteraceae), orally administered to normal and diabetic mice, showed significant hypoglycemic effects.

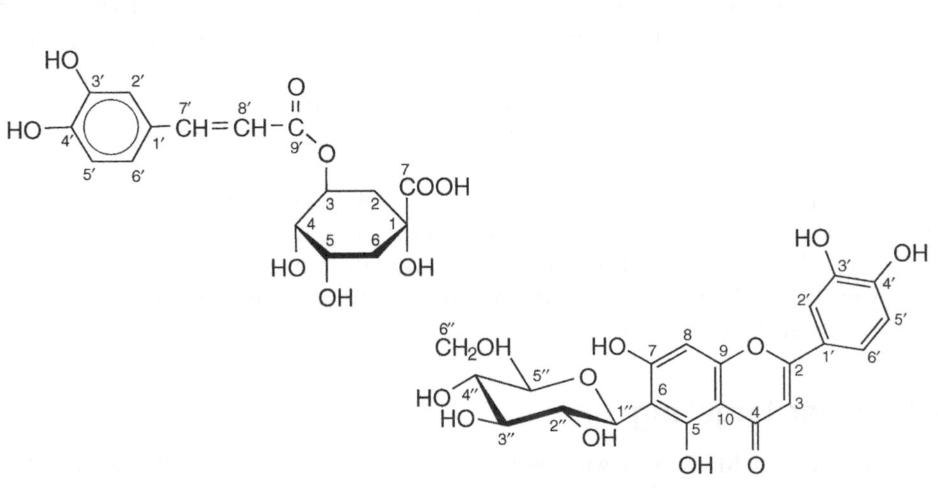

**Figure 20.1**   Chlorogenic acid (left) and isoorientin (right) isolated from *Cecropia Obtusifolia*.

The extract attenuated postprandial hyperglycemia in diabetic mice during oral glucose and sucrose tolerance tests. The extract also showed potent inhibitory activity ($IC_{50} = 0.169$ mg/ml vs 1.12 mg/ml for acarbose) towards yeast $\alpha$-glucosidase. The bioassay-guided fractionation of the active extract using the $\alpha$-glucosidase inhibition assay led to the isolation of several compounds, including three chromenes, three sesquiterpene lactones, several flavonoids and a coumarin. One of these chromenes is a new chemical entity and was identified by spectroscopic techniques. Moreover, all the compounds were tested *in vitro* against $\alpha$-glucosidase activity; the active products were a flavonoid (isorhamnetin), a sesquiterpene lactone (calein C) and the new chromene (Figure 20.2) ($IC_{50}$ = 0.16, 0.28 and 0.42 mM, respectively, vs 1.7 mM for acarbose). Enzyme kinetic analysis of these compounds revealed that calein C ($Ki$ 1.91 mM) and isorhamnetin ($Ki$ 0.41 mM) behaved as mixed inhibitors, whereas the new chromene (Ki 0.13) was a non-competitive inhibitor. Docking analysis predicted that the flavonoids and sesquiterpene lactones but not the chromene bind to the enzyme at the catalytic site (Mata *et al.*, 2013).

## 20.4.3 Insulin targeting

The fruit of *Momordica charantia* L. (bitter gourd, Cucurbitaceae) is used in the Ayurveda for treating diabetes. Unripe fruits, seeds and aerial parts of the plant have a widespread use as a phytomedicine in various parts of the world to treat diabetes. Several clinical studies have been performed with the plant since the 1970s. Rahman *et al.*, 2009 compared the effects of the plant juice (55 ml/day for 5 months) and rosiglitazone, in 25 patients. The results showed that the plant was more effective in the management of fasting blood glucose and total cholesterol, and in some diabetes-related complications (retinopathy and myocardial infarction) than rosiglitazone.

The plant's effects on glucose uptake were assessed in adipose tissue, a key link between obesity (as observed in MS) and diabetes. Additionally, uptake was assessed in the classic insulin target tissues – hepatocytes, adipose tissue and skeletal muscle – as these tissues play important roles in glucose homeostasis after glucose uptake. A protein extract of the fruit at 5 and 10 µg/ml was tested in perfused islet cells, incubated C2C12 myocytes and 3T3-L1

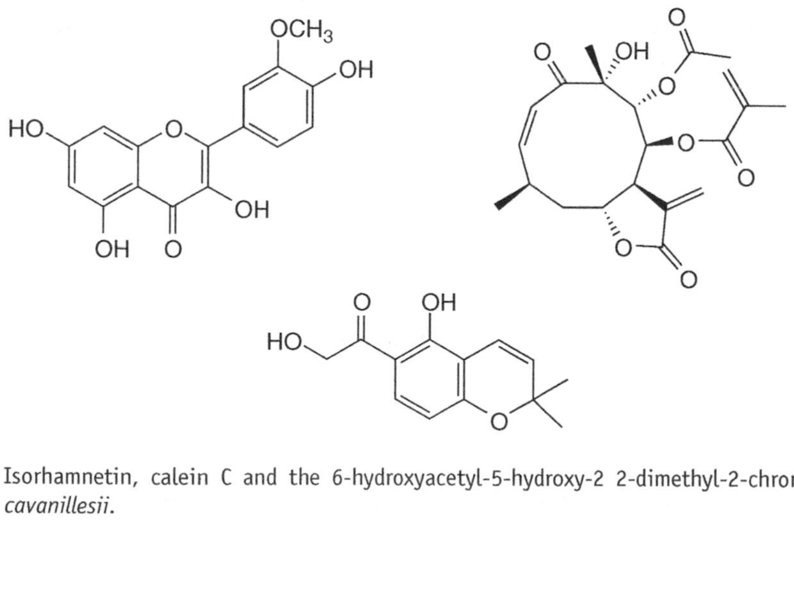

**Figure 20.2**  Isorhamnetin, calein C and the 6-hydroxyacetyl-5-hydroxy-2 2-dimethyl-2-chromene isolated from *Brickellia cavanillesii*.

adipocytes, and the authors reported an increase in insulin secretion and an increase in glucose uptake in myocytes and adipocytes (Yibchok-anun *et al.*, 2006).

The saponin-rich fraction (125 µg/ml) of the total ethanolic extract from *M. charantia* stimulated insulin secretion in MIN6 pancreatic β-cells and monodesmoside, and a bidesmoside (Figure 20.3) and cucurbitanes (0.05 and 0.010 mg/ml) were identified as active substances. The plant lowers blood glucose by promoting insulin secretion and this mechanism may contribute substantially to the plant's overall hypoglycemic effect (Keller *et al.*, 2011).

*Cinnamomun cassia* J. Presl. (Lauraceae) also targets insulin, possibly linked to enhanced insulin action, increased phosphorylation of the insulin receptor and overall facilitation of the insulin signalling system, inhibition of α-glucosidase activity and a possible activation of peroxisome proliferator activated receptors. The main active ingredients are procyanidin type-A polymers. A meta-analysis of clinical trials involving 282 people indicated that doses of 1–6 g/day of *C. cassia* resulted in decreased fasting glucose and lipid levels. Furthermore, a 3-month study in 102 people with T2D found a significant decrease in Hb1Ac of 0.83% using 1 g/day. A meta-analysis of six clinical trials involving 435 patients found that the plant improved fasting glucose by 15 mg/dl and only slightly decreased Hb1Ac in short-term studies. It remains controversial whether the whole powdered spice has an effect because a possibly combination of different types of cinnamon or an aqueous extract will be used (Shane-McWhorter, 2013).

## 20.4.4   Obesity and insulin resistance

*Cordyceps* species (Hypocreaceae) (a genus of endoparasitic ascomycete fungi, mainly on insects and other arthropods) have a long history of use in traditional medicine. One of the earliest clear records is a 15th-century Tibetan medical text, and there are claims of thousands of years of use in TCM (Winkler, 2008). *Cordyceps* has been used in tonics and stimulants to enhance energy, thus revealing potential effects on energy metabolism. Clinical trials have suggested beneficial effects on lipid metabolic disorders such as hyperlipidemia. The effect of *Cordyceps militaris* on metabolic parameters using obese C58BL/6J mice induced by a high-fat diet were studied, including body and organ weight measurements, stained sections of epididymal adipose tissue, fat accumulation in frozen liver sections and the plasma biochemical parameters (Kim *et al.*, 2014). Two active new compounds, cordyrroles A and B (Figure 20.4), together with 12 known compounds, including pyrrole alkaloids and nucleotide derivatives, were identified. The administration of the extract (100 mg/kg and 300 mg/kg) the body weight gain and food efficiency ratio induced by the diet. The amount of epididymal fat and the size of adipocytes were also decreased. Liver weight and fat deposition in the liver

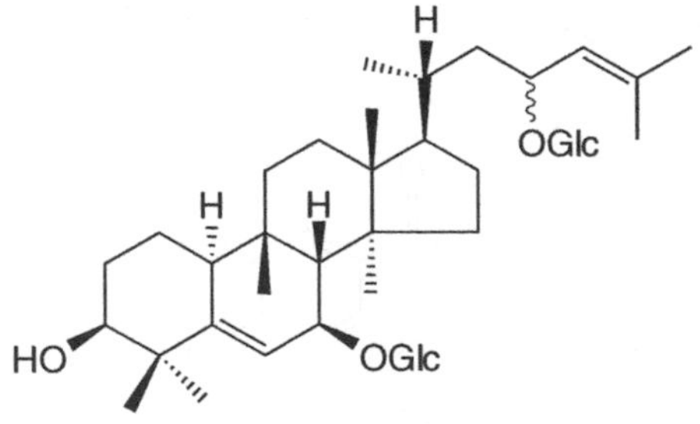

**Figure 20.3**  Kuguaglycoside isolated from *Momordica charantia*.

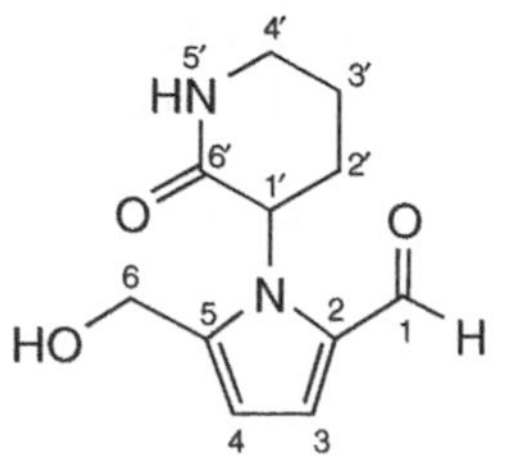

**Figure 20.4** Cordyrrole A isolated from *Cordyceps militaris*.

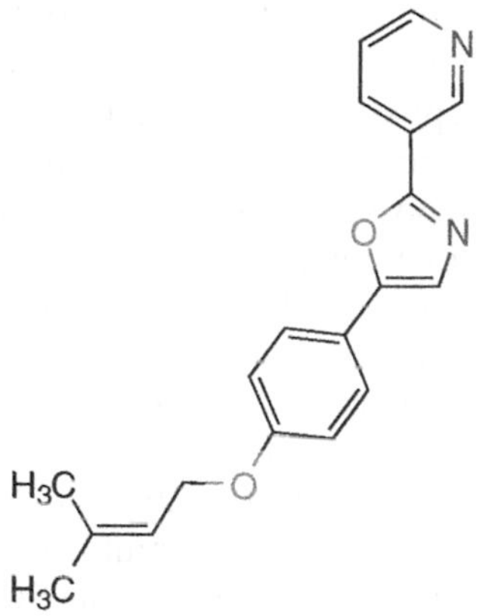

**Figure 20.5** (3,3-dimethylallyl) halfordinol isolated from *Aegle marmelos*.

were dramatically reduced, and the lipid profiles were also reduced. Among the isolated compounds, cordyrrole A significantly inhibited adipocyte differentiation in 3T3-L1 preadipocytes and pancreatic lipase activity, whereas cordyrrole B was more effective at inhibiting pancreatic lipase. Cordycepin, a characteristic compound of *Cordyceps militaris*, decreased the rate of adipocyte differentiation.

A plant widely used in South-East Asia for the treatment of T2D and obesity is *Aegle marmelos* Correa. (Rutaceae). Lipolytic and antiadipogenic effects of (3,3-dimethylallyl) halfordinol (Hfn) (Figure 20.5) isolated from the leaves have only been shown recently (Saravanan *et al.*, 2014). The authors measured the intracellular lipid accumulation by Oil Red O staining and glycerol secretion. They analysed the expression of genes related to adipocyte differentiation by reverse transcriptase-polymerase chain reaction (PCR). The isolated compound dose-dependently (5–20 µg/ml) decreased intracellular triglyceride accumulation and increased glycerol release in differentiated 3T3-L1 adipocytes. Furthermore, they tested Hfn in high-fat diet-fed C57/BL 6J mice; treatment with 50 mg/kg for 4 weeks reduced plasma glucose, insulin and triglyceride levels, and significantly reduced total adipose tissue mass by 37.85% and visceral adipose tissue mass by 62.99%.

The PCR analyses indicated that Hfn decreased the expression of peroxisome proliferator-activated receptor γ (PPARγ) and CCAAT enhancer binding protein α (CEBPα) and increased the expression of sterol regulatory enzyme binding protein (SREBP-1c), peroxisome proliferator-activated receptor α (PPARα), adiponectin and glucose transporter protein 4 (GLUT4) compared to the high-fat diet group. These results suggested that Hfn decreased adipocyte differentiation and stimulated the lipolysis of adipocytes. The main conclusion of this study was that Hfn showed lipolytic and antiadipogenic effects in *in vitro* and *in vivo* models. The reduced adipocyte size and decreased circulating triglyceride levels showed decreased insulin resistance in the treated animals.

## 20.5    Conclusions

T2D and MS are rapidly growing worldwide health problems. Although the aid of a physician and laboratory testing are required for diagnosis, patients seek alternative treatments, including traditional medicines. Why? Because when people realize that they will need extended treatment for these perpetual conditions, they look for treatments they believe will be less harmful. It is beyond the scope of this chapter to discuss the side effects of medicinal plants, but certainly if a plant has a pharmacological effect, it will also have side effects.

As we saw in the examples, flavonoids, coumarins, alkaloids, terpenes and nearly all types of structures have been reported to possess hypoglycemic effects.

The good news is that at least one compound, n,n-dimethylguanidine, isolated from the European lilac *Galega officinalis* L., was used to produce metformin, a modern first-line treatment of choice for T2D, especially in overweight and obese individuals (MS). This provides hope for the discovery of new natural compounds or chemically well-characterized extracts with a therapeutic profile similar to metformin.

There are many options for the treatment of T2D and MS, and several possible targets. We can increase the incretin levels in the gut or inhibit the enzymes that destroy them to increase insulin levels. We can instead delay the ingestion of carbohydrates by inhibiting alpha glucosidases; these only represent a broad approach to gut targeting. We can target the liver via several enzymatic and genetic targets to limit excessive glucose production due to the lack of insulin activity, or we can improve the insulin resistance in the liver.

There is a close relationship between obesity and T2D, and insulin resistance bridges them. It is important to note that not all patients with insulin resistance and obesity become diabetic; these conditions can be lifelong and accompanied by blood sugar levels in normal ranges. However, this relationship provides us with the tools for the study of new compounds in nature. Even if traditional medicine does not recognize MS, we can look for plants traditionally used to reduce glucose levels (hypoglycemic) and/or plants used to control weight (obesity), and there certainly are examples from traditional medicines for such uses.

Until now, there has been no phytomedicine available to treat MS or T2D, so ethnopharmacological field studies in places where medicinal plants are still at the top range of use can provide us with opportunities for discovering unknown hypoglycemic agents. More and better clinical studies are needed on the hypoglycemic plants discussed here.

As a final reflection, why must we search for treatments for people with T2D and MS? We know that the origin of these problems is in many cases obesity produced by poor nutrition. Why do we not learn to eat correctly instead? Perhaps, in time, we can stop this growing epidemic in a better and more far-reaching way.

## Acknowledgments

Thanks to Dr Prof. Michael Heinrich for his help editing the manuscript. This work was partially supported by grants from DGAPA, PAPIIT (project IN214413) and CONACyT CB-0151264.

# References

Alsahli, M. and Gerich, J.E. (2012) Pathogenesis of type 2 diabetes, in *Atlas of Diabetes* (ed. J.S. Skyler), Diabetes Research Institute University of Miami Miller School of Medicine Miami, FL, pp. 149–166.

American Heart Association (2014) *Metabolic Syndrome*, http://www.heart.org/.

Andrade-Cetto, A. (2012) Effects of medicinal plant extracts on gluconeogenesis. *Botanics, Targets and Therapy*, **2**, 1–6.

Andrade-Cetto, A. and Heinrich, M. (2005) Mexican plants with hypoglycaemic effect used in the treatment of diabetes. *Journal of Ethnopharmacology*, **99**, 325–348.

Boden, G. (2006) Fatty acid-induced inflammation and insulin resistance in skeletal muscle and liver. *Current Diabetes Reports*, **6**, 177–181.

Clark, C. and Newgard, C.B. (2003) Hepatic regulation of fuel metabolism, in *Mechanisms of Insulin Action* (eds A.R. Saltiel and J.E. Pessin), Springer Science + Business Media, New York, pp. 90–109.

Courtney, C.H. and Olefsky, J.M. (2003) Insulin resistance, in *Mechanisms of Insulin Action* (eds A.R. Saltiel and J.E. Pessin), Springer Science + Business Media, New York, pp. 185–209.

Expert Committee (2003) Report of the Expert Committee on the Diagnosis and Classification of Diabetes Mellitus. *Diabetes Care* **26**, S5.

Gordon, C., Weier, C.G., Bonner-Weier, S. and Sharma, A. (2012) Regulation of insulin secretion and islet cell function, in *Atlas of Diabetes* (ed. J.S. Skyler), Diabetes Research Institute, University of Miami, Miller School of Medicine, Miami, FL, pp. 1–17.

International Diabetes Federation (2014) *Diabetes*, http://www.idf.org.

Keller, A.C., Mab, J., Kavalier, A., *et al.* (2011) Saponins from the traditional medicinal plant *Momordica charantia* stimulate insulin secretion in vitro. *Phytomedicine*, **19**, 32–37.

Kim, S.B., Ahn, B., Kim, M., *et al.* (2014) Effect of *Cordyceps militaris* extract and active constituents on metabolic parameters of obesity induced by high-fat diet in C58BL/6J mice. *Journal of Ethnopharmacology*, **151**, 478–484.

National Library of Medicine (2014) *Metabolic Disorders*, http://www.nlm.nih.gov/medlineplus/.

Rahman, I., Malik, S.A., Bashir, M., *et al.* (2009) Serum sialic acid changes in non-insulin-dependant diabetes mellitus (NIDDM) patients following bitter melon (*Momordica charantia*) and rosiglitazone (Avandia) treatment. *Phytomedicine*, **16**, 401–405.

Revilla-Monsalve, M.C., Andrade-Cetto, A., Palomino, M., *et al.* (2007) Hypoglycemic effect of *Cecropia obtusifolia* Bertol aqueous extracts on type 2 diabetic patients. *Journal of Ethnopharmacology*, **111**, 636–640.

Saravanan, M., Pandikumar, P., Saravanan, S., *et al.* (2014) Lipolytic and antiadipogenic effects of (3,3-dimethylallyl) halfordinol on 3T3-L1 adipocytes and high fat and fructose diet induced obese C57/BL6J mice. *European Journal of Pharmacology*, **740**, 714–721.

Shane-McWhorter, L. (2013) Dietary supplements for diabetes are decidedly popular: help your patients decide. *Diabetes Spectrum*, **26**, 259–266.White, M. (2012) Mechanisms of insulin action, in *Atlas of Diabetes* (ed. J.S. Skyler), Diabetes Research Institute, University of Miami, Miller School of Medicine, Miami, FL, pp. 1–17.

Winkler, D. (2008) Yartsa Gunbu (*Cordyceps sinensis*) and the fungal commodification of the rural economy in Tibet AR. *Economic Botany*, **63**, 291–306.

World Health Organization (2014) *Diabetes*, http://www.who.org.

Yibchok-anun, S., Adisakwattana, S., Yao, C.Y., *et al.* (2006) Slow acting protein extract from fruit pulp of *Momordica charantia* with insulin secretagogue and insulinomimetic activities. *Biological and Pharmaceutical Bulletin*, **29**, 1126–1131.

# 21

# The Ethnopharmacology of the Food–Medicine Interface: The Example of Marketing Traditional Products in Europe

Gunter P. Eckert

*Goethe-University, Campus Riedberg, Department of Pharmacology, Frankfurt, Germany*

## 21.1   Introduction

In the past ethnopharmacology identified numerous plant species and botanical products that are consumed by certain population groups because of their health benefits. These findings could be of utmost interest also for other populations and the translation into new products seems to be a meaningful transfer of results into practice, for instance population ageing is a growing socioeconomic burden, not only in western societies, that goes along with a dramatic increase in age-related brain disorders (Qiu *et al.*, 2009). Using the example of Alzheimer's disease (AD) the development of botanical preparations traditionally used in aged-related brain disorders (Adams *et al.*, 2007; Stafford *et al.*, 2008; Eckert, 2010) into medicinal products may lead to new therapeutic options for a disease that currently has no cure. Although the exact underlying cause initiating the onset of AD is still unclear, an imbalance in oxidative and nitrosative stress, intimately linked to mitochondrial dysfunction, characterizes early stages of AD pathology (Friedland-Leuner *et al.*, 2014).

A variety of AD-related medicine originates from traditionally used botanical preparations, of which *Ginkgo biloba* L. (Ginkgoaceae) (Kumar, 2006) and galantamine, an alkaloid known form several members of *Amaryllidaceae* (Heinrich, 2010), are the best known. A special extract (EGb761) from *Ginkgo biloba* L. leaves (Lautenschlager *et al.*, 2012) and galantamine were successfully introduced as medicines into the therapy of AD. Because of the major hurdle of extensive clinical approval, traditionally used plants are marketed as food, which seems to be a less regulated alternative, therefore products of *Ginkgo biloba* L. can be found in food markets while galantamine was exclusively developed as drug. Another example is Holy Basil, *Ocimum tenuiflorum* L. (also known as *Ocimum sanctum* L., Tulsi), which has been used for thousands of years in Ayurveda for its diverse healing properties (Pattanayak *et al.*, 2010). It has been reported that traditionally used plant-derived products and their extracts exert activities on AD-related drug targets, including AChE activity, antioxidant activity, modulation of Aβ-producing secretase activities, Aβ-degradation, heavy metal chelating, induction of neurotrophic factors and cell death mechanisms (Eckert, 2010).

This article introduces the legislative regulations for the marketing of traditionally used products in Europe. Other countries such as the USA have similar regulations that differ in details and are not discussed here.

A large number of botanical materials (e.g. whole, fragmented or cut botanical preparations, algae, fungi, lichens) and botanical preparations obtained from these materials by various processes (e.g. extraction, distillation, purification, concentration and fermentation) readily find their way onto the food supplement market. These materials are also often labelled as natural foods, largely organic, and foods specifically intended to support sport activities. Personal care products and the so-called 'traditional herbal medicinal products' represent additional sources of exposure of consumers to botanical products. New products are also emerging consisting of substances that commonly occur at low levels in botanical components of the diet, which are then extracted and re-introduced at much higher levels in specific products (EFSA Scientific Committee, 2009).

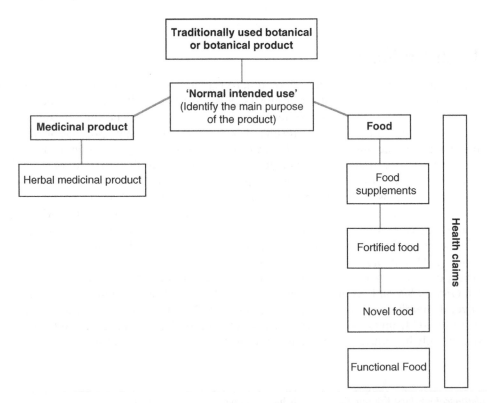

**Figure 21.1**   Decision tree for the medicine–nutrition interface. Please refer to text for more details.

Botanical preparations are widely available to consumers through several distribution channels in the EU and elsewhere. In particular, they are sold over the counter in pharmacies, health food shops, supermarkets, herbalist's shops or via the internet. They are currently available and used in such a way that they are almost becoming part of the common diet, thus from a public health point of view have significant human exposure (EFSA Scientific Committee, 2009).

Because botanical preparations can have many uses it may not always be clear whether the product containing them will fall within the definition of a medicinal product or a food. Thus it is important to determine first which legal framework – medical or food law – would be applicable to an individual product (Coppens *et al.*, 2006).

Depending on their use botanical preparations are classified in the legal categories shown in Figure 21.1. The category a product is classified as is determined primarily by its intended normal use, which will be discussed later in the chapter.

## 21.2  Medicinal products for human use

To guarantee the highest possible level of public health and to secure the availability of medicinal products to citizens across the EU, all medicinal products for human use have to be authorised either at the Member State or the Community level before they can be placed on the EU market. Special rules exist for the authorization of medicinal products for paediatric use, orphan medicines, traditional herbal medicines, vaccines and clinical trials. Furthermore, to ensure that medicinal products are consistently produced and controlled against the quality standards appropriate to their intended use, the EU has set quality standards. In addition, once a medicinal product has been approved in the European Community and placed on the market, its safety is monitored throughout its entire lifespan to ensure that in case of adverse reactions that present an unacceptable level of risk under normal conditions of use, it is rapidly withdrawn from the market. This is done through the EU system of pharmacovigilance. In order to help the EU ensure the highest possible level of public health protection, the European Medicines Agency (EMA) was established in 1994, with the main task of coordinating the scientific evaluation of the quality, safety and efficacy of medicinal products which undergo an authorization procedure, and providing scientific advice of the highest possible quality (European Commission, 2014a).

### 21.2.1  Legal framework

The requirements and procedures for the marketing authorization for medicinal products for human use, as well as the rules for the constant supervision of products after they have been authorized, are primarily laid down in Directive 2001/83/EC and in Regulation (EC) No 726/2004. These texts additionally lay down harmonized provisions in related areas such as the manufacturing, wholesaling or advertising of medicinal products for human use.

### 21.2.2  Definition of medicinal products

Directive 2001/82/EC defines a medicinal product as any substance or combination of substances presented as having properties for treating or preventing disease in human beings or which may be used in or administered to human beings either with a view to restoring, correcting or modifying physiological functions by exerting a pharmacological, immunological or metabolic action, or to making a medical diagnosis (European Commission, 2001). Thus, medicinal products are intended to be taken with the aim to bring back into 'the normal average limits' any physiological process that is out of normality and hence considered as pathological. Products which block or alter normal physiological processes in unphysiological ways are also medicines. In this respect all these products have a 'therapeutic activity' (Coppens *et al.*, 2006).

## 21.2.3  Herbal medicinal products

In general EU legislation on pharmaceutical products for human use also applies to traditional herbal medicines. However, in order to overcome difficulties encountered by Member States in applying pharmaceutical legislation to traditional herbal medicinal products in a uniform manner, in 2004 a simplified registration procedure for such medicines was introduced (European Commission, 2014b).

The simplified procedure was introduced by Directive 2004/24/EC of the European Parliament and of the Council of 31 March 2004 amending, as regards traditional herbal medicinal products, Directive 2001/83/EC on the Community code relating to medicinal products for human use (European Commission, 2014b).

The simplified registration procedure aims to safeguard public health, remove the differences and uncertainties about the status of traditional herbal medicinal products that existed in the past in the Member States and facilitate the free movement of such products by introducing harmonized rules in this area. Herbal medicinal products are defined as any medicinal product exclusively containing as active ingredients one or more herbal substances or one or more herbal preparations, or one or more such herbal substances in combination with one or more such herbal preparations.

The simplified registration procedure is intended for herbal medicinal products with a long tradition, which do not fulfil the requirements for a marketing authorization, in particular those requirements whereby an applicant can demonstrate by detailed references to published scientific literature that the constituent or the constituents of the medicinal products has or have a well-established medicinal use with recognized efficacy and level of safety (European Commission, 2014b).

The simplified procedure allows the registration of herbal medicinal products without requiring particulars and documents on tests and trials on safety and efficacy, provided that there is sufficient evidence of the medicinal use of the product throughout a period of at least 30 years, including at least 15 years in the Community (European Commission, 2014b).

With regard to the manufacturing of these products and their quality, applications for registration of traditional herbal medicinal products have to fulfil the same requirements as applications for a marketing authorization (European Commission, 2014b).

In view of the peculiarities of herbal medicinal products, a Committee for Herbal Medicinal Products (HMPC) has been established at the European Medicines Agency (EMA). A major task for the HMPC is to establish Community monographs for traditional herbal medicinal products and, with the objective of further facilitating registration and harmonization in the field of traditional herbal medicinal products, prepare a draft list of herbal substances that have been in medicinal use for a sufficiently long time, and hence are considered not to be harmful under normal conditions of use (European Commission, 2014b).

With a view to further facilitating the registration of certain traditional herbal medicinal products in the EU, a list of herbal substances, preparations and combinations thereof for use in traditional herbal medicinal products has been established on the basis of the scientific opinion of the HMPC. As regards the safety and efficacy of a traditional herbal medicinal product, applicants can refer to the list. However, they would still need to demonstrate the quality of the medicinal products they seek to register. The list was established by Commission Decision 2008/911/EC of 21 November 2008 on the basis of Commission Decision 2004/24/EC. The decision has been amended to include *Calendula officinalis* L. and *Pimpinella anisum* L., *Eleutherococcus senticosus* (Rupr. et Maxim.) Maxim and *Echinacea purpurea* (L.) Moench, *Mentha × piperita* L., *Hamamelis virginiana* L., *Thymus vulgaris* L. and *Thymus zygis* Loefl. ex L., and *Vitis vinifera* L. It is suspected that Commission Decision 2004/24/EC, which was enforced in order to offer an option for traditional medicinal products to stay on the market, bears the risk that a locked-up-system is created by this Directive. In this environment any incentives for innovations are minimized, but specific traditions like Ayurveda or TCM may be excluded (Wiesner *et al.*, 2014). Only a limited number of herbal medicinal products from non-European traditions commonly used in Europe have been registered (Qu *et al.*, 2014), for instance of the 109 adopted Community herbal monographs, only 10 are herbal substances used in TCM. The main reasons have been identified as due to unfulfilled requirements of Directive 2004/24/EC. The most common reasons that botanical preparations from non-European traditions were not accepted for inclusion in the Community herbal monographs were the lack of evidence to demonstrate a 15-year minimum medicinal use period in the EU and evidence of absence of health risk (Qu *et al.*, 2014). As a consequence many products might be forced into the food supplement environment where they are less controlled, which is regarded as a risk for the patient/consumer (Wiesner *et al.*, 2014).

## 21.3  Food

### 21.3.1  Definition of food

Food law in the EU includes for the most part general specifications but also very specific rules for individual food groups. The definition of requirements for certain foods is to define an instrument to relevant markets. The main regulation in EU food law is Regulation 178/2002/EC (European Commission, 2002a). In this regulation food is defined as 'any substances that is intended to be ingested and that does not belong to an exclusion list'. Thus, everything is regarded as food unless it is not included in the exclusion list. This way, new products can enter the market much more easily, which follows the aim of the EU to reduce trade barriers. The exclusion list includes feed, live animals unless they are prepared for placing on the market for human consumption, botanical preparations prior to harvesting, medicinal products, cosmetics, tobacco, narcotic or psychotropic substances, and residues and contaminants (European Commission, 2002a). According to this definition food supplements, fortified food and novel food also belong to the food group, but these items are specifically regulated.

### 21.3.2  Food supplements

According to Directive 2002/46/EC food supplements are concentrated sources of nutrients or other substances with a nutritional or physiological effect whose purpose is to supplement the normal diet (European Commission, 2002b). Food supplements are intended to be taken with the 'aim to improve, support or optimize the normal physiological processes within the boundaries of homeostasis without modifying, altering or blocking any physiological process outside these boundaries' (Coppens *et al.*, 2006). This could be referred to as 'physiological activity' (Coppens *et al.*, 2006).

Food supplements are marketed in dose form, i.e. as pills, tablets, capsules or liquids in measured doses. So far nutrients have been defined as vitamins and minerals. Other substances have to be legally defined in future based on adequate and appropriate scientific data. As a consequence, no community-specific roles have been adapted in the past. Permitted vitamin or mineral preparations that may be added for specific nutritional purposes in food supplements are listed in the annexes to the Directive (European Commission, 2002b). Although the Directive does not address all aspects of food supplements, it does set general legal requirements for all food supplements in Articles 6 to 9. These general requirements focus on the labelling and presentation of food supplements, and apply to all food supplements, i.e. they apply also to those supplements for which no specific rules have yet been established (Schwitters *et al.*, 2007).

## 21.3.3  Fortified food

In the past there has been no specific harmonized way for the European Community to control the use of ingredients that represent a potential risk to health (Department of Health, 2011). Regulation 1925/2006/EC (Food Fortification Regulation) sets a requirement for the addition of vitamins, minerals and other substances to food (European Commission, 2006a). The Regulation puts in place a mechanism to allow such ingredients to be assessed, including a safety assessment by the European Food Safety Authority (EFSA), and where necessary prohibited or restricted. Detailed rules on how this will be implemented are yet to be adopted (Department of Health, 2011). The Regulation will only control other substances that present a potential risk to consumers' health. The Regulation defines 'other substances' as a substance other than a vitamin or mineral that has a nutritional or physiological effect. The substance must also have been added to a food or used as an ingredient in a food, which results in more of that substance being ingested than under normal conditions or via a balanced diet (Department of Health, 2011). If there is concern that a substance may represent a potential risk to consumers the EFSA will carry out an assessment of available information. Based on this assessment the European Commission will take a decision on its use in foods, which will be summarized in Annex III to Regulation 1925/2006/EC. Substances will be listed that are deemed to be allowed under specified conditions. Substances that could have a harmful effect on health, but where there is some uncertainty, will also be listed in this annex. Substances and ingredients deemed safe can continue to be used in food without control (Department of Health, 2011).

## 21.3.4  Novel food

The Commission considers foods and food ingredients that have not been used for human consumption to a significant degree in the EU before 15 May 1997 novel foods and novel food ingredients. Novel foods can be classified in one of the following categories:

- foods and food ingredients with a new or intentionally modified primary molecular structure (e.g. fat substitutes)
- foods and food ingredients consisting of or isolated from micro-organisms, fungi or algae (e.g. oil made from microalgae)

- foods and food ingredients consisting of or isolated from plants (e.g. phytosterols) and food ingredients isolated from animals.

Food and food ingredients obtained by traditional propagating or breeding practices with a history of safe food use do not come under the scope of the Regulation. Furthermore, additives, flavourings and extraction solutions are not covered by the scope of the Regulation either. Other legal provisions of the EU apply to them to the extent that they have to comply with the safety level stipulated in the Novel Foods Regulation. To market a novel food or ingredient, companies must apply to an EU country authority for authorization, presenting the scientific information and safety assessment report. A novel food or ingredient may be marketed through a simplified procedure called 'notification'. The company notifies the Commission about their marketing a novel food or ingredient based on the opinion of a food assessment body that has established 'substantial equivalence'.

The Commission sends decisions on a novel food or ingredient likely to affect public health to the Scientific Committee for Food. The authorization procedure laid down in Articles 4 and 6 of the Novel Foods Regulation must always be applied if the novel food or feed is not essentially similar to conventional products. The procedure is compulsory in the case of foods and ingredients whose molecular structure has been modified and for products where a novel process was used in their production if this leads to a major modification of their composition or structure. Although following one common scheme, authorization procedures differ between countries (Federal Institute for Risk Assessment, 2014a), for example the authorization procedure for Germany can be found on the website of the Federal Institute for Risk-Assessment (Federal Institute for Risk Assessment, 2014a).

## 21.3.5 Functional food

The term 'functional food' is increasingly being used for foods which in addition to their nutritional function seek to influence the major health-related, physiological parameters in consumers in a long-term and targeted manner. Functional foods are not nutrient concentrates like food additives but reach the market in typical food forms. Terms like 'designer foods' or 'nutraceuticals' are sometimes used as synonyms for functional foods (Federal Institute for Risk Assessment, 2014b). There is not, as such, a regulatory framework for functional foods or nutraceuticals in EU food law. The rules to be applied are numerous and depend on the nature of the foodstuff. The rules of the General Food Law Regulation, including responsibility for food safety, traceability, recall and notification, definitely are applicable to all foods. The regulatory frameworks, i.e. of dietetic foods, food supplements or fortified food, may be applicable to some functional foods. The Novel Food Regulation will be applicable to 'new' functional foods depending on if they have been used to a significant degree in the EU before 15 May 1997 (see above) (Coppens *et al.*, 2006). The regulations on health claims are also important factors for the marketing of functional foods in Europe.

## 21.4 Consumer protection - security and protection against fraud

Regulation (EC) No 178/2002 ensures the quality of foodstuffs intended for human consumption. In addition, the European Union's food legislation protects consumers against fraudulent or deceptive commercial practices (European Commission, 2014c).

## 21.4.1    Food safety

The objective of the EU's food safety policy is to protect consumer health and interests while guaranteeing the smooth operation of the single market. In order to achieve this objective, the EU ensures that control standards are established and adhered to as regards food and food product hygiene, animal health and welfare, plant health and preventing the risk of contamination from external substances. It also lays down rules on appropriate labelling for these foodstuffs and food products. This policy underwent reform in the early 2000s, in line with the 'from farm to fork' approach, thereby guaranteeing a high level of safety for foodstuffs and food products marketed within the EU at all stages of the production and distribution chains. This approach involves both food products produced within the EU and those imported from other countries (European Commission, 2014d).

Food safety is to be warranted in all steps of production and processing along the food value chain from farm to fork. In 2002, the EFSA was founded as an independent scientific centre for expertise on risk assessment (Federal Institute for Risk Assessment, 2014c). It provides independent scientific advice, and scientific and technical support in all areas impacting on food safety. It also ensures that the general public is kept informed. The EFSA is responsible for coordinating risk assessments and identifying emerging risks, providing scientific and technical advice to the Commission, including in connection with crisis management, collecting and publishing scientific and technical data in areas relating to food safety, and establishing European networks of organizations operating in the field of food safety (European Commission, 2014c).

A compendium of botanical preparations reported to contain toxic, addictive, psychotropic or other substances of concern was made available to assist risk assessors responsible for the evaluation of specific ingredients in food supplements in more easily identifying the compound(s) of concern on which to focus the assessment. Meanwhile, a second version of that compendium has been published, considering botanical preparations that appear on a negative list or subject to restricted use (e.g. maximum level or certain parts allowed only) in at least one European Member State. Two annexes have been added: the first one lists botanical preparations for which insufficient information on possible substances of concern is available, or for which the information present could not be verified, and the second one lists botanical preparations for which, although some data were available, the Scientific Committee could not identify substances of concern, or other reasons for the inclusion in the compendium (Authority, 2012).

Contrary to the approach for conventional foods, individuals consciously and voluntarily choose to purchase and consume food supplements and/or fortified foods. Consumers expose themselves to the ingredients contained in those products, therefore consumers expect those products to be safe. Food supplements and fortified food that come to the market must be safe not only in terms of safety of the ingredients used and the ways in which they are embodied in the relevant products, but also in terms of carrying clear, simple and product-specific indications for normal use, such as recommended daily intake (Schwitters *et al.*, 2007).

## 21.4.2    Health claims

On 1 July 2007, the EU Regulation 1924/2006 on nutrition and health claims made on foods came into force (European Commission, 2006b). Thus, the legal regulations concerning the use of such statements changed. Food manufacturers may make statements on nutrition under Article 4 of this Regulation and use health claims on foods only if they are listed on a positive

EU list, and if the food corresponds to a given nutritional profile. Anything (in terms of uses) not permitted is prohibited ('prohibition principle'). The Regulation aims to protect consumers from being misled and is intended to give consumers ownership and responsibility for choosing a healthy and balanced diet.

Two types of health claims are distinguished. Statements about the role of a nutrient (or another substance) for growth, development and body functions or their physiological function, such as 'calcium is important for healthy bones', are regulated in Article 13 of the regulation (Federal Institute for Risk Assessment, 2014d). Article 14 regulates statements indicating a reduction of disease risk (e.g. 'an adequate calcium intake can help reduce the risk of osteoporosis') or related to the development and health of children. Statements suggesting a therapeutic effect or curing of a disease are prohibited ('vitamin C – for relief of colds').

The European Commission is responsible for the approval of health claims. According to the EU Health Claims Regulation claims may be used only if they are based on generally accepted scientific evidence and well understood by the average consumer (Federal Institute for Risk Assessment, 2014d).

For health claims pursuant to Article 13 a positive list of health claims is created that can be used in the future. To this end, Member States were invited to submit proposals for this list at the EU Commission. The proposed statements were reviewed by the EFSA to assess whether they are supported by scientific evidence and then published (Federal Institute for Risk Assessment, 2014d).

Manufacturers claiming a reduction of disease risk and targeting child health need to submit scientific data validating these claims (Article 14). The EFSA verifies that the statements are scientifically correct and proposes acceptance or rejection of the claims to the European Commission. The approval is again the responsibility of the European Commission. (Federal Institute for Risk Assessment, 2014d) (for the positive lists according to Articles 13 and 14 see http://ec.europa.eu/nuhclaims/).

## 21.5 Intended normal use: the distinction between medicinal products and foods

The use of functional plant products in foodstuffs is well established and includes the use of vegetables and fruits, herbs and spices such as garlic or rosemary, herbal teas, and herbs added to foods and beverages for taste or functional purpose such as guarana or gentian. Moreover, botanical food supplements with functional ingredients are used for health-promoting properties such as carotenoids, flavonoids or phytosterols (Coppens et al., 2006). Supplements containing botanical preparations or botanical preparations can be defined as food supplements. Such products may at first glance look very similar to medicinal products, but the intended use is quite different. While medicinal products are intended to *prevent or treat* a disease or modify the way in which the body functions, food supplements are intended to *complement* the diet, with substances possessing health-maintenance or promoting properties. The most practical element to distinguish between these classes of products to determine what legal framework is applicable is therefore their intended use. Internationally it is regulatory and legal practice to define products for their intended normal use. This is especially relevant for those botanical preparations that are used in both food supplement and medicinal products, such as garlic, artichoke and ginkgo (Coppens et al., 2006). Intended normal use is a remarkably simple concept that serves to regulate products and to organize and harmonize relevant markets (Schwitters et al., 2007). In formulating a product's intended normal use, scientific evidence and the safety that has been established as a result of long-term widespread use are different yet complementary and need to be internalized and/or explained by the producer through experimental scientific research, literature studies or both (Schwitters *et al.*, 2007).

## 21.6   Conclusion

It is clear that the translation of scientific evidence from ethnopharmacological research into products cannot simply follow Hippocrates's advice 'let your food be your medicine and medicine your food'. Finding the correct dividing line between foods and medicines is a challenge for all market participants, a challenge which predates the Europe-wide regulations of food supplements and fortified foods. Although the question What is a food and what is a medicine?' is not easy to answer, for the benefit of consumers the right decision has to be made.

## References

Adams, M., Gmunder, F. and Hamburger, M. (2007) Plants traditionally used in age related brain disorders – a survey of ethnobotanical literature. *Journal of Ethnopharmacology*, **113**, 363–381.

Authority, E.F.S. (2012) Compendium of botanicals reported to contain naturally occurring substances of possible concern for human health when used in food and food supplements. *EFSA Journal*, **10**, 2663.

Coppens, P. and Fernandes da Silva, M.S.P. (2006) European regulations on nutraceuticals, dietary supplements and functional foods: A framework based on safety. *Toxicology*, **221**, 59–74.

Department of Health (2011) Fortified Foods – Guidance to compliance with European Regulation (EC) No. 1925/2006 on the addition of vitamins and minerals and certain other substances to food, http://www.dh.gov.uk/publications, accessed 2 September 2014.

Eckert, G.P. (2010) Traditionally used plants against cognitive decline and Alzheimer's disease. *Frontiers in Pharmacology*, **1**, 138.

EFSA Scientific Committee (2009) Guidance on safety assessment of botanicals and botanical preparations intended for use as ingredients in food supplements. *EFSA Journal* **7**, 1249.

European Commission (2001) Directive 2001/83/EC of the European Parliament and of the Council of 6 November 2001 on the Community code relating to medicinal products for human use. *Official Journal of the European Communities*, **54**, 67–128.

European Commission (2002a) Regulation (EC) No 178/2002 of the European Parliament and of the Council of 28 January 2002 laying down the general principles and requirements of food law, establishing the European Food Safety Authority and laying down procedures in matters of food safety. *Official Journal of the European Communities*, **45**, 1–24.

European Commission (2002b) Directive 2002/46/EC of the European Parliament and of the Council of 10 June 2002 on the approximation of the laws of the Member States relating to food supplements. *Official Journal of the European Communities*, **45**, 51–57.

European Commission (2006a) Regulation (EC) No 1925/2006 of the European Parliament and of the Council of 20 December 2006 on the addition of vitamins and minerals and of certain other substances to foods. *Official Journal of the European Communities*, **49**, 26–38.

European Commission (2006b) Regulation (EC) No 1924/2006 of the European Parliament and of the Council of 20 December 2006 on nutrition and health claims made on foods. *Official Journal of the European Communities*, **49**, 9–25.

European Commission (2014a) *Medicinal Products for Human Use*, http://ec.europa.eu/health/human-use/index_en.htm, accessed 2 September 2014.

European Commission (2014b) *Herbal Medicinal Products*, http://ec.europa.eu/health/human-use/herbal-medicines/index_en.htm, accessed 2 September 2014.

European Commission (2014c) *Food and Feed Safety*, http://europa.eu/legislation_summaries/ consumers/consumer_information/f80501_en.htm, accessed 2 September 2014.

European Commission (2014d) *Food Safety – Summaries of EU Legislation*, http://europa.eu/ legislation_summaries/food_safety/index_en.htm, accessed 1 September 2014.

Federal Institute for Risk Assessment (2014a) *Authorisation Procedure*, http://www.bfr.bund.de/ en/health_assessment_of_novel_foods-1809.html, accessed 20 November 2014.

Federal Institute for Risk Assessment (2014b) *Health Assessment of Functional Foods*, http://www. bfr.bund.de/en/health_assessment_of_functional__foods-735.html, accessed 20 November 2014.

Federal Institute for Risk Assessment (2014c) *EU Food Safety Almanac*, Federal Institute for Risk Assessment (BfR), Berlin.

Federal Institute for Risk Assessment (2014d) *Heath Claims*, http://www.bfr.bund.de/de/health_claims-9196.html, accessed 2 September 2014.

Friedland-Leuner, K., Stockburger, C., Denzer, I., *et al.* (2014) Mitochondrial dysfunction: cause and consequence of Alzheimer's disease. *Progresses in Molecular and Biological Translational Science*, **127**, 183–210.

Heinrich, M. (2010) Galanthamine from galanthus and other Amaryllidaceae – chemistry and biology based on traditional use. *Alkaloids Chemical Biology*, **68**, 157–165.

Kumar, V. (2006) Potential medicinal plants for CNS disorders: an overview. *Phytotherapy Research*, **20**, 1023–1035.

Lautenschlager, N.T., Ihl, R. and Müller, W.E. (2012) Ginkgo biloba extract EGb 761® in the context of current developments in the diagnosis and treatment of age-related cognitive decline and Alzheimer's disease: a research perspective. *International Psychogeriatrics*, **24**, S46–S50.

Pattanayak, P., Behera, P., Das, D. and Panda, S.K. (2010) *Ocimum sanctum* Linn. A reservoir plant for therapeutic applications: An overview. *Pharmacognosy Reviews*, **4**, 95–105.

Qiu, C., Kivipelto, M. and von Strauss, E. (2009) Epidemiology of Alzheimer's disease: occurrence, determinants, and strategies toward intervention. *Dialogues in Clinical Neuroscience*, **11**, 111–128.

Qu, L., Zou, W., Zhou, Z., *et al.* (2014) Non-European traditional herbal medicines in Europe: A community herbal monograph perspective. *Journal of Ethnopharmacology*, **156**, 107–114.

Schwitters, B., Achanta, G., van der Vlies, D. and Moriset, H. (2007) The European regulation of food supplements and food fortification. *Environmental Law and Management*, **19**, 19.

Stafford, G.I., Pedersen, M.E., van Staden, J. and Jager, A.K. (2008) Review on plants with CNS effects used in traditional South African medicine against mental diseases. *Journal of Ethnopharmacology*, **119**, 513–537.

Wiesner, J. and Knöss, W. (2014) Future visions for traditional and herbal medicinal products – A global practice for evaluation and regulation? *Journal of Ethnopharmacology*, **158**, 516–518.

# 22

# Retrospective Treatment-Outcome as a Method of Collecting Clinical Data in Ethnopharmacological Surveys

Bertrand Graz[1], Merlin Willcox[2] and Elaine Elisabetsky[3]

[1] Social and Preventive Medicine, University of Lausanne, Switzerland
[2] Nuffield Department of Primary Care Health Sciences, University of Oxford, UK
[3] Labratório de Etnofarmacologia, Universidade Federal do Rio Grande do Sul, Porto Alegre, Brazil

## 22.1   Introduction

Integration of treatments from modern biomedical (i.e. conventional western-type) and traditional medical systems is a common occurrence in current international clinical practice, with plural therapeutic itincraries adopted by increasingly larger proportions of those seeking health care. However, this process is often chaotic and defined by factors mostly extraneous to a rational choice of effective and safe treatment. Even if the very rational underlying diverse medical systems and their practices are taken into account, ultimately scientifically validated clinical studies can be helpful for patients to come to an informed decision, as well as for resource allocation from a governmental perspective.

Investigating effectiveness (the overall benefit of a treatment or drug) is not usually the aim of ethnopharmacology studies (Graz, 2013). However, ethnopharmacology studies may provide relevant data for future assessment of clinical effectiveness and safety of locally used products. A significant contribution from ethnopharmacology lies in revealing emic concepts (e.g. patient's views on health, disease, expected treatment outcomes and adverse effects) which at times may be very different from the biomedical perspectives. Such differences are

*Ethnopharmacology*, First Edition. Edited by Michael Heinrich and Anna K. Jäger.
© 2015 John Wiley & Sons, Ltd. Published 2015 by John Wiley & Sons, Ltd.

not entirely surprising given that medical systems are organized as cultural systems (Kleinman, 1978). Research on traditional medicine and the evaluation of the effectiveness of traditional medicines and practices can provide invaluable information for public health policies and programmes, which are particularly relevant for the local population (Vandebroek, 2013).

The collection and understanding of emic concepts of health/disease and treatment outcomes (i.e. clinical data) during ethnopharmacological field studies is relevant for various purposes, including defining a working hypothesis for scrutiny of specific bioactivity associated with a medicinal species or formula, adjusting laboratory research designs (dose, timing, etc.), preparing clinical studies, as well as improving local health programmes by improving communication between health authorities and target populations (Elisabetsky and Setzer, 1985). The collection of key clinical data during ethnoharmacological fieldwork may prove crucial to assess traditional medicines *per se* and plural therapeutic strategies. Recommendations from the WHO on traditional medicine (WHO, 2013) are 'to help users to make informed choices about self-health care' and to increase research efforts because 'a knowledge-based policy is the key to integrate T&CM into national health systems'.

The purpose of this chapter is to draw attention to the ways in which ethnopharmacologists can contribute to these goals, with the example of the retrospective treatment outcome study method.

## 22.2   Key concepts: clinical data, outcome and patient progress

Madame Bâ complains of back ache. Mr Zhang says his young daughter is scratching her arms all the time and has red patches on her elbows. These observations are clinical data, by which we mean 'observations about the health status of a human subject'. The outcome is the patient progress observed after a treatment, i.e. observed changes in the human subject's health status.

We will resist defining 'health status' or 'health' in general because in studies on traditional medicine we often find it more practical to work with patient's views on health, disease and progress (the emic perspective). In other words, the patient is at the centre of the research process; what will be measured is a change in health status according to the patient. This being said, patients today often mix cultural influences. Their accounts of their health status may well draw on local, traditional disease concepts as well as on laboratory results. For example, the same patient in Mauritania reported having 'creatures in the stomach' (after consulting a traditional practitioner) and 'high blood glucose' (after a blood test in the nearby health centre). Observed progress (= outcome) will encompass all reported aspects of health: the fate of the creatures in the stomach (emic perspective) and glycaemia; the latter being used, possibly with other blood tests, as a proxy for diabetes control.

Sometimes what may be seen as an adverse effect in one culture can be regarded as a necessary part of the treatment in another culture (Etkin, 1994). Detailed ethnopharmacology can be revealing, as in this example from Nigeria: 'Hausa practitioners advise that the treatment of measles be aimed at several stages, beginning with efforts to expel disease substance from the body interior' ((Etkin, 2006), p. 34). In this case, vomiting is regarded as a therapeutic step, and a vital one. If a medicine does not induce vomiting, Hausa practitioners may find it inappropriate or use it along with something that will induce vomiting. In conventional medicine, vomiting might be regarded as an adverse effect whereas for Hausa people, in this particular disease, if you do not vomit you will not properly expel the disease and will not be cured.

What kind of working hypothesis, or clinical data, would be created if the ethnopharmacological data were limited to a list of medicinal plants used to treat disease? That those plants used to induce vomiting are potential sources of antiviral compounds? What are the pharmacological and clinical consequences of western medicines taken along with plants to induce vomiting? It is the detailed understanding of both disease and treatment concepts that will ultimately allow for a sound working hypothesis. Starting from a rigorous working hypothesis is a valuable short cut for the evaluation of interesting bioactivity in a specific plant species or for the assessment of treatment effectiveness.

Here is another example: in several parts of Brazil memory loss is not considered a disease, but a normal feature of ageing, but if ethnopharmacologists ask for remedies to improve memory they may find that elderly people use medicinal plants to help them be 'tuned with things, with what is going on around us'. These treatments are often referred to as 'brain tonics'. At least one medicinal plant used as such, *Ptychopetalum olacoides* Benth (Olaceceae) used in the treatment of 'nerve weakness', was shown to possess memory improving and anti-amnesic effects (da Silva, 2004; da Silva, 2009).

What are the links between clinical data and effectiveness? It is not sufficient to be told or even to observe that many patients are healed after a certain treatment to conclude that this treatment is safe and effective because there could be many other reasons why the patients improved. Perhaps the illness would have improved just the same without any treatment, or perhaps the patients did something else (other than the treatment considered) which improved their condition (for example a change in diet or lifestyle). The collection and interpretation of clinical data requires slightly sophisticated methods in order to adjust for such confounding factors.

## 22.3  Evaluation of the effectiveness and safety of traditional medicines

Many users of traditional medicines and many practitioners say that the effect of a treatment is obvious when there is an improvement in health status. However, most ailments are self-limiting and tend to get better over time even in the absence of treatment. Even with chronic diseases there are periods of remission. Hence the general rule: clinical improvement is not proof of effectiveness. When a patient improves after using a medicinal plant preparation, the cure may well be credited to the patient's natural healing ability or the natural course of the disease. Care may also have a non-specific, 'placebo' effect, i.e. the stimulation of the patient's healing potential, for example through the endogenous pharmacy of inner secretions like endorphins (Kaptchuk *et al.*, 2010). Clinical data, i.e. details on patient status and progress, can only be informative about a treatment effect under particular conditions and with a point of comparison, otherwise they can be misleading and confusing.

There have been attempts to estimate effectiveness by counting independent authors, traditional healers or ethnobotanical studies citing the treatment. The use of the same species for treating a particular disease by different cultures might be indicative of physiological effects, since it is not bound to specific cultural contexts. However, this is not accepted as proof of effectiveness by physicians and health policy makers. Indeed, discrepancies have been often observed between strong reputation, laboratory results and clinical outcome (Bourdy *et al.*, 2008; Willcox *et al.*, 2011a). However, clinical observations documented over decades by clinicians are not devoid of value. In the WHO monographs on selected medicinal plants, data under the heading 'Uses supported by clinical data' included trials that 'may have been controlled, randomized, double-blind studies, open trials, or well-documented observations of therapeutic applications' (WHO, 1999). A careful assessment of 'well-documented observations' is indeed necessary to assess their informative value.

For clinical studies or trials (with human subjects), observations need to be organized in a way that makes it possible to compare clinical data with and without treatment, or between different treatments or treatment doses. Different outcomes can only be attributed to treatment difference if all other conditions during treatment are kept similar. This can be obtained through a diversity of study designs, including observational studies with proper adjustments through propensity scores and other statistical tools, a dose-escalating prospective study (comparing outcomes with different doses of a treatment) or a randomized controlled trial (RCT), the latter being considered the most reliable method for evidence-based medicine. RCT results give an estimate of the magnitude of a treatment's effects, as compared to effects obtained with another or no treatment.

## 22.4   The role of ethnopharmacologists and ethnobotanists

How can ethnopharmacologists and ethnobotanists contribute to the process of determining a treatment's safety and effectiveness? During ethnobotanical surveys, clinical data can be collected to provide indications (although not proof) of the effectiveness – or risk – of certain local preparations. This effort, at the end of a research-and-policy process, will help users of traditional medicine to make safer and more effective choices.

Investigating the clinical effectiveness of traditional medicine can also provide new therapeutic possibilities for modern medicine practitioners. This may happen through the discovery of new chemical compounds or through clinical validation of a traditional preparation. Even when no single active compound is found, it can be useful for modern medicine practitioners to investigate the clinical effects of a whole plant preparation. A well-known example is St John's wort (*Hypericum perforatum* L.), which was found (in randomized controlled clinical studies) to be effective and safe for treating mild to moderate depression, although the active compounds responsible for its clinical effectiveness had not yet been fully determined (Linde *et al.*, 2008). Even when the local preparation is of known clinical effectiveness and safety, discovering active compounds is still useful since it allows for precise quality control.

At the very beginning of a research process leading to a validated traditional medicine or a new modern medicine, or both, ethnopharmacologists and ethnobotanists can play an important role since preclinical clinical data collected during field surveys can enhance the chances that the end product will be safe. The safety of traditional preparations is a major concern and field studies, such as ethnobotanical and retrospective treatment-outcome (RTO) studies, are of utmost importance for this matter. If it is shown that the preparation is of common and ancient use, with no known important side effects, the preparation is deemed to be most probably safe and toxicological studies are not a regulatory requirement (Zheng and WHO, 2000). WHO guidelines state that 'If the product has been traditionally used without demonstrated harm, no specific restrictive regulatory action should be undertaken unless new evidence demands a revised risk-benefit assessment' (WHO, 1996). Toxicology studies are only required for new medicinal herbal products, or for a new formulation or dosage of traditional products. However, local regulations may have different requirements.

**Table 22.1**  Databases with results from clinical studies on herbal medicine.

- Cochrane Complementary Medicine Group: Reviews on Complementary Medicine
    http://www.thecochranelibrary.com
- Reviews on a selection of medicinal plants by a US government institution
    http://nccam.nih.gov/health/herbsataglance.htm
- Summaries of research on a number of herbal medicines, with a focus on cancer but also many other health problems
    http://www.mskcc.org/cancer-care/integrative-medicine/about-herbs-botanicals-other-products
- Help in clinical evidence search
    http://www.evidence.nhs.uk

## 22.5  Collection of clinical data during ethnopharmacological field studies

To start with, an interdisciplinary team must be established. A doctor or nurse will help to define the problem and the research question, while the main data collection will be performed by a botanist or ethnopharmacologist, sometimes helped by students, and data analysis performed with the help of a statistician or epidemiologist. Health authorities, traditional healers and local physicians may need to be involved as well.

The time spent in carefully preparing a study with the right specialists and stakeholders can save months, if not years; it can make the difference between a major medical discovery and useless research. Protocol discussions and support from statisticians/epidemiologists and clinicians (in addition to colleagues in the fields of botany and ethnopharmacology) may be possible with a local university department or through multidisciplinary groups. It is important to ensure that all partners fully agree with the chosen objectives.

Literature searches will also help to design research in line with presently unanswered questions. A lot of clinical research has already been conducted on medicinal plants and can be easily retrieved (Table 22.1).

## 22.6  Example of a method for gathering clinical data during field surveys

### 22.6.1  Defining the health problem

The health problem can be defined along local disease classification and terms, or along a syndromic description (e.g. 'hot body', a proxy for fever), allowing for further correlation with classifications from several heath systems. At this stage, collaboration between a medical anthropologist, a physician and a botanist is essential. For example, if you are in France, patients may describe a 'crise de foie', which for a physician indicates indigestion attributed to liver problems. In the UK, a man presenting with 'chest tightness' may mean that he is having symptoms of asthma (difficulty in breathing because lung movements feel 'tight') or ischaemic heart disease ('tight' chest pain). In East Africa, 'homa' may be interpreted as fever or malaria. In Mali, 'kono' ('the nightjar') refers to fever with convulsions in a child, thought to be caused by the passing of the nightjar and, in modern medicine, with a differential diagnosis of febrile seizures, cerebral malaria or meningitis. The same applies to 'deguedegue' (fever + convulsions) in Tanzania.

In many countries, childhood symptoms such as diarrhoea and fever are mistakenly ascribed to 'teething'. In Uganda, fever and diarrhoea in a young child is often called 'ebiino', which is believed to be caused by a small worm in the growing toothbud; parents therefore believe that they must take their child to a tooth extractor to remove the tooth bud, which may have unfortunate consequences.

## 22.6.2    Research question

For any ailment, there are often many different traditional medicines in use. For example, over 1200 remedies are reported worldwide for the treatment of fevers or malaria (Willcox and Bodeker, 2004). Even in two relatively small areas of Mali, 166 remedies containing 66 plant species are used to treat malaria (Willcox *et al.*, 2011b). In the bedside-to-bench approach, the main question is to know which one is the best among the many treatments used for the same ailment in a population.

A quantitative collection of outcome data from patient reports will provide two essential elements: precise clinical information on real cases and statistical analysis of correlations between treatments and outcomes (Willcox *et al.*, 2011a; Willcox *et al.*, 2011b).

## 22.6.3    Data collection: ask patients!

The RTO design is proposed here because it has proved to be feasible. It provides the indications of safety and effectiveness necessary to proceed to a formal clinical studies process. Laboratory experiments will start only after the clinical safety and effectiveness have been established.

During the whole RTO process, patients (*not* healers) are interviewed and observed. For respondents who do not know exactly what they have used (e.g. if they got it from a healer outside of the family), it might be necessary to contact the treatment provider. Healers are of course an important source of information, but not for treatment *outcome*: they are usually more aware of the good results than of the failures because patients experiencing a treatment failure tend to go away and try another treatment elsewhere. This is why, if one wants to collect informative data on a treatment effect, it is usually preferable to ask patients about their own experience.

Case reports from users are formalized with a questionnaire exploring the following questions: Who has been sick recently? What disease? Which treatment? What was the patient progress (the outcome)? If we find a statistical association with poor outcome, this may be related to an absence of effect or a detrimental effect (toxicity). If we find an association with patient cure, this could mean that the treatment is effective and this will be studied by other types of clinical studies.

## 22.6.4    Getting consent: a much debated topic

In theory, getting consent is a rather straightforward process. The study is presented to the respondent. If he/she agrees, a form is signed (or verbal consent is noted). Confidentiality is guaranteed as the data are kept separately from the consent form, then are analysed and presented in an anonymous fashion. Most ethics committees now insist on written information sheets for participants and written (signed) consent forms. In practice, however, this may prove more complicated. For example, in many study areas the respondents are illiterate, so are unable to read or understand a written form. Many illiterate people are reluctant to sign documents because they fear that maybe they are being misled. Furthermore, in some cultures a woman may not be allowed to sign a document without her husband's permission, which poses a problem when the husband is working away from home at the time of the survey.

Teams conducting ethnobotanical surveys must also consider the issue of intellectual property rights. In theory it should be simple to deal with this by the investigator accepting that the respondent may not wish to disclose some information. However, ethics committees often do not consider issues of intellectual property rights (as this is not viewed as a patient safety issue) and not all researchers may be scrupulous. There are several cases of traditional 'secrets' being developed into profitable commercial products with hot controversy on benefit sharing with traditional knowledge holders. Notorious examples include *Pelargonium sidoides DC.* and the *Hoodia* cactus (*Hoodia gordonii* (Masson) Sweet ex Decne.) from South Africa. Respondents should be fully informed of what will be done with the information they provide. In the event that a commercial product is to be developed, there should also be an access and benefit-sharing agreement such that information providers (or the community according to the agreement in place) will be given a fair share of the benefits. The International Society for Ethnobiology has published a code of ethics which ethnobotanists and ethnopharmacologists are encouraged to follow (International Society of Ethnobiology, 2006).

## 22.6.5  Sample size

By interviewing large numbers of people, it is possible to discover which plants are most commonly used and, through statistical analysis, which are the most likely to be associated with reported clinical recovery. To collect enough data for such analysis required one survey to ask 1000 respondents to find six groups of at least 20 people using the same treatment (the six most common treatments – there were many other treatments used by fewer than 20 people), thus allowing for meaningful comparisons between groups (Graz *et al.*, 2010a). A pre-test may be necessary to determine the sample size (i.e. to estimate how many people need to be asked in order to have enough treatment groups of sufficient size). In some cases, for example when most respondents use one of two plants, a sample of less than 100 may be sufficient.

A representative sample of the population makes it possible to draw a picture of the situation in a certain geographical area. To select the sample, it is sometimes not possible to use the classical method based on a recent population census; in this case there are other possibilities for reaching the population, keeping the principle that every individual of the target population should have the same chances of being interviewed (Department of Economic and Social Department of Economic and Social Affairs, 2005). When looking for the best way to compile the sample, it will be useful to ask a statistician, an epidemiologist or anybody used to preparing local population surveys such as vaccination coverage studies. When a quick and rough estimate is desired, easy but relatively biased methods could be preferred, such as having all students from a province or district high school taking the questionnaire home and finding respondents among their family and neighbours; with this sampling technique it must be clearly stated that, because of socio-educational clustering, individuals with a formal education might be over-represented.

## 22.6.6  Statistical analysis and interpretation

The basic principle is that it should be possible to quantify the number of patients using a particular plant or remedy, and the percentage of patients improving with a specific treatment

**Table 22.2**  Traditional antimalarial recipes in Mali, usages and clinical outcome (patient reported whether he/she was cured after being treated or whether the treatment failed) (from Diallo *et al.*, 2006).

| Recipe | Usage | Cured | Failed |
|---|---|---|---|
| *Argemone mexicana* L. alone | 17 | 17 | 0 |
| *Argemone mexicana* L. + *Carica papaya* L. | 9 | 9 | 0 |
| *Carica papaya* L. + *Anogeissus leiocarpus* (DC.) Guill. & Perr. | 7 | 5 | 2 |

**Table 22.3**  Correlation between plants used and reported outcome in a study on traditional treatments for malaria in Mali.

| Plant | Usage | Healed | Failed | % healed (95% CI) | P (Fisher exact) |
|---|---|---|---|---|---|
| *Argemone mexicana* L. | 30 | 30 | 0 | 100% (88–100) | (Reference) |
| *Carica papaya* L. | 33 | 28 | 5 | 85% (68–95) | 0.05 |
| *Anogeissus leiocarpus* (DC.) Guill. & Perr. | 33 | 27 | 6 | 82% (64–93) | 0.03 |

option. From this information it should be possible to test whether there is a statistically significant difference between the proportions of patients improving after taking each of the most common remedies.

Although the frequency of use of medicinal species, and especially those used for the same purpose by different cultures, has been considered as an indication of efficacy (usually reported in ethnopharmacology surveys as the 'consensus factor', see (Trotter and Logan, 1986)), the most frequently used treatment may not be the most effective. It is also possible that a treatment that is relatively rarely used in a population may be associated with the best patient progress. For example, in a study on traditional treatments for malaria in Mali, use of the RTO method resulted in a database of treatments taken for malaria cases in 952 households. A table was compiled showing every reported recipe and related information. The same plant is reportedly used in combination or alone, as in Table 22.2 (reported recipes with *Argemone mexicana* L.).

The second step of the analysis aim to determine whether or not individual plants are associated with clinical outcomes. For this, the recipes table is re-categorized according to the presence of every plant used (Table 22.3). In the Malian example, from the 66 plants used, alone or in various combinations, one was clearly associated with the best outcomes: a decoction of *A. mexicana* (Table 22.3) (Diallo *et al.*, 2007). Fisher's exact test was chosen because the numbers in the subgroups were small.

More sophisticated analyses (such as regression) might be necessary if there is a possibility that factors other than the treatment may explain the observed differences. For example, if older patients use another treatment, they might have better outcome not because of the other treatment but because they are older (and so have had more time to build immunity). In this case, age should be taken into account in the regression model. The method has the usual limitations and caveats of observational studies and regression analyses, which is why it can only be one stage in a larger research process.

In the example given above, the distribution of ages (and other potential confounders recorded) was similar across treatments. In addition, clinical outcomes were not better when the treatment was used in combination. The recipe with best outcomes, a single plant in its traditional mode of preparation and utilization, was therefore selected for further studies.

### 22.6.7  Results: a research programme leading to the validation of safe and effective phytomedicines

In the example of traditional treatments against malaria in Mali, a dose-escalating prospective study showed a dose-response phenomenon in terms of clinical progress (fever, other symptoms) and presence of malaria parasites in the blood (Willcox *et al.*, 2007), paving the way for a subsequent RCT in the form of a pragmatic non-inferiority trial that showed how the local traditional recipe was close to the standard imported drug in terms of effectiveness (Graz *et al.*, 2010b; Willcox *et al.*, 2011c). After these clinical studies, the search for active compounds was undertaken. The whole research process was labelled 'reverse pharmacology' or, more specifically, the bedside-to-bench approach.

In 2013 a new RTO study was conducted in the same area of south Mali. Most children with reported uncomplicated malaria were still first treated at home (76%), with a herbal preparation in 58% of cases (modern treatment 13%, combined 29%). Mention of a local treatment made with *A. mexicana* (extensively studied but not officially recommended) had increased from 8% of respondents in 2003 to 26% in 2013 ($p < 0.001$). *A. mexicana* use was followed by reported cure or improvement in 91% of cases (100% among those > 5 years old), compared to 71% with other traditional treatments ($p = 0.006$). A second treatment was considered necessary in 11% of patients receiving *A. mexicana*, the same as in the RCT conducted on *A. mexicana* in the area (Graz *et al.*, 2015).

In the Malian example, the whole research process cost less than a million euros. Contrary to a commonly held myth, clinical studies can be conducted at relatively low cost if the researcher works with local/regional research institutes and with doctoral students, focusing on meaningful clinical measures rather than sophisticated laboratory analyses (Graz *et al.*, 2010a).

## 22.7  Conclusion: clinical data and field surveys for a positive impact on health

The clinical effects of medicinal plants can and should be studied with sound methods that are as much as possible the same as those methods used for testing conventional medicines. If this is done, rigorous and scientifically accepted evaluation will produce results that are understandable and acceptable by the scientific community, health professionals and policy makers. In our experience traditional healers can also be efficient partners; thanks to their vast experience in providing care they can effectively help in developing and interpreting clinical studies.

A field survey can provide some knowledge of interest for the population at stake. Clinical data collected during field surveys can be beneficial for both the plant users and the researcher. If the research is conducted rigorously and results are fed back to the community, this will inform patients about which common remedies are associated with the best outcomes. Researchers may gain a better relationship and work environment when they are seen as bringing information useful for the quality of care in the community.

For further information see the online course 'The Retrospective Treatment Outcome Study (RTO) for Traditional Medicines', which is available at http://globalhealthtrials.tghn.org/elearning/the-retrospective-treatment-outcome-study/. Readers wishing to discuss these issues are encouraged to visit the online forum at https://globaltraditionalmedicine.tghn.org/key-areas/medical-anthropology-and-ethnobotany/.

# References

Bourdy, G., Willcox, M.L., Ginsburg, H., *et al.* (2008) Ethnopharmacology and malaria: new hypothetical leads or old efficient antimalarials? *International Journal for Parasitology*, **38**, 33–41.

da Silva, A.E.A. (2004) Memory retrieval improvement by Ptychopetalum olacoides in young and ageing mice. *Journal of Ethnopharmacology*, **95**, 199–203.

da Silva, A.E.A. (2009) MK-801- and scopolamine-induced amnesiaa are reversed by an Amazonian herbal locally used as a 'brain tonic'. *Psychopharmacology*, **202**, 165–172.

Department of Economic and Social Affairs (2005) *Designing Household Survey Samples: Practical Guidelines* [online]. United Nations, New York, available at http://unstats.un.org/unsd/demographic/sources/surveys/Handbook23June05.pdf, accessed 26 June 2014.

Diallo, D., Diakite, C., Mounkoro, P.P., *et al.* (2007) [Knowledge of traditional healers on malaria in Kendié (Bandiagara) and Finkolo (Sikasso) in Mali ]. *Mali Médical*, **22**, 1–8.

Elisabetsky, E. and Setzer, R. (1985) Caboclo oncepts of disease, diagnosis and therapy: Implications for ethnopharmacology and health systems in Amazonia, in *The Amazon Cacoclo: Historical and contemporary perspectives* (ed. E.P. Parker), Studies in Third World Societies, Vol, **32**, College of William and Mary, Williamsburg, pp. 243–278.

Etkin, N.L. (1994) The negotiation of 'side'effects in Hausa (northern Nigeria) therapeutics, in *Medicines: Meanings and Contexts* (eds N. Etkin and M.L. Tan), Medical Antrhopology Unit, University of Amsterdam, Amsterdam.

Etkin, N.L. (2006) *Chapter 1 in* Edible Medicines: An Ethnopharmacology of Food, Unversity of Arizona Press, Tucson.

Graz, B. (2013) What is 'clinical data'? Why and how can they be collected during field surveys on medicinal plants? *Journal of Ethnopharmacology*, **150**, 775–779.

Graz, B., Falquet, J. and Elisabetsky, E. (2010a) Ethnopharmacology, sustainable development and cooperation: the importance of gathering clinical data during field surveys. *Journal of Ethnopharmacology*, **130**, 635–638.

Graz, B., Willcox, M. L., Diakite, C., *et al.* (2010b) *Argemone mexicana* decoction versus artesunate-amodiaquine for the management of malaria in Mali: policy and public-health implications. *Transactions of the Royal Society of Tropical Medicine & Hygiene*, **104**, 33–41.

Graz, B., Willcox, M., Berthé, D., *et al.* (2015) Home treatments alone or mixed with modern treatments for malaria in Finkolo AC, South Mali: reported use, outcomes and changes over 10 years. *Transactions of the Royal Society of Tropical Medicine and Hygiene, Epub ahead of print.*

International Society of Ethnobiology (2006) The ISE Code of Ethics [online], available at http://ethnobiology.net/what-we-do/core-programs/ise-ethics-program/code-of-ethics/, accessed 23 May 2014.

Kaptchuk, T.J., Friedlander, E., Kelley, J.M., *et al.* (2010) Placebos without deception: a randomized controlled trial in irritable bowel syndrome. *PLoS ONE [Electronic Resource]*, **5**, e15591.

Kleinman, A. (1978) Concepts and a model for comparison of medical systems as cultural systems. *Social Science and Medicine*, **12**, 85–83.

Linde, K., Berner, M.M. and Kriston, L. (2008) St John's wort for major depression. *Cochrane Database Systematic Reviews*, Issue 4, Art. No. CD000448, available at http://summaries.cochrane.org/CD000448/DEPRESSN_st.-johns-wort-for-treating-depression, accessed 7 October 2014.

Trotter, R. and Logan, M. (1986) Informant consensus: a new approach for identifying potentially efffective medicinal plants, in *Indigenous Medicine and Diet: Biobehavioural approaches* (ed. N.L. Etkin), Redgrave, New York, pp. 91–112.

Vandebroek, I. (2013) Intercultural health and ethnobotany: How to improve healthcare for underserved and minority communities? *Journal of Ethnopharmacology*, **148**, 746–754.

WHO (1996) WHO Expert Committee on specifications for pharmaceutical preparations. *World Health Organization Technical Report Series*, **863**, 1–194.

WHO (1999) *WHO monographs on selected medicinal plants, Introduction, Volume 1*, Publications of the World Health Organization, Geneva, p. 3.

WHO (2013) *Traditional Medicine Strategy, 2014–2023*, World Health Organization, Geneva.

Willcox, M.L. and Bodeker, G. (2004) Traditional herbal medicines for malaria. *British Medical Journal*, **329**, 1156–1159.

Willcox, M.L., Graz, B., Falquet, J., *et al.* (2007) *Argemone mexicana* decoction for the treatment of uncomplicated falciparum malaria. *Transactions of the Royal Society of Tropical Medicine & Hygiene*, **101**, 1190–1198.

Willcox, M., Benoit-Vical, F., Fowler, D., *et al.* (2011a) Do ethnobotanical and laboratory data predict clinical safety and efficacy of anti-malarial plants? *Malaria Journal*, **10**, S7.

Willcox, M., Graz, B., Falquet, J., *et al.* (2011b) A 'reverse pharmacology' approach for developing an anti-malarial phytomedicine. *Malaria Journal*, **10**, S8.

Willcox, M.L., Graz, B., Diakite, C., *et al.* (2011c) Is parasite clearance clinically important after malaria treatment in a high transmission area? A 3-month follow-up of home-based management with herbal medicine or ACT. *Transactions of the Royal Society of Tropical Medicine & Hygiene*, **105**, 23–31.

Zheng, X. and WHO (2000) *General Guidelines for Methodologies on Research and Evaluation of Traditional Medicine*, World Health Organization, Geneva.

# Ethnopharmacology: Regional Perspectives

# 23

# Ethnopharmacology in Sub-Sahara Africa: Current Trends and Future Perspectives

Mack Moyo[1], Adeyemi O. Aremu[1] and Johannes van Staden[1]

*Research Centre for Plant Growth and Development, School of Life Sciences, University of KwaZulu-Natal, Pietermaritzburg, Scottsville, South Africa*

## 23.1   Introduction

The importance of medicinal plants in African traditional medicine (ATM) and their contribution in primary healthcare across the continent is well recognized. ATM has complemented the orthodox western medical system in the fight against various health conditions and diseases. As depicted in Figure 23.1, the incidence of some diseases, such as diabetes, has significantly increased during the period 2002–2012. The growing importance of medicinal plants in primary healthcare is based on their long-standing utilization in folk medicine and prophylactic properties (Houghton *et al.*, 2007). In essence, the therapeutic philosophy of ATM is primarily based on prevention and the promotion of good health, hence mixtures of plant extracts and herbal preparations are sometimes regularly consumed as rejuvenators, tonics and/or nutritional supplements (Amoo *et al.*, 2012). Thus, African traditional healthcare is generally characterized by a multidrug therapy philosophy, in contrast to the single-drug approach in orthodox medicine. Over the past 20 years, ATM has undergone a remarkable revival and transformation due to significant research investments, particularly in South Africa, which is arguably the epicentre of innovation in African ethnopharmacology. Most importantly, ethnopharmacology has become an integral component of university pharmacy and medical science curricula in many member states of the Economic Community of West African States (ECOWAS), Democratic Republic of Congo, South Africa and Tanzania (WHO, 2013). The vast richness and diversity of African medicinal plants is a pharmaceutical resource with the potential to rescue the crumbling healthcare systems of most African countries (Busia, 2005). The objective of this chapter is to provide a critical and updated review of ethnopharmacology in sub-Sahara Africa.

*Ethnopharmacology*, First Edition. Edited by Michael Heinrich and Anna K. Jäger.
© 2015 John Wiley & Sons, Ltd. Published 2015 by John Wiley & Sons, Ltd.

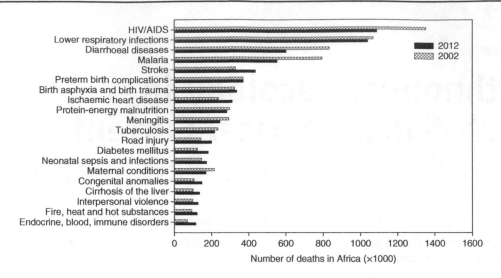

**Figure 23.1**   The 20 leading causes of death in Africa (WHO, 2014).

## 23.2   Role of traditional medicine in Africa

Globally, evidence of the vital influence of natural products, especially plant materials in drug discovery, cannot be overemphasized (Gurib-Fakim, 2006; Newman and Cragg, 2012). Africa is endowed with more than 60,000 taxa, which is equivalent to about 25% of the world's higher plant species, and a significant portion of these plants have therapeutic potential (Iwu, 1993; van Wyk, 2008). Local preparations of medicinal plants still provide the only therapeutic option for about 80% of the population (Ibrahim *et al.*, 2014), a situation aggravated by a low medical doctor-to-patient ratio of about 1:40,000 (Abdullahi, 2011). This is in contrast to the more favourable ratio of one traditional medicine practitioner per 500 patients for sub-Saharan Africa (Albertyn *et al.*, 2014). Apart from being a fundamental aspect of the culture, ATM remains the most economical and accessible system of healthcare for a large number of the African population in rural and semi-urban areas (Gurib-Fakim, 2006). Furthermore, in some places primary healthcare inaccessibility is compounded by long hospital waiting times of 6–12 hours (Busia, 2005).

As documented by Neuwinger (2000), the Continent has an estimated 5400 medicinal plant taxa with over 16,300 therapeutic uses. Recently, enormous efforts by scientists have identified several plant species with potential against common ailments, including microbial infections (Eloff and McGaw, 2006; Ndhlala *et al.*, 2013), malaria (Soh and Benoit-Vical, 2007; Zofou *et al.*, 2013; Adia *et al.*, 2014), HIV/AIDS (Kamatenesi-Mugisha *et al.*, 2014), diabetes mellitus (Mohammed *et al.*, 2014), tuberculosis (TB) (McGaw *et al.*, 2008; Bunalema *et al.*, 2014; Fomogne-Fodjo *et al.*, 2014; Ibekwe *et al.*, 2014; Madikizela *et al.*, 2014), diarrhoea (Schlage *et al.*, 2000; Madikizela *et al.*, 2012), helminthiasis (Muthee *et al.*, 2011; Aremu *et al.*, 2012), trypanosomiasis (Ibrahim *et al.*, 2014), cancer (Fouche *et al.*, 2008; Nair *et al.*, 2012; Nair and van Staden, 2014; Ochwang'i *et al.*, 2014), pain and inflammation (Agyare *et al.*, 2013), and burns (Albertyn *et al.*, 2014). The rich medicinal plant diversity represents a valuable resource from both commercial development and basic scientific perspectives. Based on their wide popularity and usage, 51 medicinal plant species were identified as important and valuable plants in ATM (Brendler *et al.*, 2010). These species only represent a marginal fraction of African medicinal plants known to possess different health-related uses against various ailments, including infectious, parasitic and non-communicable diseases. In addition, they are a source of raw materials for the pharmaceutical, herbal, food, cosmetic and essential oil industries. In particular, the pharmaceutical and herbal industries use fresh/dried plants, extracts or isolated active ingredients to manufacture medicines. Many African countries, notably Mali, Burkina Faso, Ghana, Cameroon, South Africa and Nigeria, have witnessed a drastic increase in the number of registered and unregistered cottage-level herbal enterprises which are involved in the manufacturing of herbal formulations based on ATM (Obi *et al.*, 2006; Kasilo *et al.*, 2010; Ndhlala *et al.*, 2011; Kunle *et al.*, 2012; Sanogo, 2014). Inevitably, studies aimed at establishing the scientific basis of the potential potency of these herbal medicinal products are increasing across the Continent.

## 23.3  Ethnopharmacological research in sub-Saharan Africa

In sub-Saharan Africa, popular ethnobotanical information has been gathered through surveys and provides a solid foundation for many ethnopharmacological studies. Using the ethnobotanical approach, numerous African medicinal plants have found their way into modern scientific laboratories with cutting edge drug discovery and medical research facilities and technologies, both on the African continent and developed countries. Most of the research on African medicinal plants has focused on validating their uses in traditional medicine by evaluating their corresponding pharmacological activity in both *in vitro* and *in vivo* models. As a result, many African medicinal plants have been evaluated for a range of pharmacological properties, including antimicrobial, anthelmintic, antimalarial and anti-inflammatory activities (McGaw *et al.*, 2000; Eloff and McGaw, 2006; Soh and Benoit-Vical, 2007; Agyare *et al.*, 2013; Ndhlala *et al.*, 2013; Madikizela *et al.*, 2014). The sometimes controversial subject of the antioxidative health benefits of medicinal plants has also received appreciable attention (Nafiu *et al.*, 2013; Ndhlala *et al.*, 2014). Besides the predominant focus on antimicrobial studies, ethnopharmacological research in Africa is gradually shifting towards other major diseases (Figure 23.1) affecting the Continent, such as HIV/AIDS, TB, respiratory infections, malaria, diarrhoea and sickle-cell anaemia. For instance, malaria remains a major health challenge in most parts of sub-Saharan Africa with unprecedented high mortality rates. As an indication of the severity of the disease, designated research institutes are not only found in West and East Africa with high incidence but also now in southern Africa. It is encouraging to note that the active research on new antimalarial compounds is yielding promising outcomes. In West Africa, four out of 109 medicinal plants that have been evaluated for antimalarial activity, namely *Cochlospermum tinctorium* A. Rich. (Bixaceae), *Cryptolepis sanguinolenta* (Lindl.) Schlechter (Periplocaceae), *Azadirachta indica* A. Juss (Meliaceae) and *Guiera senegalensis* J.F. Gmel (Combretaceae), had compounds with good selectivity indices and $IC_{50}$ values below 1.0 µg/ml (Soh and Benoit-Vical, 2007). Despite these promising findings, Soh and Benoit-Vical (2007) lamented the lack of adequate infrastructure in West Africa to undertake well-controlled clinical trials as a major limitation in the drug discovery process. A worrying trend is the increasing incidences of previously uncommon diseases such as cancer and dementia-related ailments in Africa (WHO, 2014). Concomitantly, there is current research into African medicinal plants with potential anticancer (Kuete *et al.*, 2013; Nair and van Staden, 2013) and acetylcholinesterase inhibitory (Nair *et al.*, 2011; Ndhlala *et al.*, 2012; Nair and van Staden, 2013; Wansi *et al.*, 2013) properties, primarily from the

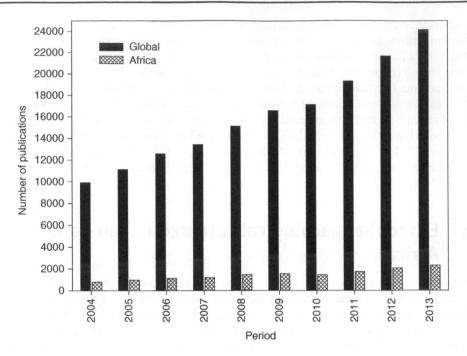

**Figure 23.2** The number of scientific publications from Africa compared to the global total in Science Direct journals over the last 10 years (January 2004 to December 2013), based on the search words 'traditional medicine' and 'traditional medicine in Africa'. The data were collected in October 2014. (Note: The analysis serves to give a general trend and is not a comprehensive study).

alkaloid-rich Amaryllidaceae family. Overall, the increased research efforts in the field of ethnopharmacology in Africa have led to a gradual rise in scientific publications from the Continent (Figure 23.2). Despite these gains, studies on the uses of medicinal plants by African cultures have been relatively scarce when compared to other regions of the world (Schlage *et al.*, 2000). The majority of the studies have been published in the *Journal of Ethnopharmacology*. Considering the WHO health statistics on leading causes of deaths in Africa (Figure 23.1), it is only logical to assume that ethnopharmacology research on the Continent should be geared towards addressing these major health challenges. Based on this assumption, scientists in Africa should play a key role in HIV/AIDS research and its associated opportunistic infections such as TB. In their review of South African medicinal plants used to alleviate TB symptoms, McGaw *et al.* (2008) reiterated the need for more research on the systematic assessment of anti-TB efficacy.

It is estimated that over 15,000 phytochemical compounds exhibiting significant pharmacological activity have been isolated from African medicinal plants (Busia, 2005). Kuete (2013) provided a comprehensive review of the chemistry and pharmacology of important plants traditionally used in ATM. Nevertheless, relatively few medicinal taxa from other parts of Africa, notably East Africa, have undergone detailed pharmacological and phytochemical studies (Schlage *et al.*, 2000). Although significant progress has been made in ethnopharmacological research, there is a conspicuous lack of scientific data on clinical studies to evaluate the efficacy of the promising extracts or compounds (Busia, 2005; Aremu *et al.*, 2012; Ibrahim *et al.*, 2014). Ironically, most of the clinical studies on African medicinal plants have been done outside the continent, mainly in Europe. *Pelargonium sidoides* DC. (Geraniaceae), a popular southern African medicinal plant used in the treatment of respiratory infections, for which 16 clinical studies have been conducted, is a case in point (Moyo and van Staden, 2014). Exceptions to this trend include the clinical evaluation of Niprisan®, a phytomedicine used in Nigeria for the management of sickle cell disorder (Wambebe *et al.*, 2001).

The practice of ATM has been sustained largely through oral transmission of indigenous knowledge, making it highly susceptible to loss of information from generation to generation. Thus, this mode of knowledge transfer accentuates the fragility of ATM. Citing this challenge, Light *et al.* (2005) advocated the urgent need for scientific documentation of African indigenous knowledge. To curb the ever-increasing loss of ethnopharmacology knowledge, a variety of forums are being used. Recently, special issues on ethnobotany in South Africa (*Journal of Ethnopharmacology*, Vol. 119, 2008), economic botany (*South African Journal of Botany*, Vol. 77, 2011) and quality control (*South African Journal of Botany,* Vol. 82, 2012) have been published covering various aspects of ethnopharmacology research in South Africa. A number of countries, notably Benin, Burkina Faso, Cameroon, Cote d'Ivoire, Guinea, Madagascar, Mali, Senegal and South Africa, have developed monographs on their respective medicinal and aromatic plants (Kasilo *et al.*, 2010). In addition, the *Ghananian Herbal Pharmacopoeia* (2nd edition, 2007), *Nigerian Herbal Pharmacopoeia* (2008) and *African Herbal Pharmacopoeia* (2010) have been published. In particular, the *African Herbal Pharmacopoeia* provides comprehensive botanical, commercial and phytochemical information on 51 medicinal plants considered to be the most important in ATM (Brendler *et al.*, 2010). The number of books entirely devoted to ethnopharmacology in Africa has also increased over the past two decades to complement classical reference materials such as Watt and Breyer-Brandwijk (1962), Iwu (1993), Kokwaro (1976, 1993) and Hutchings *et al.* (1996), including recent ones (van Wyk *et al.*, 2002; van Wyke, 2008; Kokwaro, 2009; Kuete, 2013; Iwu, 2014; Kuete, 2014) which are likely to generate renewed interest in medicinal plant research. These detailed and comprehensive scientific publications on African medicinal plants constitute valuable reference material for guiding future research. Based on the current momentum of research on African ethnopharmacology, this encouraging trend is likely to intensify.

# 23.4 Challenges of traditional medicine in Africa

The increasing popularity, acceptance and demand as well as rise in the market value of medicinal plants in Africa is well recognized and documented (Dzoyem *et al.*, 2013). As a result of the continuously increasing reliance on medicinal plants, major stakeholders have intensified efforts geared towards overcoming major challenges that have been associated with the practice of ATM. Often, these challenges are related to regulatory status, assessment of safety and efficacy, quality control and lack of knowledge about ATM within national drug regulatory authorities (Fennell *et al.*, 2004a,2004b; WHO, 2005; Street *et al.*, 2008; Kunle *et al.*, 2012). In the last few years, concerted efforts among African countries have resulted in significant progress on the development of national policies and regulations on ATM (WHO, 2005). In fact, African regional data compared favourably with global data with regard to commitment aimed at promoting, developing and establishing the scientific basis for ATM. However, the development of national policies and regulation for herbal medicines is much more limited among African countries when compared to global data (WHO, 2005). In order to gain better insights and identify the existing knowledge gaps, an overview of common challenges affecting ATM is highlighted below.

## 23.4.1   Efficacy, toxicology and safety concerns

Most African countries are still behind in the development and control of their medicinal plant industry when compared to China, which is renowned for its excellent traditional medicine. African researchers frequently investigate several aspects required for the development of ATM, especially the pharmacology and toxicology of the medicinal plants (Fennell *et al.*, 2004b). Even though there is no shortage of (preliminary) data demonstrating the pharmacological effects of many African medicinal plants against different diseases (Kuete, 2013), the main concern remains the significance or reliability of the majority of these findings, which are often *in vitro*-based assays (Aremu *et al.*, 2012; Ibrahim *et al.*, 2014). Ideally, *in vitro* assays providing promising results should be followed up with *in vivo* and ultimately clinical studies (Houghton *et al.*, 2007). As emphasized by these authors, it is essential that the processes underlying the disease state should be known, explored and investigated to determine the best battery of tests as this will justify the basis for taking an extract or preparation into *in vivo* or clinical tests.

In many African countries, adverse effects and even death associated with medicinal plant ingestion still remain largely unreported and poorly documented (Stewart *et al.*, 1998; Steenkamp *et al.*, 2002; Kunle *et al.*, 2012). Despite a general assumption that commonly used medicinal plants are safe (Gurib-Fakim, 2006), recent scientific research has shown that some plants commonly used as food or diet supplements as well as in ATM are potentially toxic, mutagenic and carcinogenic (Verschaeve and van Staden, 2008; Akinmoladun *et al.*, 2014). The availability of relatively few studies focusing on the safety of ATM is associated with the inadequate and/or lack of resources for forensic investigation as well as the relative paucity of methods for the detection of herbal toxins (Stewart *et al.*, 1998; Kamsu-Foguem and Foguem, 2014a). Often, misidentification, inadvertent or deliberate substitution of herbal materials, incorrect preparation, inappropriate administration and non-standardized dosages are key causes of the toxicity of herbal medicine (Stewart *et al.*, 1998; Street *et al.*, 2008). Based on a study by Stewart *et al.* (1999) in South Africa, poisoning resulting from consumption of traditional remedies was caused by plant materials and heavy metals, which accounted for more than 70% of the toxicity. A study in Nigeria by Obi *et al.* (2006) indicated that of 25 herbal remedies tested, all had elevated amounts of heavy metals. Similar incidences of heavy metal contamination have been documented in other African countries (Street, 2012). In terms of agri-chemical contamination, Elgorashi *et al.* (2004) isolated captan (a pesticide) from *Cyrtanthus suaveolens* Schönland (Amaryllidaceae). This commercial pesticide, used on a large scale on agricultural crops, is known to possess mutagenic, genotoxic and teratogenic activity. Environmental sources have also been implicated in the contamination of medicinal plants (Street, 2012). For instance, the physical conditions and infrastructure in medicinal plant markets are generally poor, with most plant material displayed in the open (mostly situated close to both pedestrian and motor vehicle traffic), where they are exposed to microbial and insect attack as well as the effects of light, gases and temperature (Govender *et al.*, 2006; Katerere *et al.*, 2008; Kaume *et al.*, 2012; van Vuuren *et al.*, 2014). In addition, traders in ATM often keep these medicinal plants in old recycled containers previously used for dangerous chemicals, and these practices pose a great health risk to the consumers due to cross-contamination (Street *et al.*, 2008). Owing to the increasing necessity to provide consumers with the correct information about the medicinal products they consume, an urgent requirement for a concerted effort to enlarge forensic and toxicological databases to include methods for the detection of toxicity in traditional remedies in Africa remain crucial (Steenkamp *et al.*, 2002; Obi *et al.*, 2006; Street *et al.*, 2008; Kunle *et al.*, 2012).

## 23.4.2 Shelf-life, post-harvest physiology and storage

While literature pertaining to the botany, bioactivity and chemistry of medicinal plants is not in short supply, relatively limited information exists on other equally important aspects such as shelf-life, post-harvest physiology and storage (Street *et al.*, 2008). For instance, shelf-life basically indicates the point at which a product no longer meets the requirements that it is supposed to, and may even be considered hazardous when consumed. Furthermore, heightened collection of high-demand plant species leads to unsustainable harvesting, resulting in longer storage periods of plant materials than would normally be projected (Fennell *et al.*, 2004a; Stafford *et al.*, 2005). However, the lack of storage facilities and trading infrastructure frequently results in the spoiling of medicinal plant materials, causing wastage and/or a decrease in product quality (Mander, 1997). The post-harvest phase may induce chemical changes in the collected material emanating from the effects of oxidizing enzymes, environmental conditions and pre-storage processing procedures such as mode of drying and storage (Fennell *et al.*, 2004a). Even though much can be learned and adapted from research on food crops (Fennell *et al.*, 2004a), there is less emphasis on commercial or sensory values (physical appearance, odour and taste) with medicinal plants. Rather the phytochemicals which are responsible for the biological activity of the plant are paramount. Although knowledge of storage aspects of medicinal plants in Africa is almost non-existent, a few scientific studies have been conducted by South African researchers (Eloff, 1999; Stafford *et al.*, 2005; Amoo *et al.*, 2012, 2013; Laher *et al.*, 2013). As indicated by these authors, storage methods and duration of storage influence the pharmacological and phytochemical activity of medicinal plants. In addition, the chemical changes are not always detrimental or undesired. The bioactivity of some plant species may actually increase with storage/ageing. Given the increasing importance of ATM, it will be highly valuable for researchers and other stakeholders to intensify efforts leading towards the documentation of the effects of storage and shelf-life on the dynamics of the phytochemical and subsequent pharmacological activity of medicinal plants.

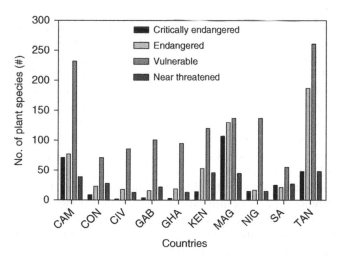

**Figure 23.3** An overview of conservation status of plant species in some sub-Sahara countries. CAM, Cameroon; CON, Congo; CIV, Côte d'Ivoire; GAB, Gabon; GHA, Ghana; KEN, Kenya; MAG, Madagascar; NIG, Nigeria; SA, South Africa; TAN, Tanzania. Source of data: IUCN (2014).

### 23.4.3   Conservation challenges of protecting plant resources

Countries such as Madagascar, South Africa, Tanzania and Congo are among the well-recognized biodiversity hotspots in Africa (IUCN, 2014). These areas, especially Madagascar, which is endowed with a high level of endemism (about 90% of plant taxa), provide inestimable treasures that require stringent laws and regulations to ensure their protection. However, such laws and regulations are either non-existent or poorly implemented and enforced in many Africa countries (Cunningham, 1993). Currently, a number of medicinal plant species are severely threatened in the wild and are often difficult to find outside protected areas (Stuart *et al.*, 1990; Affolter and Pengelly, 2007; Williams *et al.*, 2013). Current data from IUCN (2014) provide an indication of the severity of these biodiversity losses in sub-Saharan Africa (Figure 23.3). The majority of critically endangered plant species are found in Madagascar, Cameroon and Tanzania. In addition to these countries, Nigeria and Kenya are also faced with a high number of vulnerable plant species.

## 23.5   Future perspectives

Following the adoption of policy and legislative frameworks to regulate, promote, develop and standardize the practice of ATM by some countries, it is becoming increasingly clear that provision of healthcare in the 21st century will be driven by a preventative approach based on natural products and healthy lifestyles. Successful integration of herbal medicine into mainstream healthcare in Africa will partially depend on interdisciplinary research in ethnopharmacology that encompasses various disciplines, namely ethnobotany, pharmacology, phytochemistry and toxicology. Several authors (Busia, 2005; Light *et al.*, 2005; Albertyn *et al.*, 2014; Kamsu-Foguem and Foguem, 2014b) have lamented the dearth of comprehensive toxicology studies for commonly used herbal medical products in ATM, therefore for herbal medicines to be fully integrated in African healthcare systems there is an urgent need to improve their quality and safety through stricter regulatory controls (Busia, 2005).

Amongst the complex challenges pertaining to the use of indigenous plants as herbal medicines is the issue of intellectual property rights (George and van Staden, 2000). In a study of medicinal plant use in East Africa, Schlage *et al.* (2000) reiterated that local communities ought to be financially rewarded in terms of royalties for sharing their knowledge with scientists and other outsiders. Such issues can be addressed through a comprehensive policy and legal framework on ATM, for example the Biodiversity Act 2004 in South Africa. However, such legislation has been criticized for stifling innovation and the commercialization of South African medicinal plants (Myburgh, 2011). Depending on their unique circumstances, African countries also need to seriously focus on conservation of medicinal plants. The increasing commercial demand for some plants to supply both the local and international markets has led to localized uncontrolled, indiscriminate and sometimes illegal harvesting of wild populations, even driving some taxa into extinction. Whether done out of ignorance or greed, the long-term impacts of the current over-harvesting practices and habitat destruction are real and frightening. Consequently, there is a dire need for conservation strategies and the promotion of sustainable use of medicinal plants. In this regard, recent calls for the systematic cultivation of many more medicinal plant species (van Staden, 1999; Canter *et al.*, 2005; Lubbe and Verpoorte, 2011) require serious consideration.

## 23.6 Conclusions

The importance of medicinal plants and their contribution to the provision of primary health-care in Africa is well recognized. Equally profound is the scale of scientific advances in the field of ethnopharmacology emanating from numerous research endeavours across the African continent. The phenomenal increase in the number of scientific publications produced over the past few decades testifies to the renewed interest in the field of medicinal plant research. The same period has also witnessed the unprecedented efforts of numerous African countries to regularize the practice of traditional medicine. However, the paradox of ethnopharmacology in Africa is that despite the immensely unique floral richness and diversity, and its inherent potential for the discovery of novel pharmaceutical compounds, most of the research, which is largely based on *in vitro* models, remains preliminary and incomplete. Landmark plant-derived drug discoveries in other parts of the world, such as galanthamine, quinine and arteminisin, should provide inspiration in the search for the next generation of novel pharmaceuticals. In the future it is almost inevitable that nature-inspired molecules will again rescue humankind from some of the world's most daunting health challenges.

## Acknowledgements

We thank the University of KwaZulu-Natal, Claude Leon Foundation (Cape Town) and the National Research Foundation (NRF), Pretoria, South Africa for financial support. We thank Dr L.J. McGaw for valuable suggestions and advice.

## References

Abdullahi, A.A. (2011) Trends and challenges of traditional medicine in Africa. *African Journal of Traditional, Complementary and Alternative Medicines*, **8**, 115–123.

Adia, M.M., Anywar, G., Byamukama, R., *et al.* (2014) Medicinal plants used in malaria treatment by Prometra herbalists in Uganda. *Journal of Ethnopharmacology*, **155**, 580–588.

Affolter, J.M. and Pengelly, A. (2007) Conserving medicinal plant biodiversity, in *Veterinary Herbal Medicine* (eds S.G. Wynn and B.J. Fougère), Mosby, St Louis, pp. 257–263.

Agyare, C., Obiri, D.D., Boakye, Y.D. and Osafo, N. (2013) Anti-inflammatory and analgesic activities of African medicinal plants, in *Medicinal Plant Research in Africa* (ed. V. Kuete), Elsevier, Oxford, pp. 725–752.

Akinmoladun, A.C., Olaleye, M.T. and Farombi, E.O. (2014) Cardiotoxicity and cardioprotective effects of African medicinal plants, in *Toxicological Survey of African Medicinal Plants* (ed. V. Kuete), Elsevier, London, pp. 395–421.

Albertyn, R., Berg, A., Numanoglu, A. and Rode, H. (2014) Traditional burn care in sub-Saharan Africa: A long history with wide acceptance. *Burns*, 10.1016/j.burns.2014.06.005.

Amoo, S.O., Aremu, A.O., Moyo, M. and van Staden, J. (2012) Antioxidant and acetylcholinesterase-inhibitory properties of long-term stored medicinal plants. *BMC Complementary and Alternative Medicine*, **12**, 87.

Amoo, S.O., Aremu, A.O., Moyo, M. and van Staden, J. (2013) Assessment of long-term storage on antimicrobial and cyclooxygenase-inhibitory properties of South African medicinal plants. *Phytotherapy Research*, **27**, 1029–1035.

Aremu, A.O., Finnie, J.F. and van Staden, J. (2012) Potential of South African medicinal plants used as anthelmintics – Their efficacy, safety concerns and reappraisal of current screening methods. *South African Journal of Botany*, **82**, 134–150.

Brendler, T., Eloff, J.N., Gurib-Fakim, A. and Phillips, L.D. (2010) *African Herbal Pharmacopoeia*, Association for African Medicinal Plants Standards (AAMPS), Port Louis, Mauritius.

Bunalema, L., Obakiro, S., Tabuti, J.R.S. and Waako, P. (2014) Knowledge on plants used traditionally in the treatment of tuberculosis in Uganda. *Journal of Ethnopharmacology*, **151**, 999–1004.

Busia, K. (2005) Medical provision in Africa – past and present. *Phytotherapy Research*, **19**, 919–923.

Canter, P.H., Thomas, H. and Ernst, E. (2005) Bringing medicinal plants into cultivation: opportunities and challenges for biotechnology. *Trends in Biotechnology*, **23**, 180–185.

Cunningham, A.B. (1993) *African medicinal plants: Setting priorities at the interface between conservation and primary healthcare*, United Nations Educational, Scientific and Cultural Organisation (UNESCO).

Dzoyem, J.P., Tshikalange, E. and Kuete, V. (2013) Medicinal plants market and industry in Africa, in *Medicinal Plant Research in Africa* (ed. V. Kuete), Elsevier, Oxford, pp. 859–890.

Elgorashi, E., Stafford, G., Mulholland, D. and van Staden, J. (2004) Isolation of captan from *Cyrtanthus suaveolens*: the effect of pesticides on the quality and safety of traditional medicine. *South African Journal of Botany*, **70**, 512–514.

Eloff, J.N. (1999) It is possible to use herbarium specimens to screen for antibacterial components in some plants. *Journal of Ethnopharmacology*, **67**, 355–360.

Eloff, J.N. and McGaw, L.J. (2006) Plant extracts used to manage bacterial, fungal, and parasitic infections in Southern Africa, in *Modern Phytomedicine* (eds I. Ahmad, F. Aqil and M. Owais), Wiley-VCH Verlag GmbH & Co., KGaA, pp. 97–121.

Fennell, C.W., Light, M.E., Sparg, S.G., *et al.* (2004a) Assessing African medicinal plants for efficacy and safety: agricultural and storage practices. *Journal of Ethnopharmacology*, **95**, 113–121.

Fennell, C.W., Lindsey, K.L., McGaw, L.J., *et al.* (2004b) Assessing African medicinal plants for efficacy and safety: pharmacological screening and toxicology. *Journal of Ethnopharmacology*, **94**, 205–217.

Fomogne-Fodjo, M.C.Y., van Vuuren, S., Ndinteh, D.T., *et al.* (2014) Antibacterial activities of plants from Central Africa used traditionally by the Bakola pygmies for treating respiratory and tuberculosis-related symptoms. *Journal of Ethnopharmacology*, **155**, 123–131.

Fouche, G., Cragg, G.M., Pillay, P., *et al.* (2008) *In vitro* anticancer screening of South African plants. *Journal of Ethnopharmacology*, **119**, 455–461.

George, J. and van Staden, J. (2000) Intellectual property rights: plants and phytomedicinals – past history, present scenario and future prospects in South Africa. *South African Journal of Science*, **96**, 433–443.

Govender, S., Du Plessis-Stoman, D., Downing, T. and van de Venter, M. (2006) Traditional herbal medicines: microbial contamination, consumer safety and the need for standards. *South African Journal of Science*, **102**, 253–255.

Gurib-Fakim, A. (2006) Medicinal plants: traditions of yesterday and drugs of tomorrow. *Molecular Aspects of Medicine*, **27**, 1–93.

Houghton, P.J., Howes, M.J., Lee, C.C. and Steventon, G. (2007) Uses and abuses of *in vitro* tests in ethnopharmacology: visualizing an elephant. *Journal of Ethnopharmacology*, **110**, 391–400.

Hutchings, A., Scott, A.H., Lewis, G. and Cunningham, A. (1996) *Zulu Medicinal Plants*. An Inventory, University of Natal Press, Pietermaritzburg.

Ibekwe, N.N., Nvau, J.B., Oladosu, P.O., *et al.* (2014) Some Nigerian anti-tuberculosis ethnomedicines: A preliminary efficacy assessment. *Journal of Ethnopharmacology*, **155**, 524–532.

Ibrahim, M.A., Mohammed, A., Isah, M.B. and Aliyu, A.B. (2014) Anti-trypanosomal activity of African medicinal plants: A review update. *Journal of Ethnopharmacology*, **154**, 26–54.

IUCN (2014) *The IUCN Red List of Threatened Species*, Version 2014.2, http://www.iucnredlist.org/about/summary-statistics#Tables_5_6, accessed on 20 September 2014.

Iwu, M.M. (1993) *Handbook of African Medicinal Plants*, CRC Press, Boca Raton.

Iwu, M.M. (2014) *Handbook of African Medicinal Plants*, 2nd edn, CRC Press, Boca Raton.

Kamatenesi-Mugisha, M., Asiimwe, S., Namutebi, A., *et al.* (2014) Ethnobotanical study of indigenous knowledge on medicinal and nutritious plants used to manage opportunistic infections associated with HIV/AIDS in western Uganda. *Journal of Ethnopharmacology*, **155**, 194–202.

Kamsu-Foguem, B. and Foguem, C. (2014a) Adverse drug reactions in some African herbal medicine: literature review and stakeholders' interview. *Integrative Medicine Research*, **3**, 126–132.

Kamsu-Foguem, B. and Foguem, C. (2014b) Could telemedicine enhance traditional medicine practices? *European Research in Telemedicine/La Recherche Européenne en Télémédecine*, **3**, 117–123.

Kasilo, O.M., Trapsida, J.-M., Mwikisa, C. and Lusamba-Dikassa, P.S. (2010) An overview of the traditional medicine situation in the African region, in *The African Health Monitor*, (ed. WHO), pp. 1–15.

Katerere, D., Stockenström, S., Thembo, K., *et al.* (2008) A preliminary survey of mycological and fumonisin and aflatoxin contamination of African traditional herbal medicines sold in South Africa. *Human and Experimental Toxicology*, **27**, 793–798.

Kaume, L., Foote, J.C. and Gbur, E.E. (2012) Microbial contamination of herbs marketed to HIV-infected people in Nairobi (Kenya). *South African Journal of Science*, **108**, 4 pp, 10.4102/sajs.v108i9/10.563.

Kokwaro, J.O. (1976) *Medicinal Plants of East Africa*, East African Literature Bureau, Kampala.

Kokwaro, J.O. (1993) *Medicinal Plants of East Africa*, 2nd edn, Kenya Literature Bureau, Nairobi.

Kokwaro, J.O. (2009) *Medicinal Plants of East Africa*, University of Nairobi Press, Nairobi.

Kuete, V. (2013) *Medicinal Plant Research in African: Pharmacology and Chemistry*, Elsevier, Oxford.

Kuete, V. (2014) *Toxicological Survey of African Medicinal Plants*, Elsevier, London.

Kuete, V., Viertel, K. and Efferth, T. (2013) Antiproliferative potential of African medicinal plants, in *Medicinal Plant Research in Africa* (ed. V. Kuete), Elsevier. Oxford, pp. 711–724.

Kunle, O.F., Egharevba, H.O. and Ahmadu, P.O. (2012) Standardization of herbal medicines – A review. *International Journal of Biodiversity and Conservation*, **4**, 101–112.

Laher, F., Aremu, A.O., van Staden, J. and Finnie, J.F. (2013) Evaluating the effect of storage on the biological activity and chemical composition of three South African medicinal plants. *South African Journal of Botany*, **88**, 414–418.

Light, M.E., Sparg, S.G., Stafford, G.I. and van Staden, J. (2005) Riding the wave: South Africa's contribution to ethnopharmacological research over the last 25 years. *Journal of Ethnopharmacology*, **100**, 127–130.

Lubbe, A. and Verpoorte, R. (2011) Cultivation of medicinal and aromatic plants for specialty industrial materials. *Industrial Crops and Products*, **34**, 785–801.

Madikizela, B., Ndhlala, A.R., Finnie, J.F. and van Staden, J. (2012) Ethnopharmacological study of plants from Pondoland used against diarrhoea. *Journal of Ethnopharmacology*, **141**, 61–71.

Madikizela, B., Ndhlala, A.R., Finnie, J.F. and van Staden, J. (2014) Antimycobacterial, anti-inflammatory and genotoxicity evaluation of plants used for the treatment of tuberculosis and related symptoms in South Africa. *Journal of Ethnopharmacology*, **153**, 386–391.

Mander, M. (1997) *Medicinal Plants Marketing and Strategies for Sustaining the Plant Supply in the Bushbuckridge Area and Mpumalanga Province, South Africa*, Department of Water Affairs and Forestry, Pretoria.

McGaw, L.J., Jäger, A.K. and van Staden, J. (2000) Antibacterial, anthelmintic and anti-amoebic activity in South African medicinal plants. *Journal of Ethnopharmacology*, **72**, 247–263.

McGaw, L.J., Lall, N., Meyer, J.J.M. and Eloff, J.N. (2008) The potential of South African plants against *Mycobacterium* infections. *Journal of Ethnopharmacology*, **119**, 482–500.

Mohammed, A., Ibrahim, M.A. and Islam, M.S. (2014) African medicinal plants with antidiabetic potentials: A review. *Planta Medica*, **80**, 354–377.

Moyo, M. and van Staden, J. (2014) Medicinal properties and conservation of *Pelargonium sidoides* DC. *Journal of Ethnopharmacology*, **152**, 243–255.

Muthee, J.K., Gakuya, D.W., Mbaria, J.M., *et al.* (2011) Ethnobotanical study of anthelmintic and other medicinal plants traditionally used in Loitoktok district of Kenya. *Journal of Ethnopharmacology*, **135**, 15–21.

Myburgh, A.F. (2011) Legal developments in the protection of plant-related traditional knowledge: An intellectual property lawyer's perspective of the international and South African legal framework. *South African Journal of Botany*, **77**, 844–849.

Nafiu, M.O., Salawu, M.O. and Kazeem, M.I. (2013) Antioxidant activity of African medicinal plants, in *Medicinal Plant Research in Africa* (ed. V. Kuete), Elsevier, Oxford, pp. 787–803.

Nair, J.J. and van Staden, J. (2013) Pharmacological and toxicological insights to the South African Amaryllidaceae. *Food and Chemical Toxicology*, **62**, 262–275.

Nair, J.J. and van Staden, J. (2014) Cytotoxicity studies of lycorine alkaloids of the Amaryllidaceae. *Natural Product Communications*, **9**, 1193–1210.

Nair, J.J., Aremu, A.O. and van Staden, J. (2011) Isolation of narciprimine from *Cyrtanthus contractus* (Amaryllidaceae) and evaluation of its acetylcholinesterase inhibitory activity. *Journal of Ethnopharmacology*, **137**, 1102–1106.

Nair, J.J., Rárová, L., Strnad, M., *et al.* (2012) Apoptosis-inducing effects of distichamine and narciprimine, rare alkaloids of the plant family Amaryllidaceae. *Bioorganic and Medicinal Chemistry Letters*, **22**, 6195–6199.

Ndhlala, A.R., Stafford, G.I., Finnie, J.F. and van Staden, J. (2011) Commercial herbal preparations in KwaZulu-Natal, South Africa: The urban face of traditional medicine. *South African Journal of Botany*, **77**, 830–843.

Ndhlala, A.R., Aremu, A.O., Moyo, M., *et al.* (2012) Acetylcholineterase inhibitors from plant sources: friends or foes? in *Cholinesterase: Production, Uses and Health Effects* (eds C.J. White and J.E. Tait), Nova, New York, pp. 67–98.

Ndhlala, A.R., Amoo, S.O., Ncube, B., *et al.* (2013) Antibacterial, antifungal, and antiviral activities of African medicinal plants, in *Medicinal Plant Research in Africa: Pharmacology and Chemistry* (ed. V. Kuete), Elsevier, Oxford, pp. 621–659.

Ndhlala, A., Ncube, B. and van Staden, J. (2014) Antioxidants versus reactive oxygen species – A tug of war for human benefits? in *Systems Biology of Free Radicals and Antioxidants* (ed. I. Laher), Springer, Berlin and Heidelberg, pp. 3987–4002.

Neuwinger, H.D. (2000) *African Traditional Medicine*. A Dictionary of Plant Use and Applications, Medpharm Scientific Publishers, Stuttgart.

Newman, D.J. and Cragg, G.M. (2012) Natural products as sources of new drugs over the 30 years from 1981–2010. *Journal of Natural Products*, **75**, 311–335.

Obi, E., Akunyili, D.N., Ekpo, B. and Orisakwe, O.E. (2006) Heavy metal hazards of Nigerian herbal remedies. *Science of the Total Environment*, **369**, 35–41.

Ochwang'i, D.O., Kimwele, C.N., Oduma, J.A., *et al.* (2014) Medicinal plants used in treatment and management of cancer in Kakamega County, Kenya. *Journal of Ethnopharmacology*, **151**, 1040–1055.

Sanogo, R. (2014) Development of phytodrugs from indigenous plants: The Mali experience, in *Novel Plant Bioresources* (ed. A. Gurib-Fakim), John Wiley & Sons, Ltd, pp. 191–203.

Schlage, C., Mabula, C., Mahunnah, R.L.A. and Heinrich, M. (2000) Medicinal plants of the Washambaa (Tanzania): Documentation and ethnopharmacological evaluation. *Plant Biology*, **2**, 83–92.

Soh, P.N. and Benoit-Vical, F. (2007) Are West African plants a source of future antimalarial drugs? *Journal of Ethnopharmacology*, **114**, 130–140.

Stafford, G.I., Jäger, A.K. and van Staden, J. (2005) Effect of storage on the chemical composition and biological activity of several popular South African medicinal plants. *Journal of Ethnopharmacology*, **97**, 107–115.

Steenkamp, V., Stewart, M.J., Curowska, E. and Zuckerman, M. (2002) A severe case of multiple metal poisoning in a child treated with a traditional medicine. *Forensic Science International*, **128**, 123–126.

Stewart, M.J., Steenkamp, V. and Zuckerman, M. (1998) The toxicology of African herbal remedies. *Therapeutic Drug Monitoring*, **20**, 510–516.

Stewart, M.J., Moar, J.J., Steenkamp, P. and Kokot, M. (1999) Findings in fatal cases of poisoning attributed to traditional remedies in South Africa. *Forensic Science International*, **101**, 177–183.

Street, R.A. (2012) Heavy metals in medicinal plant products – An African perspective. *South African Journal of Botany*, **82**, 67–74.

Street, R.A., Stirk, W.A. and van Staden, J. (2008) South African traditional medicinal plant trade – challenges in regulating quality, safety and efficacy. *Journal of Ethnopharmacology*, **119**, 705–710.

Stuart, S.N., Adams, R.J. and Jenkins, M.D. (1990) *Biodiversity in Sub-Saharan Africa and its Islands Conservation, Management, and Sustainable Use. A Contribution to the Biodiversity Conservation Strategy Programme*, IUCN – The World Conservation Union, Cambridge.

van Staden, J. (1999) Medicinal plants in southern Africa: utilization, sustainability, conservation – can we change the mindsets? *Outlook on Agriculture*, **28**, 75–76.

van Vuuren, S., Williams, V.L., Sooka, A., *et al.* (2014) Microbial contamination of traditional medicinal plants sold at the Faraday muthi market, Johannesburg, South Africa. *South African Journal of Botany*, **94**, 95–100.

van Wyk, B.-E. (2008) A broad review of commercially important southern African medicinal plants. *Journal of Ethnopharmacology*, **119**, 342–355.

van Wyk, B.-E., van Heerden, F.R. and van Oudtshoon, B. (2002) *Poisonous Plants of South Africa*, Briza Publications, Pretoria.

Verschaeve, L. and van Staden, J. (2008) Mutagenic and antimutagenic properties of extracts from South African traditional medicinal plants. *Journal of Ethnopharmacology*, **119**, 575–587.

Wambebe, C., Khamofu, H., Momoh, J.A.F., *et al.* (2001) Double-blind, placebo-controlled, randomised cross-over clinical trial of NIPRISAN® in patients with sickle cell disorder. *Phytomedicine*, **8**, 252–261.

Wansi, J.D., Devkota, K.P., Tshikalange, E. and Kuete, V. (2013) Alkaloids from the medicinal plants of Africa, in *Medicinal Plant Research in Africa* (ed. V. Kuete), Elsevier, Oxford, pp. 557–605.

Watt, J.M. and Breyer-Brandwijk, M.G. (1962) *The Medicinal and Poisonous Plants of Southern and Eastern Africa*, 2nd edn, Livingstone, London.

WHO (2005) *National policy on traditional medicine and regulation of herbal medicines: report of a global WHO survey*, WHO, Geneva.

WHO (2013) WHO traditional medicine strategy *2014–2023*, 1–78, WHO, Geneva.

WHO (2014) *Global health estimates 2014 summary tables: Death by cause, age and sex, by WHO region, 2000–2012*, WHO, Geneva.

Williams, V.L., Victor, J.E. and Crouch, N.R. (2013) Red Listed medicinal plants of South Africa: Status, trends, and assessment challenges. *South African Journal of Botany*, **86**, 23–35.

Zofou, D., Kuete, V. and Titanji, V.P.K. (2013) Antimalarial and other antiprotozoal products from African medicinal plants, in *Medicinal Plant Research in Africa* (ed. V. Kuete), Elsevier, Oxford, pp. 661–709.

# 24
# Ethnopharmacology and Integrative Medicine: An Indian Perspective

Pulok K. Mukherjee[1], Sushil K. Chaudhary[1], Shiv Bahadur[1] and Pratip K. Debnath[2]

[1]School of Natural Product Studies, Department of Pharmaceutical Technology, Jadavpur University, Kolkata, India
[2]Gananath Sen Institute of Ayurveda and Research, Kolkata, India

## 24.1 Ethnopharmacology and the development of traditional medicine in India

India is recognized amongst the 12-mega diverse regions in the world, including 15 agro-climatic zones. It is the world's richest sources of biodiversity in terms of medicinal plants. It has been estimated that about 15,000–20,000 plant species with high medicinal value (out of approximately 47,000 plant species) are found in India and these are the backbone of our indigenous systems of medicine, such as Ayurveda, Unani and Siddha (Mukherjee *et al.*, 2012). Medicinal plants and products derived from them have a tremendous impact in India because of their wide-ranging biological activities, higher safety margin and lower costs compared to synthetic drugs (Nema *et al.*, 2011).

Today, evidence-based uses of such preparations receive significant acceptance in India. The concept and methods of ethnopharmacological research incorporate elements from diverse medical practices like Ayurveda and Siddha, and scientific disciplines like ethnobotany/ethnomedicine, anthropology, chemistry, pharmacognosy, pharmacology, biochemistry, molecular biology, pharmacy etc. (Raza, 2006). The main objective of ethnopharmacology is to develop appropriate techniques to evaluate local and traditional remedies in line with the medical concepts of the respective medical traditions, like Ayurvedic medicine. Importantly, any evaluation of traditional remedies, particularly those of classical traditions, has to be

*Ethnopharmacology*, First Edition. Edited by Michael Heinrich and Anna K. Jäger.
© 2015 John Wiley & Sons, Ltd. Published 2015 by John Wiley & Sons, Ltd.

ॐ सर्वे भवन्तु सुखिनः सर्वे सन्तु निरामयाः ।
सर्वे भद्राणि पश्यन्तु मा कश्चिद्दुःखभाग्भवेत् ।
ॐ शान्तिः शान्तिः शान्तिः ॥

*"Om Sarve Bhavantu Sukhinah Sarve Santu Nir-Aamayaah ।*
*Sarve Bhadraanni Pashyantu, Maa Kashcid-Duhkha-Bhaag-Bhavet ॥*
*Om Shaantih Shaantih Shaantih"*

(May all remain happy, May all remain disease free, May All See what
is Auspicious, May no one Suffer, Let Peace prevail)
*Brihadaaranyaka Upanisad 1.4.14*

**Figure 24.1**  The goals of Ayurveda.

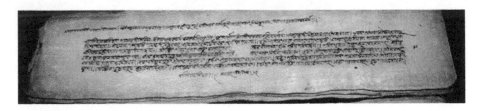

प्रयोजनं चास्य स्वस्थस्य स्वास्थ्यरक्षणमातुरस्य विकारप्रशमनं च

*'Prayojanang  Chhasya Swasthaasya*
*Swasthaarakshanamaaturashya Vikaraprasanamang Cha'*

**It is a prerequisite to protect health of the healthy
and to alleviate the disorders in the diseased.**
**(*Charaka Samhita, Sutra Sthana* 30/26)**

**Figure 24.2**  The objective of Ayurveda in *Charaka Samhita*.

based on the theoretical and conceptual foundation of these classical systems of medicine (Mukherjee *et al.*, 2009a).

India has a strong base of many systems of medicines, including Ayurveda, Unani, Siddha and other local health practices. The earliest mention of medicinal plants in India is found in different *vedas* (Sanskrit *ved* = 'knowledge') dating back to roughly 1500–1000 BCA. *Vedas* are ancient Indian religious treaties described in a large written body of knowledge. Four *vedas* are known: Rig veda, Yajur veda, Atharva veda and Sama veda. Diseases and cures by medicinal plants are important elements in some *vedas*. Rig veda (67 medicinal plants), Yajur veda (81 medicinal plants) and Atharva veda (290 medicinal plant species) with Charak Samhita (700 BC) and Sushruta Samhita (200 BC) are the traditional databases (Sinha, 2002).

Ayurveda – the science and art of life or living – is accepted as one of the ancient documented comprehensive medical systems. The Vedic literature (Brihadaaranyaka Upanisad, 1.4.14), the most ancient written document of India, presents the perception of health of that time (Figure 24.1). It reveals that *nirmaya* (disease-free healthy living) can only be attained through happiness (*sarve sukhina bhabantu*) and peace (*shaantih*). Later on this belief-based medical philosophy transformed to reason-based Ayurveda, which is considered as an Upaveda (or branch of the original *veda*), which just like any other science has been created on the basis of knowledge-based observations, evidence and logical deductions (Debnath *et al*, 2015).

Ayurveda based on herbal remedies has always played a key role in Indian healthcare systems (Figure 24.2). Modern treatment facilities do not reach marginalized indigenous people or people who live far away from towns (WHO, 2002). Although the therapeutic usefulness of these medicinal plants and the preparations derived from them is reported by traditional practitioners, such uses have not been validated scientifically. Thus, ethnopharma-cologists typically develop working hypotheses derived from field observations. One of the main research goals is to enhance the knowledge of local communities incorporating scientific findings into traditional practice (Gertsch, 2009).

## 24.2   Biological wealth and ancient wisdom

Approximately 15,000 medicinal plants species are used in different systems of medicine, such as popular practice (44%), Ayurveda (19%), Siddha (12%), Unani (10%), homeopathy (8%), Tibetan (5%) and modern medicine (2%) (Mukherjee and Wahile, 2006).

The knowledge about the cultivation, management, processing and utilization of medicinal plant products is inadequate primarily due to lack of research and awareness. In addition, the supply of selected seeds and manufacturing processes to produce world-class products with a very high standard of quality control should be ensured (Mukherjee *et al.*, 2012).

## 24.3   Indian systems of medicine

Today Ayurveda, yoga and naturopathy, Unani, Siddha and homeopathy are the official Indian traditional systems of medicine (AYUSH, 2011a). In March 1995 the Department of Indian Systems of Medicines and Homeopathy (ISM&H) was established as a separate department in the Indian Ministry of Health and Family Welfare. It was re-named the Department of Ayurveda, Yoga & Naturopathy, Unani, Siddha and Homoeopathy (AYUSH) in November 2003, with a vision to provide quality control and standardization of drugs, and to facilitate the generation of awareness about these systems by upgrading national and international educational standards (Mukherjee, 2002). Within this department there are five research councils, two statutory councils, three subordinate offices, eleven national institutes and one drug manufacturing unit established at national level for promoting current research, clinical practices and related aspects (Nema *et al.*, 2011).

Contributions are made by historians of science, clinicians, ethnographers, agronomists, biochemists and researchers in veterinary medicine and other disciplines. The constituents and activities of medicinal plants and the effects of the variations in the collection and storage of plants and the preparation and administration of medicines, which affects pharmacologic profiles, are a key focus of the Department of AYUSH (Mukherjee *et al.*, 2012).

It is important to identity the medicinal plants suitable for specific soil and climatic conditions and promote them among farmers. The farmers and villagers of areas with large indigenous populations play a major role in social entrepreneurship initiatives for cultivating various medicinal plants required by the pharmaceutical industry. Farmers should be left to cultivate while independent organizations should focus on post-harvest processing and storage together with the network for marketing. Business opportunities in this sector are enormous due to the diversified uses of plant-derived molecules and compounds in the pharmaceuticals, nutrition and agro-chemical industries (Mukherjee *et al.*, 2010a). There is a need to understand the possible pharmacological uses of medicinal plants and encourage pharmaceutical industries to utilize natural molecules from the medicinal plants in their products. This will also encourage the export of products derived from medicinal plants (Dutt, 2014).

## 24.4   Ayurveda: the Indian system of medicine

Ayurveda, accepted as one of the oldest treatises on medical systems, came into existence in about 900 BC. According to Indian Hindu mythology, there are four *vedas* written by the Aryans: Rigveda, Shamaveda, Yajurveda and Atharvaveda. Among these, Rigveda, the oldest, was written after 1500 BC. The Ayurveda is said to be an Upaveda (part) of Atharvaveda, whereas the Charaka Samhita (1900 BC) is the first recorded treatise fully devoted to the concept of the practice of Ayurveda (Mukherjee *et al.*, 2010b).

According to Ayurveda, all matters consist of five basic elements (*panchamahabhutas*) (Anonymous, 2001): the first element is space (*aakash*) and the others are earth (*prithivi*), air (*vayu*), water (*jala*) and fire (*agni*), which exist within the space (Atreya, 2002). Both the human (microcosm) and universal (macrocosm) systems are linked permanently, since both are built from the same elements. According to Ayurveda, a human being is a replica of nature and everything that affects the human being also influences the macrocosm (Heyn, 1990). Along with these panchamahabhutas, the functional aspects of movement, transformation and growth are governed by three biological humours: *vata* (space and air), *pitta* (fire and water) and *kapha* (water and earth) (Atreya, 2002). Ayurveda is widely respected for its uniqueness and global acceptance as it offers natural ways to treat diseases and promote healthcare (Mukherjee and Houghton, 2009).

### 24.4.1   Panchakarma

Panchakarma is a specialty of Ayurveda, which has diversified defensive healing and support for wide range of diseases and health conditions. It is a personalized medicine concept where a therapeutic regimen is designed according to the Prakriti of individual patients (individual characteristics). Every individual is born with his/her own basic constitution, termed *Prakriti*, which is important to determine the inter-individual variability in susceptibility to diseases and response to external environment, diet and drugs (Mukerji and Prasher, 2011). These therapeutic procedures are employed to get rid of the impurities of various systems of the human body and force toxic metabolites from the body by maintaining the normal functions of the system. They also enhance the acceptability of the body to various dietary regimens and use rejuvenation therapy for promoting health as well as for specific therapeutics. The group of five major detoxification measures comprising *Vamana* (therapeutic emesis), *Virechana* (therapeutic purgation), *Anuvasana vasti* (induced enema with medical oils), *Niruha vasti* (induced enema with decoction of plants) and *nasya* (nasal administration of medicaments) are technically termed *panchakarma*, which has its basis in the basic principles and practices of Ayurveda. It comprises *deepana-Pachana* (enhances enzyme activities), *Snehana* (oleation, i.e. lubricating the system using unctuous substances like oil or ghee externally and internally) and *Swedana* (applying heat over the body to stimulate the action of sweat glands to secrete sweat, as well as to increase body temperature and circulation). There are many procedures to perform depending on the conditions (Mukherjee *et al.*, 2010c).

*Vamana karma* is one of the *panchakarma* procedures indicated for Kapha disorders as mentioned in the Ayurvedic pathology. The oral administration of emetic drugs in particular dosages with large amounts of liquid, such as milk, or a decoction of madhuka (*Glycerhizza glabra* L. - Fabaceae) is regarded to be effective in bronchial asthma, psoriasis and other chronic skin diseases. *Virechana karma* (therapeutic purgation) is done by the oral administration of specific purgative drugs in specific dosage form. This treatment is highly appreciated in *pitta* and *vata* predominant diseases such as skin diseases, urinary disorders, diabetes, ano-rectal diseases, arthritis, hemiplegia, etc.

*Anuvasana* (induced enema with oils) and *Niruha vasti* (induced enema with decoction of plants) are indicated in *vata* predominant diseases, such as arthritis, constipation, sciatica, hemiplegia, amenorrhea etc. *Nasya karma* (nasal application of drugs) is especially employed in specific disease conditions in headache, brachial neuralgia, ear ache, chronic sinusitis, facial palsy etc. The regimen after completion of the principle therapy is very important in *panchakarma*. This is done to revitalize the *Agni* (metabolic enzyme system), which becomes imbalanced due to the processes. This regimen should be followed strictly. Commonly *peyadi samsarjana karma* (medicated drink therapy) is widely practiced in all cases of *pradhan karma*, causing the enhancement of enzyme activities in the patient. In this procedure no oral medicine(s) targeting the disease is administered, but a diet schedule including liquid, semisolids and solids is given successively. These therapies encompass the original fundamental essence of Ayurvedic treatment and are regarded as highly effective in different diseases, lifestyle disorders and degenerative diseases (Mitra *et al.*, 2011).

There are many well-known books dealing with compound formulations in Ayurveda. While *Sarngadhara Samhita*, *Chakradatta*, *Bhaisajya Ratnavali*, *Sahasrayogum*, *Bharat Bhaishajya Ratnakara* and others deal with both single or groups of formulations, others like *Rasendra Sarasangraha*, *Rasarathna Samuccaya*, *Rasaprakasam Sudhakara*, *Ayurveda prakasa*, *Rasatarangini* and *Rasayogasagara* deal only with the Rasausadhi group of formulations. Ayurveda is based on experiences and as such on the observation of therapeutic outcomes. It has been divided into eight major disciplines known as *Astanga ayurveda*, a major component of which includes *kaya chikitsa* (medicine), *sulya chikitsa* (surgery), *salakya chikitsa* (ear, nose and throat treatment), *bala chikitsa* (pediatric treatment), *jara chikitsa* (treatment related to genetics), *rasayana chikitsa* (treatment with chemicals), *vajikarama chikitsa* (treatment with rejuvenation and aphrodisiacs), *graham chikitsa* (planetary effects) and *visha chikitsa* (toxicology), as shown in Figure 24.3 (Mukherjee *et al.*, 2009a).

## 24.4.2 Validation of classical Ayurvedic formulation

Reserpine is an alkaloid from *Rauvolfia serpentina* Benth. (Apocynaceae) that received international attention for the twin effect of lowering high blood pressure and acting as a tranquillizer (Woodson *et al.*, 1957). Shatavarin-I, a glycoside isolated from the Ayurvedic drug obtained from the roots of *Asparagus racemosus* Willd. (Liliaceae, s.l.), is recommended as a treatment to prevent miscarriage (Gaitunde and Jetmalani, 1969).

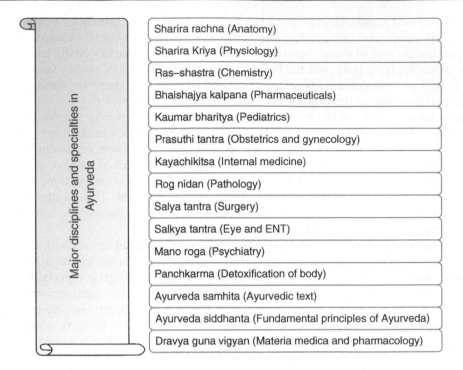

**Figure 24.3**   Major disciplines and specialties in Ayurveda.

### 24.4.2.1  Triphala

*Triphala* is a classic example of a polyherbal formulation in Ayurveda that has synergistic and counter-balancing properties. It contains dried fruits of *Emblica officinalis* Gaertn. (Euphorbiaceae), *Terminalia belerica* Roxb. and *T. chebula* Retz. (Combretaceae) in equal proportions (1:1:1). This formulation has been prescribed for many ailments, for example as a laxative in chronic constipation, a detoxifying agent of the colon, for digestive problems and as a rejuvenator of the body. Standardization and marker profiling of *triphala* formulations have been established through the quantitative determination of gallic acid and ellagic acid using HPLC (Mukherjee *et al.*, 2008) and RP-HPLC (Figure 24.4) (Ponnusankar *et al.*, 2011).

### 24.4.2.2  Trikatu

*Trikatu* is a very well-known polyherbal *Rasayana* formulation. It is a mixture of three acrid tasting drugs, *Piper longum* L., *P. nigrum* L. (Piperaceae) and *Zingiber officinale* Rosc. (Zingiberaceae), in a ratio of 1:1:1. It has been prescribed for cough, cold, fever, asthma, respiratory problems and improvement of digestive disorders. Marker profiling and standardization of *trikatu* through RP-HPLC for the identification and quantification of piperine and 6-gingerol has been reported (Harwansh *et al.*, 2014) (Figure 24.5).

## 24.4.3  Ayurgenomics

Pharmacogenomics is the study of the hereditary basis for differences in the response of populations to a drug. In Ayurveda the therapeutic regimen is designed according to the *prakriti* of individual patients and individual characteristics governed by what is today termed

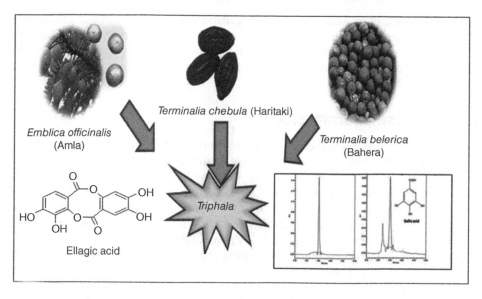

**Figure 24.4** Validation of an Ayurvedic formulation *triphala* by HPLC.

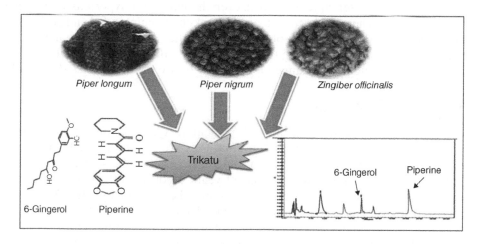

**Figure 24.5** Validation of an Ayurvedic formulation *trikatu* by HPLC.

ayurgenomics. Every individual has his/her own basic constitution, termed *prakriti*, which is important to determine inter-individual variability (Mukerji and Prasher, 2011).

Better understanding of the human genome has helped in understanding the scientific basis of individual variation. The same dose of a drug will result in elevated plasma concentrations for some patients and low concentrations for others. Some patients will respond well to a drug, while others will not. A drug might show adverse effects in some patients, but not in others. The importance of such individual variations in health and disease is a basic principle of Ayurveda and was underlined by *charaka* some 4000 years ago as every individual is different from another and hence should be considered as a different entity (Mukherjee, 2001).

Ayurgenomics focuses on understanding the possible relationship between *prakruti* (nature) and genome. Functionally, this will involve creation of three organized databases that are capable of intelligently communicating with each other to give a customized prescription: these are human constitution (genotype), disease constitution (phenotype) and drug constitution (Mukherjee *et al.*, 2009b).

### 24.4.4   Reverse pharmacology

Reverse pharmacology is a research strategy based on observations of traditional treatments that is a trans-disciplinary approach integrating traditional knowledge, experimental observations and clinical experiences with the aim of reversing from the classical laboratory to clinic process to a clinic to laboratory approach (Simoes-Pires *et al.*, 2014). Ayurveda-based drug discovery uses this reverse pharmacology approach, in which drugs are first identified based on large-scale use in the population and validated in clinical trials. Time and cost are reduced for drug discovery from traditional medicine by reverse pharmacology (Patwardhan, 2007).

The Ayurvedic knowledge database allows drug researchers to start from a well-tested and safe botanical material. By using this knowledge the conventional drug discovery begins from patients instead of laboratories. The reverse pharmacology approach first confirms the activity of a drug (like an Ayurvedic drug), after which further studies should link the activity to bioactive components (Mukherjee *et al.*, 2011). This method emphasizes safety and efficacy, and is an alternative path for drug discovery. Drugs like reserpine, obtained from *Rauvolfia serpentina*, emerged only after 20 years of work even though its antihypertensive property was demonstrated long ago. There is a need to document unknown, unintended and desirable novel prophylactic and therapeutic effects in observational studies. Since not many new molecules are being developed, the scope of using this approach for validating traditional knowledge is tremendous and many studies are planned for the near future (Mukherjee *et al.*, 2009b).

### 24.4.5   Ayurinformatics

There is a need to build libraries of compounds present in Ayurvedic preparations. Although some institutions have small plant extract libraries, they are not in the public domain. Such libraries could serve as a powerful tool and a source of extracts to be screened for biological activities using high-throughput assays. In recent years, a considerable body of information has accumulated on the chemical constituents of Ayurvedic medicinal plants. This is reflected in the appearance of a number of new electronic databases that contain both structural details of several thousand herbal constituents and accompanying information on their uses in Ayurveda. Although obscure at first, many of the therapeutic categories found in the Ayurvedic *Materia Medica* are interpretable in western terminology and a variety of texts are now available in English. All the main classical works on Ayurveda, such as *Charaka Samhita*, *Sushruta Samhita*, *Ashtanga Sangraha* and *Astanga Hrdaya*, deal with drugs, their composition and action in addition to the other aspects of the medical system. Some of the Ayurvedic books, known as Nighantugranthas, such as *Dhanvantarinighantu*, *Kaiyadevanighantu*, *Bhavaprakasanighantu*, *Rajanighantu* and so on, deal mainly with a single drug, describing its characteristics and therapeutic action.

## 24.5   Siddha

This system was developed in the southern part of India, particularly in Tamil Nadu. Siddha refers to a being who has achieved a high degree of physical as well as spiritual perfection or enlightenment. Siddha science is the oldest traditional treatment system generated from Dravidian culture. Siddha flourished in the period of the Indus Valley civilization (c. 3300–1300 BCE). The Siddha system is almost analogous to Ayurveda, which was developed by 18 Siddhars, who glorified human beings as the highest form of birth and believed that preserving the human body was essential to achieving eternal bliss. Siddha drugs are derived from minerals, metals and plants. Processes like calcination of mercury, minerals, metals and the preparation of a super salt, *muppu* (animated mercury pills), with high potency are ample testimony of such medical concepts (Mukherjee *et al.*, 2009a). The preparations in which Siddhars specialize are metallic preparations (*chunnam*), which are alkaline, waxy preparations (*mezhugu*) and preparations that are impervious to water and flames (*kattu*). These preparations have a long shelf-life and their potency and efficacy improve with time. The use of metals and minerals forms an integral part of the Siddha system of therapy to cure diseases (Mukherjee *et al.*, 2007).

## 24.6  Unani

Unani medicine owes its origin to the ancient Greek culture. The Greek philosopher–physician Hippocrates (460–377 BCE) freed medicine from the realm of superstition and magic, and gave it the status of science. The Unani system of medicine is known in different parts of the world by various names, such as Arat medicine, Greco-Arab medicine, Loniah medicine, Islamic medicine and Oriental medicine. In this traditional system, single drugs or their combinations in raw form are preferred over a compound formulation. Unani medicine is the result of the fusion of various thoughts and experience of nations and countries with ancient cultural heritages, such as Egypt, Arabia, India, Iraq, Iran and other Middle East and Far East countries. Unani medicine had its heyday during the 13th and 17th centuries in India. At present, the Unani system of medicine, with its own recognized practitioners, hospitals and educational research institutions, forms an integral part of the national healthcare system in India.

Key elements of Unani medicine given in the formularies (Mukherjee *et al.*, 2009a) include:

- ethnopharmacological relevance for the selection of various medicinal plants, minerals, animal products etc.
- adverse drug–drug or food–drug interactions
- the use of various preservatives
- defined methods of administration
- the inclusion of restriction, avoidance and abstinence of certain foods (*parhez*)
- considerations of adverse drug effects
- guidelines for prescribing in extremes of age or in the presence of altered organ function or in pregnancy or lactation.

## 24.7  Traditional knowledge digital library

India is one of the 12 mega bio-diversity zones covering 2.4% of world's area but with 8% of global biodiversity (WHO, 2007). Providing information on traditional knowledge through databases is one of the approaches for the protection of traditional knowledge. Databases like the Traditional Knowledge Digital Library (TKDL) of India act as a bridge between traditional knowledge and patent examiners at the International Patent Offices. The Ethno-Medicinal Plants of Western Ghats database project in India safeguards the claims of the local communities on intellectual property right issues (Upadhya *et al.*, 2010). The TKDL databases that store traditional knowledge are seen as a medium for legal protection. However, the archiving of medicinal information should not just have the legal framework as its prime objective, but it should also be seen as a means of using traditional knowledge in the service of humanity. Databases on traditional knowledge should be the medium for hybridization of scientific and indigenous knowledge for sustainable use of bioresources (Ningthoujam *et al.*, 2012).

The TKDL for Ayurveda, Unani, Siddha and yoga is a collaborative project between the Council of Scientific and Industrial Research, the Ministry of Science and Technology, the Department of AYUSH and the Ministry of Health and Family Welfare. TKDL is an original proprietary database that is fully protected under national and international intellectual property rights. About 212,000 medicinal formulations (Ayurveda 82,900, Unani 115,300, Siddha 12,950) from 148 books are available in the public domain, and the database documents this information in a patent-compatible format in five international languages (English, French, German, Spanish and Japanese) (AYUSH, 2011a). The traditional medicinal knowledge exists in various local languages, such as Sanskrit, Urdu, Arabic, Persian and Tamil. TKDL aims to break the language and format barrier with the help of information technology tools and a novel classification system, i.e. traditional knowledge resource classification. This is an innovative approach that facilitates conversion to make the knowledge available for patent examiners in patent application format and an understandable language (Mukherjee *et al.*, 2010d). In 2003 the Inter-Governmental Committee of the World Intellectual Property Organization (WIPO) on intellectual property and genetic resources, traditional knowledge and expression of local culture adopted the international specifications and standards of traditional knowledge databases. A TKDL access agreement was concluded with the European patent office in February 2009, as a mutual beneficial agreement, since it enhances the quality of examination for traditional knowledge-based patent applications for the European patent office. It has been recognized by the Director General of WIPO (AYUSH, 2011b).

## 24.8   Integrated approaches for the development of Indian traditional medicine

There is a need to integrate traditional and modern (biomedical) medicine and several integrated approaches have been developed (Figure 24.6). Although traditional systems of medicine are recognized, their integration and mainstreaming in healthcare delivery systems, including in national programmes, remains a challenge (Mukherjee *et al.*, 2013).

Several schemes have been produced for the promotion, cultivation and regeneration of Indian medicinal plants as per pharmacopoeial standards. The National Medicinal Plant Board (NMPB) has been constituted to deal with different issues like conservation and cultivation, demand and supply, research and development, trade and export, quality control and standardization of medicinal plants (AYUSH, 2011a). The NMPB also takes initiatives to ensure the status of medicinal plants in respect of policy support, infrastructure, legislation and regulation, research and development, courses of study, quality control and standardization at national and international levels.

### 24.8.1   Strategies and innovations

Applications of ethnographic field methodologies have advanced over the last few decades and will continue to improve our understanding of the cultural construction and social transaction of healing in diverse cultures. An integrated, theory and issue-driven ethnopharmacology

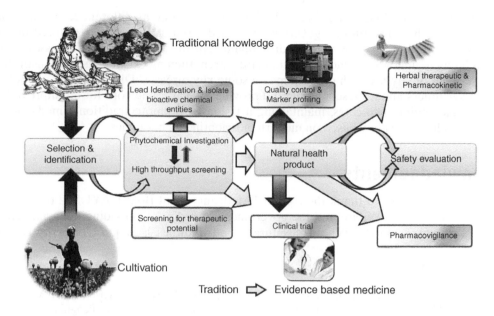

**Figure 24.6** Integrated approaches towards the development of Ayurveda.

will move from multidisciplinary to interdisciplinary to transdisciplinary methodologies that integrate the perspectives, objectives and tools of diverse disciplines (Mukherjee *et al.*, 2010d).

In order to bridge the demand gap for public health professionals in India, the plan is to step up the activities further to ensure AYUSH mainstreaming by developing/upgrading traditional medicine. AYUSH has started various training programmes for experts and officers to facilitate international exchange facilities, including providing incentives to manufacturers and entrepreneurs, the establishment of several institutions for international propagation of AYUSH, the development of a uniform policy, establishing AYUSH information cells in foreign countries, organizing international fellowships for undertaking AYUSH courses in premier institutions in India, conducting community-based research to assess the scope of AYUSH, and involving pharmacists in the implementation of various strategies (Singh, 2011; Kumar *et al.*, 2012).

The development of high-quality phyto-pharmaceutical product practices like good agriculture practice, good harvesting practice, good storage practice, good clinical practice, good therapeutic practice, good manufacturing practice and good laboratory practice is are urgently needed to meet global market expectations (Mukherjee *et al.*, 2009a).

The Society for Ethnopharmacology, India (SFE, www.ethnopharmacology.in) aims to disseminate knowledge on natural health products through globalization of local knowledge and localizing global technologies.

## 24.9 Conclusion

India has an ancient heritage of traditional medicine and India's *Materia Medica* provides a wealth of information on the local practices and traditional aspects of therapeutically important natural products. The major challenges of herbal medicine are quality, safety and efficacy. The government of India has taken several initiatives for the promotion and development of traditional medicine and ethnopharmacology at different levels, including establishing teaching institutions, government-funded research institutes, registered medical practitioners, hospitals, dispensaries and drug-manufacturing units. AYUSH addresses the key issues relating to upgrading educational standards, strengthening existing research institutions and ensuring a timely research programme on some key diseases. Different national policies increase awareness about these systems and provide a legal framework for an improved use of traditional Indian medicines, maintaining a vision to promote traditional medicine and ascertain quality and safety based on modern bioscientific technologies.

## Acknowledgements

The authors would like to thank the National Medicinal Plant Board, AYUSH, the Ministry of Health and Family Welfare and the government of India for providing financial support through a project grant to the School of Natural Product Studies, Jadavpur University, Kolkata.

## References

Anonymous (2001) *Caraka Samhita-Sharira Sthanam*, Chaukhamba Sanskrit Series Office, Varanasi.

Atreya (2002) *Perfect Balance: Ayurvedic Nutrition for Mind, Body, and Soul*, Penguin Putnam Inc., New York.

AYUSH (2011a) AYUSH in India, Planning & Evaluation Cell, Department of Ayurveda, Yoga & Naturopathy, Unani, Siddha and Homoeopathy, Ministry of Health and Family Welfare, Government of India.

AYUSH (2011b) *Traditional Knowledge Digital Library*, Department of AYUSH, Ministry of Health and Family Welfare, Government of India, New Delhi.

Debnath, P.K., Banerjee, S., Debnath, P., Mitra, A. and Mukherjee, .K. (2015) Ayurveda opportunities for developing safe and effective treatment choices for the Future, in *Evidence-based Validation of Herbal Medicine* (ed. P.K. Mukherjee), Elsevier, Netherlands/USA, pp. 427–451.

Dutt, S. (2012) Development of traditional medicine – A review, in *Traditional Medicine and Globalization – The Future of the Ancient System of Medicine* (ed. P.K. Mukherjee), Maven Publishers, Kolkata, pp. 8–11.

Gaitunde, B.B. and Jetmalani, M.H. (1969) Antioxytocic action of saponin isolated from Asparagus racemosus Willd. (Shatavari) on uterine muscle. *Archives Internationales de Pharmacodynamie et de Therapie*, **179**, 121–129.

Gertsch, J. (2009) How scientific is the science in ethnopharmacology? Historical perspectives and epistemological problems. *Journal of Ethnopharmacology*, **122**, 177–183.

Harwansh, R.K., Mukherjee, K., Bhadra, S., *et al.* (2014) Cytochrome P450 inhibitory potential and RP-HPLC standardization of trikatu – A Rasayana from Indian Ayurveda. *Journal of Ethnopharmacology*, **153**. 674–681.

Heyn B. (1990) *Ayurveda: The Ancient Indian Art of Natural Medicine & Life Extension*, Inner Traditions/Bear & Co, Vermont.

Kumar, D., Raina, S.K., Bhardwaj, A.K. and Chander, V. (2012) Capacity building of AYUSH practitioners to study the feasibility of their involvement in non-communicable disease prevention and control. *Ancient Science of Life*, **32**, 116–119.

Mitra, A., Banerjee, M., Das, B., *et al.* (2011) Acquiscence of Ayurvedic principles and practices in kitibha (Psoriasis) and excellent clinical responses – A case study. *Indian Journal of Traditional Knowledge*, **10**, 689–692.

Mukherjee, P.K. (2001) Evaluation of Indian traditional medicine. *Drug Information Journal*, **35**, 631–640.

Mukherjee, P.K. (2002) *Quality Control of Herbal Drugs – An Approach to Evaluation of Botanicals*, Business Horizons, New Delhi, pp. 604–608.

Mukherjee, P.K. (2003) Medicinal Plants for Indian System of Medicine, in *GMP for Botanicals* (eds R. Verpoorte and P.K. Mukherjee), Business Horizons Ltd, New Delhi, pp. 99–112.

Mukherjee, P.K. and Houghton, P.J. (2009) The worldwide phenomenon of increased use of herbal products: Opportunity and threats, in *Evaluation of Herbal Medicinal Products – Perspectives on Quality, Safety and Efficacy* (eds P.J. Houghton and P.K. Mukherjee), Pharmaceutical Press, Royal Pharmaceutical Society of Great Britain, pp. 3–12.

Mukherjee, P.K. and Wahile, A. (2006) Integrated approaches towards drug development from Ayurveda and other Indian system of medicines. *Journal of Ethnopharmacology*, **103**, 25–35.

Mukherjee, P.K., Rai, S., Kumar, V., *et al.* (2007) Plants of Indian origin in drug discovery. *Expert Opinion in Drug Discovery*, **2**, 633–657.

Mukherjee, P. K., Rai, S., Bhattacharya, S., *et al.* (2008) Marker analysis of polyherbal formulation, Triphala – A well-known Indian traditional medicine. *Indian Journal of Traditional Knowledge*, **7**, 379–383.

Mukherjee, P.K., Sahoo, A.K., Narayanan, N., *et al.* (2009a) Lead finding from medicinal plants with hepatoprotective potentials. *Expert Opinion on Drug Discovery*, **4**, 545–576.

Mukherjee, P.K., Venkatesh, M. and Gantait, A. (2009b) Ayurveda in Modern Medicine: Development and Modification of Bioactivity, in *Comprehensive Natural Products. II Chemistry and Biology, Vol 3* (eds L. Mander and H.-W. Lui), Elsevier Science, Oxford, pp. 479–507.

Mukherjee, P.K., Venkatesh, M. and Gantait, A. (2010a) Ayurveda in modern medicine: development and modification of bioactivity, in *Comprehensive Natural Products. II Chemistry and Biology* (eds L. Mander and H.-W. Lui), Elsevier Science, Oxford, pp. 479–507.

Mukherjee, P.K., Ponnusankar, S. and Venkatesh, M. (2010b) Ethnomedicine in complementary therapeutics, in *Ethnomedicine: A Source of Complementary Therapeutics* (ed. D. Chattopadhyay), Research Signpost, Trivandrum, pp. 29–52.

Mukherjee, P.K., Venkatesh, P., Venkatesh, M., *et al.* (2010c) Strategies for the revitalization of traditional medicine. *Chinese Herbal Medicines*, **2**, 1–15.

Mukherjee, P.K., Venkatesh, P. and Ponnusankar., S. (2010d) Ethnopharmacology and integrative medicine – let the history tell the future. *Journal of Ayurveda and Integrative Medicine*, **1**, 100–109.

Mukherjee, P.K., Ponnusankar, S. and Venkatesh, P. (2011) Synergy in herbal medicinal products: concept to realization. *Indian Journal of Pharmaceutical Education and Research*, **45**, 210–217.

Mukherjee, P.K., Nema, N.K., Venkatesh, P. and Debnath, P.K. (2012) Changing scenario for promotion and development of Ayurveda – way forward. *Journal of Ethnopharmacology*, **143**, 424–434.

Mukherjee, P.K., Bahadur S., Harwansh, R.K., *et al.* (2013) Development of traditional medicines: Globalizing local knowledge or localizing global technologies. *Pharma Times*, **45** (9).

Mukerji, M. and Prasher, B. (2011) Ayurgenomics: a new approach in personalized and preventive medicine. *Science and Culture*, **77**, 10–17.

Nema, N.K., Dalai, M.K. and Mukherjee, P.K. (2011) Ayush herbs and status que in herbal industries. *The Pharma Review*, **141–148**.

Ningthoujam, S. S., Talukdar, A.D., Potsangbam, K.S. and Choudhury, M.D. (2012) Challenges in developing medicinal plant databases for sharing ethnopharmacological knowledge. *Journal of Ethnopharmacology*, **141**, 9–32.

Patwardhan, B. (2007) Drug discovery and development: Traditional medicine and ethnopharmacology, New India Publishing Agency, New Delhi, pp. **284**, 307.

Ponnusankar, S., Pandit, S., Babu, R., *et al.* (2011) Cytochrome P450 inhibitory potential of Triphala – a rasayana from Ayurveda. *Journal of Ethnopharmacology*, **133**, 120–125.

Raza, M. (2006) A role for physicians in ethnopharmacology and drug discovery. *Journal of Ethnopharmacology*, **104**, 297–301.

Simoes-Pires, C., Hostettmann, K., Haouala, A., *et al.* (2014) Reverse pharmacology for developing an anti-malarial phytomedicine. *The example of Argemone mexicana. International Journal for Parasitology: Drugs and Drug Resistance*, **4**, 338–346.

Singh, R.H. (2011) Perspectives in innovation in the AYUSH sector. *Journal of Ayurveda and Integrated Medicine*, **2**, 52–54.

Sinha, P. (2002) Overview on diseases of medicinal plants and their management, in *Recent Progress in Medicinal Plants – Diseases and their Management* (eds J.N. Govil and V.K. Singh), Scientific and Technical Publishing LLC, pp. 1–212.

Upadhya, V., Hegde, H.V., Mesta, D., *et al.* (2010) Digital database on ethno-medicinal plants of Western Ghats. *Current Science*, **99**, 1658–1659.

WHO (2002) *Traditional Medicinal Strategy*, World Health Organization, Geneva, pp. 2002–2005.

WHO (2007) Country Cooperation Strategy 2006–2011 India. *Supplement on traditional medicine*, World Health Organization, Country Office for India, New Delhi.

Woodson, R.E., Youngken, H.W., Schlitter, E. and Schneider, J.A. (1957) Rauwolfia: Botany, *Pharmacognosy, Chemistry and Pharmacology*, Little Brown & Co, Boston.

# 25
# Chinese Medicine: Contentions and Global Complexities

Anthony Booker

*Research Cluster Biodiversity and Medicines' / Centre for Pharmacognosy and Phytotherapy, UCL School of Pharmacy, London, UK*

## 25.1 Introduction

Chinese medicine (CM) covers a wide range of treatment modalities originating in China and now practised widely in many countries (although often not in their original form). Most Asian countries have a long history of using traditional herbal medicines, which more recently are becoming popular in the USA and in Europe (NIH, 2007; IpsosMORI, 2009; UOM, 2011). The different types of CM practised, i.e. acupuncture, moxibustion and herbal medicine, share an underlying medico-philosophy that distinguishes them from biomedical and other practices. This philosophy has a theoretical base rooted within the wider concepts of Chinese Daoism, a naturalistic philosophy that focuses on the harmonious balance ever present within nature and regards disease as emanating from a disconnect with this balance. This more Eastern way of viewing illness has struck a resonance with a section of the general public outside China who often are looking for an alternative to orthodox medicine, although of course there is also a large section of the public who may purely use CM because they think it might help rather than having any connection to its theory. However, it is very much the theory and lack of evidence with regard to potential effectiveness that puts CM at odds with many of those within the established medical and scientific fields. This transdisciplinary tension, together with the lack of evidence, variability of practitioner training and poor safety and quality profile of many of the medicinal products are the main focus of this chapter.

According to many of the world's medical traditions, including CM, disease begins with minor imbalances within the body's systems. Often the body will correct these imbalances naturally through homeostasis and physiological regulatory processes. However, if the body is weak or continually subject to external influences that can prevent a return to a healthy state, then over time disease processes will manifest, eventually leading to symptoms that will also be well recognised through biomedical diagnostics. The primary focus of CM therefore is to

*Ethnopharmacology*, First Edition. Edited by Michael Heinrich and Anna K. Jäger.
© 2015 John Wiley & Sons, Ltd. Published 2015 by John Wiley & Sons, Ltd.

treat the individual before any major symptoms have arisen. In CM philosophy, no-one is considered in perfect health, some people are just less sick than others. This sentiment is summed up in an ancient Chinese text:

> 'Trying to cure disease once symptoms have arisen is like digging a well once you are already thirsty or forging a warrior's spear once the battle has already begun.'
>
> *Yellow Emperor's Classic of Internal Medicine* (Anon., 947–951 CE)

This is not to infer practitioners of CM only deal with healthy individuals, but that the emphasis is ideally on prevention rather than on cure. This thread of traditional medical philosophy continues when treating those with symptoms, where a practitioner of CM will attempt to establish the underlying cause of disease based on traditional medico-philosophical principles.

This, what is often perceived by the general public as a more preventative, holistic way of treating human beings has become increasingly popular in Europe, North America and Austral-Asia, and has led to significant increases in exports of traditional Asian remedies, including Chinese herbal medicinal products (CHMPs) (Vasisht and Kumar, 2002) along with other non-plant based practices such as acupuncture, tai chi, yoga and various forms of Asian massage and physical therapy.

## 25.2   Ancient concepts meet scientific understanding

CM is reputed to be one of the world's oldest medical systems, originating over 4000 years ago. Throughout the centuries different theories of practice have been presented and medicines (including flora, fauna and minerals) added to the *materia medica*. Probably the most famous of these is the Ben Cao Gang Mu 本草纲目 (*Compendium of Materia Medica*) written by Li Shizhen (1518–1593) over a period of 27 years, with the first draft appearing in 1578. It contains 1892 entries for medicines derived from plant, animal and mineral origin, and includes 11,096 different formulae.

Throughout the diversity of knowledge that contributes to CM, one unifying factor is that it derives from a body of written historical texts, e.g. the Shang Han Lun,傷寒論 (*Treatise on Cold Damage*) and the Wen Bing Xue, 溫病學 (*Warm Disease Theory*). However, the extent that these texts are used in the modern teaching curriculum of different educational establishments throughout the world may vary.

In China, the simplification of the written Chinese language during the latter half of the 20th century aimed to increase access to information and raise the literacy level of the population. While this was achieved, one negative impact of this simplification process was the loss of some of the complex meanings and nuances that the traditional characters yielded. Practitioners outside China have often relied on translations of Chinese texts and consequently their understanding of important concepts has been inextricably linked to the skill and understanding of the translator and whether the original material has been simplified. A good example of this is the meaning of one of the key concepts of CM, the concept of qi (chi).

The understanding of the simplified character for qi 气 can be interpreted as the manifestation of breath becoming visible on a cold day, or steam. The traditional character for qi 氣 is made up of the character for steam 气 rising from rice 米 through cooking, suggesting a transformative process of the material into something more energetic. Another interpretation of the traditional character is that it represents a bursting grain of rice that is acted on by an upward energy. This may suggest a potential energy brought into being by a divine force.

Whatever the true meaning, it can be observed readily that the traditional character is far more open to individual interpretation, discussion, debate and even disagreement. The traditional character also lends itself far more to scholarly study in order to reveal its original meaning. This thread is applicable to the entire body of CM and from the very early stages of study, beginning with a clear appreciation and understanding of the word for a medicine or cure (yào 藥). This character in turn is made from elements of two other characters, the character for grass or plant 草 and the character for happiness or music 樂.

Therefore, conceptually medicines (or cures) derive from the music or harmonious nature of plants or that medicines are natural substances that restore harmony to the individual (Zhang, 2005).This concept of harmony within an individual is distinct from the dominant biomedical viewpoint of health and disease but is perhaps more in tune with a systems biology approach to medicine.

In the field of drug discovery it has become popular to use Chinese herbal medicine (CHM) as a reservoir for potential new drug candidates but so far very few of the investigations have led to any new drug being marketed (e.g. Artemisinin; Wright *et al.*, 2010). This reductionist approach runs the danger of missing some good opportunities for the development of new treatments in the search for simple single compounds that are readily patentable. An interesting parallel can be drawn here with the simplification of Chinese characters – another reductionist approach that inevitably led to less effective practice (of communication).

There may well be novel effective treatments to be identified but these may come not as simple single active ingredients but in the form of more complex poly-phytomedicines and to add another level of complexity, often prescribed on an individual basis. In this area 'omics' techniques (metabolomics, proteomics, transcriptomics, genomics) have begun to provide a greater understanding of the way in which complex herbal formula affect biomolecular pathways in different diseases and conditions (Buriani *et al.*, 2012).

Using an 'omics' approach it is possible to identify a complex range of molecular targets, typically using human fluid samples, e.g. blood plasma or urine, and map these against different stages of health and disease, including in those people receiving treatment. Through this methodology it is possible to identify which medicinal plants and medicinal formulae have the most beneficial effect in each individual. Moreover, the traditional Chinese diagnosis (pattern differentiation) can be used to guide the choice of formulas used and then omics techniques can be used to investigate the outcomes through a detailed analysis of primary and secondary metabolites and the multiple molecular targets that they act on (Buriani *et al.*, 2012). This relatively new strategy for investigating the potential of CHM may help to confirm the underlying theories and diagnostic methods of CM and at the same time help to guide further research into the molecular basis and mechanistic action responsible for any therapeutic effect.

Apart from monitoring and evaluating clinical effectiveness, plant metabolomics is able to provide data on a wide range of plant metabolites (van der Kooy *et al.*, 2009) and so has applications in different scientific disciplines, including drug discovery and quality assurance. Rather than relying on one or two marker compounds, using a metabolomic approach, it is possible to investigate small differences in metabolite content between different crude raw materials and herbal medicinal products (HMPs). A more detailed understanding of these phytochemical differences help us to appreciate the complexities involved in producing HMPs along different value chains and help us to evaluate quality from a different perspective (Booker *et al.*, 2014a,2014b). This has direct implications for CHMPs, which are often constructed from many different medicinal plants, and need novel analytical methods to assure their quality and monitor their use in laboratory experiments and clinical intervention studies.

## 25.3   Traditional and modern dosage forms and application

Traditionally, herbal prescriptions came in the form of powders, pills, aqueous decoctions or medicinal wines. Today, the preferred dosage forms are aqueous decoctions or the concentrated powders and granules produced from aqueous extraction. This change in the way medicinal plants are taken gives rise to some interesting questions with regard to the effectiveness and safety of these products.

*Artemesia annua* L. is a good example of this, showing only limited efficacy in treatment outcome when the dried material is used in the form of an aqueous decoction. Through careful exploration of ancient texts it was established that the juice of the fresh plant should be the dosage form used medically. Using this preparation the antiparasitic effects against the malaria parasite rose considerably (Wright *et al.*, 2010). One question arising from this is how many other CHM formulas are taken according to convenience or cost rather than how they were originally prescribed?

Another example can be seen with reference to the Chinese medicinal plant Jiāng Huáng 姜黄 (ginger yellow), more commonly known as turmeric, *Curcuma longa* L., which is chiefly used for its blood-moving and pain-relieving qualities. It contains anti-inflammatory metabolites (Funk *et al.*, 2010; Kim *et al.*, 2012), most notably the curcuminoids (Jurenka, 2009) only found naturally within *Curcuma* species. Pharmacological evidence substantiating its use for gastritis, osteo-arthritis and age-related cognitive diseases is of particular relevance (Goel *et al.*, 2008; Mishra and Palanivelu, 2008). However, these compounds are insoluble in water and so, taken as aqueous decoction, are of limited value compared with other dosage forms (Shoba *et al.*, 1998). Examination of the classical texts reveals that many of the formulas containing this drug were previously taken as whole powders of the crude drug material rather than decoctions (Scheid *et al.*, 2009), which from a phytochemical-pharmacokinetic perspective makes perfect sense.

This not only applies to *C. longa* but to all species that contain predominantly lipophilic compounds with low water solubility. Moreover, often these more lipophilic compounds are more pharmacologically active and, therefore, are more likely to have a therapeutic effect. This often seems to be overlooked by practitioners, producers and suppliers of CHMPs. This lack of attention to the bioavailability of particular compounds has far-reaching consequences, both for individual patients receiving CM and on a wider scale when attempting to justify the legitimacy of CM through intervention studies. It is vitally important that not only has an ethnopharmacological link been made for the use of a particular plant or formula to be used to treat a particular illness or condition, but also the dosage form and method of delivery has been thoroughly researched also.

## 25.4   Medicinal plant production in China

China has a long history of using plants for medicinal purposes (Petrovska, 2012). There are hundreds of state-owned and increasingly shared ownership companies producing traditional Chinese medicines, many of which export their products internationally (PMMI, 2001). Botanical drugs used for other purposes, e.g. as cosmetics, supplements or as 'European' herbal medical products, are also produced widely.

There have been numerous instances of poor-quality and adulterated medicines being produced, particularly originating from small manufacturing operations. China has partly addressed these difficulties relating to the manufacture and supply of TCM products[1], including CHMPs, by modernising its traditional medicines industry with the help of government-sponsored strategies aimed at improving good agricultural and collection practice (GACP) and good manufacturing practice (GMP). All manufacturers of TCM products must comply with standards set down by the China Food and Drug Administration (CFDA) in order to gain GMP certification.

Taiwan has become a major exporter of concentrated herbal powders and granules. These products are normally aqueous extractions that are then dried and manufactured into a product that is relatively easy to take compared with conventional decoctions. Some companies add the crude medicinal plant powder to these extracts, which often improves the range of metabolite content. The Taiwanese companies which export internationally generally operate to a high standard of GMP and typically hold GMP certification issued by the Australian regulatory authorities.

## 25.5   Quality and safety

Instances of poor-quality and adulterated TCM products are commonly reported, e.g. in the UK (MHRA, 2008, 2013). The safety of CHMPs has been under the spotlight since the 1990s. Probably the greatest concern for the day-to-day safety of consumers is the purchase of CHMPs over the internet. Particular concerns regarding adulteration with pharmaceutical products exist for products marketed as skin treatments, slimming products and alleged aphrodisiacs.

It could be argued that these products are not part of CM and are in fact pharmaceutical products. However, these products are mainly marketed as TCM products and mainly originate from the Chinese mainland and therefore they are part of the current Chinese pharmaceutical market.

The EU standards for chemical and microbiological quality, and the limits set for chemical and microbiological contamination often exceed those laid down by the regulatory authorities of less economically developed countries. This can lead to difficulties for international importing companies who import their products through legitimate means, leading to the temptation to circumnavigate official routes of supply. This is particularly true in the case of pesticides, where China and other Asian countries may use pesticides prohibited in the EU and other countries. Moreover, with the increase of pollution caused by heavy industry there is an increase in heavy metal contamination within some medicinal plants, particularly those that have a tendency to store these contaminants within their plant matrix (Tangahu, 2011).

Adulteration and contamination, however, do not represent the only safety risks connected with the use of CHMPs. Some medicinal plants used in CM are intrinsically toxic and should only be used clinically for acute conditions for short periods of time. Other medicinals that may have some toxicity might only be used in very small quantities. Probably the most concerning additions are those of heavy metals, traditionally used in Chinese and other medicinal traditions (Wijenayake et al., 2014) for their effects on calming the mind, e.g. cinnabar. Although these products are still used in China, in the EU it is illegal for practitioners or retailers to prescribe or sell any mineral or animal-derived product to treat a medical condition.

---

[1] TCM products may include those that are derived from or include animal or mineral substances.

## 25.6  Aristolochic acids

Aristolochic acid nephropathy and urothelial cancers have been unequivocally linked to the ingestion of aristolochic acid and its derivatives found in *Aristolochia* and some other species of plants used in traditional medicine. Although *Aristolochia* species have been banned in Europe and other countries since the 1990s there have been continued instances of CHMPs containing aristolochic acids being found for sale (especially on the internet). The current testing requirements are aimed at ensuring that products are free from aristolochic acids 1 and 2, but research has indicated that there may be a much larger range of toxic and potentially carcinogenic aristolochic acid derivatives (Michl *et al.*, 2013). Current testing techniques are unlikely to identify these potentially harmful compounds.

There is also some confusion regarding the dangers of using related species containing aristolochic acid derivatives, e.g. *Asarum* species. Species from the *Asarum* genus have some usage in CM and many practitioners regard them as essential for the treatment of certain painful conditions, e.g. arthritis. Although *Asarum* species have been shown to contain aristolochic acids, they are still available to buy in the UK. Most worryingly a formula containing this medicinal plant (du huo sheng ji wan) was recommended to arthritis sufferers by a UK arthritis charity (ARUK, 2012). This not only presented a danger to the public but highlights a lack of any harmonisation of knowledge or expertise throughout the scientific and herbal medicine communities.

Without doubt the quality and safety of TCMs is variable. The European Traditional Herbal Registration (THR) scheme has been brought in to tackle deficiencies regarding over-the-counter (OTC) medicines but the availability of these medicines outside the EU and particularly from the internet continues to present a danger to the public. Moreover, unlicensed medicines as used by practitioners can be of variable quality and a well-defined and well-regulated quality system is urgently required in all countries where TCM products are used.

## 25.7  Regulatory requirements

Introducing non-conventional practice into a well-defined regulatory system is inevitably problematic. The UK provides an excellent example of the problems and dangers associated with practising complementary and alternative medicine (CAM) within a non-regulated environment (both practitioners and products) and also the arguments presented by those already within the system for keeping disciplines that cannot demonstrate an acceptable evidence-base outside of the regulatory bubble. Without statutory regulation, and with that more effective regulation of therapeutic products, there are no legal constraints preventing someone from practising 'alternative' medicine (like TCM). The result is numerous safety concerns, including the use of dangerous practices, treatment of diseases that need to be treated by a medical doctor, poor training in diagnosis and a lack of an effective pharmacovigilance strategy in the case of adverse reactions to herbal medicinal products (HMPs).

In the UK, for example, there are several voluntary regulatory bodies that are in place to provide both professional support, e.g. continuing professional development (CPD), access to reputable suppliers, herb safety updates, accreditation of educational courses and professional conferences, and at the same time provide the public with information on herbal medicine and a place to bring any complaint against a practitioner, but these are voluntary schemes totally reliant on the goodwill of their members and so can only offer limited protection to the public.

This has led to the UK government proceeding with plans to subject herbal medicine practitioners to further regulation and a new regulatory framework. On 16 February 2011 the then

Secretary of State for Health Andrew Lansley announced in a written statement to the UK Parliament that all UK practitioners prescribing herbal medicines are to be statutorily regulated via the Health Professions Council. The Health Secretary went on to explain that:

'This would ensure that practitioners would meet specified registration standards, giving practitioners and consumers continuing access to unlicensed manufactured herbal medicines to meet individual patient needs after the introduction of new EU legislation after April 30th this year.'

(Lansley, 2011).

This further regulation of herbal practitioners and their supporting industry will come with some expectations attached and the Medicines and Healthcare Products Regulatory Agency (MHRA), the UK's medicines' regulators, have indicated that they would like to see a positive list of plant medicines established that can be used safely in daily practise (MHRA, 2006). The plants and plant products that make up this list will be required to satisfy standards of quality and safety appropriate to the UK. For plant material obtained from outside the EU this is likely to present some challenges but also some opportunities for Asian producers to benefit from a regulated and quality-driven medicinal plant industry.

Statutory regulation would bring the UK in line with more regulated countries. However, there has been some opposition to the statutory regulation of UK herbalists, including TCM practitioners, with objections being raised that it lacks a credible evidence base and may give false credibility to the profession (Ernst, 2012). This opposition, coupled with a lack of a single voice from the profession, with a proportion of herbalists themselves being 'anti-regulation' (Jones and Evans, 2013), has led to a delay in the process. With further consultation planned, the prospect of full statutory regulation is far from being assured, with 'softer' regulatory options being considered. The government's stance in May 2013 was:

'The legislation around this policy is complex and there are a number of issues that have arisen which the government needs to work through. I appreciate that the delay in going out to consult on this matter is causing concern, but it is important that any new legislation is proportionate and fit for purpose.'

(Hansard, 2013)

The outcome of these proposals was announced in early 2015 and the government chose not to go ahead with full statutory regulation. This will have a direct impact on the herbal profession and the HMP manufacturing industry in the UK and, to a lesser extent, the rest of Europe. This in turn will impact on both home producers of medicinal plants and suppliers outside Europe, particularly in Asia and the USA, where many CM products are manufactured for the European market.

## 25.8  Training practitioners of TCM

The UK provides a clear example of how educational standards can be developed and implemented to satisfy national standards of health care and uses a model similar to the one found in many states of the USA. There is currently (2014) no undergraduate training in CHM available in the UK. There are BSc degree courses that offer a combined training in TCM over four years, which includes some training in medicinal plants, or it is possible to take a three-year training in acupuncture at undergraduate level, followed by a one- to two-year postgraduate training in CHM, some of which is offered at MSc level. These courses have come in for some criticism for teaching subjects that according to some commentators have little scientific credibility and are not evidence-based. However, these courses are validated at BSc or MSc level by universities and must demonstrate through the university's quality system that they have appropriate content and are taught at the correct level. Much of the syllabus at BSc level concerns the study of the medical sciences, including anatomy, physiology and pathology. There is a strong emphasis on recognising the warning signs of serious pathologies (red flags) so that patients can be referred to other specialists when necessary. Postgraduate courses in CHM fulfil the requirements necessary at this level. On these taught masters courses students are required to develop their skills in independent thinking and be able to analyse critically complex problems. A weakness of these courses is possibly the amount of time allocated to the study of the adjunct sciences related to herbal medicine, i.e. pharmacology, toxicology and pharmacognosy.

One reason that the courses are lacking in this area, compared to conventional medicine or even training in western herbal medicine, is because of the historical route that CM took in being established in the UK. When more formalised CM education first came to the UK in the early 1970s, only acupuncture was taught and this acupuncture typically used theories of medicine that were acupuncture-specific and did not provide the theoretical framework for the practice of CHM. As more information was gradually disseminated from educational establishments and the medical profession in China, and more books began to be published, the practice of CHM followed the prevailing approach as was practised in China, i.e. modern TCM, and little attention was paid either to the Chinese classical literature or to conventional medical sciences.[2] Moreover in China today acupuncture and herbal medicine are usually practised as separate disciplines, giving the practitioner more time to specialise in one form of treatment. Even herbal medicine can be divided into those who diagnose and treat (TCM doctors) and those who make and dispense medicines (TCM pharmacists). This is a different situation generally for practitioners outside China, who often combine different disciplines and who are required to be both doctor and pharmacist.

To some extent the role of CM pharmacist has been undertaken by the TCM supply companies in the UK. These companies typically import medicinal plants from mainland China or Taiwan and supply CM practitioners with small quantities of medicinal plants for the treatment of individual patients. Sometimes practitioners will run their own pharmacy, and this is more common amongst Chinese immigrants who have set up small high street businesses in the UK offering treatments in TCM. Both of these methods of practice have certain limitations compared with practices in mainland China, where pharmacists are responsible for the safety and quality of medicines.

## 25.9   Future prospects

CM is available in the UK probably more than in any other European country, with acupuncture being a particular success. A large number of biomedically trained professionals use it in daily practice, i.e. medical doctors and physiotherapists, as well as a strong body of traditionally trained acupuncturists. CHM, however, has struggled to be accepted in the same way. This is probably due to the lack of credible evidence-base, the many negative reports associated with adverse reactions to Chinese medicinal plants, the lack of proper quality controls and the lack of standardised training across the profession. Without statutory regulation and an accompanying well-regulated system governing the quality of CHMPs, it is difficult to imagine how public confidence can be restored.

---

[2] The modernisation of Chinese medicine, instigated by Mao in the early 1950s included less emphasis on either science or the Chinese classics.

For manufactured CHMPs, the only route to market available in the UK and in the rest of Europe is via the Traditional Herbal Medicinal Products Directive and registration as a traditional herbal medicinal product. However, this requires considerable investment from companies, and the treatment indications available is only on offer for the treatment of relatively minor, self-limiting conditions. This may be commercially less attractive, but it would allow the public access to Chinese herbal remedies of acceptable quality and safety.

In the USA it is still possible to obtain many of these manufactured products as unlicensed 'food supplements' and there are fewer restrictions on the use of animal and mineral components. This designation of CHMPs as foods is less than ideal and it remains to be seen how this system can be sustained for the longer term.

In hospitals throughout China the practice of internal medicine (using Chinese *materia medica*) is regarded as the main treatment modality for most illnesses, with acupuncture being reserved mainly for musculo-skeletal conditions. It is interesting how in the west the use of Chinese medicinals (including flora, fauna and minerals) have yet to be used in the same way. A strong evidence base for herbal treatments, including pharmacokinetic and pharmacodynamic studies, is an essential prerequisite. In parallel, quality assurance systems need to be put into place that will assure the quality and safety of CHMPs in line with the regulatory requirements of the user countries. The third piece of this jigsaw is to ensure that personnel in different sectors of CM have an equivalent level of training and regulation to that of any other healthcare provider.

Ethnopharmacology can lead us to a better appreciation of the complex processes that underpin the modern practice of CM. A detailed and correct understanding of how plant-derived medicines are cultivated, processed and administered will help to ensure that best practices are employed in the contemporary delivery of these traditional medicines. The use of technologies such as medical and plant metabolomics can help to unravel some of this complexity and can be applied to quality assurance and clinical studies. Using this approach the quality and safety of traditional medicines can be monitored more satisfactorily and a more robust evidence base can be established.

# References

Anon. (947–951 CE) 0000 *The Yellow Emperor's Classic of Internal Medicine*, Hungdi Neijing.

ARUK (2012) Complementary and alternative medicines for the treatment of rheumatoid arthritis, osteoarthritis and fibromyalgia, http://www.arthritisresearchuk.org/arthritis-information/complementary-and-alternative-medicines/cam-report/complementary-medicines-for-osteoarthritis.aspx.

Booker, A., Frommenwiler, D., Johnston, D., *et al.* (2014a) Chemical variability along the value chains of turmeric (*Curcuma longa*): A comparison of nuclear magnetic resonance spectroscopy and high performance thin layer chromatography. *Journal of Ethnopharmacology*, doi: 10.1016/j.jep.2013.12.042.

Booker, A., Suter, A., Krnjic, A., *et al.* (2014b) A phytochemical comparison of saw palmetto products using gas chromatography and $^1$H nuclear magnetic resonance spectroscopy metabolomic profiling. *Journal of Pharmacy and Pharmacology*, doi: 10.1111/jphp.12198.

Buriani, A., Garcia-Bermejo, M.L., Bosisio, E., *et al.* (2012) Omic techniques in systems biology approaches to traditional Chinese medicine research: Present and future. *Journal of Ethnopharmacology*, **140**, 535–544.

Ernst, E. (2012) *Regulating alternative practitioners may give them false credibility*, Notes and theories: Dispatches from the science desk, *The Guardian science blog*, http://www.theguardian.com/profile/edzardernst.

Funk, J.L., Frye, J.B., Oyarzo, J.N., *et al.* (2010) Anti-arthritic effects and toxicity of the essential oils of turmeric (*Curcuma longa* L.). *Journal of Agricultural and Food Chemistry*, **58**, 842–849.

Goel, A., Kunnumakkara, A.B. and Aggarwal, B.B. (2008) Curcumin as 'Curecumin': from kitchen to clinic. *Biochemistry and Pharmacology*, **75**, 787–809.

Hansard (2013) *Commons debates, Parliamentary Business*, http://www.publications.parliament.uk/pa /cm201213/cmhansrd/cm130417/text/130417w0002.htm.

IpsosMORI (2009) *Public Perceptions of Herbal Medicines*, https://www.ipsos-mori.com /researchpublications/researcharchive/2307/Public-Perceptions-of-Herbal-Medicines.aspx.

Jones, L. and Evans, P. (2013) *Afraid of statutory regulation not going ahead? Reassurance for you*, http://www.herbal-practitioners.co.uk/regulation-anti.htm.

Jurenka, J.S. (2009) Anti-inflammatory properties of curcumin, a major constituent of *Curcuma longa*: A review of preclinical and clinical research. *Alternative Medicine Review*, **14**, 141–153.

Kim, J.H., Gupta, S.C., Park, B., *et al.* (2012) Turmeric (*Curcuma longa*) inhibits inflammatory nuclear factor (NF)-kB and NF-kB-regulated gene products and induces death receptors leading to suppressed proliferation, induced chemosensitization, and suppressed osteoclastogenesis. *Molecular Nutrition and Food Research*, **56**, 454–465.

Lansley, A. (2011) *Practitioners of acupuncture, herbal medicine and traditional Chinese medicine*, http://www.publications.parliament.uk/pa/cm201012/cmhansrd/cm110216/wmstext/110216m0001 .htm.

MHRA (2006) *Discussion paper: No 3. Reforms of s12(1) of the Medicines Act 1968: Safety issues*, http://ehtpa.eu/pdf/medicines_legislation/3%20SafetyDiscussiondocdrFinalDec06.pdf.

MHRA (2008) *Public health risk with herbal medicines: An overview, Herbal Documents*. MHRA Policy Division, http://www.mhra.gov.uk/home/groups/es-herbal/documents/websiteresources/ con023163.pdf.

MHRA (2013) *Warning over dangerous traditional Chinese medicines*. Press release, http://www.mhra .gov.uk/home/groups/comms-po/documents/news/con307406.pdf.

Michl, J., Jennings, H.M., Kite, G.C., *et al.* (2013) Is aristolochic acid nephropathy a widespread problem in developing countries? A case study of *Aristolochia indica* L. in Bangladesh using an ethnobotanical–phytochemical approach. *Journal of Ethnopharmacology*, **149**, 235–244.

Mishra, S. and Palanivelu, K. (2008) The effect of curcumin (turmeric) on Alzheimer's disease: An overview. *Annals of Indian Academy of Neurology*, **11**, 13–19.

Petrovska, B.B. (2012) Historical review of medicinal plants' usage. *Pharmacognosy Review*, **6**, 1–5.

PMMI (2001) *China Industry Sector Report: Outlook on China's Pharmaceutical Industry*, Packaging Machinery Manufacturers Institute, http://pmmi.files.cms-plus.com/uploads/ChinaPharm.pdf.

Scheid, V., Bensky, D., Ellis, A. and Barolet, R. (2009) *Chinese Herbal Medicine: Formulas and Strategies*, 2nd edn, Eastland Press, Washington.

Shoba, G., Joy, D., Joseph, T., *et al.* (1998) Influence of piperine on the pharmacokinetics of curcumin in animals and human volunteers. *Planta Medica*, **64**, 353–356.

Tangahu, B.V., Rozaimah, S., Hassan Basri, A. *et al.* (2011) A review on heavy metals (As, Pb, and Hg) uptake by plants through phytoremediation. *International Journal of Chemical Engineering*, doi: 10.1155/2011/939161.

UOM (2011) *Herbal Medicine*. University of Maryland.

van der Kooy, F., Maltese, F., Hae Choi, Y., *et al.* (2009) quality control of herbal material and phytopharmaceuticals with MS- and NMR-based metabolic fingerprinting. *Planta Medica*, **75**, 763–775.

Vasisht, K. and Kumar, V. (2002) *Trade and Production of Herbal Medicines and Natural Health Products*, United Nations Industrial Development Organization and the International Centre for Science and High Technology, pp. 1–86.

Wijenayake, A., Pitawala, A., Bandara, R. and Abayasekara, C. (2014) The role of herbometallic preparations in traditional medicine – A review on mica drug processing and pharmaceutical applications. *Journal of Ethnopharmacology*, **155**, 1001–1010.

Wright, C.W., Linley, P.A., Brun, R., *et al.* (2010) Ancient Chinese methods are remarkably effective for the preparation of artemisinin-rich extracts of Qing Hao with potent antimalarial activity. *Molecules*, **15**, 804–812.

Zhang, H. (2005) The art of applying Chinese herbs. *Journal of Chinese Medicine*, **79**, 36–41.

# 26

# Chinese Medicinal Processing: A Characteristic Aspect of the Ethnopharmacology of Traditional Chinese Medicine

Ping Guo, Eric Brand and Zhongzhen Zhao

*School of Chinese Medicine, Hong Kong Baptist University, Kowloon Tong, Hong Kong, China*

## 26.1   Introduction

The extensive use of processed medicinals is a distinctive feature of traditional Chinese medicine (TCM). Standardizing processing methods of Chinese medicinals is as important as authentication for maintaining their quality and ensuring their safe use (Zhao *et al.*, 2006).

Before being used in clinical applications, Chinese medicinal materials are first processed into 'decoction pieces' (small pieces or slices ready for decocting). In the *Chinese Pharmacopoeia* (Chinese Pharmacopoeia Commission, 2010), a total of 591 raw medicinal materials are recorded. Among them, decoction pieces standards of 446 raw medicinal materials are established, involving 672 individual decoction pieces. It has been clarified in the *Chinese Pharmacopoeia* that medicinal properties, channel tropisms, functions, indications, usage and dosage are attributed to decoction pieces. The *British Pharmacopoeia* (British Pharmacopoeia Commission, 2009) also lists processed medicinal materials such as processed astragalus root (*huangqi, Astragalus propinquus* Schischkin[*]). Only small amounts of processed medicinal materials are listed in the pharmacopoeias of other eastern and western countries (Society of Japanese Pharmacopoeia, 2006; British Pharmacopoeia Commission, 2009; European Pharmacopoeia Commission, 2007; United States Pharmacopoeial Convention, 2007).

[*]*Astragalus membranaceus* (Fisch.) Bge. and *Astragalus membranaceus* (Fisch.) Bge. var. *mongholicus* (Bge.) Hsiao are recorded in the *Chinese Pharmacopoeia* (2010) as the botanical origins of the Chinese medicinal *huangqi*. The

*Ethnopharmacology*, First Edition. Edited by Michael Heinrich and Anna K. Jäger.
© 2015 John Wiley & Sons, Ltd. Published 2015 by John Wiley & Sons, Ltd.

former is now treated as a synonym of *Astragalus propinquus* Schischkin and the latter a synonym of *Astragalus mongholicus* Bunge.

It is well known that there is a close relationship between the processing and safety of Chinese medicinals. Some poisonings and side effects are caused by improper processing methods. For example, improperly processed aconite lateral root (*fuzi, Aconitum carmichaeli* Debx.) has caused poisoning in nearly 5000 people in the past 20 years (Zou and Wang, 2005). Similar poisoning incidents have been reported in Hong Kong due to the intake of incompletely processed aconite root (*chuanwu, Aconitum carmichaeli* Debx.) or wild aconite root (*caowu, Aconitum kusnezoffii* Reichb.) (Chan *et al.*, 1994).

The processing of Chinese medicinals started early in the history of TCM and has developed along with its practice. In recent years, there has been considerable confusion of the processed products in both Chinese and overseas herbal markets. In this chapter, the present state and problems of Chinese medicinal processing as well as the recent progress in research are documented, the development of processing methods and possible approaches to solve those problems are explored and the most urgent work needed is proposed.

## 26.2   Definition, methods and historical changes in Chinese medicinal processing

### 26.2.1   Definition

Chinese medicinal processing is a pharmaceutical technique that meets different therapeutic, dispensing and preparation requirements based on TCM theory. In short, it is a technique that transforms raw medicinal materials into decoction pieces. In commerce, Chinese medicinals include raw medicinal materials, decoction pieces, proprietary TCM products and herbal concentrated powders, which have emerged in recent years. Of these, decoction pieces are most frequently used in clinical applications. Most raw medicinal materials also need to undergo certain processing procedures before they are manufactured into proprietary TCM products.

### 26.2.2   Methods

A variety of methods are used to process Chinese medicinals. The main purpose is to enhance the efficacy and/or reduce the toxicity. Chinese medicinal processing methods are basically divided into simple preparation (such as cleaning and cutting) and elaborate processing (such as stir-frying, stir-frying with liquid adjuvants, steaming, boiling and calcining). The main processing methods recorded in the *Chinese Pharmacopoeia* are shown in Table 26.1 (Chinese Pharmacopoeia Commission, 2010) and several commonly used methods are described below.

#### 26.2.2.1   Stir-frying (*chao*)

Cleaned and cut medicinal materials are put in a pot, with or without solid adjuvants, heated with certain types of fire (low, moderate or strong fire), and are constantly stirred until the medicinal materials reach a certain state. For example, dried ginger (*ganjiang*, rhizome of *Zingiber officinale* Rosc.) is known as blast-fried ginger (*paojiang*) when it is stir-fried with sand until it becomes puffy and brown externally. When it is stir-fried until the surface becomes scorched black and the interior brown, it is known as charred ginger (*jiangtan*). Dried ginger (*ganjiang*) warms the spleen and stomach, dissipates cold, restores yang, unblocks the channels, dries dampness and eliminates phlegm. Blast-fried ginger (*paojiang*) specifically warms

**Table 26.1**  Main medicinal processing methods listed in the *Chinese Pharmacopoeia* (2010).

| Processing methods | Adjuvants | Examples |
|---|---|---|
| Stir-frying till yellow, scorched and carbonized | | Hawthorn fruit (*shanzha*, *Crataegus pinnatifida* Bge./*C. pinnatifida* Bge. var. *major* N.E. Br.) stir-fried till yellow (*chaoshanzha*), hawthorn fruit (*shanzha*) stir-fried till scorched (*jiaoshanzha*), charred ginger (*ganjiang*, rhizome of *Zingiber officinale* Rosc.) (*jiangtan*) |
| Stir-frying with solid adjuvants | Oven earth | Ovate atractylodes rhizome (*baizhu*, *Atractylodes macrocephala* Koidz.) stir-fried with oven earth (*tubaizhu*) *Chinese Pharmacopoeia (2005) |
| | Bran | Atractylodes rhizome (*cangzhu*, *Atractylodes lancea* (Thunb.) DC. /*A. chinensis* (DC.) Koidz.*) stir-fried with bran (*fuchaocangzhu*) *Atractylodes chinensis (DC.) Koidz. is now treated as a synonym of Atractylodes lancea (Thunb.) DC |
| | Rice | Codonopsis root (*dangshen*, *Codonopsis pilosula* (Franch.) Nannf./*C. pilosula* Nannf. var. *modesta* (Nannf.) L.T. Shen*/*C. tangshen* Oliv.) stir-fried with rice (*michaodangshen*) *Codonopsis pilosula Nannf. var. modesta (Nannf.) L.T. Shen is now treated as a synonym of Codonopsis pilosula (Franch.) Nannf. |
| | Sand | Blast-fried ginger (*paojiang*) |
| Stir-frying with liquid adjuvants | Wine | Chinese angelica root (*danggui*, *Angelica sinensis* (Oliv.) Diels) processed with wine (*jiudanggui*) |
| | Vinegar | Bupleurum root (*chaihu*, *Bupleurum chinense* DC./*B. scorzonerifolium* Willd.) processed with vinegar (*cuchaihu*) |
| | Salt water | Eucommia bark (*duzhong*, *Eucommia ulmoides* Oliv.) processed with salt water (*yanduzhong*) |
| | Honey | Licorice (*gancao*, root and rhizome of *Glycyrrhiza uralensis* Fisch. / *G. inflata* Bat./*G. glabra* L.) processed with honey (*zhigancao*) |
| | Ginger juice | Coptis rhizome (*huanglian*, *Coptis chinensis* Franch./*C. deltoidea* C.Y. Cheng et Hsiao/*C. teeta* Wall.) processed with ginger juice (*jianghuanglian*) |
| | Suet oil | Epimedium leaf (*yinyanghuo*, *Epimedium brevicornu* Maxim./*E. sagittatum* (Sieb. et Zucc.) Maxim./*E. pubescens* Maxim./*E. koreanum* Nakai) processed with suet oil (*zhiyinyanghuo*) |
| Steaming | | Red ginseng (*renshen*, root and rhizome of *Panax ginseng* C.A. Mey.) (*hongshen*) |
| | Salt water | Morinda root (*bajitian*, *Morinda officinalis* How) steamed with salt water (*yanbajitian*) |
| | Medicinal juices | Processed fleeceflower root (*heshouwu*, *Polygonum multiflorum* Thunb.) (*zhiheshouwu*) |
| | Vinegar | Schisandra berry (*wuweizi*, *Schisandra chinensis* (Turcz.) Baill.) steamed with vinegar (*cuwuweizi*) |
| | Wine | Polygonatum rhizome (*huangjing*, *Polygonatum kingianum* Coll. et Hemsl./*P. sibiricum* Red./*P. cyrtonema* Hua) steamed /stewed with wine (*jiuhuangjing*) |

*(Continued overleaf)*

**Table 26.1**   (*Continued*)

| Processing methods | Adjuvants | Examples |
|---|---|---|
| Calcining | | Calcined gypsum (*duanshigao*) |
| Boiling | | Processed aconite root (*chuanwu, Aconitum carmichaeli* Debx.) (*zhichuanwu*) |
| | Edible mother solution of mineral salts | Sliced aconite lateral root (*fuzi, Aconitum carmichaeli* Debx.) (*fupian*) |
| | Alumen and fresh ginger | Processed arisaema rhizome (*tiannanxing, Arisaema erubescens* (Wall.) Schott/*A. heterophyllum* Bl./*A. amurense* Maxim.) (*zhitiannanxing*) |
| | Fresh ginger and alumen | Pinellia rhizome (*banxia, Pinellia ternata* (Thunb.) Breit.) processed with ginger (*jiangbanxia*) |

the spleen and stomach, relieves pain, warms the channels and arrests bleeding. Charred ginger (*jiangtan*) stabilizes and binds to arrest bleeding.

### 26.2.2.2  Stir-frying with liquid adjuvants (*zhi*)

Cleaned and cut medicinal materials are stir-fried with liquid adjuvants so that the latter gradually infuse into their interior. Commonly used liquid adjuvants include wine, vinegar, salt water, honey, ginger juice and suet oil. For example, slices of licorice (*gancao*, root and rhizome of *Glycyrrhiza uralensis* Fisch./*G. inflata* Bat./*G. glabra* L.) are mixed with a diluted solution of honey and moistened thoroughly in a closed container. They are stir-fried with a low fire until they become deep yellow and no longer sticky to touch. They are then removed and allowed to cool. Licorice (*gancao*) clears heat, resolves toxicity, dispels phlegm and relieves cough. After processing with honey, it is good at tonifying the spleen, harmonizing the stomach, benefiting qi and restoring the pulse.

### 26.2.2.3  Steaming (*zheng*)

Cleaned and cut medicinal materials are placed in a suitable container and are cooked in steam. Sometimes adjuvants such as medicinal juices (e.g. black bean juice), vinegar and wine are added. For example, fleeceflower root (*heshouwu, Polygonum multiflorum* Thunb.*) slices or pieces are mixed with black bean juice, put in a non-ferrous container and stewed until the black bean juice is completely absorbed and the fleeceflower root (*heshouwu*) slices or pieces become brown. They are then removed and dried. After this processing, it is known as processed fleeceflower root (*zhiheshouwu*). Fleeceflower root (*heshouwu*) resolves toxicity, eliminates carbuncles, moistens the intestines and promotes defecation. Its processed form tonifies the liver and the kidney, benefits the essence and the blood, blackens the hair, and strengthens the tendons and bones.

*\*Polygonum multiflorum* Thunb. is now treated as a synonym of *Fallopia multiflora* (Thunb.) Haraldson.

### 26.2.2.4  Calcining (*duan*):

Medicinal materials are calcined directly in a smokeless flame or indirectly in a suitable container with a strong fire. This method is mainly applicable to minerals, shells and fossils with firm and hard texture, and other medicinal materials that need to be charred. For example, gypsum (*shigao*) pieces are calcined directly in a smokeless flame or indirectly in a suitable container with a strong fire until they are red hot. They are then removed, allowed to cool and ground into powders. Gypsum (*shigao*) clears heat, drains fire, relieves restlessness and quenches thirst, while calcined gypsum (*duanshigao*) astringes damp discharge, engenders flesh, constrains sores and arrests bleeding.

Among the list of 31 toxic and potent Chinese medicinal materials described by the Department of Health of Hong Kong (Xia *et al.*, 2007), most are raw medicinal materials. Once processed, they can be applied clinically by qualified TCM practitioners. Examples include processed forms of aconite lateral root (*fuzi*) and pinellia rhizome (*banxia, Pinellia ternata* (Thunb.) Breit.).

Some medicinal materials can be processed in different ways, giving them different medicinal properties. For example, the medicinal properties of Chinese angelica root (*danggui, Angelica sinensis* (Oliv.) Diels) processed with wine are different from those of charred Chinese angelica root (*dangguitan*). Aconite lateral root (*fuzi*) can be processed into black sliced aconite lateral root (*heishunpian*), white sliced aconite lateral root (*baifupian*), blast-fried sliced aconite lateral root (*paofupian*) and desalted sliced aconite lateral root (*danfupian*) (Table 26.2, Figure 26.1).

**Table 26.2**  Processing methods of Chinese angelica root (*danggui, Angelica sinensis* (Oliv.) Diels) and aconite lateral root (*fuzi, Aconitum carmichaeli* Debx.).

| Decoction pieces | Main processing methods |
|---|---|
| Chinese angelica root (*danggui, Angelica sinensis* (Oliv.) Diels) | Raw medicinal material → remove foreign matter → clean → moisten thoroughly → cut into thin slices → dry |
| Chinese angelica root processed with wine (*jiudanggui*) | Chinese angelica root (*danggui*) slices → mix with yellow rice wine → moisten in a sealed container → stir-fry with a low fire until they become dark yellow → remove → allow to cool |
| Charred Chinese angelica root (*dangguitan*) | Chinese angelica root (*danggui*) slices → stir-fry with a moderate fire until they become slightly black → remove → sun-dry |
| Black sliced aconite lateral root (*fuzi, Aconitum carmichaeli* Debx.) (*heishunpian*) | Unprocessed lateral root (*nifuzi*) → clean → soak in edible mother solution of mineral salts → boil thoroughly → rinse in water → cut longitudinally into slices about 0.5 cm in thickness → rinse in water again → stain into dark brown → steam → bake to half-dryness → sun-dry or bake to complete dryness |
| White sliced aconite lateral root (*baifupian*) | Unprocessed lateral root (*nifuzi*) → clean → soak in edible mother solution of mineral salts → boil thoroughly → peel the skin → cut longitudinally into slices about 0.3 cm in thickness → rinse in water → steam thoroughly → sun-dry |
| Blast-fried sliced aconite lateral root (*paofupian*) | Put black sliced aconite lateral root (*heishunpian*) or white sliced aconite lateral root (*baifupian*) into hot sand → stir-fry with strong fire till they are inflated and become yellow-brown → sift out the sand → allow to cool |
| Desalted sliced aconite lateral root (*danfupian*) | Unprocessed lateral root (*nifuzi*) → clean → soak in edible mother solution of mineral salts → add salt → soak again → sun-dry/air-dry → salted aconite lateral root (*yanfuzi*) → rinse in water → boil thoroughly together with licorice (*gancao*) and black bean until the cut slice does not cause numbness to the tongue → cut into slices → sun-dry |

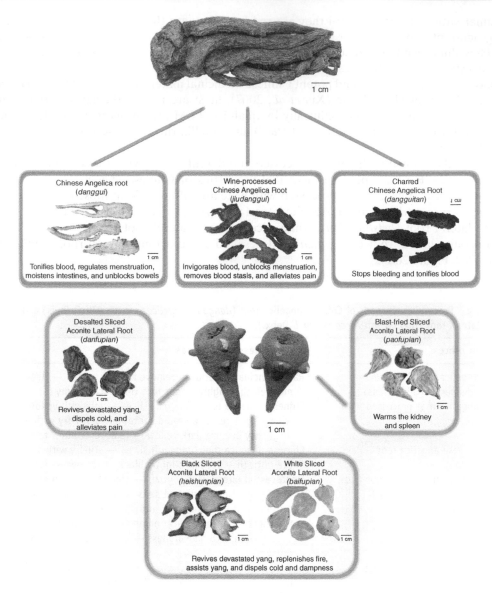

**Figure 26.1**   Processed Chinese angelica root (*danggui, Angelica sinensis* (Oliv.) Diels) and aconite lateral root (*fuzi, Aconitum carmichaeli* Debx.) products.

## 26.2.3   Historical changes

Chinese medicinal processing has a long history. Some processing methods, such as burning, calcining, decocting, and soaking with wine and vinegar, are recorded in *Prescriptions for 52 Diseases (Wu Shi Er Bing Fang)*, which was written in approximately 200 BC (Wang, 1992). *Grandfather Lei's Treatise on Herbal Processing (Lei Gong Pao Zhi Lun)*, written in about 500 AD, sums up documentations and experiences of the ancient practice of processing. It is the first monograph on Chinese medicinal processing (Lei, 1991). *Methods of Herbal Processing (Pao Zhi Da Fa)*, published in 1662, is another monograph on Chinese medicinal processing

(Miao, 1992). In the Qing dynasty, *A Guide to Herbal Processing* (*Xiu Shi Zhi Nan*), written by Zhang Zhongyan, was the third monograph on Chinese medicinal processing. Information related to processing from various ancient herbal medicine literature is cited in this book, especially from *Compendium of Materia Medica* (*Ben Cao Gang Mu*) and *Materia Medica Arranged According to Pattern* (*Zheng Lei Ben Cao*) (Zhang, 2000). Additionally, the contents of processing are also recorded in a large number of other classic texts on Chinese *materia medica* and medicinal formulas. These records include the condensed clinical experiences of ancient TCM practitioners, which are worthy of further research. Having disappeared for 400 years, the 14-volume *Concise Addendum to Grandfather Lei's Treatise on Herbal Processing* (*Bu Yi Lei Gong Pao Zhi Bian Lian*) of the Ming dynasty reappeared recently. This book records 1193 elaborate colour illustrations (including 219 illustrations of medicinal processing scenes) and thus provides valuable information for us to better understand ancient Chinese medicinal processing. As shown in Figures 26.2A (medicinal processing scenes and equipments such as chopper, mortar and pestle, boiler, stove and jar) and 26.2B (the steps of processing aconite lateral root (*fuzi*), such as cutting, mixing with adjuvants, boiling, sun-drying and rinsing in running water), this book can be considered as an illustrated standard operation procedure manual for Chinese medicinal processing (Zheng and Qiu, 2004). Experiences of Chinese medicinal processing are also scattered in some 4000 ancient medicinal formula books. Modern scholars such as X.T. Wang and X.Z. Zhang have published monographs that partially sum up medicinal processing methods recorded in ancient Chinese medicinal literature (Zhang and Cai, 1984; Wang, 1998). Chinese medicinal processing is now an academic subject that studies the theory, technique, specification, standard, historical change and prospective of medicinal processing.

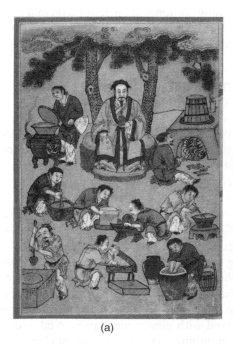 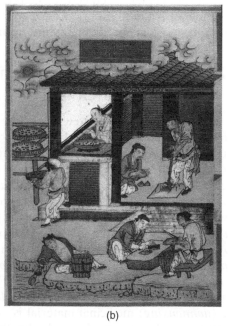

(a)                                          (b)

**Figure 26.2** Medicinal processing scenes and equipments (A) and steps of processing aconite lateral root (*fuzi, Aconitum carmichaeli* Debx.) (B) in *Concise Addendum to Grandfather Lei's Treatise on Herbal Processing (Bu Yi Lei Gong Pao Zhi Bian Lian)*.

## 26.3   Present state of Chinese medicinal processing

In TCM education and industry circles there is a common view of Chinese medicinal processing: 'process (medicinal materials) according to ancient processing methods'. With the passage of time, Chinese medicinal processing techniques have changed greatly. 'Process (medicinal materials) according to ancient processing methods' just embodies a principle. Which processing method should be used as the standard has evoked much controversy.

### 26.3.1   Inconsistency of ancient and current processing methods

In some cases, the current processing methods are inconsistent with the ancient ones. For example, in ancient times the processing methods of fleeceflower root (*heshouwu*) included cleaning, cutting and processing with or without adjuvants, as described in the *Compendium of Materia Medica* (*Ben Cao Gang Mu*) from the Ming dynasty: 'Peel off the coarse bark with a bamboo knife, soak overnight in rice rinse water, and then cut into slices. Put one layer of water soaked black beans and one layer of fleeceflower root (*heshouwu*) slices in a pot, repeat the layers, and then steam. When the black beans become cooked, take out fleeceflower root (*heshouwu*) slices and dry in the sun. Repeat this steaming and sun-drying procedure 9 times. This is known as processing with rice rinse water and black bean, and steaming and sun-drying 9 times.' This method emphasizes 'steaming 9 times and sun-drying 9 times' (Li, 1985). Nowadays, the main processing methods of fleeceflower root (*heshouwu*) include steaming with black bean juice, stewing with black bean juice, steaming alone, steaming with black bean juice and yellow rice wine, and pressure steaming. The processing of fleeceflower root (*heshouwu*) lasts for 3–40 hours. Clearly the present processing methods do not completely match those in ancient times. As mentioned before, the processing contents in ancient medicinal literature include condensed clinical experiences of ancient TCM practitioners. Until further comparative studies have been carried out, discarding ancient processing methods is not appropriate.

### 26.3.2   Inconsistency of processing practice in different provinces of China

Currently, there are no harmonized processing practices for all regions of China. Apart from the national standard, various local standards are still in practice in different provinces and districts. Although decoction pieces standards of 446 raw medicinal materials are established in the *Chinese Pharmacopoeia*, they do not cover all processed medicinal products. For example, as described in the *Chinese Pharmacopoeia*, gastrodia tuber (*tianma*, rhizome of *Gastrodia elata* Bl.) is 'cleaned, moistened thoroughly or steamed soft, cut into thin slices, and dried', while in *Fujian Provincial Standards of Chinese Medicinal Processing*, gastrodia tuber (*tianma*) processed with ginger and wine is recorded (Fujian Provincial Public Health Bureau, 1988). Another example is that the processing method of arisaema rhizome (*tiannanxing*, *Arisaema erubescens* (Wall.) Schott/*A. heterophyllum* Bl./*A. amurense* Maxim.) recorded in *Hunan Provincial Standards of Chinese Medicinal Processing* is different from that recorded in *Fujian Provincial Standards of Chinese Medicinal Processing*. In the former, arisaema rhizome (*tiannanxing*) medicinal material is mixed with ginger juice, preserved and soaked with alumen, then boiled until it is only slightly numbing to the tongue when chewed. In the latter, arisaema rhizome (*tiannanxing*) medicinal material is mixed with fresh ginger slices, and then boiled with alumen until it is thoroughly cooked (Hunan Provincial Public Health Bureau, 2000).

Besides the differences in processing methods, the use of adjuvants also differs. For example, in the preparation of cooked rhubarb (*dahuang*, root and rhizome of *Rheum palmatum* L./*R. tanguticum* Maxim. ex Balf./*R. officinale* Baill.) (*shudahuang*), alcohol is used as the adjuvant in *Hunan Provincial Standards of Chinese Medicinal Processing*, but yellow rice wine is used as the adjuvant in the standards of Chinese medicinal processing of other provinces such as Fujian, Anhui and Guangxi (Fujian Provincial Public Health Bureau, 1988; Hunan Provincial Public Health Bureau, 2000; Food and Drug Administration of Guangxi Zhuang Autonomous Region, 2007; Food and Drug Administration of Anhui Province, 2006). Commonly used adjuvants in Chinese medicinal processing, such as wine, vinegar and honey, are often in different concentrations, specifications and quantities according to different standards. However, decoction pieces processed with the above adjuvants are indiscriminately prescribed as ingredients in proprietary TCM products and in prescriptions given by TCM practitioners.

The above phenomenon of 'one medicinal material with different processing methods in different places' should undergo scientific evaluation so that consistent practice can be established.

## 26.3.3 Differences in decoction pieces between Hong Kong and mainland China

According to our previous investigation on 356 common Chinese medicinals sold in Hong Kong herbal markets, most of them are in processed forms. However, the processing methods in Hong Kong and mainland China are not exactly the same (Table 26.3) (Zhao, 2004). A large number of Chinese medicinals in overseas herbal markets are imported from Hong Kong, therefore the situation of the Hong Kong herbal market reflects that of overseas herbal markets.

## 26.3.4 Differences in national pharmacopoeias regarding medicinal processing

Although botanical substances (including some Chinese medicinals) are listed in the pharmacopoeias of European countries and North America, information regarding their processing methods is absent. Among the 384 traditional medicinals listed in the *Korean Herbal Pharmacopoeia* only the following nine contain processing contents: agkistrodon (*qishe*), alumen (*baifan*), complanate astragalus seed (*shayuanzi, Astragalus complanatus* R. Br.), human placenta (*ziheche*), magnetitum (*cishi*), clam shell (*geqiao*), fish air bladder (*yubiao*), pyritum (*zirantong*) and boat-fruited sterculia seed (*pangdahai, Sterculia lychnophora* Hance\*). For example, magnetitum (*cishi*) is processed with the calcining method in the *Korean Herbal Pharmacopoeia*, while it is processed with the calcining method followed by quenching in vinegar in the *Chinese Pharmacopoeia* (Korea Food and Drug Administration, 2002). Similarly, a small number of processed medicinal materials are also recorded in the Vietnamese and Japanese pharmacopoeias (Vietnamese Pharmacopoeia Commission, 2005), but the processing methods of some medicinal materials are different from those in the *Chinese Pharmacopoeia* (Table 26.4).

\**Sterculia lychnophora* Hance is now treated as a synonym of *Scaphium affine* (Mast.) Pierre.

**Table 26.3**   Comparison of processing methods in mainland China and Hong Kong.

| Decoction Pieces | Mainland China | Hong Kong |
| --- | --- | --- |
| Chinese angelica root (*danggui*, *Angelica sinensis* (Oliv.) Diels) | Head : cut into pieces<br>Body: cut length-wise into slices<br>Tail: tie into a bundle and cut into slices<br>Process with wine<br><br>1 cm | Head: cut length-wise and strike into thin slices<br>Process with wine or simply steam<br><br>1 cm |
| Notoginseng (*sanqi*, root and rhizome of *Panax notoginseng* (Burk.) F.H. Chen) | Cut, or grind into fine powders<br><br>1 cm | Give the medicinal material a black stain and a polished look<br><br>1 cm |
| Danshen (*danshen*, root and rhizome of *Salvia miltiorrhiza* Bge.) | Transversely cut into slices or segments<br><br>1 cm | Compress and cut length-wise<br><br>1 cm |
| Phellodendron bark (*huangbo*, *Phellodendron chinense* Schneid.) | Transversely cut into thin strips<br><br>1 cm | Longitudinally cut into rectangular plates and then cut into thin slices<br><br>1 cm |
| Bitter orange (*zhiqiao*, immature fruit of *Citrus aurantium* L.) | Cut into slices<br><br>1 cm | Strike flat (with a hammer) and cut<br><br>1 cm |
| Fleeceflower root (*heshouwu*, *Polygonum multiflorum* Thunb.) | Cut into irregular and thick slices or segments<br>Process with black bean juice or simply steam<br><br>1 cm | Cut length-wise into slices after processing<br>Simply steam or steam with sugar, or boil with black bean<br><br>1 cm |

## 26.3.5   Lack of objective quality control standards

Quality control is extremely important for the safety of Chinese medicinals. However, quality control standards in Chinese medicinal processing practices are weak. The techniques used Chinese medicinal processing often depend on the practitioner's experience, which is strongly subjective and lacks objective criteria. For example, processed aconite root (*zhichuanwu*) is boiled until it 'hardly causes numbness to the tongue', whereas processed fleeceflower root (*zhiheshouwu*) is steamed until it 'becomes brown internally and externally'.

**Table 26.4**  Comparison of processing methods described in the Vietnamese, Japanese and Chinese pharmacopoeias.

| Medicinal materials | Vietnam | Japan | China |
|---|---|---|---|
| Chinese angelica root (*danggui, Angelica sinensis* (Oliv.) Diels) | Stir-fry with 40% aqueous alcohol. For each 100 kg of Chinese angelica root (*danggui*), 10 kg of 40% aqueous alcohol is used | Scald (dip into boiling water) *Root of *Angelica acutiloba* (Sieb. & Zucc.) Kitag. | Stir-fry with yellow rice wine. For each 100 kg of Chinese angelica root (*danggui*), 10 kg of yellow rice wine is used |
| Rehmannia root (*dihuang, Rehmannia glutinosa* Libosch.) | Three methods: steam with wine and ginger juice, steam with wine, simply steam | With or without the application of steaming | Two methods: stew with yellow rice wine, simply steam |
| Dried ginger (*ganjiang*, rhizome of *Zingiber officinale* Rosc.) | Clean, sun-dry or dry at a low temperature | Scald (dip into boiling water) | Clean and dry. Process into charred ginger (*jiangtan*) and blast-fried ginger (*paojiang*) |
| Cornus fruit (*shanzhuyu, Cornus officinalis* Sieb. et Zucc.) | Stew with wine. For each 10 kg of cornus fruit (*shanzhuyu*), 0.6–1 litre of wine is used | No records of processing | Stew or steam with yellow rice wine. For each 100 kg of cornus fruit (*shanzhuyu*), 20 kg of yellow rice wine is used |
| Nux vomica (*maqianzi*, seed of *Strychnos nux-vomica* L.) | Two methods: stir-fry with sand, process with sesame oil. | No records of processing | Stir-fry with sand |

## 26.3.6  Progress in research

The main objectives of medicinal processing are enhancing the efficacy and reducing the toxicity of Chinese medicinals. When a medicinal material is heated and treated with such adjuvants as wine, vinegar and medicinal juices (e.g. black bean juice), its chemical components change. Modern research has proved that after processing, the contents of some chemical components in a medicinal material may increase while others may decrease, and their chemical structures may alter. In some cases, the contents and structures of chemical components may change at the same time. This is mainly because structural transformation in some chemical components may occur during processing. For example, raw aconite lateral root (*fuzi*) contains toxic diterpenoid alkaloids such as aconitine, mesaconitine and hypaconitine. Processing causes hydrolysis of these toxic alkaloids into less toxic compounds (benzoylaconine, benzoylmesaconine and benzoylhypaconine). Thus, the processed form of aconite lateral root (*fuzi*) is less toxic than its unprocessed form (Lin *et al.*, 1999). After the steaming procedure, ginseng (*renshen*, root and rhizome of *Panax ginseng* C.A. Mey.) is processed into red ginseng (*hongshen*). During the heating process in steam, primary glycosides (ginsenosides) are transformed into secondary glycosides by losing malonic acids, and parts of ginsenosides with $S$ structure are transformed into those with $R$ structure. As a result, characteristic chemical components are generated in red ginseng (*hongshen*) (Li, 1990).

In addition, processing also has certain influences on the dissolution of chemical components of medicinal materials. For example, the dissolution of alkaloids in a decoction made from wine-processed coptis rhizome (*huanglian, Coptis chinensis* Franch./*C. deltoidea* C.Y. Cheng et Hsiao/*C. teeta* Wall.) is higher than that in a decoction made from the unprocessed form of coptis rhizome (*huanglian*) (Fan *et al.*, 2006).

Because changes in chemical components occur after processing, the functions and pharmacological activities of a Chinese medicinal may change accordingly. One current focus of research is the comparative study of the pharmacological activities of Chinese medicinals before and after processing.

Research on medicinal processing techniques has also been conducted. These research efforts include the optimization of medicinal processing techniques and the improvement of traditional facilities and methods for medicinal processing. Improvement and innovation of traditional medicinal processing techniques are beneficial to the industrialized production of Chinese medicinal decoction pieces.

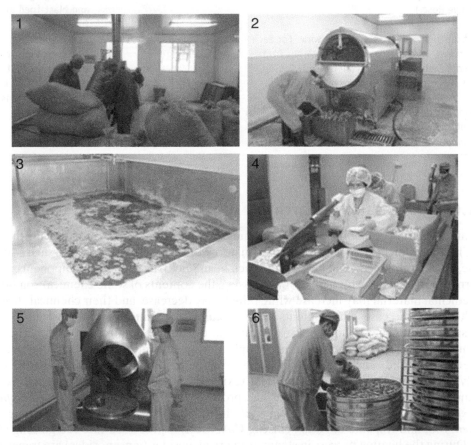

**Figure 26.3**  A sketch of Chinese medicinal processing procedures: 1, storage; 2, cleaning; 3, soaking; 4, cutting; 5, stir-frying; 6, steaming.

## 26.4 Prospect for future developments in Chinese medicinal processing

Decoction pieces standards of 446 raw medicinal materials are established in the *Chinese Pharmacopoeia* (Chinese Pharmacopoeia Commission, 2010). However, these standards are not sufficient when compared with quality evaluation standards for raw medicinal materials listed in the *Chinese Pharmacopoeia*. As mentioned before, changes in chemical components in a Chinese medicinal occur after processing. The quality evaluation standard of the processed form of a Chinese medicinal should be different from that of its unprocessed form. Different marker compounds should also be determined where necessary. Research on quality standards for the processed forms of Chinese medicinals therefore needs to be increased.

With the development of modern technology, facilities in traditional Chinese medicinal processing manufacturing have gradually improved (Figure 26.3). Modern research on medicinal processing techniques provides the necessary scientific basis for the standardization of Chinese medicinal processing. However, a comprehensive evaluation method combining marker compounds, chemical fingerprints and pharmacological activities should be used when research on the optimization of medicinal processing techniques is carried out. As a unique characteristic in the practice of TCM, Chinese medicinal processing has a close relationship with the safety and efficacy of Chinese medicinals. Standardization of Chinese medicinal processing techniques and the establishment of criteria for processed forms of Chinese medicinals are urgently needed.

In conclusion, the establishment of united and scientific standards of Chinese medicinal processing is one of the key steps in the standardization of Chinese *materia medica* (Zhao *et al.*, 2010).

## References

British Pharmacopoeia Commission (2009) *British Pharmacopoeia, 2009 edition*, The Stationery Office on Behalf of the Medicines and Healthcare Products Regulatory Agency, London.

Chan, T.Y., Tomlinson, B., Tse, L.K., *et al.* (1994) Aconitine poisoning due to Chinese herbal medicines: a review. *Veterinary and Human Toxicology*, **36**, 452–455.

Chinese Pharmacopoeia Commission (2010) *Pharmacopoeia of the People's Republic of China, 2010 edition*, China Medical Science Press, Beijing.

European Pharmacopoeia Commission (2007) *European Pharmacopoeia*, 6th edn, European Directorate for the Quality of Medicines & Healthcare of the Council of Europe, Strasbourg.

Fan, D.L., Liao, Q.W., Yan, D., *et al.* (2006) A comparative study on the alkaloids in different processed forms of *huanglian* (Coptidis Rhizoma). *Pharmaceutical Journal of Chinese People's Liberation Army*, **22**, 276–279.

Food and Drug Administration of Anhui Province (2006) *Anhui Provincial Standards of Chinese Medicinal Processing, 2005 edition*. Anhui Science and Technology Press, Hefei.

Food and Drug Administration of Guangxi Zhuang Autonomous Region (2007) *Standards of Chinese Medicinal Processing of Guangxi Zhuang Autonomous Region*, Guangxi Science and Technology Press, Nanning.

Fujian Provincial Public Health Bureau (1988) *Fujian Provincial Standards of Chinese Medicinal Processing*, Fujian Science and Technology Press, Fuzhou.

Hunan Provincial Public Health Bureau (2000) *Hunan Provincial Standards of Chinese Medicinal Processing, 1983 edition*, Hunan Science and Technology Press, Changsha.

Korea Food and Drug Administration (2002) *Korean Pharmacopoeia*, 8th edn, Yakup Daily, Seoul.

Lei, X. (1991) *Grandfather Lei's Treatise on Herbal Processing (Lei Gong Pao Zhi Lun)*, Anhui Science and Technology Press, Hefei.

Li, S.Z. (1985) *Compendium of Materia Medica (Ben Cao Gang Mu)*, People's Medical Publishing House, Beijing.

Li, X.G. (1990) Progress in research of the processing mechanism of ginseng. *Chinese Traditional and Herbal Drugs*, **13**, 22–25.

Lin, W.F., Zhang, X.L. and Wang, L. (1999) Modern research on the processing of aconite root. *Journal of Shandong University of Traditional Chinese Medicine*, **23**, 232–234.

Miao, X.Y. (1992) *Methods of Herbal Processing (Pao Zhi Da Fa)*, Cathay Book Shop, Beijing.

Society of Japanese Pharmacopoeia (2006) *Japanese Pharmacopoeia*, 15th edn, Yakuji Nippo, Ltd, Tokyo.

United States Pharmacopoeial Convention (2007) *The United States Pharmacopoeia, 30th revision/National Formulary*, 25th edn, The United States Pharmacopoeial Convention, Rochville.

Vietnamese Pharmacopoeia Commission (2005) *Pharmacopoeia Vietnamica*, 3rd edn, *Hanoi*.

Wang, X.T. (1992) The view on the research of historical changes of Chinese medicinal processing. *China Journal of Chinese Materia Medica*, **17**, 211–212.

Wang, X.T. (1998) *A Collection of Chinese Medicinal Processing Methods in Past Dynasties (Ancient Times)*, Jiangxi Science and Technology Press, Nanchang.

Xia, L., Bai, L.P., Yi, L., *et al.* (2007) Authentication of the 31 species of toxic and potent Chinese Materia Medica (T/PCMM) by microscopic technique, Part 1: three kinds of toxic and potent animal CMM. *Microscopy Research Technique*, **70**, 960–968.

Zhang, R. (2000) *A Guide to Herbal Processing (Xiu Shi Zhi Nan)*, Hainan Publishing House, Haikou.

Zhang, X.Z. and Cai, G.H. (1984) *Chinese Medicinal Processing*. China Medical College, Taichung, Taiwan.

Zhao, Z.Z. (2004) *An Illustrated Chinese Materia Medica in Hong Kong*, Chung Hwa Book Co., (H.K.) Ltd, Hong Kong.

Zhao, Z.Z., Hu, Y.N., Liang, Z.T., *et al.* (2006) Authentication is fundamental for standardization of Chinese medicines. *Planta Medica*, **72**, 865–874.

Zhao, Z.Z., Liang, Z.T., Chan, K., *et al.* (2010) A unique issue in the standardization of Chinese Materia Medica: Processing. *Planta Medica*, **76**, 1975–1986.

Zheng, J.S. and Qiu, J. (2004) A preliminary study on newly appeared *Concise Addendum to Grandfather Lei's Treatise on Herbal Processing (Bu Yi Lei Gong Pao Zhi Bian Lian)*. *Chinese Pharmaceutical Journal*, **39**, 389–391.

Zou, J.M. and Wang, L.S. (2005) Analysis of the situation of the processing of Chinese Materia Medica. *Chinese Traditional and Herbal Drugs*, **36**, 620–623.

# 27

# A South-East Asian Perspective on Ethnopharmacology

Pravit Akarasereenont[1,3], Marianne J.R. Datiles[2,3], Natchagorn Lumlerdkij[2,4], Harisun Yaakob[5], Jose M. Prieto[2] and Michael Heinrich[2]

[1]Department of Pharmacology, Faculty of Medicine Siriraj Hospital, Mahidol University, Bangkok, Thailand
[2]Centre for Pharmacognosy and Phytotherapy/Research Cluster 'Biodiversity and Medicines', UCL School of Pharmacy, London, UK
[3]Department of Botany, US National Museum of Natural History, US Smithsonian, Washington DC, USA
[4]Center of Applied Thai Traditional Medicine, Faculty of Medicine Siriraj Hospital, Mahidol University, Bangkok, Thailand
[5]Institute of Bioproduct Development, Universiti Teknologi Malaysia, Johor, Malaysia

## 27.1 Introduction

South-East Asia consists of Brunei Darussalam, Cambodia, Indonesia, Lao PDR, Malaysia, Myanmar, the Philippines, Singapore, Thailand and Vietnam – collectively known as the Association of South-East Asian Nations (ASEAN). TM along with biomedicine has been used to maintain people's health in this region for a long time. The diversity of ASEAN TM is shown in Table 27.1. In 2004, following the Asian financial crisis (1997–98), ASEAN members agreed to implement the WHO's TM strategy (WHO, 2002) and drive the use of TM, especially herbal medicine, into their healthcare systems to reduce the cost of imported drugs and improve access to healthcare. The ASEAN member states declared the integration safe, effective and quality TM into their national healthcare systems. The ASEAN member states declared the integration of safe, effective and quality TM into their national healthcare systems (ASEAN Secretariat, 2009) to be a political priority. They put particular emphasis on the conservation and restoration of TMs (Ministers of Health of ASEAN Member Countries, 2004). This agreement is expected to positively impact the primary healthcare system of each country, as well as many other areas of national concern, including household economic status, social and cultural preservation and promotion efforts, and the discovery of substances with pharmacological action leading to new drug development.

**Table 27.1**   Summary of TM systems in ASEAN countries (Chuthaputti and Boonterm, 2010a).

| Countries | National TM | TCM | Indian TM* | Others |
|---|---|---|---|---|
| Brunei Darussalam | – | + | + | Malay TM, Indonesian TM (*Jamu*), Thai TM |
| Cambodia | Khmer | – | – | |
| Indonesia | *Jamu* | + | + | |
| Lao PDR | Yaphurnmeung | – | – | |
| Malaysia | Malay | + | + | Malay TM, Indonesian TM (*Jamu*), Islam TM (*Ruqyah*) |
| Myanmar | Myanmar | + | + | |
| Philippines | Hilots | + | + | |
| Singapore | – | + | + | Malay TM, *Jamu*, Thai TM |
| Thailand | Thai | + | + | |
| Vietnam | Vietnamese | + | + | |

*Indian TM is Ayurveda, Siddha, Unani.

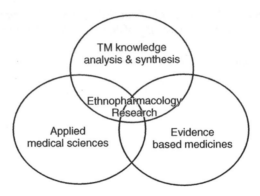

**Figure 27.1**   The main dimensions of ethnopharmacology research in ASEAN countries.

Ethnopharmacology includes the study of the pharmacology of TM, particularly of active substances and their pharmacological action. Within the context of healthcare systems based on evidence-based medicine, the integration of TM into the national healthcare systems of ASEAN countries requires continued research on the quality, safety and efficacy of herbal medicines used within TM. In this chapter we consider three dimensions of ethnopharmacology research in ASEAN countries (Figure 27.1). Each country utilizes these differently, but each maintains the same core dimensions based on ASEAN policy and TM strategies. Some examples are provided in Table 27.2.

The use of TM in national healthcare systems has been limited, especially by biomedicine. This is largely due to the lack of data on the quality, safety and efficacy of TM, therefore in order to promote the use of TM and herbal drugs, the ASEAN has established the Traditional Medicines and Health Supplements Product Working Group (TMHSPWG) and five member states were assigned to lead five key actions (Table 27.2). To accomplish the aim, the working group has set the following objectives and action plans (ASEAN Ministers on Agriculture and Forestry, 2004):

1.   Establishment of databases on ASEAN herbal products and medicinal plants by:
     1.1   Submission of species of medicinal plants and profile of selected families.

**Table 27.2** Ethnopharmacology in ASEAN countries – implications of policy on political targets and main scientific aims.

| Coordinating country | Main dimensions of ethnopharmacology research | Aim |
| --- | --- | --- |
| Thailand | Evidence-based medicines | Integration of TM into primary health care |
| Vietnam | Evidence-based medicines | Development of TM clinical services |
| Myanmar | TM knowledge analysis and synthesis | Provision of TM education and training |
| Malaysia | Applied medical sciences | Creating plant databases |
| Indonesia | Applied medical sciences | Conducting TM research |

    1.2   Compilation and consolidation of the submitted information.

    1.3   Publication of the databases.

2.  Coordination of research and development (R&D) and sharing of scientific information by:

    2.1   Documentation of R&D information/directory (project brief and institution).

    2.2   Compilation and consolidation of the submitted information.

    2.3   Publication of the R&D activities on herbal and medicinal plants.

    2.4   Organization of workshops on the activities on herbal and medicinal plants.

3.  Development of training programme in appropriate areas by:

    3.1   Scientist exchange programme.

4.  Organization of workshops on:

    4.1   Registration and licensing in TM.

    4.2   Extraction of essential oils and marketing of medicinal plants.

5.  Transfer in herbal and medicinal plant technologies by:

    5.1   Implementation of projects on biological and chemical investigation, and selected ASEAN medicinal plant standardization.

6.  Provision of technical inputs for trade promotion in herbal and medicinal plants by:

    6.1   Collaboration on the development of guidelines for quality control of raw materials, such as good agriculture practices (GAP) and good collection practices (GCP).

    6.2   Establishment of a directory of products and companies (herbal hub).

## 27.2 Ethnopharmacology in Thailand

Thai traditional medicine (TTM) is considered a holistic medicine. The practice of TTM can be divided into four areas, including medical practice involving diagnosis and treatment, pharmacy practice involving the use and production of herbal medicine, traditional midwifery and traditional Thai massage (*Nuad Thai*). A decline in TTM acceptance occurred during the period 1916–77 due to the influence of western medicine. However, the revival began in 1978 after WHO urged its members to implement TM and herbal medicine in their primary health-care systems. Since 1977, every Thai government has supported medicinal plants research and development (R&D) by provision of research funding for Thai researchers. As a result, R&D in herbal medicines has been performed in most universities. However, most research involved preclinical studies of single herbs. During 2000–2003 only 31 out of 395 publications

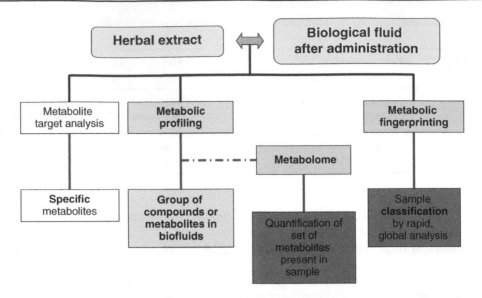

**Figure 27.2**   The metabolomic study network in Thailand and its approach in herbal medicine research.

with Thai authors were clinical trials (Chuthaputti and Boonterm, 2010b). The extensive study of single herbs led to success in medicinal plants databases creation, such as MedPlant Online by the Faculty of Pharmacy, Mahidol University (http://www.medplant.mahidol.ac.th) and Thaicrudedrug.com by Faculty of Pharmaceutical Sciences, Ubon Ratchathani University (http://www.thaicrudedrug.com).

Recently, the trend of TM research has shifted to clinical trials assessing the efficacy and safety of herbal medicines. Subsequently, studies on the mechanism of action and pharmacokinetics of traditional medicines with proven efficacy and safety will follow. At the moment ethnopharmacology (e.g. Siriwatanametanon *et al.*, 2010) and reverse pharmacology (Vaidya, 2006) has been employed. For instance, Thongpraditchote *et al.* (2001) studied the antipyretic activity of Chantaleela, a Thai traditional drug for relief of fever containing eight herbal ingredients, including *Gymnopetalum chinense* (Lour.) Merr., *Myristica fragrans* Houtt., *Dracaena loureiri* Gagnep, *Tinospora crispa* (L.) Hook. f. & Thomson, *Eurycoma longifolia* Jack, *Atractylodes lancea* (Thunb.) DC., *Angelica sylvestris* L. and *Artemisia vulgaris* L. The result showed that 400 mg/kg Chantaleela exhibited antipyretic properties similar to 200 mg/kg paracetamol

**Figure 27.3**   Example of systematic analysis of *A. paniculata* effects on platelet function in Thai healthy volunteers (unpublished data). Gene expression and protein measurements of cyclooxygenase-1 (COX-1), COX-2, P-selectin and thromboxane $A_2$ were measured to examine patient-to-patient variability in platelet aggregation. Data at 0 hour represents baseline measurement whereas data for 2 and 24 h represent relative changes normalized by the 0-hr baseline. A, Two-way hierarchical clustering of patient-to-patient variations and the relationship of parameters. B, Score plot from the principal component analysis (PCA) showing similarity of platelet function among all patients. Results were illustrated using different marker types for the different agonists, including ADP at 5 μM, collagen at 1 μg/ml, epinephrine at 1 and 25 μM. Platelet status of the volunteers are as follows; disaggregated- 8, hyperaggregated- 1, 2, 4, 6, normal—3, 5, 7, 9. C, Loading plot from the PCA analysis showing contributions of the measured parameters towards each principal component 1 and 2. D, Linear discriminant analysis of the measured parameters by genders; female—1, 2, 4, 5, 10, male—3, 6, 7, 8, 9.

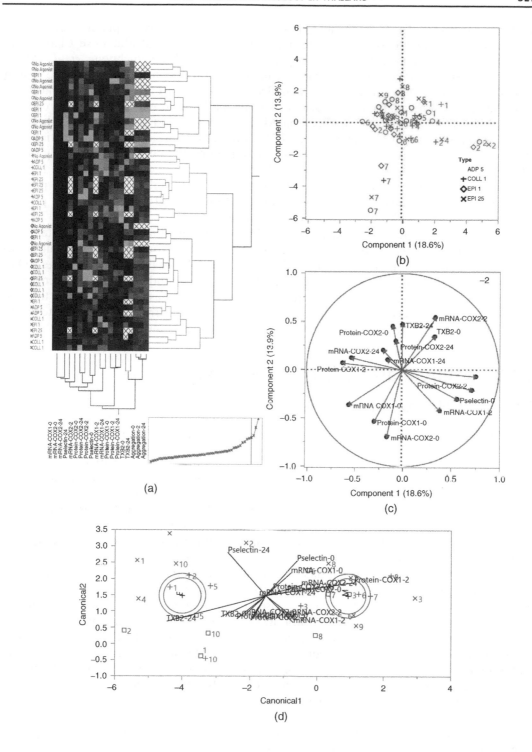

(a)

(b)

(c)

(d)

in an animal model (Thongpraditchote *et al.*, 2001). Later, its effect on platelet aggregation was assessed in 12 healthy volunteers to evaluate its safety. At normal adult dose, Chantaleela did not affect platelet aggregation and platelet numbers (Itthipanichpong *et al.*, 2010). Although these data are not grade A evidence in the general evidence-based medicine system (Ebell *et al.*, 2004) that can confirm Chantaleela's safety and efficacy, these publications reflect the trend of herbal medicine research in Thailand. Moreover, a group of researchers at Mahidol University's Center of Applied Thai Medicine in Thailand is creating a metabolomic (Figure 27.2) and system biology (Figure 27.3) study network to integrate information into practice and rational use. An example of research done by the network is the study of the effect of *Andrographis paniculata* (Burm.f.) Nees on platelet aggregation in Thai healthy volunteers. As shown in Figure 27.3, a difference was observed in response on platelet aggregation after *A. paniculata* intake that depended on induced agonists, sex and platelet status (Akarasereenont/Lumlerdkij/Heinrich? *et al.*, unpublished).

In addition, to accelerate the integration of TM into the national healthcare system, the government has in 1999 established the national essential herbal drug list containing traditional drugs and herbal items for many health conditions (National Drug Committee, 2006). The prescribed items can be reimbursed from the government under the universal coverage scheme. However, physicians have not prescribed them as much as expected due to the lack of clinical data on safety and efficacy. Thus we hope that our current research strategy will encourage Thai physicians to prescribe more traditional drugs in the near future.

## 27.3   Ethnopharmacology in Malaysia

### 27.3.1   Malay traditional medicine

Current Malay traditional medicine is a truly rich complex heritage due to the huge biological diversity and multiethnic–multicultural origins of the country. The *Orang Asli* (indigenous people) who have lived in the region from 40,000 BC adopted – and adapted – Indonesian traditional practices to their own needs. The *bomoh* (Malay traditional healer) diagnosed the disease and administered the traditional treatment, and therefore these people are important in the life of many Malay villagers (Raden Sanusi & Werner, 1985). Chinese and Indian immigrants bringing in their own traditions as early as 1 AD subsequently influenced the aboriginal culture. After the creation of the Malacca Sultanate in the early 15th century, the Malay traditional medical system was repositioned in the context of Arabic Unani medicine and Galenic philosophy. As a result of so many influences Malay traditional medicine today, uses a holistic approach for the purpose of treating and preventing illnesses, and for rehabilitation and health promotion. Diagnosis is based on the examination of physical conditions, which comprise four elements, namely *suprawi* (fire), *suddawi* (earth), *dammawi* (wind) and *balpawi* (water), and spiritual influences, namely bad spirits and ghosts. The prescription may include single- or multi-ingredient medicines compounded from plant, animal, microorganism and/or mineral drugs as well as chants (*jampi*), prayers (*doa*), massage, abstinence (*pantang*) and other practices (Jamal, 2006; Zakaria and Mohd, 2010). Malay medicinal plants can either be collected from home gardens or the neighbouring forests, or purchased from retail stores or local herbal suppliers.

A characteristic of many remedies in Malay traditional herbal medicines is that they are important from both a nutritional and a medicinal point of view. In terms of indications, Malay medicine pays particular attention to two gender-related groups of preparations. On the one hand, women's health before, during and after childbirth is maintained and/or restored with the help of *Jamu* and/*or Meroyan* remedies, respectively. On the other hand, tonics or *makjun* contribute to men's health by 'cleansing the blood' and improving virility (Zakaria and Mohd, 2010).

Regarding women's health, postnatal care is indeed an important aspect in Malay traditional medicines. A recent survey of medicinal plants used for postnatal care in just two Southern districts (Muar and Kuala Pilah) unveiled an impressive list of 23 different preparations making use from 52 species (Jamal *et al.*, 2011). The plants were used by the mother as *Jamu*, to treat infant's common conditions such as eye infections and to prevent skin conditions. The species found to occur most frequently were *Curcuma longa* L. (Zingiberaceae), *Zingiber officinale* Roscoe (Zingiberaceae), *Cinnamomum zeylanicum* Blume (Lauraceae), *Kaempferia galanga* L. (Zingiberaceae), *Piper cubeba* Bojer (Piperaceae), *Zingiber cassumunar* Roxb. (Zingiberaceae), *Acorus calamus* L. (Acoraceae), *Piper nigrum* Beyr. ex Kunth (Piperaceae), *Alyxia stellata* (J.R.Forst. & G.Forst.) Roem. & Schult. (Apocinaceae), *Coriandrum sativum L* (Apiaceae), *Foeniculum vulgare* Mill. (Apiaceae), *Nigella sativa* L. (Ranunculaceae) and the lichen *Usnea barbata* Fries (Parmeliaceae). All can be locally sourced except black cumin, suggesting that this is an influence of Prophetic medicine rather than a pre-Muslim Malay tradition because it is described as a panacea in the Quran. This shortlist is dominated by common spices, thus stressing the strong link between food and medicine in Malay traditions. Indeed, dietary interventions are part of the health management of Malay women, who avoid most fruits and vegetables during the postpartum period and eat foods considered 'hot', such as eggs, dairy, and salty and spicy meals (Naser *et al.*, 2012).

Tonics (*makjun*) consist of decoctions of tree roots usually taken daily, and most of them are especially for men such as Tongkat Ali (*Eurycoma longifolia* Jack, Simaroubaceae) and Tongkat Ali Hitam (*Polyalthia bullata* King, Annonaceae). Others are Bodilalat (*Diospyros discolor* Willd., Ebenaceae) and Bunga tanjung (*Mimusops elengi* L., Sapotaceae) (Ong and Norzalina, 1999; Ong and Nordiana, 1999). Interestingly, Kacip Fatimah – *Marantodes pumilum* (Blume) Kuntze; (*syn. Labisia pumila* (Blume) Mez) – is considered as providing the equivalent of Tongkat Ali for women, and its consumption alone or in the form of various food supplements is hugely popular in Malaysia. This, together with it being considered a gynaecological panacea justifies its common alias of 'Queen of Herbs' (Bodeker, 1999).

## 27.3.2  Clinical integration of the Malay traditional medicines

In line with other ASEAN countries, since 2000 Malaysia has adopted a coordinated approach to integration. It is based on self-regulation by complementary professions which include Malay, Chinese and Indian traditional health systems, complementary therapies and homoeopathy. Dedicated councils recognize, accredit and register their own practitioners while developing standardized training programmes, guidelines, accreditation standards and codes of ethics (Bodeker, 2001).

Furthermore, in 2006 the Malaysian cabinet approved a proposal to set up an integrated medicine programme that incorporates into the health system selected traditional and CAM practices such as traditional Malay massage and acupuncture for chronic and post-stroke management, herbal therapy as an adjuvant treatment for cancer and Malay postnatal care, with the aim of ensuring the safety and quality of these practices to the patients. As of 2012, a total of 10 hospitals have integrated these traditional and CAM practices as an outpatient service only. However, the hospitals require patients to be seen by the allopathic practitioners before opting for traditional therapies. This has resulted in setting up detailed guidelines on Malay massage and postnatal care, acupuncture, reflexology, and herbal therapies as an adjunct treatment for cancer (Farooqui, 2013).

## 27.3.3   Modern phytotherapeutic products and food supplements from Malay traditional medicinal plants

Recent studies confirm that the use of plants for healing, consumption as health foods, beautification, utilities and rituals are still very important in Malay culture, even in urban environments (Adnan and Othman, 2012). However, the use of TM is decreasing as literacy increases among the population (Naser *et al.*, 2012), and the use of traditional food is also in danger as new generations do not pass traditional culture onto their descendants (Nor *et al.*, 2012).

Furthermore, with the global resurgence in interest in natural remedies as a commodity, Malaysia is looking towards capitalizing on its megabiodiversity, which includes the oldest rainforest in the world and an estimated 1200 medicinal plants. To harness this potential, a Herbal Development Office has been formed under the Ministry of Agriculture (MoA). It outlines the strategic direction, policies and regulation of R&D clusters, focusing on discovery, crop production and agronomy, standardization and product development, toxicology/pre-clinical and clinical studies, and processing technology. Preference has been given to a subset of 10 traditional plant species with high economic potential (Table 27.3). Given that Malaysia is mostly an agricultural country, sufficient supply of raw materials for R&D is ensured. Moreover, its multiethnic population facilitates clinical trials whose results can be extrapolated to many other markets. With this in mind, and to promote and protect the growth of a local herbal industry, endemic species and varieties of these medicinal plants are under active study to derive high-value herbal supplements and remedies (Malaysian Ministry of Agriculture, 2011).

**Table 27.3**   Top traditional herbs under current R&D focus in Malaysia.

| Latin name | Family | Malay name | Part used | Targeted Indications |
|---|---|---|---|---|
| *Androgaphis paniculata* (Burm.f.) Nees | Acanthaceae | Hempedu Bumi | Leaves | Antidiabetic tonic and supplement |
| *Centella asiatica* (L.) Urb. | Apiaceae | Pegaga | Leaves, stem | Skin care ingredients, herbal drink |
| *Clinacanthus nutans* (Burm.f.) Lindau | Acanthaceae | Belalai gajah | Leaves | Herbal drink, anticancer supplement |
| *Eurycoma longifolia* Jack | Simaroubaceae | Tongkat Ali | Roots | Male's tonic, coffee, energy drink |
| *Ficus deltoidea* Jack | Moraceae | Mas Cotek | Fruit, roots and leaves | Afterbirth tonic, whitening serum |
| *Hibiscus sabdariffa* L. | Malvaceae | Roselle | Fruit, leaves | Functional drink, skin care |
| *Marantodes pumilum* (Blume) Kuntze (*syn. Labisia pumila* (Blume) Mez) | Primulaceae | Kacip Fatimah | Leaves and roots | Gynecological, antiaging serum, women tonic and supplement |
| *Morinda citrifolia* L. | Rubiaceae | Mengkudu | Fruits, leaves and roots | Herbal drink, coffee |
| *Orthosiphon aristatus* (Blume) Miq. | Lamiaceae | Misai Kucing | Stem and leaves | Diuretic, Tea, herbal supplement for kidney disease |
| *Phyllanthus niruri* L. | Phyllanthaceae. | Dukung Anak | Whole plant | Liver tonic |

### 27.3.4   The future direction of Malay TM

From the many traditional herbal medicines used by Malay TM, *Jamu* and *Makjun* stand out as the most popular remedies used both in rural and urban areas. They are widely and regularly consumed, and may contribute to promote the health of the Malaysian population. However, because of this frequent and prolonged consumption, the natural occurrence of contaminants and possible herb–drug interactions with allopathic medicine are an important concern. Steps are being taken in terms of quality control (Ali *et al.*, 2005), but pharmacovigilance has to start to actively monitor for their adverse effects. Nonetheless, Malaysia is an example of how the potential of a rich ethnopharmacological heritage is being actively used to boost both the wealth and wellness of its society.

## 27.4   Ethnopharmacology in Indonesia

TMs in Indonesia has been used for hundreds years and are part of the national culture. Indonesia has the second largest biodiversity in the world expressed by the high number of indigenous medicinal plants. Because of its rich source of medicinal plants and poor facilities in the primary healthcare system, 70–80% of Indonesian people still use TM, known as *Jamu* (herbal medicine in Javanese) (Elfahmi *et al.*, 2014). In 2007, *Jamu* was declared to be an Indonesian brand (Figure 27.4) by the President of the Republic of Indonesia, Susilo Bambang Yudhoyono (Chuthaputti and Boonterm, 2010c). Although there has been much data from *in vitro* and *in vivo* studies that support the traditional use of many *Jamu* products, there is still too little clinical information on its effectiveness and safety to recommend uses on an evidence-based approach.

As Indonesia is clearly an important source of herbal medicines in the world and its people are still relying on its TM, the government established a policy for national TMs to achieve several important objectives, such as to promote the sustainable use of natural resources and to ensure the availability of quality, safe and effective TM. It launched 11 principles and measures of policy (Prapti, 2011) as follows:

1.  ethnobotanical-medical survey
2.  cultivation and conservation of herbal medicinal plants
3.  safety, efficacy and quality of herbal medicines
4.  accessibility for self-medication and formal health services
5.  rational use
6.  control of herbal medicine usage
7.  research and development
8.  industrialization of herbal medicines
9.  documentation and database

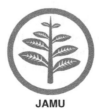

**JAMU**

**Figure 27.4**   Jamu brand.

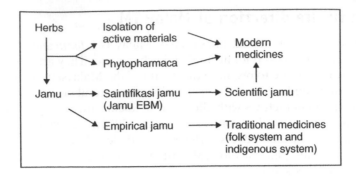

**Figure 27.5**    Plan for the development of Jamu.

10. development of human resources
11. monitoring and evaluation.

These lead to the plan for the development of *Jamu* (Figure 27.5), which is based on *Jamu*, Obat Herbal Terstandar (standardized herbal medicines) and Fitofarmaka (phytopharmaca) (National Agency of Drug and Food Control, 2007).

Thus, key tasks in the future include the evaluation of *Jamu* as a rational phytotherapy, which covers different areas of research, including clinical, social, cultural and economic studies, as well as ethical issues. In addition, pharmacological studies in the preclinical phase of herbal extracts and isolated compounds would be performed extensively to obtain standardized herbal medicines and phytopharmaca.

## 27.5    Ethnopharmacology in the Philippines

The use of medicinal plants in the Philippines is influenced by a complex variety of historical, cultural and political economic factors. The country consists of over 7000 islands and, due to centuries of influence from three separate continents as well as from neighbouring islands, healthcare in the Philippines can be understood as a reflection of Philippine identity: a mix of indigenous, Malay, Spanish, Chinese and American practices that vary from *barangay* (village) to *barangay*, coupled with a decentralized healthcare system that reinforces this heterogeneity (Kadetz, 2011, pers. comm. 13 Apr 2014; Galvez-Tan, 2013).

Local practitioners include the *hilots*, traditional Filipino healers known for their touch therapy techniques, and *albularyos*, herbalists or rural 'medicine men'. These terms are often interchangeable depending on locality, and both are locally understood to be an alternative to 'western' biomedicine.

In recent years the Philippine government has taken measures to regulate plant-based medicines for safer use. Republic Act No. 8423, the Traditional and Alternative Medicine Act of 1997, was enacted in 1999 and resulted in the formation of the Philippine Institute of Traditional and Alternative Health Care (PITAHC). One of PITAHC's major objectives is to 'promote and advocate the use of traditional, alternative, preventive and curative health care modalities that [have] been proven safe, effective, cost-effective and consistent with government standards on medical practice' (RA No. 8423). In 2004, the Department of Health of the Philippines (DOH)'s Bureau of Food and Drugs (BFAD) published the first Philippine pharmacopoeia (PP1). Prior to 2004, the major references for botanical

**Table 27.4** First 10 Herbal Plants Approved by the Department of Health (DOH) for Traditional Use in the Philippines.

| Latin name | Family | Filipino name | Part used | Targeted Indications |
|---|---|---|---|---|
| *Vitex negundo* L. | Piperaceae | Lagundi | Leaves | Cough and asthma |
| *Blumea balsamifera* (L.) DC. | Asteraceae | Sambong | Leaves | Anti-urolithiasis (kidney stones) |
| *Momordica charantia* L. | Rubiaceae | Ampalaya | Leaves | Anti-diabetes and lowering blood sugar |
| *Allium sativum* L. | Amaryllidaceae | Bawang | Bulbs | Anti-cholesterol |
| *Psidium guajava* L. | Myrtaceae | Bayabas | Leaves | Oral and skin antiseptic |
| *Carmona microphylla* (Lam.) G. Don | Boraginaceae | Tsaang-gubat | Leaves | Oral antiseptic |
| *Mentha arvensis* L. | Lamiaceae | Yerba-buena | Leaves | Analgesic or ant-pyretic |
| *Combretum indicum* (L.) DeFilipps | Combretaceae | Niyug-niyogan | Fruits | Anti-helminthic |
| *Senna alata* (L.) Roxb. | Fabaceae | Akapulko | Leaves | Anti-fungal |
| *Peperomia pellucida* (L.) Kunth | Piperaceae | Ulasimang-bato | All aerial parts | Anti-hyperurisemia |

uses in Philippine medicine were an 84-monograph government national formulary in 1978, Eduardo Quisumbing's 1935 *Medicinal Plants of the Philippines*, and Spanish and American colonial-period documents (BFAD, 2004). Also before 2004, medicinal plant regulations had been based on other countries' models, including those of the US, UK and Japan, and were inconsistently enforced (JICA, 2001).

The PP1 contains monographs for 32 medicinal plant species, 10 of which have now been officially endorsed by the DOH for traditional use (Table 27.4). The PP1 monographs serve as models that provide uniformity for future pharmaceutical product and medicinal plant additions to the pharmacopoeia, and contain information concerning morphology, botanical descriptions, histology, laboratory identification methods, major chemical constituents and specific medicinal uses of each plant, but exclude usage history and ethnobotanical diversity.

The endorsement process for these first 10 plants required, in some cases, decades. The development of *lagundi*, for example, began in the 1970s under the National Integrated Research Program on Medicinal Plants led by the University of the Philippines–Manila, where the National Institutes of Herbal Medicine (NIHM) was formed and is now based. While researchers from the NIHM and other research institutions have continued to produce new research to scientifically validate known traditional uses of plant species, the DOH has been unable to confirm an additional 10 plants from the PP1 to endorse every five years as originally planned due to limited government funds (Feria, 2007).

The Philippines is also home to approximately 25 ethnolinguistically distinct indigenous peoples of Afro-Asian descent called the Negritos, who have traditionally been known to have extensive knowledge and use of local medicinal plants (e.g. Sia *et al.*, 2002; Datiles and Heinrich, 2013). There is a lack of internationally published research and documentation of this knowledge, likely due to the strict regulations put in place by the government to protect indigenous knowledge, but the NIHM is compiling ethnopharmacological studies in the Philippines online (http://www.tkdlph.com/) and has been working to produce a publicly available database of medicinal plant uses with inputs from members of indigenous groups (http://www.katutubolokal.com/).

The future of ethnopharmacology in the Philippines will rely on the successful collaboration of scientific researchers, both within the country and internationally, local community *hilots* and *albularyos,* and the existing government agencies, as well as the continued growth in new research on local ethnopharmacological knowledge that respects and complies with the protection of indigenous plant knowledge in the Philippines.

## 27.6   Ethnopharmacology in Vietnam

Vietnamese TM has evolved under the shadows of TCM, Chinese culture and Chinese rule for several thousand years. Now it is almost impossible to distinguish traditional Vietnamese medicine (Thuoc Nam or southern medicine) from TCM (Thuoc Bac or northern medicine) (Thai, 2011). For this reason, the future of ethnopharmacology in Vietnam is likely to follow TCM development.

## 27.7   Ethnopharmacology in Myanmar, Lao PDR and Cambodia

As research in these countries is still under development, the trend of TM research may focus on quality control of herbal medicine under GMP in order to serve primary healthcare and to expand the economic scale of herbal medicinal plants.

In Myanmar, the Department of Traditional Medicine established a research unit to ensure the authenticity, safety, efficacy, toxicity and quality of TM. The Ministry of Health established the Department of Medical Research to implement research activities for new traditional medicines, especially for six common diseases, namely diarrhoea, dysentery, malaria, tuberculosis, hypertension and diabetes (Chuthaputti and Boonterm, 2010a). The future of ethnopharmacology in these countries is to serve the clinical use of these six common diseases.

## 27.8   Ethnopharmacology in Singapore and Brunei

There is no autochthonous TM in Singapore and Brunei. Singapore was separated from Malaysia, and Brunei was separated from the UK, who governed Malaysia during that time. Both countries are therefore influenced by Malay culture, as well as the TM which they use, TCM and Indian TM (Chuthaputti and Boonterm, 2010a). For this reason, the future of ethnopharmacology in Singapore is likely to follow TCM development. For Brunei, the future of ethnopharmacology is likely to follow mixed knowledge from TCM, Indian TM and Malay TM, where research in the quality control of herbal materials would be the focus.

## 27.9   Conclusion

Ethnopharmacological research in ASEAN countries is, in general, both a governmental priority and a key interest of the healthcare sector. The increasing use of TM in ASEAN countries has led to the development of many strategies in order to integrate it into national healthcare systems where biomedicine is the main form. The need for scientific evidence supporting TM use is one of the strategies. As a result of the 2004 ASEAN agreement, there has been an increase in ethnopharmacological research within South-East Asia, which each ASEAN country applies differently based on its individual strategies.

In the future, additional approaches such as reverse pharmacology may prove to be a key element of new research and development strategies on TM in most ASEAN countries.

## Acknowledgement

The authors would like to thank Dr Anchalee Chuthaputti, Director, Office of International Cooperation, Department for Development of Thai Traditional and Alternative Medicine, Ministry of Public Health, for information on ASEAN countries. We also appreciate Dr Somponnat Sampattavanich, Department of Pharmacology, Faculty of Medicine Siriraj Hospital, Mahidol University, for providing system biology information and Professor Isidro Sia, Director of the National Institute of Herbal Medicine, Republic of the Philippines, for providing information for the manuscript preparation.

## References

Adnan, N. and Othman, N. (2012) The relationship between plants and the Malay culture. *Procedia – Social and Behavioral Sciences*, **42**, 231–241.

Ali, N., Hashim, N.H., Saad, B., *et al.* (2005) Evaluation of a method to determine the natural occurrence of aflatoxins in commercial traditional herbal medicines from Malaysia and Indonesia. *Food Chemistry and Toxicology*, **43**, 1763–1772.

ASEAN Ministers on Agriculture and Forestry (2004) Strategic plan of action on ASEAN cooperation in food, agriculture and forestry, http://www.asean.org/communities/asean-economic-community/item/strategic-plan-of-action-on-asean-cooperation-in-food-agriculture-and-forestry, accessed 20 September 2014.

Bodeker, G. (1999) *Health and Beauty from the Rainforest: Malaysian Traditions of Ramuan*, Didier Millet, Kuala Lumpur.

Bodeker, G. (2001) Lessons on integration from the developing world's experience. *British Medical Journal*, **322**, 164–167.

Chuthaputti, A. and Boonterm, B. (2010a) Traditional Medicine in ASEAN, based on country report presentations in the *"Conference on Traditional Medicine in ASEAN Countries"*. WVO Office of Printing Mill, Bangkok, p. 136.

Chuthaputti, A. and Boonterm, B. (2010b) Traditional medicine in the Kingdom of Thailand: the integration of Thai traditional medicine in the national health care system of Thailand. In: *Traditional Medicine in ASEAN, based on country report presentations in the "Conference on Traditional Medicine in ASEAN Countries"*, WVO Office of Printing Mill, Bangkok, pp. 97–120.

Chuthaputti, A. and Boonterm, B. (2010c). Traditional medicine in the Republic of Indonesia: Indonesian traditional medicine – national strategy and scope of cooperation. In: *Traditional Medicine in ASEAN, based on country report presentations in the "Conference on Traditional Medicine in ASEAN Countries"*, WVO Office of Printing Mill, Bangkok, pp. 23–36.

Datiles, M.J.R. and Heinrich, M. (2013) Living on a volcano: medicinal plant uses of the Nabuclod Aeta, Mount Pinatubo, Philippines. *Planta Medica*, **79** (13), doi: 10.1055/s-0033-1352382.

Ebell, M.H., Siwek, J., Weiss, B.D., *et al.* (2004) Simplifying the language of evidence to improve patient care: Strength of recommendation taxonomy (SORT): a patient-centered approach to grading evidence in medical literature. *Journal of Family Practice*, **53**, 111–120.

Elfahmi , Woerdenbag, H.J. and Kayser, O. (2014) Jamu: Indonesian traditional herbal medicine towards rational phytopharmacological use. *Journal of Herbal Medicine*, **4**, 51–73.

Farooqui, M. (2013) The current situation and future direction of traditional and complementary medicine (T and CM) in Malaysian health care system. *Alternative and Integrated Medicine*, **1**, e101.

Feria, M. (2007) *Ten Medicinal Plants*, Philippine Council for Health Research and Development, http://www.pchrd.dost.gov.ph/index.php/2012-05-23-07-46-36/2012-05-24-00-03-06/713-10-medicinal-plants, accessed 24 April 2014.

Galvez-Tan, J.Z. (2013) *Health in the Hands of the People: Framework and Action*, JZ Galvez-Tan Health Associates, Inc., Quezon City.

Itthipanichpong, R., Lupreechaset, A., Chotewuttakorn, S., *et al.* (2010) Effect of Ayurved Siriraj herbal recipe Chantaleela on platelet aggregation. *Journal of the Medical Association of Thailand*, **93**, 115–122.

Jamal, J.A. (2006) Malay traditional medicine: An overview of scientific and technological progress. *Tech Monitor*, **23**, 37–49.

Jamal, J.A., Ghafar, Z.A. and Husain, K. (2011) Medicinal plants used for postnatal care in Malay traditional medicine in the peninsular Malaysia. *Pharmacognosy Journal*, **3**, 15–24.

Kadetz, P. (2011) Assumptions of global beneficence: Health-care disparity, the WHO and the outcomes of integrative health-care policy at local levels in the Philippines. *BioSocieties*, **6**, 88–105.

Malaysian Ministry of Agriculture (2011) *Agriculture NKEA: Herbs sub-sector entry point project (EPP) high value herbal products*.

Ministers of Health of ASEAN Member Countries (2004) *Declaration of the 7th ASEAN Health Ministers meeting: Health without frontiers*, http://www.asean.org/communities/asean-socio-cultural-community/item/declaration-of-the-7th-asean-health-ministers-meeting-health-without-frontiers-22-april-2004-penang-malaysia, accessed 30 September 2014.

National Agency of Drug and Food Control (2007) *Traditional medicine in Indonesia*, http://www.ayurveda.hu/2007102628conf_arogya/speech%209%20%20traditional%20medicines%20in%20indonesia.pdf, accessed 15 August 2014.

National Drug Committee (2006) *List of Herbal Medicinal Products A.D.2006*, http://drug.fda.moph.go.th:81/nlem.in.th/sites/default/files/binder3.pdf, accessed 20 September 2014.

Naser, E., Mackey, S., Arthur, D., *et al.* (2012) An exploratory study of traditional birthing practices of Chinese, Malay and Indian women in Singapore. *Midwifery*, **28**, e865–e871.

Nor, N.M., Sharif, M.S.M., Zahari, M.S.M., *et al.* (2012) The transmission modes of Malay traditional food knowledge within generations. *Procedia – Social Behavior Science*, **50**, 79–88.

Ong, H. and Norzalina, J. (1999) Malay herbal medicine in Gemencheh, Negri Sembilan, Malaysia. *Fitoterapia*, **70**, 10–14.

Ong, H.C. and Nordiana, M. (1999) Malay ethno-medico botany in Machang, Kelantan, Malaysia. *Fitoterapia*, **70**, 502–513.

Prapti, I.Y. (2011) Implementation of herbal medicine (JAMU) networking, http://herbalnet.healthrepository.org/bitstream/123456789/2461/1/Djamoe%20Revisi%203.pdf, accessed 17 August 2014.

Raden Sanusi, H. and & Werner, R. (1985) The role of traditional healers in the provision of health care and family planning services: Malay traditional and indigenous medicine. *Malaysian Journal of Reproductive Health*, **3** (1 Suppl.), S82–S89.

Sia, I.C., Sur A.L.D., Co, L., *et al.* (2002) *Ethnopharmacological study of the Philippine ethno-linguistic groups: the Bugkalot people of Talbec, Dupax del Sur, Nueva Vizcaya*, Complementary and Traditional Medicine Study Group Report, National Institutes of Health, University of Manila, http://herbs.ph/attachments/article/5460/Bugkalots_of_Nueva_Viscaya_final_report_.pdf, accessed 25 August 2014.

Siriwatanametanon, N., Fiebich, B.L., Efferth, Th., *et al.* (2010) Traditionally used Thai medicinal plants: *In vitro* anti-inflammatory, anticancer and antioxidant activities. *Journal of Ethnopharmacology*, **130**, 196–207.

Thai, S.C. (2011) *Traditional Vietnamese medicine: Historical perspective and current usage*, EthnoMed, https://ethnomed.org/clinical/traditional-medicine/traditional-vietnamese-medicine-historical-perspective-and-current-usage, accessed 17 June 2014.

Thongpraditchote, S., Wongkrajang, Y., Temsiririkkul, R., *et al.* (2001) The antipyretic activity of Chantaleela formula. *Thai Journal of Phytopharmacy*, **8**, 20–26.

Vaidya, A. (2006) Reverse pharmacological correlates of ayurvedic drug actions. *Indian Journal of Pharmacology*, **38**, 311–315.

WHO (2002) *WHO Traditional Medicine Strategy 2002–2005*, WHO, Geneva, http://herbalnet.health repository.org/bitstream/123456789/2028/1/WHO_traditional_medicine_strategy_2002-2005.pdf.

Zakaria, M. bin, and Mohd, M.A. (2010) *Traditional Malay Medicinal Plants*, Institut Terjemahan & Buku Malaysia.

# 28
# Historical Approaches in Ethnopharmacology

Andreas Lardos

*Research Cluster Biodiversity and Medicines/Centre for Pharmacognosy and Phytotherapy, UCL School of Pharmacy, London, UK*

## 28.1   Introduction

This chapter focuses on ethnopharmacological research based on the investigation of historical texts. The term 'historical texts' is used in this chapter in its broadest sense and includes various kinds of written sources from the past which contain information about (medicinal) plant usage, as, for example, codices of the great medical traditions from antiquity, scholarly herbals and lay handbooks of plant lore from medieval times or ethnographic literature from more recent centuries which document local or indigenous traditions.

Various cultures from around the globe have documented their knowledge about the use of plants in an extensive body of writing. Because many of these cultures have already vanished, their herbals or texts on *materia medica* that have come down to us represent a unique gateway to access knowledge which otherwise would be lost. However, historical texts can also be invaluable for the study of contemporary cultures which largely rely on oral traditions of knowledge transmission. Because cultures evolve and people make choices (McClatchey, 2005) much of the knowledge about plants which local or indigenous communities have acquired in the course of time would no longer be available without the existence of historical written records in which this information has been preserved.

From an ethnopharmacological perspective it is this context which makes historical texts interesting. It has been suggested, for example, that a careful investigation of medicinal plants mentioned in historical texts can lead to the discovery of new therapeutic agents (Holland, 1994; Riddle, 1996; Buenz *et al.*, 2004) and that a comparative analysis of these texts may not only bring new insight into plant usage but also the development of the related medicinal systems (Heinrich, 2005). However, the potential pitfalls linked with the investigation of historical texts have also been pointed out (Piomelli and Pollio, 1994; Heinrich *et al.*, 2006).

*Ethnopharmacology*, First Edition. Edited by Michael Heinrich and Anna K. Jäger.
© 2015 John Wiley & Sons, Ltd. Published 2015 by John Wiley & Sons, Ltd.

Based on this framework, the aim of the present contribution is to provide an overview of recent developments in ethnopharmacological research involving a historical approach, highlight essential methodological aspects linked to such an investigation and outline some of the opportunities and challenges in using historical texts as a tool for the study of medicinal plant knowledge.

## 28.2  Historical texts in ethnopharmacological research

What are the core interests in today's ethnopharmacological studies which in terms of their methodology largely relied on the investigation of historical texts? To pursue this question I have used the *Journal of Ethnopharmacology* (Elsevier) as an example and searched its archive for corresponding studies that were published in the last ten years (2003–2013). The search yielded 33 publications, which provide a snapshot of the available research on the topic. These studies were concerned with diverse subjects of investigation regarding the human interactions with plants (or other natural products) recorded in historical texts and approached the topic not only from the perspective of ethnobotany, ethnopharmacology or ethnozoology but also ecology, history, history of medicine, history of pharmacy, medical and social anthropology, pharmacognosy, philology or phytochemistry. Based on the primary focus of each of these studies, they can be assigned to three major groups, which will be addressed in the following sections.

### 28.2.1  Documentation of (mainly) medicinal plant knowledge

In the majority of the studies in this group the subject of investigation was a specific historical text or body of literature and the principle aim was documenting the plants or other natural products and their uses mentioned in these resources (Moussaieff *et al.*, 2005; Lardos, 2006; Lev and Amar, 2006, 2008; López-Muñoz *et al.*, 2006; Lev, 2007; Voultsiadou, 2010; Jarić *et al.*, 2011; Medeiros and Albuquerque, 2012; Breitbach *et al.*, 2013). In other studies a specific condition was the centre of interest and the aim was to document plants that were used in this context based on information in historical written sources (Campos-Navarra *et al.*, 2013; Tagarelli *et al.*, 2013).

### 28.2.2  Evaluation of medicinal plant knowledge and identification of potential plant candidates

Most of the studies in this group concentrated on the analysis of herbals, texts on *materia medica* and ethnographic literature with the aim of evaluating medicinal plant uses by applying empirical concepts and at the same time identifying interesting plant candidates for further pharmacological or phytochemical investigations (Buenz *et al.*, 2005; Giorgetti *et al.*, 2007; Mendes and Carlini, 2007; Brandão *et al.*, 2008, 2012; Lansky *et al.*, 2008; Adams *et al.*, 2009, de Vos, 2010; Adams *et al.*, 2011a, 2012; Cosenza *et al.*, 2013).

### 28.2.3  Development of (medicinal) plant knowledge

This group includes studies with diverse conceptual approaches linked to the topic of the development of (medicinal) plant knowledge. Some of the studies placed a particular plant or group of species in the centre of their interest and conducted a comparison of historical to present-day uses (Fiore *et al.*, 2005; Pardo de Santayana *et al.*, 2005; Heinrich *et al.*, 2006; Pollio *et al.*, 2008; Obón *et al.*, 2012). Other studies investigated the consistency in the use of drug substances mentioned in texts on *materia medica* (de Vos, 2010), the changes in the use of plants based on information from ethnographic collections (Łuczaj, 2010; Sõukand and Kalle, 2011), the transmission of knowledge about natural drugs between different regions of the world (Touwaide and Appetiti, 2013) or the influence of historical texts on present-day medicinal plant knowledge (Leonti *et al.*, 2009, 2010; Leonti, 2011). Two further studies explored how medicinal plant knowledge changes over time (Heinrich *et al.*, 2006; Lardos and Heinrich, 2013).

## 28.3 Methodological aspects

Before any text analysis can be started the written sources of interest need to be defined, located and made accessible. While in many cases an *in situ* study of original manuscripts or documents in libraries and archives is required, technical advances in uploading texts into electronic format have greatly improved availability and an increasing number of historical texts can now be accessed via the internet. Because access to original texts is not always possible, inventories in print or electronic databases containing data that was extracted from earlier written sources can also in principle be included in the text analysis.

Specific protocols for analysing historical texts have been developed with the aim of identifying plant candidates for drug discovery (Buenz *et al.*, 2004) or conducting a systematic analysis of medicinal plant usage (Lardos *et al.*, 2011). Several of the process steps described in these protocols are essential in every analysis of historical written sources from an ethnopharmacological perspective, including (i) extraction of information, (ii) translation or transcription, (iii) identification of plants and (iv) interpretation of symptoms or diseases. The extraction of information linked to the medicinal use of plants (or other natural products) is usually at the beginning of the process. In many cases this information first needs to be made accessible through translation or transcription from an ancient language or dialect. As an option to streamline data extraction from previously digitized texts the application of natural language processing solutions has been suggested (Buenz *et al.*, 2004), but it seems this has not been explored systematically.

Perhaps the most crucial steps in the ethnopharmacological analysis of historical texts concerns the identification of the plant or plant substances and the interpretation of the symptoms or diseases (see section below). In most cases this requires the collaboration of experts from different disciplines, making it a truly interdisciplinary effort. The result of the procedure is a basic inventory of data about plants or plant uses which can then be subjected to specific analysis depending on the aim of the study. This is often linked to some quantification of the data in order to better appraise the information and can include descriptive or other statistical methods (e.g. de Vos, 2010; Leonti *et al.*, 2010; Lardos *et al.*, 2011).

## 28.4 Challenges in the analysis of historical texts

Accessibility and legibility of original manuscripts, language, plant identifications, terminology of diseases or the labourious extraction of information through reading of the entire text are challenges inherent to most investigations of historical texts on *materia medica* (e.g. Oritz de Montellano, 1975; Riddle, 1996; Buenz *et al.*, 2004; Adams *et al.*, 2009; Lardos *et al.*, 2011).

The identification of plants or plant substances is one of the most difficult and complex issues in the analysis of historical texts (Riddle, 1996; Lev and Amar, 2006). In many instances the only information available about the botanical identity of a species is the plant name. Unless the written source has a more recent and scientific background, the plant names mentioned do not follow the Linnaean binomial nomenclature but are stated in the local vernacular of the respective culture and time. The situation can be further complicated by the fact that the same plant or substance may have several names, often as a consequence of the influence of different routes of knowledge transmission (Lardos, 2006; Lev and Amar, 2006; Lardos *et al.*, 2011).

Depending on the type and language of the historical text, its cultural background and age, the difficulties linked to the identification of plants or substances vary considerably. In many herbals of the European Renaissance, for example, botanical illustrations and morphological details in combination with plant names corresponding to modern nomenclature are available, which often can facilitate the identification procedure (Adams *et al.*, 2009; Leonti *et al.*, 2010). However, although it is usually possible to identify the great majority of the plants mentioned in historical texts down to the level of the genus or even the species, there are problems on various levels, as illustrated by examples from different cultures and eras (Piomelli and Pollio, 1994; Riddle, 1996; Heinrich *et al.*, 2006; Lev and Amar, 2006; Brandão *et al.*, 2012). This particularly applies to the identification of specific substances as, for example, plant exudates (Lardos *et al.*, 2013).

The procedure of identifying plant names in historical texts primarily relies on linguistic, pharmacognostic and botanical criteria, and essentially consists of cross-referencing the name mentioned in the text with the botanical name of the species stated in appropriate literature (e.g. Lev and Amar, 2006; Pollio *et al.*, 2008; Lardos *et al.*, 2011). The determination of the botanical identity requires not only a careful study of the relevant pharmacognostic or taxonomic literature but also the verification of the botanical scientific nomenclature stated in the references used (Buenz *et al.*, 2004). To achieve a fair degree of reliability for the identity established, it is often indispensable to consider aspects of plant distribution as well as the cultural historical context of plant or substance names (Lardos *et al.*, 2011). Phytogeographical and philological considerations also belong to the key criteria highlighted by Stannard (1961) in the identification of the plants mentioned in the *Corpus Hippocraticum* (mainly 5th to 4th century BCE).

Apart from a careful study of the references available, the quality of the literary sources used in the plant identification procedure is a factor which plays a central role. Problems exist in this regard and the unreliability of certain plant identifications in authoritative dictionaries of plant names mentioned in historical texts has been highlighted by the example of ancient Greek plant names (Raven *et al.*, 2000).

A challenge that is similar to the identification of plants or substances is the correct interpretation of symptoms or diseases mentioned in historical texts and the linking of this information with modern concepts of nosology (Buenz *et al.*, 2004; Lardos *et al.*, 2011). Pre-modern societies often had a different concept of anatomy (as have present-day local and indigenous cultures) and the medical terminology in historical texts usually differs from modern clinical terminology. Also, it is often problematic to draw direct conclusions on certain conditions based on the symptoms stated because of a potentially differing understanding of the aetiology behind the observable physiological reactions of the body (Riddle, 1996; Pollio *et al.*, 2008). It is therefore essential to consider the medical concepts and beliefs of the particular culture or period of time, not only for the interpretation of the uses of the remedies but also when evaluating their efficacy (Oritz de Montellano, 1975; Adams *et al.*, 2009; Uehleke *et al.*, 2012).

# 28.5 Opportunities offered by a historical approach

What are the opportunities offered by an investigation of historical texts from an ethnopharmacological perspective and how can the information gained through such an approach be exploited or put in a wider context?

The documentation of ethnobiological or ethnomedical knowledge contained in historical written sources, as prioritized in many of the recently published studies cited above, may lead to the re-evaluation and utilization of this knowledge. First, when the topic of the text is linked to one of today's cultural communities, such an approach can contribute to the preservation of the local or indigenous knowledge of the respective culture. This might be of potential value in connection with the safeguarding of intangible cultural heritage as promoted by UNESCO (www.unesco.org). Second, it may have important implications in terms of the protection of the rights of holders of traditional knowledge as defined in the Convention on Biological Diversity (www.cbd.int) and embraced by the Intergovernmental Committee on Intellectual Property and Genetic Resources, Traditional Knowledge and Folklore of the World Intellectual Property Organization (http://www.wipo.int/tk/en/igc/). Since property rights over traditional knowledge can only be exercised if the particular knowledge is available in a carefully documented and accessible form, researchers have pointed to the potential importance of such a work in this context and the conservation of biological diversity in general (Breitbach *et al.*, 2013).

Access to the documented ethnomedical knowledge contained in these sources might also become useful in the context of developing a regulatory framework for herbal medicines. It has been suggested that traditional uses recorded in historical medical texts should be implemented as an evidence criterion in the registration of phytopharmaceuticals (Helmstädter and Staiger, 2014) and that a careful study of these sources could provide important clues about the safety of a medicinal plant (Riddle, 1999). Of course access to this kind of information might also contribute to the safe and efficacious use of herbal medicines on a community level, especially in societies largely relying on the surrounding flora for the preparation of their medicines. The underlying consideration is based on the notion that traditional or local knowledge recorded in historical texts will enable the reconstruction of medicinal plant usage in the past and that, based on this, important information for consolidating the claims for an herbal medicine can be gained. If a consistent use of a plant for the treatment of a specific condition over an extended period of time can be demonstrated, this may be evidence for a therapeutic efficacy. This evidence is further corroborated if the same information is available in sources from different practices and schools of thought (Crellin, 2008).

Historical consistency in a certain range of indications also represents an important criterion in evaluating plant candidates from historical texts in terms of their qualification for further investigations (Hunt, 1996; Anagnostou, in press). The isolation of lines of tradition for specific therapeutic applications of medicinal plants and their subsequent scientific evaluation provides a rational approach in knowledge-guided drug discovery (Anagnostou, 2005, in press).

The potential value of historical texts as a starting point in drug discovery is underscored by examples of plant uses described in ancient medical texts which suggest that some of the discoveries of modern medicine are in fact re-discoveries of what was once known (Riddle, 1996). By making reference to Greek and Latin medical text Holland (1994) argued that a re-examination of the medicinal plant knowledge contained in these sources might be a useful approach in the search for new therapeutic agents. Meanwhile systematic ethnopharmacological investigations of several writings of these traditions have become available and they also underscore the value of historical texts in this context (Adams *et al.*, 2009, 2011a, 2012; de Vos, 2010; Lardos *et al.*, 2011).

One of the circumstances which makes historical texts a highly relevant tool for natural product research in general emanates from the view that the medicinal plant knowledge contained in these sources is largely based on empirical concepts, as suggested for the case of Dioscorides' *De Materia Medica* (Riddle, 1985). This is supported by various studies which corroborated the validity of numerous ancient plant uses from diverse traditions around the globe by comparing them with relevant pharmacological, clinical or therapeutic data (Oritz de Montellano, 1975; Buenz *et al.*, 2005; Adams *et al.*, 2009; Lardos *et al.*, 2011; Brandão *et al.*, 2012; Uehleke *et al.*, 2012). The application of such empirical approaches also enabled researchers to identify plant candidates which deserve further investigation (Buenz *et al.*, 2005; Adams *et al.*, 2011a, 2012). Finally, some of the plants which had been identified as candidates in the text analysis have already been tested and in fact exhibited a pharmacological activity that corresponded to the historical use (Buenz *et al.*, 2006; Adams *et al.*, 2011b).

A further focal point in ethnopharmacological research with a historical approach that has gained increasing attention in recent years concerns the study of the development of (medicinal) plant knowledge. This approach is based on the view that 'traditional' knowledge is cumulative and dynamic (Johnson, 1992) and from a methodological point of view refers to the above-mentioned context, which highlighted the possibility of tracing plant usage diachronically through time. Recent studies have included a systematic comparative analysis of data from different points in time with the aim of exploring the evolution of medicinal plant use in local or indigenous knowledge systems; They demonstrate a causal dependence of present-day medicinal plant use on historical texts (Leonti *et al.*, 2010), a change in the importance of plants based on ecological factors (Sõukand and Kalle, 2011), continuity and change in medicinal plant knowledge as well as the adoption of new knowledge (Kufer *et al.*, 2005; Lardos and Heinrich, 2013) or the existence of a constant body of medicinal plant knowledge since ancient times (Dal Cero *et al.*, 2014). While the potential of considering dynamic and evolving aspects in human plant use has been highlighted earlier (Heinrich *et al.*, 2006), the findings of the above studies illustrate that a systematic diachronic approach can facilitate the understanding of the complex processes involved in the development of (medicinal) plant knowledge.

## 28.6  Conclusions

Modern ethnopharmacological research involving the study of historical written sources is characterized by diversity not only in terms of the subject of investigation or the perspective taken but also regarding the opportunities which may arise from such an approach.

As suggested by a representative selection of publications from the last 10 years, the core interests of corresponding studies include the documentation of medicinal plant knowledge, the evaluation of this knowledge together with the identification of potential plant candidates for further investigation as well as the development of medicinal plant knowledge. The consideration of methodological aspects concerning the analysis of historical written sources highlights some of the challenges inherent to this type of work, especially the identification of the plants or the interpretation of symptoms and diseases. Apart from the need for a conceptually sound approach for addressing the relevant research question, an adequate understanding of the ethnopharmacognostic background of the (herbal) drugs described in the historical text and also the medical concepts and beliefs of the respective culture and time are essential prerequisites in most studies of this kind.

An outline of some of the opportunities offered by an ethnopharmacological investigation of historical texts points to the potential importance of such a work in terms of the protection of the world's biocultural diversity or the safe and efficacious use of herbal medicines. The validity of using historical texts as a starting point in the search for new medicines is underscored by increasing evidence for the rational basis and pharmacological relevance of many of the remedies described in these sources. Recent studies which included a systematic diachronic analysis highlight the significance of a historical approach from an evolutionary perspective, specifically in facilitating the understanding of the complex processes involved in the development of medicinal plant knowledge. Much of the potential of using historical written sources in ethnopharmacological research has not yet been realized and further scientific insight can be expected from this research approach, which finally contributes to the mutlidisciplinary nature of ethnopharmacology.

# References

Adams, M., Berset, C., Kessler, M., and Hamburger, M. (2009) Medicinal herbs for the treatment of rheumatic disorders – a survey of European herbals from the 16th and 17th century. *Journal of Ethnopharmacology*, **121**, 343–359.

Adams, M., Alther, W., Kessler, M., *et al.* (2011a) Malaria in the Renaissance: remedies from European herbals from the 16th and 17th century. *Journal of Ethnopharmacology*, **133**, 278–288.

Adams, M., Gschwind, S., Zimmermann, S., *et al.* (2011b) Renaissance remedies: Antiplasmodial protostane triterpenoids from *Alisma plantago-aquatica* L. (Alismataceae). *Journal of Ethnopharmacology*, **135**, 43–47.

Adams, M., Schneider, S.V., Kluge, M., *et al.* (2012) Epilepsy in the Renaissance: A survey of remedies from 16th and 17th century German herbals. *Journal of Ethnopharmacology*, **143**, 1–13.

Anagnostou, S. (in press). Forming, transfer and golbalization of medical-pharmaceutical knowledge in South East Asia missions (17th to 18th c.) – Historical dimensions and modern perspectives. *Journal of Ethnopharmacology*.

Anagnostou, S. (2005) Missionsarzneien des 16. bis 18. Jahrhunderts, Ein Forschungsansatz zur Entwicklung von Phytotherapeutika. *Zeitschrift für Phytotherapie*, **26**, 66–71.

Brandão, M.G.L., Zanetti, N.N.S., Oliveira, P., *et al.* (2008) Brazilian medicinal plants described by 19th century European naturalists and in the Official Pharmacopoeia. *Journal of Ethnopharmacology*, **120**, 141–148.

Brandão, M.G.L., Pignal, M., Romaniuc, S., *et al.* (2012) Useful Brazilian plants listed in the field books of the French naturalist Auguste de Saint-Hilaire (1779–1853). *Journal of Ethnopharmacology*, **143**, 488–500.

Breitbach, U.B., Niehues, M., Lopes, N.P., *et al.* (2013) Amazonian Brazilian medicinal plants described by C.F.P. von Martius in the 19th century. *Journal of Ethnopharmacology*, **147**, 180–189.

Buenz, E.J., Schnepple, D.J., Bauer, B.A., *et al.* (2004) Techniques: Bioprospecting historical herbal texts by hunting for new leads in old tomes. *Trends in Pharmacological Sciences*, **25**, 494–498.

Buenz, E.J., Johnson, H.E., Beekman, E.M., *et al.* (2005) Bioprospecting Rumphius's Ambonese Herbal: Volume I. *Journal of Ethnopharmacology*, **96**, 57–70.

Buenz, E.J., Bauer, B.A., Johnson, H.E., *et al.* (2006) Searching historical herbal texts for potential new drugs. *British Medical Journal*, **333**, 1314–1315.

Campos-Navarro, R. and Scarpa, G.F. (2013) The cultural-bound disease 'empacho' in Argentina A comprehensive botanico-historical and ethnopharmacological review. *Journal of Ethnopharmacology*, **148**, 349–360.

Cosenza, G.P., Somavilla, N.S., Fagg, C.W. and Brandão, M.G.L. (2013) Bitter plants used as substitute of *Cinchona* spp. (quina) in Brazilian traditional medicine. *Journal of Ethnopharmacology*, **149**, 790–796.

Crellin, J.K. (2008) 'Traditional use' claims for herbs: The need for competent historical research. *Pharmaceutical Historian*, **38**, 34–40.

Dal Cero, M., Saller, R. and Weckerle, C.S. (2014) The use of the local flora in Switzerland: A comparison of past and recent medicinal plant knowledge. *Journal of Ethnopharmacology*, **151**, 253–264.

de Vos, P. (2010) European *materia medica* in historical texts: longevity of a tradition and implications for future use. *Journal of Ethnopharmacology*, **132**, 28–47.

Fiore, C., Eisenhut, M., Ragazzi, E., *et al.* (2005) A history of the therapeutic use of liquorice in Europe. *Journal of Ethnopharmacology*, **99**, 317–324.

Giorgetti, M., Negri, G. and Rodrigues, E., 2007. Brazilian plants with possible action on the central nervous system – A study of historical sources from the 16th to 19th century. *Journal of Ethnopharmacology*, **109**, 338–347.

Heinrich, M. (2005) Challenges and Threats to Interdisciplinary Medicinal Plant Research, in *Handbook of Medicinal Plants* (eds Y. Zohara and U. Bachrach), Food Products Press and The Harworth Mecial Press, New York, London, Oxford, pp. 447–464.

Heinrich, M., Kufer, J., Leonti, M. and Pardo-de-Santayana, M. (2006) Ethnobotany and ethnopharmacology – interdisciplinary links with the historical sciences. *Journal of Ethnopharmacology*, **107**, 157–160.

Helmstädter, A. and Staiger, C. (2012) Traditional use of medicinal agents: a valid source of evidence. *Drug Discovery Today*, **19**, 4–7.

Holland, B.K. (1994) Prospecting for drugs in ancient texts. *Nature*, **369**, 702.

Hunt, T. (1996) From plant lore to pharmacy: A prototype of the process, in *Prospecting for Drugs in Ancient and Medieval European Texts: A scientific approach* (ed. B.K. Holland), Harwood Academic Publishers GmbH, Amsterdam, pp. 91–96.

Jarić, S., Mitrović, M., Djurdjević, L., *et al.* (2011) Phytotherapy in medieval Serbian medicine according to the pharmacological manuscripts of the Chilandar Medical Codex (15–16th centuries). *Journal of Ethnopharmacology*, **137**, 601–619.

Johnson, M. (ed.) (1992) *Lore: Capturing Traditional Environmental Knowledge*, Dene Cultural Institute and International Development Research Centre, Ottawa.

Lansky, E.P., Paavilainen, H.M., Pawlus, A.D. and Newman, R.A. (2008) *Ficus* spp. (fig): Ethnobotany and potential as anticancer and anti-inflammatory agents. *Journal of Ethnopharmacology*, **119**, 195–213.

Lardos, A. (2006) The botanical *materia medica* of the *Iatrosophikon* – a collection of prescriptions from a monastery in Cyprus. *Journal of Ethnopharmacology*, **104**, 387–406.

Lardos, A. and Heinrich, M. (2013) Continuity and change in medicinal plant use: The example of monasteries on Cyprus and historical *iatrosophia* texts. *Journal of Ethnopharmacology*, **150**, 202–214.

Lardos, A., Prieto, J.M. and Heinrich, M. (2011) Resins and gums in historical *iatrosophia* texts from Cyprus – a botanical and medico-pharmacological approach. *Frontiers in Pharmacology*, **2**, 1–26.

Leonti, M. (2011) The future is written: Impact of scripts on the cognition, selection, knowledge and transmission of medicinal plant use and its implications for ethnobotany and ethnopharmacology. *Journal of Ethnopharmacology*, **134**, 542–555.

Leonti, M., Casu, L., Sanna, F. and Bonsignore, L. (2009) A comparison of medicinal plant use in Sardinia and Sicily-De Materia Medica revisited? *Journal of Ethnopharmacology*, **121**, 255–267.

Leonti, M., Cabras, S., Weckerle, C.S., *et al.* (2010) The causal dependence of present plant knowledge on herbals – Contemporary medicinal plant use in Campania (Italy) compared to Matthioli (1568). *Journal of Ethnopharmacology*, **130**, 379–391.

Lev, E. (2007) Drugs held and sold by pharmacists of the Jewish community of medieval (11–14th centuries) Cairo according to lists of *materia medica* found at the Taylor–Schechter Genizah collection, Cambridge. *Journal of Ethnopharmacology*, **110**, 275–293.

Lev, E. and Amar, Z. (2006) Reconstruction of the inventory of *materia medica* used by members of the Jewish community of medieval Cairo according to prescriptions found in the Taylor-Schechter Genizah collection, Cambridge. *Journal of Ethnopharmacology*, **108**, 428–444.

Lev, E. and Amar, Z. (2008) 'Fossils' of practical medical knowledge from medieval Cairo. *Journal of Ethnopharmacology*, **119**, 24–40.

López-Muñoz, F., Alamo, C. and García-García, P. (2006) 'The herbs that have the property of healing ... ,': the phytotherapy in Don Quixote. *Journal of Ethnopharmacology*, **106**, 429–441.

Łuczaj, L. (2010) Changes in the utilization of wild green vegetables in Poland since the 19th century: A comparison of four ethnobotanical surveys. *Journal of Ethnopharmacology*, **128**, 395–404.

McClatchey, W.C. (2005) Exorcizing misleading terms from ethnobotany. *Ethnobotany Research & Applications*, **3**, 001–004.

Medeiros, M.F.T. and Albuquerque, U.P. de (2012) The pharmacy of the Benedictine monks: The use of medicinal plants in Northeast Brazil during the nineteenth century (1823–1829). *Journal of Ethnopharmacology*, **139**, 280–286.

Mendes, F.R. and Carlini, E.A. (2007) Brazilian plants as possible adaptogens: An ethnopharmacological survey of books edited in Brazil. *Journal of Ethnopharmacology*, **109**, 493–500.

Moussaieff, A., Fride, E., Amar, Z., *et al.* (2005) The Jerusalem Balsam: From the Franciscan Monastery in the old city of Jerusalem to Martindale 33. *Journal of Ethnopharmacology*, **101**, 16–26.

Obón, C., Rivera, D., Verde, A., *et al.* (2012) *Árnica*: A multivariate analysis of the botany and ethnopharmacology of a medicinal plant complex in the Iberian Peninsula and the Balearic Islands. *Journal of Ethnopharmacology*, **144**, 44–56.

Oritz de Montellano, B. (1975) Empirical Aztec Medicine. *Science*, **188**, 215–220.

Pardo-de-Santayana, M., Blanco, E. and Morales, R. (2005) Plants known as *té* in Spain: An ethno-pharmaco-botanical review. *Journal of Ethnopharmacology*, **98**, 1–19.

Piomelli, D. and Pollio, A. (1994) Medicinal plants. *Nature*, **371**, 9.

Pollio, A., Natale, A. de, Appetiti, F., *et al.* (2008) Continuity and change in the Mediterranean medical tradition: Ruta spp. (Rutaceae) in Hippocratic medicine and present practices. *Journal of Ethnopharmacology*, **116**, 469–482.

Raven, J., Lindsell, A. and Raven, F. (2000) *Plants and Plant Lore in Ancient Greece*, Leopard's Head, Oxford.

Riddle, J.M. (1985) *Dioscorides on Pharmacy and Medicine*, University of Texas Press, Austin.

Riddle, J.M. (1996) The medicines of Greco-Roman antiquity as a source of medicines for today, in *Prospecting for Drugs in Ancient and Medieval European Texts: A scientific approach* (ed. B.K. Holland), Harwood Academic Publishers GmbH, Amsterdam, pp. 717.

Riddle, J.M. (1999) Historical data as an aid in pharmaceutical prospecting and drug safety determination. *Journal of Alternative and Complementary Medicine*, **5**, 195–201.

Sõukand, R. and Kalle, R. (2011) Change in medical plant use in Estonian cthnomedicine: A historical comparison between 1888 and 1994. *Journal of Ethnopharmacology*, **135**, 251–260.

Stannard, J. (1961) Hippocratic pharmacology. *Bulletin of the History of Medicine*, **35**, 497–518.

Tagarelli, G., Tagarelli, A., Liguori, M. and Piro, A. (2013) Treating epilepsy in Italy between XIX and XX century. *Journal of Ethnopharmacology*, **145**, 608–613.

Touwaide, A. and Appetiti, E. (2013) Knowledge of Eastern *materia medica* (Indian and Chinese) in pre modern Mediterranean medical traditions: A study in comparative historical ethnopharmacology. *Journal of Ethnopharmacology*, **148**, 361–378.

Uehleke, B., Hopfenmueller, W., Stange, R. and Saller, R. (2012) Are the correct herbal claims by Hildegard von Bingen only lucky strikes? A new statistical approach. *Forschende Komplementärmedizin*, **19**, 187–190.

Voultsiadou, E. (2010) Therapeutic properties and uses of marine invertebrates in the ancient Greek world and early Byzantium. *Journal of Ethnopharmacology*, **130**, 237–247.

# 29
# Medical Ethnobotany and Ethnopharmacology of Europe

Manuel Pardo-de-Santayana[1], Cassandra L. Quave[2], Renata Sõukand[3] and Andrea Pieroni[4]

[1] Departamento de Biología (Botánica), Universidad Autónoma de Madrid, Madrid, Spain
[2] Center for the Study of Human Health, Emory University, Atlanta, USA
[3] Estonian Literary Museum, Vanemuise, Tartu, Estonia
[4] University of Gastronomic Sciences, Piazza Vittorio Emanuele, Bra/Pollenzo, Italy

## 29.1   Introduction

European medicinal plants have attracted scholars since ancient times and continue to be a central interest of ethnographers, anthropologists, ethnobiologists, pharmacologists and other scholars interested in wider health questions (Kołodziejska-Degórska, 2012; Lardos and Heinrich, 2013; Shikov *et al.*, 2014). Medicinal plant knowledge in Europe is rooted in a long history of health traditions dating back to ancient Greek, Roman and Arabic medical systems and over the centuries has been passed down via both written and oral pathways (see Chapters 28 and 30). Over time, Sumerian, Chinese, Indian or American medicines have entered into the European pharmacopoeia. While some of these traditions have survived throughout the centuries, many others have changed or disappeared, and new uses of plants have emerged either from local experience or imported from other traditions. The result is a very rich pharmacopoeia and a profound local knowledge about medicinal plants. However, in fast-changing environments many traditions are disappearing. An alarming rate of decline of traditional medical knowledge has been highlighted by most European ethnobotanical field studies (Quave *et al.*, 2012b).

While numerous studies address the increasing importance of medicinal plant use in Europe, many of the medicinal plants that are widely used and marketed in Europe today do not belong to its historical medical tradition. The mainstream popularization of complementary and alternative medicines is promoting the use of plants and plants products originating from outside Europe or popularizing others that were previously consumed only in some parts of the continent. These studies show that medicinal plants are being combined with the use

*Ethnopharmacology*, First Edition. Edited by Michael Heinrich and Anna K. Jäger.
© 2015 John Wiley & Sons, Ltd. Published 2015 by John Wiley & Sons, Ltd.

of pharmaceuticals for curing an incredibly wide range of illnesses and medical symptoms. Indeed, this spans simple conditions such as catarrh to the extensively more complex, such as cancer and HIV/AIDS (e.g. Du *et al.*, 2014; Engdal *et al.*, 2008).

This chapter focuses on the local and regional medical traditions in Europe and is based on ethnobotanical studies provided that they adopt a proper botanical methodology and address the ethnographic and anthropological context of human–plant relationships. We have updated and reinterpreted our previous review of recent original medico-ethnobotanical field studies conducted in Europe (Quave *et al.*, 2012b), therefore many pre-2012 references that appeared in this paper have not been included in the chapter. After a brief presentation of the history of ethnobotanical studies in Europe, we present the current state of such studies, highlighting the richness of the European ethnomedicinal flora and its importance for promoting our understanding of traditional healthcare and self-medication practices. Specifically, ethnobiological data are useful to medical practitioners charged with the care of rural, migrant and other populations that still use their own knowledge for curing themselves and other members of the community (Maxia *et al.*, 2014).

## 29.2   A brief history of European medicinal plants studies

Europe represents a melting pot of cultures and has a long history of medical knowledge transmission across geographic, cultural and linguistic borders. Medical knowledge appears in the earliest written records and fortunately some of these texts have been preserved until today. Greek and Roman authors reported an incredible amount of data about medicinal plants used at their times. Famously, the physician Pedanius Dioscorides (AD 40–90) wrote *De Materia Medica*, which heavily influenced early medicine in Europe and inspired the production of herbal texts, especially during the Middle Ages (AD 500–1400) until the renaissance and can be considered the most important European herbal.

Monasteries became essential during the Middle Ages since monks and nuns wrote herbals and their physic gardens were used to grow medicinal species (Furniss, 1968). Medieval herbals maintained the Greco-Latin tradition by updating and adding new data to the old texts. Arab and Andalusian authors such as Ibn Sina (Avicenna, c. 980–1037) and Ibn Al-Baytar (c. 1180–1248) were also highly influential. Ibn Al-Baytar, for instance, compiled a book of food and medicinal plants based on his own observations and more than 200 sources (including Dioscorides), presenting uses for 1400 simples. The plant materials used were gathered or grown locally while exotic medicines, including spices like black pepper (*Piper nigrum* L.) and nutmeg (*Myristica fragrans* Houtt.), became accessible through trade routes (Pols, 2009).

The invention and diffusion of Gutenberg's printing press in the late 15th century fostered a revolution for the diffusion of written medicinal plant knowledge. For instance, Leonhart Fuchs' herbal *Neu Kreüterbuch* (1543) catalogued more than 400 plants native to what is now known as Germany and Austria, as well as about 100 exotic plants. Other herbals, for example by Henrick Smid (1546), William Turner (1551), Remberd Dodoens (1554), Andrés Laguna (1555), Pietro Andrea Mattioli (1568), Juhász Melius (1578), Marcin z Urzędowa (1595), John Gerard (1597) and Simon Syrennius (1613), were also widely read.

Later, during the mid-1700s, a wealth of data concerning local medicinal plant uses was gathered by Carl Linnaeus and many of his contemporaries. From his travels in Dalecarlia, Linnaeus reported on the long-distance trade in medicinal plants. Bitterwort (*Gentiana purpurea* L.) roots were imported by peasant peddlers into Sweden from Norway. Harvesting was so intense that the species eventually disappeared from many localities and the trade collapsed. His works inspired a whole generation of scholars. For instance, Peter Kalm (1716–1779) compiled very interesting first-hand data from south-western Sweden (1741), Russia (1744) and North America (1749–1752), while Johan Peter Falck (1732–1774), recorded animal and plant knowledge among several Russian ethnic groups (Svanberg *et al.*, 2011). Other relevant works were those of Jens Christian Svabo (1746–1824) on the Faroes, John Lightfoot (1735–1788) in Scotland, José Quer y Martínez (1695–1764) in Spain, Félix de Avelar Brotero (1744–1828) in Portugal andr Krzysztof Kluk (1739–1796) in Poland.[1]

# 29.3  Modern European medico-ethnobotanical studies

Europe is a complex continent where over the last century industrialization developed at varying rates and to a varying degree. Transhumance livestock-keeping, gathering wild food and medicinal plants for humans or livestock as well as hand-crafting utensils for the household were common activities in many parts of Europe until only a few decades ago and remain so in some regions (Svanberg *et al.*, 2011), therefore at the beginning of the 21st century a very rich body of traditional knowledge concerning the European flora continues to attract ethnobiologists.

## 29.3.1  The development of ethnobotanical studies in Europe

Many European scholars have contributed to the field of medicinal plant research. However, ethnobotanical studies in a modern sense, substantiated by clear methods, aims and appropriate documentation, were not introduced in Europe until the mid-19th century, a time of increasing scientific exploration in the world.

An early example is the German doctor Johann Wilhelm Ludwig von Luce (1756–1842), who, after working for several decades as a practicing physician among local peasants, wrote one of the very first systematic medico-ethnobotanical surveys within a specific area in Europe, the Estonian island of Saaremaa. Another relevant author was Leopold Glück (1856–1907), who at the end of the 19th century gathered popular remedies based on 108 taxa in Bosnia and Herzegovina, and recognized the importance of an emic perspective (Svanberg *et al.*, 2011).

The first proper ethnobotanical study in Italy was probably that of Giuseppe Ferraro (1845–1907). His work describes the traditional plant uses of his hometown, Carpeneto d'Acqui (Piedmont), and includes an early attempt to conceptualize the relevance of ethnobotanical studies. However, it lacks a clear indication of the methods used. A few years later the ethnologist Giuseppe Pitrè (1843–1916) described many popular remedies still in use in various areas of Sicily in his *Medicina Popolare Siciliana* (*Sicilian Popular Medicine*) (1896). His medico-anthropological approach can be considered a further step towards the development of ethnomedical studies despite it being more an overview of information than a proper survey, with methods not being clearly spelled out. In Spain, the botanist José Pardo Sastrón (1822–1909) published a catalogue with the popular names and uses of plants in his hometown (Torrecilla de Alcañiz, Teruel, Aragon) where more than 400 species were identified (Pardo Sastrón, 1895).

Other interesting examples are the Polish authors Oskar Kolberg (1814–1990) and Józef Rostafiński (1850–1928). The former spent his life travelling around Poland recording various

---

[1] For a through overview of the history of medicinal plant use in Europe see Svanberg *et al.* (2011).

aspects of local culture, including many references to medicine. The latter used a 70-question questionnaire about the traditional use of plants through some print media of the period and received a few hundred letters from Poles inhabiting the present area of Poland, Ukraine, Belarus and Lithuania. The results of his research concerning wild food plants have only recently been published (Łuczaj, 2010; Łuczaj *et al.*, 2013).

Over the period 1920–1967, with the help of 1500 correspondents (including pupils), the botanist Gustav Vilbaste (1885–1967) collected more than 100,000 Estonian plant names and 17,000 uses, 10,000 of which pertained to medical uses. He identified plants based on herbarium specimens sent along with the reports and this was complemented by several fieldtrips to collect popular plant names (Kalle and Sõukand, 2014). Only one small part of his collection concerning medicinal plants has been analysed to date (Sõukand and Kalle, 2012; for other similar approaches see Chapter 10).

## 29.3.2   Recent medico-ethnobotanical studies in Europe

We have updated an exhaustive review (Quave *et al.*, 2012b) of original medico-ethnobotanical field studies conducted in Europe over the period since 1992, incorporating details concerning the popular medicinal uses of plants, written in English (or which have an English abstract) and that have been indexed by Scopus. We did not consider reviews or meta-analyses of pre-existing data nor works conducted on a single species or a group of related species, field market surveys (unless the study involved studies of local or small-scale medicinal plant gathering and trade) or reports on large-scale trade of medicinal plants (i.e. on commodities). Given the importance of review papers, books, papers published in journals not included in Scopus, and less accessible studies such as local publications or unpublished PhD theses (e.g. Mamedov *et al.*, 2004; Aceituno-Mata, 2010; Shikov *et al.*, 2014), some of these studies were also considered, although they were not included in our overall numerical analysis. Over this period a total of 182 references were included (based on Quave *et al.*, 2012b and later studies summarized here, Figure 29.1). Turkey, Italy and Spain clearly dominate in terms of the number of papers (65%). The number of papers (30) concerning south-eastern European

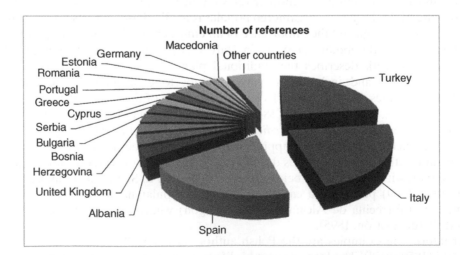

**Figure 29.1**   Countries where medico-ethnobotanical studies were conducted (1992–2014, based on data retrieved from Scopus, 30 August 2014).

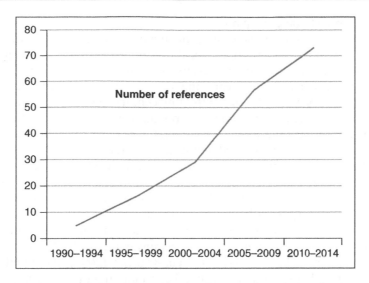

**Figure 29.2**   Number of papers published annually on medico-ethnobotanical studies in Europe (1992–2014, based on data retrieved from Scopus, 30 August 2014).

countries is also very high, but as the region includes many small countries their importance is not clearly highlighted in Figure 29.1. In the last three years a clear increase is apparent, with 25% of the papers having been published between 2011 and 2014 (Figure 29.2).

While Central Europe has recently gained more attention (Leporatti and Ivancheva, 2003; Grasser *et al.*, 2012), modern medical ethnobotanical studies are still quite rare in northern Europe, the Baltic States, Russia and other former Soviet Bloc countries. The reason for this lies in differences in the disciplinary approach. In north-eastern Europe, data regarding the use of plants and people's perceptions of plants has been mostly studied within the periphery of disciplines in the humanities (e.g. ethnology and folkloristics). A few recent publications from the region mainly concern the historical use of plants and are based on ethnographic and folkloric sources (e.g. Łuczaj, 2010; Sõukand and Kalle, 2011). A few, still unpublished, ethnobotanical field studies are ongoing in Estonia, Lithuania and Ukraine. Also, a review on medicinal plants in the *Russian Pharmacopeia* was published recently (Shikov *et al.*, 2014), being so far the only recent ethnopharmacological publication in English concerning the territory of the present Russian Federation. However, this work did not have as a goal the assessment of the current plant use at a household level. Some other studies have addressed the medicinal plant-use systems of migrants in this part of Europe in comparison to other continents, for example Polish migrants in Misiones, Argentina (Kujawska and Hilgert, 2014) and Russian phytomedicine in the USA (Domarew *et al.*, 2002). Recent studies on medicinal plants used by migrant communities in northern Europe have found that most plants used in a popular medical context are actually dried materials imported from their cultural homeland (i.e. Africa, Asia, South America, Middle East etc.) and incorporation of the local flora is very uncommon (e.g. Pieroni *et al.*, 2007; van Andel and Westers, 2010).

Given the large number of publications in Spain, Italy and south-east Europe, we present here a more detailed review of the current state of medico-ethnobotanical research in these countries. Turkey is not included here in detail as most studies belong to Anatolia, its Asian part.

### 29.3.2.1   Medical ethnobotany in Spain

Spain has a striking climatic, geological, geographical, biological, cultural and linguistic diversity complemented by rich ethnobiological traditions. Until the 1950s, industrialization was concentrated in a few regions, and it was still an agrarian and rural country. Many people could not afford professional medical care and self-care prevailed until the national health system spread in the 1980s. Since the end of the 19th century this extensive traditional lore has attracted many researchers, but systematic ethnobotanical studies with reliable botanical identification did not appear until the 1980s. Since then, the number of studies has grown steadily and there is an increasing social, political and scientific interest in traditional knowledge and specifically medical ethnobotany. Spanish legislation has affirmed the need to promote and conserve traditional knowledge as it appears in the principles of the CBD, the Nagoya Protocol on Access and Benefit Sharing, the law on Natural Heritage and Biodiversity and in the Royal Decree that regulates the Spanish Inventory of Traditional Knowledge of Biodiversity. This Inventory consists of a database and monographs that summarize the traditional knowledge concerning each species or ecosystem (Pardo-de-Santayana *et al.*, 2014).

According to Fernández-López and Amezcúa-Ogayar (2007) the number of species employed as medicinal plants in Spain is around 1200, more than 15% of the Iberian flora, but the number of taxa used is certainly higher. More than 400 plants were used in areas of the Catalan Pyrenees such as Pallars. Medicinal plants were used for humans and animals, with the human pharmacopoeia usually being richer than the ethnoveterinary *materia medica*. For instance, 154 and 86 taxa were used in human and animal medicine in Campoo, Cantabria or 229 and 60 to the west of the Granada province, respectively. Medicinal plants were mainly used for common digestive, respiratory and skin disorders such as catarrh, sore throat, diarrhoea and other stomach and intestinal disorders, furuncles or wounds. Blood complaints, bruises and muscle-skeletal pains were also commonly self-treated (see Quave *et al.*, 2012b and references therein).

Households commonly kept a few species for treating the most common disorders, serving as a sort of traditional first aid kit. Their contribution was essential to a family's well-being and health. This group of species is specific to each geographic area and reflects its idiosyncrasy, being very different even among neighbouring territories (Menendez-Baceta *et al.*, 2014). For instance, in the Sierra Norte de Madrid this traditional medical repository contained: *Malva sylvestris* L. and *Origanum vulgare* L. for respiratory disorders, *Chamaemelum nobile* (L.) All. and *Mentha pulegium* L. for digestive conditions and with a wide rank of other uses, and *Sambucus nigra* L. mainly used for respiratory, digestive and skin disorders (Aceituno-Mata, 2010).

Apart from commonly shared knowledge, there were also remedies which were the specialized knowledge of local healers (Rivera and Obón, 1996). Some of these local experts were extraordinarily wise and had an extensive traditional knowledge. For instance, in the popular medicine in the Aragonese Pyrenees, Palacín (1994) showed that three women used more than 100 medicinal plants. One of them could prepare more than 1450 remedies with 230 medicinal plant species, 31 animals and 29 minerals. This is a clear example of the extensive ethnomedical knowledge of women, as has also been reported in many other studies (e.g. Molares and Ladio, 2009).

Recent studies have highlighted the importance of the unsafe use of medicinal plants since poisonings (Vallejo *et al.*, 2009) and interactions with pharmaceuticals (Carrasco *et al.*, 2009) have recently been described. While many people perceive that medicinal plants are always safe and free of side-effects, many patients hide their use when they visit their doctor in order to avoid reprimand, since many allopathic practitioners tend to exhibit a sense of disdain towards traditional medicine. It is therefore essential that health professionals adopt a culturally sensitive attitude towards herbal medicine.

### 29.3.2.2   Medical ethnobotany in Italy

The Italian peninsula and islands (including Sardinia and Sicily) comprise a landmass of around $300,000 \text{ km}^2$. The vascular flora includes 6711 species (Conti *et al.*, 2005), which are distributed across geographic regions of mountains, hills and plains. Much like the Iberian peninsula, from the 19th to the first half of the 20th century the rich lore and popular medical traditions of Italy attracted the attention of many scholars (e.g. see Giuseppe Ferraro (1884, 1885), Giuseppe Pitrè (1896) or Oreste Mattirolo (1918)). However, it has only been in the past 40 years or so that more systematic ethnobotanical surveys throughout Italy have emerged (see Quave *et al.*, 2012b and references therein).

Ethnobotanical studies undertaken in the past in Italy have also revealed a rich traditional ethnopharmacopoeia that utilizes both local flora and fauna. For example, in one study focused only on the topical use of plants for the treatment of skin and soft tissue infection, conducted in Basilicata, 116 distinct remedies coming from 38 medicinal plant species were documented. Another study conducted in Campania shows similar richness. All of the traditional medicinal applications of plants were recorded and they found the use of 95 medicinal species, representing roughly 24% of the entire local flora. In Liguria, a total of 82 medicinal species were recorded along with reports of high levels of wild edible species consumption that were likely serving as functional or medicinal foods. A study of the popular phytotherapy along the Amalfi coast revealed that 102 medicinal plants are used for medicinal purposes, with a total of 276 distinct uses. One of the most interesting findings of this study was that 62% of the recorded uses were still in common practice, showing that many Italians still commonly use medicinal plants (see Quave *et al.*, 2012b and references therein).

### 29.3.2.3   Medical ethnobotany in south-eastern Europe

Over the last three decades, south-eastern Europe has been subject to major political turmoil and also economic shifts that have heavily influenced local lifestyles, foodways, links to nature and, as a consequence, transmission of traditional knowledge regarding health and local medical practices. The rural regions of south-eastern Europe represent some of the most vibrant scenarios for conducting medical ethnobotanical studies (see studies in Croatia, Bosnia and Herzegovina, Albania, Serbia, Kosovo, Turkey and Greece in Quave *et al.*, 2012b and references therein; Pieroni *et al.*, 2013, 2014). The reasons are numerous:

1. This largely mountainous area is a hotspot for both biodiversity and cultural/ethnic/religious diversities.
2. The area has historically provided the botanical materials that were sold in the western European herbal markets (especially during the last few centuries).
3. A remarkable number of locally gathered medicinal plants are still widely used in many households for local healthcare.
4. Local wild medicinal and food plants are central to many economic initiatives and programmes devoted to rural development and food security (Quave and Pieroni, 2014).

Moreover, medico-ethnobotanical studies in the western Balkans (e.g. Pieroni *et al.*, 2013) provide a unique arena for cross-cultural analysis of local uses of medicinal plants, which can contribute to the identification and development of a better understanding of factors that affect changes in plant uses and perceptions.

The ethnopharmacopeia of south-eastern Europe shares some similarities with that of south-western Europe, especially with regard to some of the most common medicinal species, including *Allium* spp., *Hypericum* spp., *Mentha* spp., *Olea europaea* L. and *Urtica dioica* L. Besides these few common species, however, there are many examples of medicinal plants being used in very distinct ways in different Balkan areas, even in areas sharing a similar flora, but a different cultural or linguistic heritage, highlighting the importance of documenting the traditional ecological knowledge unique to diverse areas in Europe.

## 29.4  European ethnomedicinal flora

Given the complex geography and cultural diversity of Europe, a great number of species have been used. Lamiaceae, Asteraceae and Rosaceae are always among the most important families referred to (Quave *et al.*, 2012b and references therein) as also happens in many other ethnopharmacopoeias around the world (Moerman *et al.*, 1999; Molares and Ladio, 2009).

Most species traditionally used are abundant species that are obtained locally, gathered from the wild or cultivated in home gardens. These species have the essential characteristics for being used in elementary healthcare: they are widespread, easily gathered and have a vast array of medicinal properties and pharmacological effects (Carvalho and Morales, 2010). As highlighted by Stepp and Moerman (2001), many are weeds abundant in disturbed habitats.

Here we provide a non-exhaustive list of species classified according to the distribution of use and the origin of the plant species. These examples show that there are species widely used through the continent while others are only used regionally in one or a few countries.

1. *Common and abundant wild species with a wide distribution area.* This group includes examples such as *Chelidonium majus* L., *Crataegus monogyna* Jacq., *Equisetum arvense* L. and other species of the genus, *Hypericum perforatum* L., *Malva sylvestris* L., *Marrubium vulgare* L., *Mentha pulegium* L., *Plantago major* L., *P. lanceolata* L. and other species of the genus, *Origanum vulgare* L., *Sambucus nigra* L., *Urtica dioica* L. and *Thymus vulgaris* L. This group includes the most common species, widely used throughout Europe.

2. *Species used in one or small number of countries.* This group includes common, widely used and highly valued species at a regional scale such as *Chamaemelum nobile* (L.) All., *Jasonia glutinosa* DC., *Centaurea ornata* Willd., *Santolina chamaecyparissus* L., *Sideritis hirsuta* L., *Sideritis hyssopifolia* L., *Thymus mastichina* L. and *Sorbus aucuparia* L.

3. *Regional and restricted endemisms* such as *Lilium pyrenaicum* Gouan, *Lithodora fruticosa* (L.) Griseb. and *Phlomis lychnitis* L. More restricted endemisms include *Artemisia granatensis* Boiss., *Erodium petraeum* Willd., *Santolina oblongifolia* Boiss. and *Thymus moroderi* Pau ex Martinez.

4. *Cultivated widely used species.* This group includes *Allium cepa* L., *A. sativum* L., *Aloe* spp., *Citrus limon* (L.) Osbeck, *Hylotelephium telephium* (L.) H. Ohba, *Juglans regia* L., *Matricaria recutita* L., *Melissa officinalis* L., Mentha × piperita L., *Olea europaea* L., *Pelargonium* spp., *Ruta chalepensis* L., *Salvia officinalis* L., *Tilia platyphyllos* Scop., *Vitis vinifera* L. and *Zea mays* L.

## 29.5 Adaptation, syncretism and resilience of traditional pharmacopoeias

Local knowledge is not static; rather it is highly dynamic and adaptive. It is open to adopt new species and techniques and to reject others (Gómez-Baggethun and Reyes-Garcia, 2013; Leonti and Casu, 2013). Transhumant shepherds, schoolteachers or migrants who return to their communities often facilitate the introduction of new plants and therapies. For example, remnants of ancient Albanian medicinal plant uses and names can still be found today amongst the Arbëreshë diaspora in Italy, who are descendants of Albanians that fled to southern Italy following the Ottoman occupation about 500 years ago (e.g. Pieroni *et al.*, 2002).

Most European ethnobotanical studies report a downward trend in the use of traditional medicinal plants since they have been replaced with pharmaceuticals following the dramatic social and economic changes of the past few decades (Parada *et al.*, 2009; Carvalho and Morales, 2010). However, this erosion process is not homogeneous since some species (e.g. *Chamaemelum nobile* (L.) All., *Matricaria recutita* L. *Cichorium intybus* L. and *Malva sylvestris* L.) are still widely used in different European regions (Pieroni *et al.*, 2002; Quave *et al.*, 2012b; Menendez-Baceta *et al.*, 2014).

In Estonia, changes in use illustrate the tendency for using weeds, i.e species, which grow in disturbed environments (Sõukand and Kalle, 2011). Newly introduced species and practices, sometimes as commercial herbal products, are also entering into local pharmacopeias, demonstrating the highly dynamic nature of traditional medical practices. Concerns about the health risks of consuming industrial foods and pharmaceuticals are promoting a revitalization of traditional medical practices (Carvalho and Morales, 2010). The interest in pursuing a more 'natural' or 'healthier' lifestyle as an alternative to the mainstream western system has emerged and allochthonous medical systems such as acupuncture are being syncretized with local traditional health self-care practices. For example, commercial dietary supplements and nutraceuticals containing non-native species like *Aloe vera* (L.) Burm. F., *Echinacea* spp. and *Panax ginseng* C.A. Mey have become popular elements of these traditions (Bonet *et al.*, 1992; Rivera and Obón, 2002).

## 29.6 Pharmacological studies of European medicinal plants

Bioprospecting, or searching for new drugs among plants and other remedies used by indigenous people, has been part of the European scholars' interest in economic plants at least since Linnaeus' time, who as a physician tried the plant remedies he learnt about from peasants during his travels. Marsh rosemary (*Ledum palustre* L.) was praised by him as a remedy against scurvy, whooping cough, laryngitis and leprosy (Svanberg *et al.*, 2011). He and his contemporaries had great confidence in finding new medicaments among popular medicine. Another well-known example concerns the English physician William Withering (1741–1799), who analysed a herbal remedy used by a local female healer in Shropshire for patients suffering from 'dropsy' (edema). He concluded that the key ingredient was foxglove (*Digitalis purpurea* L.), prepared an extract of the plant and examined its effect on patients. The treatment successfully reduced the fluid build-up in the tissues by its effects in strengthening contractions of the cardiac tissue (Wilkins *et al.*, 1985).

This interest in using medico-ethnobotanical field studies as a basis for phytochemical and pharmacological research still continues in Europe (e.g. Adsersen *et al.*, 2006; Jäger *et al.*, 2013; Vogl *et al.*, 2013). For example, the elm leaf blackberry (*Rubus ulmifolius* Schott.) known in the popular treatment of skin and soft tissue infections in southern Italy (Quave *et al.*, 2008) contains ellagic acid glycoside-rich fractions with potent antibacterial properties, especially against *Staphylococcus aureus* (Quave *et al.*, 2012a) and *Streptococcus pneumoniae* (Talekar *et al.*, 2014) biofilm-associated infections. In addition to the search for new antimicrobial drugs, other areas of high interest include drug targets related to cancer, chronic disease, mental health and skin health. Local ethnopharmacopoeias play a critical role in providing researchers with guidance as to which genera (or even specific taxa) merit additional analysis with regard to these high-priority targets in drug discovery.

## 29.7    Concluding remarks

Medical ethnobotanical studies in Europe have illuminated the dynamic nature of traditional knowledge concerning medicinal plants. While in some cases a resilience of local medical practices has been observed, most studies report a significant loss of knowledge that parallels transculturation processes and loss of cultural diversity.

Pluralistic and culturally appropriate approaches, which include emic views of newcomers' health-seeking strategies, are increasingly considered a crucial element of our public health policies. In fact these are often considered the only approaches that can build a genuine understanding of the holistic essence of health as a composite of physical, psychological and social aspects of well-being. Understanding migrants' use of medical plants can therefore offer a unique arena for fostering this aim and for implementing the safe use of medicinal plants within the multicultural framework of diversity in Europe.

Medical ethnobotanical field studies can provide useful, but hitherto often overlooked information to the allopathic medical community as they sought to reconcile existing and emerging therapies with conventional biomedicine. This is of great importance not only for phyto-pharmacovigilance and managing the risk of herb–drug interactions in mainstream patients that use herbal medicines, but also for informing the medical community about ethnomedical systems and practices so that they can better serve the society at large that includes a growing migrant population.

These studies are also important sources of guidance in the search for new medicines to address globally relevant diseases, such as antibiotic resistant infections, metabolic syndrome, cancer and diabetes. Thus, medical ethnobotany in Europe promises to continue to develop as a highly relevant scientific field in the future with diverse topics at the centre of research, such as:

- cultural competency in the delivery of healthcare to migrants;
- biocultural conservation initiatives;
- phyto-pharmacovigilance;
- drug discovery.

Research into medicinal plants that are presently underused may lead to the development of the pharmaceuticals, food supplements and complementary medicines of tomorrow (Quave *et al.*, 2012b).

## References

Aceituno-Mata, L. (2010) *Estudio etnobotánico y agroecológico de la Sierra Norte de Madrid*, Facultad de Ciencias, Universidad Autónoma de Madrid, Madrid.

Adsersen, A., Gauguin, B., Gudiksen, L. and Jäger, A.K. (2006) Screening of plants used in Danish folk medicine to treat memory dysfunction for acetylcholinesterase inhibitory activity. *Journal of Ethnopharmacology*, **104** (3), 418–422.

Bonet, M.A., Blanche, C. and Xirau, J.V. (1992) Ethnobotanical study in River Tenes valley (Catalonia, Iberian Peninsula). *Journal of Ethnopharmacology*, **37**, 205–212.

Carrasco, M.C., Vallejo, J.R., Pardo-de-Santayana, M., *et al.* (2009) Interactions of *Valeriana officinalis* L. and *Passiflora incarnata* L. in a patient treated with lorazepam. *Phytotherapy Research*, **23** (12), 1795–1796.

Carvalho, A.M. and Morales, R. (2010) Persistence of wild food and wild medicinal plant knowledge in a northeastern region of Portugal, in *Ethnobotany in the new Europe: people, health and wild plant resources* (eds M. Pardo de Santayana, A. Pieroni, and R. Puri), Berghahn, New York, Oxford, pp. 147–171.

Conti, F., Abbate, G., Alessandrini, A. and Blasi, C. (2005) *An annotated checklist of the Italian vascular flora, University of Roma la Sapienza*, Dip. Biologia Vegetale.

Domarew, C.A., Holt, R.R. and Snitkoff, G.G. (2002) A study of Russian phytomedicine and commonly used herbal remedies. *Journal of Herbal Pharmacotherapy*, **2** (4), 31–48.

Du, Y., Wolf, I.-K., Zhuang, W., *et al.* (2014) Use of herbal medicinal products among children and adolescents in Germany. *BMC Complementary and Alternative Medicine*, **14**, 218.

Engdal, S., Steinsbekk, A., Klepp, O. and Nilsen, O.G. (2008) Herbal use among cancer patients during palliative or curative chemotherapy treatment in Norway. *Supportive Care in Cancer*, **16** (7), 763–769.

Fernández-López, C. and Amezcúa-Ogayar, C. (2007) *Plantas medicinales y útiles en la Península Ibérica. 2.400 especies y 37.500 aplicaciones*, Herbario JAEN, Jaén.

Ferraro, G. (1884) Botanica popolare. Appunti presi a Carpeneto d'Acqui, Provincia di Alessandria. *Archivio per lo Studio delle Tradizioni Popolari*, **3**, 596–604.

Ferraro, G. (1885) Botanica popolare di Carpeneto d'Acqui. *Archivio per lo Studio delle Tradizioni Popolari*, **4**, 405–420.

Furniss, D.A. (1968) The monastic contribution to mediaeval medical care. *Journal of the Royal College of General Practitioners*, **15**, 244–250.

Gómez-Baggethun, E. and Reyes-García, V. (2013) Reinterpreting change in traditional ecological knowledge. *Human Ecology*, **41** (4), 643–647.

Grasser, S., Schunko, C. and Vogl, C.R. (2012) Gathering 'tea' – from necessity to connectedness with nature. Local knowledge about wild plant gathering in the Biosphere Reserve Grosses Walsertal (Austria). *Journal of Ethnobiology and Ethnomedicine*, **8**, 31.

Jäger, A.K., Gauguin, B., Andersen, J., *et al.* (2013) Screening of plants used in Danish folk medicine to treat depression and anxiety for affinity to the serotonin transporter and inhibition of MAO-A. *Journal of Ethnopharmacology*, **145** (3), 822–825.

Kalle, R. and Sõukand, R. (2014) A schoolteacher with a mission: Gustav Vilbaste (1885–1967) and ethnobotany in Estonia, in *Pioneers in European Ethnobiology* (eds I. Svanberg and Ł. Łuczaj), Royal Gustavus Adolphus Academy, Uppsala, pp. 201–218.

Kołodziejska-Degórska, I. (2012) Mental herbals – a context-sensitive way of looking at local ethnobotanical knowledge: examples from Bukovina (Romania). *Trames. Journal of the Humanities and Social Sciences*, **16** (3), 287–301.

Kujawska, M. and Hilgert, N.I. (2014) Phytotherapy of Polish migrants in Misiones, Argentina: Legacy and acquired plant species. *Journal of Ethnopharmacology*, **153** (3), 810–830.

Lardos, A. and Heinrich, M. (2013) Continuity and change in medicinal plant use: The example of monasteries on Cyprus and historical iatrosophia texts. *Journal of Ethnopharmacology*, **150** (1), 202–214.

Leonti, M. and Casu., L. (2013) Traditional medicines and globalization: current and future perspectives in ethnopharmacology. *Frontiers in Pharmacology*, **25**, 4–92.

Leporatti, M.L. and Ivancheva, S. (2003) Preliminary comparative analysis of medicinal plants used in the traditional medicine of Bulgaria and Italy. *Journal of Ethnopharmacology*, **87**, 123–142.

Łuczaj, Ł. (2010) Changes in the utilization of wild green vegetables in Poland since the 19th century: a comparison of four ethnobotanical surveys. *Journal of Ethnopharmacology*, **128**, 395–404.

Łuczaj, Ł., Köhler, P., Pirożnikow, E., *et al.* (2013) Wild edible plants of Belarus: from Rostafiński's questionnaire of 1883 to the present. *Journal of Ethnobiology and Ethnomedicine*, **9**, 21.

Mamedov, N., Gardner, Z. and Craker, L.E. (2004) Medicinal plants used in Russia and Central Asia for the treatment of selected skin conditions. *Journal of Herbs, Spices and Medicinal Plants*, **11** (1–2), 191–222.

Mattirolo, O. (1918) *Phytoalimurgia Pedemontana ossia Censimento delle Specie vegetali alimentari della Flora spontanea del Piemonte*, Vincenzo Bona, Turin.

Maxia, A., Demurtas, A., Kasture, S., *et al.* (2014) Medical ethnobotany survey of the Senegalese community living in Cagliari (Sardinia, Italy). *Indian Journal of Traditional Knowledge*, **13** (2), 275–282.

Menendez-Baceta, G., Aceituno-Mata, L., Molina, M., *et al.* (2014) Medicinal plants traditionally used in the northwest of the Basque Country (Biscay and Alava), Iberian Peninsula. *Journal of Ethnopharmacology*, **152** (1), 113–134.

Moerman, D.E., Pemberton, R.W., Kiefer, D. and Berlin, B. (1999) A comparative analysis of five medicinal floras. *Journal of Ethnobiology*, **19**, 49–67.

Molares, S. and Ladio, A. (2009) Ethnobotanical review of the Mapuche medicinal flora: Use patterns on a regional scale. *Journal of Ethnopharmacology*, **122**, 251–260.

Palacín, J.M. (1994) *La* ≪*medicina popular*≫: fuentes para su estudio y método de trabajo, in *Metodología de la Investigación Científica sobre Fuentes Aragonesas>*, Instituto de Ciencias de la Educación, Universidad de Zaragoza, pp. 363–418.

Parada, M., Carrió, E., Bonet, M.A. and Vallès, J. (2009) Ethnobotany of the Alt Empordà region (Catalonia, Iberian Peninsula). *Plants used in human traditional medicine. Journal of Ethnopharmacology*, **124**, 609–618.

Pardo Sastrón, J. (1895) *Catálogo ó enumeración de las plantas de Torrecilla de Alcañiz, así espontaneas como cultivadas*, Cuatro de Agosto, 5. Tip. de E. Casañal y Compañía, Zaragoza.

Pardo-de-Santayana, M., Morales, R., Aceituno, L. and Molina, M. (eds) (2014) *El Inventario Español de los Conocimientos Tradicionales relativos a la biodiversidad*, MAGRAMA, Madrid.

Pieroni, A., Quave, C., Nebel, S. and Heinrich, M. (2002) Ethnopharmacy of the ethnic Albanians (Arbereshe) of northern Basilicata, Italy. *Fitoterapia*, **73**, 217–241.

Pieroni, A., Houlihan, L., Ansari, N., *et al.* (2007) Medicinal perceptions of vegetables traditionally consumed by South-Asian migrants living in Bradford, Northern England. *Journal of Ethnopharmacology*, **113** (1), 100–110.

Pieroni, A., Rexhepi, B., Nedelcheva, A., *et al.* (2013) One century later: The folk botanical knowledge of the last remaining Albanians of the upper Reka Valley, Mount Korab, Western Macedonia. *Journal of Ethnobiology and Ethnomedicine*, **9**, 22.

Pieroni, A., Nedelcheva, A., Hajdari, A., *et al.* (2014) Local knowledge on plants and domestic remedies in the mountain villages of Peshkopia (Eastern Albania). *Journal of Mountain Science*, **11** (1), 180–193.

Pitrè, G. (1896) *Medicina Popolare Siciliana*, Clausen, Turin.

Pols, H. (2009) European physicians and botanists, indigenous herbal medicine in the Dutch East Indies, and colonial networks of mediation. *East Asian Science, Technology and Society*, **3**, 173–208.

Quave, C.L. and Pieroni, A. (2014) Fermented foods for food sovereignty and food security in the Balkans: A case study of the Gorani people of northeastern Albania. *Journal of Ethnobiology*, **34** (1), 28–43.

Quave, C.L., Carmona, M.E., Compadre, C.M., *et al.* (2012a) Ellagic acid derivatives from *Rubus ulmifolius* inhibit *Staphylococcus aureus* biofilm formation and improve response to antibiotics. *PLoS ONE*, **7** (1), e28737, doi: 10.1371/journal.pone.0028737.

Quave, C.L., Pardo-de-Santayana, M. and Pieroni, A. (2012b) Medical ethnobotany in Europe: from field ethnography to a more culturally-sensitive evidence-based CAM? *Evidence-based Complementary and Alternative Medicines*, **2012**, Article ID 156846, 17 pages. doi: 10.1155/2012/156846.

Rivera, D. and Obón, C. (1996) Phytotherapie in Spanien. *Zeitschrift für Phytotherapie*, **5**, 284–299.

Rivera, D. and Obón, C. (2002) El contexto etnobotánico mediterráneo y la fitoterapia. *Revista de Fitoterapia*, **2**, 47–55.

Shikov, A.N., Pozharitskaya, O.N., Makarov, V.G., *et al.* (2014) Medicinal plants of the Russian pharmacopoeia; their history and applications. *Journal of Ethnopharmacology*, **154** (3), 481–536.

Sõukand, R. and Kalle, R. (2011) Change in medical plant use in Estonian ethnomedicine: A historical comparison between 1888 and 1994. *Journal of Ethnopharmacology*, **135**, 251–260.

Sõukand, R. and Kalle, R. (2012) Personal and shared: the reach of different herbal landscapes. *Estonian Journal of Ecology*, **61** (1), 20–36.

Stepp, J.R. and Moerman, D.E. (2001) The importance of weeds in ethnopharmacology. *Journal of Ethnopharmacology*, **75**, 19–23.

Svanberg, I., Łuczaj, Ł., Pardo-de-Santayana, M. and Pieroni, A. (2011) History and current trends of ethnobiological research in Europe, in *Ethnobiology* (eds E.N. Anderson, D. Pearsall, E. Hunn and N. Turner), Wiley-Blackwell, Hoboken, New Jersey, pp. 189–212.

Talekar, S.J., Chochua, S., Nelson, K., *et al.* (2014) 220D-F2 from *Rubus ulmifolius* kills *Streptococcus pneumoniae* planktonic cells and pneumococcal biofilms. *PLoS ONE*, **9** (5), e97314, doi: 10.1371/journal.pone.0097314.

Vallejo, J.R., Peral, D., Gemio, P., *et al.* (2009) *Atractylis gummifera* and *Centaurea ornata* in the Province of Badajoz (Extremadura, Spain). *Ethnopharmacological importance and toxicological risk. Journal of Ethnopharmacology*, **126**, 366–370.

van Andel, T. and Westers, P. (2010) Why Surinamese migrants in the Netherlands continue to use medicinal herbs from their home country. *Journal of Ethnopharmacology*, **127**, 694–701.

Vogl, S., Picker, P., Mihaly-Bison, J., *et al.* (2013) Ethnopharmacological in vitro studies on Austria's folk medicine – An unexplored lore in vitro anti-inflammatory activities of 71 Austrian traditional herbal drugs. *Journal of Ethnopharmacology*, **149** (3), 750–771.

Wilkins, M.R., Kendall, M.J. and Wade, O.L. (1985) William Withering and digitalis, 1785 to 1985. *British Medical Journal*, **290**, 7–8.

# 30

# Ethnopharmacology in the Eastern Mediterranean and the Middle East: 'The Sun Rises from the East, but Shines on the Eastern Mediterranean'

Erdem Yesilada

*Yeditepe University, Faculty of Pharmacy, Atasehir, Istanbul, Turkey*

## 30.1   Introduction

The eastern Mediterranean, including the Balkans and the Middle East, occupies only a small fraction of the world's terrestrial territories, but has had a great impact on the human history. It is the cradle of many celestial religions, and also of the basic fundamentals of contemporary medicine. Historical evidence demonstrates that first records on therapeutic uses of plants date back over 4000 years to Mesopotamia. The oldest Egyptian medicinal record is the Ebers Papyrus, dating from 1550 BC. Moreover, the canons of medicine have also lived in the Eastern Mediterranean: Asclepius (the god of medicine), Hippocrates (c. 460–c. 370 BC) from Kos (Greece), Dioscorides (c. 40–90 AD) from Anazarba (Turkey), Galen (129–c. 200/c. 216 AD) from Pergamon (Turkey) and others. During the Abbasid period (750–945 AD) the works of the early Greek physicians were translated into Arabic. Accordingly, their treatise and corpus of medicine met with the sages of Islamic medicine, i.e. Al-Razi (c. 865–930 AD) from Rey (Iran), Avicenna (Ibn-Sīnā, c. 980–1037 AD) from Bukhara (Uzbekistan) and others. Their interpretation of the Hippocratic corpus with their own experience gave birth to Greco-Islamic medicine. When Avicenna wrote *The Canon of Medicine*, he was not only influenced by Greek and Islamic medicine, but also incorporated the wisdom of Indian medical teachings. He combined Galen's humoral system with teachings of Aristotle on life directives, namely nature, psyche and humanity, emphasizing the harmony between the two. By the end of 16th century Unani medicine influenced the old world. Later the Syrian physician/pharmacists Ibn al-Baitar (1197–1248) and Dawud Ibn Umar al-Antaki (?–1599) published books on therapy which describe the use of herbal- and mineral-based medicines by compiling and interpreting the wisdom of their predecessors.

The Silk Road was the other crucial link between the eastern (Chinese and Indian) and Mediterranean cultures. The corpus of the eastern wisdom of medicine had blended with that of Hippocratic in the eastern Mediterranean well before the sovereignty of the Muslims and thus contributed to the genesis of Unani medicine (cf. Touwaide and Appetiti (2013) on the possible consequences of this interaction). Today natural materials available in *attars* (medicinal plant and spice shops and sellers) in several Islamic societies include turmeric, ginger, ginseng, black pepper, senna etc., which do not grown in Middle Eastern or Mediterranean countries and are derived from the eastern tradition (Yesilada, 2005). However, recent methodological ethnobotanical field surveys have revealed that the list of herbal materials commercially available in these stores was found not to be very similar to the popular medical cultures in these societies (Yesilada, 2005).

There is a small body of work reporting plants available on markets in the Eastern Mediterranean, e.g. the herbal markets in Thessaloniki (Greece) (Hanlidou *et al.*, 2004) and Cyprus (Karousou and Deirmentzoglou, 2011). In the latter study, the authors also discuss the resemblance of the list of plants in the herbal shops of Cyprus with those reported for Greece, Turkey and two Middle Eastern countries (Israel and Jordan), and observe a higher affinity to Greece and Turkey, possibly due to long-lasting cultural exchanges as well as the similarity of local floras. It is noteworthy that several plants which acquired reputation only recently had also been introduced into these lists of herbal shops/markets, i.e. Echinacea (*Echinacea angustifolia* DC. (Asteraceae)), fewerfew (*Tanacetum parthenium* (L.) Sch. Bip. (Asteraceae)) and Ginkgo (*Ginkgo biloba* L. (Ginkgoaceae)). On the other hand, the natural materials lists in herbalists or *attars* may also include several herbal remedies based on the empiric knowledge of the local indigenous population. These reports have demonstrated that Unani medicine is the primary influence on the list of herbal materials in herbal shops/markets or *attars* in the Eastern Mediterranean societies, while religion, local flora, local medicine and consumer demand have had less of an impact. In other words, based on the impact of Unani medicine in Christian (Greek or Cypriots), Jewish (Israel) and Muslim societies (Turkey, Jordan, etc.) the lists of herbal remedies are quite similar.

## 30.2  Ethnobotany and ethnopharmacology in the Balkan region

The Balkan Peninsula in the eastern Mediterranean region is one of the prominent biodiversity centres of Europe. Out of 10,500 vascular plant species recorded in the *Flora Europaea*, 6340 have been reported to grow in the Balkans (Zlatkovic *et al.*, 2014). Along with the floristic richness, diversified ethnicity due to the Balkan region's historical and cultural background has enriched the traditional medical systems. However, due to periods of prolonged political instability after the disintegration of the Republic of Yugoslavia, until recently the number of ethnobotanical field surveys was scarce. During the period between the Second World War and before the collapse of Yugoslavia a small number of publications reporting some popular uses of the plants in some restricted areas in the region were published in local languages.

In the last decade, however, an increasing number of ethnobotanical field surveys has been carried out, reporting the present situation of traditional medicine in the region and particularly focusing on the mountainous remote parts of Serbia, Montenegro, Kosovo, Croatia, Bosnia and Herzegovina, Albania and Macedonia (Mustafa *et al.*, 2012). Recently, several field surveys have been conducted comparing medicinal plant use within these communities. These comparative surveys have revealed that, despite the prolonged historical togetherness of the societies in the western Balkans and similarities in the medicinal plants used, the local ethnobotanical knowledge seems to be quite specific to each community (Pieroni *et al.*, 2011, 2014; Mustafa *et al.*, 2012a,2012b; Rexhepi *et al.*, 2013).

This point was also highlighted by Hadjichambis *et al.* (2008). Because of the impact of culture, history, personal attitudes and philosophy, local popular medicine shows great variation from region to region. Field surveys documenting the wild food plants traditionally used in seven of the Mediterranean countries (Albania, Greece, Cyprus, Egypt, Italy, Spain and Morocco) led the authors to conclude that, 'the collection of wild plants is inextricably embedded in cultural concepts describing the traditional management of natural sources and the spatial organization of the natural-cultural landscape, and therefore it is difficult to speak about Mediterranean ethnobotany as a whole' (p. 410). Also, the most frequently quoted wild food plants of each surveyed area differed significantly. This may be explained by the preference of people to use plants that are easily available to them and to collect plants growing in their vicinity (Yesilada, 2005). The frequent use of taxa belonging to Asteraceae, Lamiaceae and Rosaceae might be due to their widespread distribution in Mediterranean countries and merits further investigation.

Using the genus *Helleborus* and its uses in ethnoveterinary medicine as an example, one can demonstrate the diversity of such uses. Among the traditional practices, an uncommon ethnoveterinary application was quite striking. In Serbia, the stem of *Helleborus odorus* Waldst and Kit. (Ranunculaceae) is inserted into a hole opened with a knife in sheep's ear to treat an unspecified disease (Jaric *et al.*, 2007). In Macedonia, however, the root of *Helleborus* species (unspecified) was applied on the breast for treating muscular weakness (possibly due to inflammation) in horses (Pieroni *et al.*, 2013). Interestingly, we have recorded a similar application in Marmara region (Turkey) restricted to a few localities, where local people use the sharpened root of *Helleborus orientalis* Lam. by piercing the earlobe of the animal for the treatment of oedema in the legs of cattle. Correspondingly, in an ethnopharmacological investigation carried out by our group, the hexane extract exerted a significant *in vivo* anti-inflammatory activity, supporting this traditional use (Erdemoglu *et al.*, 2003). Although all these utilizations addressed animal health, an external application of *H. odorus* root was also prescribed for humans against several inflammatory conditions, i.e. eczema, skin redness and itching in Montenegro (Menkovic *et al.*, 2011).

## 30.3  Modern ethnobotany and ethnopharmacology in the Middle East

Traditional practitioners, including local healers, midwifes and *attars*, are the main group of professional healers in the Middle East countries. Currently, these institutions are a family matter and the skills have been passed on by oral transmission over generations. They mainly practice Unani medicine. However, since they apply local plants as well as specific recipes formulated based on their own experience, the list of herbal materials may show variations. There are several ethnobotanical field surveys reporting on the present situation; i.e. in Israel

(Lev and Amar, 2000), Lebanon (El-Beyrouthy *et al.*, 2008), Iraq (Mati and De Boer, 2011) and Jordan (Lev and Amar, 2002). Between 2002 and 2007 successive field surveys were carried out by El-Beyrouthy and colleagues in localities selected from the different regions of Lebanon. They interviewed local healing professionals, namely. *attars*, folk healers and midwives, for their recipes against rheumatic and neuralgic complaints (El-Beyrouthy *et al.*, 2008). Among the recorded 231 plant species 53.3% were indigenous, while 19.2% were cultivars and 17.5% were imported. On the other hand, due to the recently increased public interest and demand for herbal medicines, unauthorized vendors have swung into action and set up herbal shops. However, most of these false practitioners have very limited knowledge about herbal remedies in the gathering and identification of correct species as well as the appropriate processing of medicinal remedies, which increases the efficacy and safety concerns. In fact, they are using 'mystical' or 'magical' methods of healing, which could injure the reputation of traditional institutions (Saad *et al.*, 2005).

Apart from the above-mentioned traditional institutions, there are healing practices applied by local healers, whose practice is also based on orally transmitted knowledge, i.e. elderly people in remote areas and the uplands and/or nomads, who generally inhabit the desert and some areas of the steppe. Unfortunately, the number of ethnobotanical surveys reporting the medical cultures in such Middle Eastern communities still seems quite limited (cf. Yesilada, 2005). Fortunately, several field surveys have recently become available focusing on popular medicine in such localities, particularly from Jordan.

Aburjai *et al.* (2007) investigated popular medicine in the Ajloun Heights region in Jordan by direct interviewing of elderly people and a few local practitioners. They listed 46 plants that are used for the treatment of various disorders and highlighted two important points:

(a)   Many medicinal plants well-known in Unani medicine were not mentioned at all by the locals. Instead species native to the study area were important.

(b)   Most of the locals interviewed dealt with well-known safe medicinal plants, while moderately unsafe or toxic plants were noted to be used by traditional practitioners rather than locals.

One such study was also carried out in Egypt (Eissa *et al.*, 2014). From 2006 to 2011 they visited 117 settlements of 17 Bedouin nomadic groups in the Sinai Peninsula region of Egypt and interviewed 700 people. The authors compiled 491 plant remedies used for treating various disorders, particularly emphasizing the central nervous disorders, namely with acclaimed sedative, analgesic, stimulating and anticonvulsant effects. Accordingly, it is evident that the nomadic Bedouins also use plants provided from the vicinity of their settlements for the treatment of their health problems. As a result of their widespread distribution in the region, 35% of the recorded medicinal plants were from the Asteraceae and Lamiaceae. Among these, *Haplophyllum tuberculatum* (Forssk.) A Juss. (Rutaceae), *Mentha longifolia* (L.) Hudson and *Teucrium polium* L. (Lamiaceae) were the most cited species.

Among the herbal remedies used in the eastern Mediterranean one of the most characteristic species for the region is *Ecbalium elaterium* A.Rich. (Cucurbitaceae), squirting cucumber. Because of the widespread distribution of the plant in the eastern Mediterranean region, the fruits and roots have been reported frequently for treating various disorders. In fact, Elatérion sediment, which is simply obtained from the fruit juice by filtering through muslin, was recorded in the old books of Hippocrates, Dioscorides and Avicenna, particularly for purging (Núñez *et al.*, 2011). In current popular practice in Turkey, on the Greek Islands and in Middle-Eastern countries (Jordan, Iraq, Syria, Israel, Palestine) the fruit juice of the plant has been used to treat sinusitis and liver diseases (jaundice or hepatitis) by dropping it into the nostrils directly or diluted (Al-Qura'n, 2009; Núñez *et al.*, 2011). Similar utilizations were also recorded in the *Materia Medica* of Dioscorides. The clinical efficacy of the fruit juice in the treatment of sinusitis was demonstrated and a potent anti-inflammatory compound cucurbitacin B, a tetracyclic triterpen, was isolated by *in vivo* bioassay-guided processing as the active principle responsible in both pathologies (Yesilada *et al.*, 1988; Sezik and Yesilada, 1995; Agil *et al.*, 1999).

The seeds of *Nigella sativa* L. (Ranunculaceae), black seed or black cumin, is one of the most commonly used herbal remedies throughout eastern Mediterranean societies for the treatment of a wide range of diseases as well as having culinary uses. In the ancient documents of Egyptian, Assyrian, Hittites and Greek physicians it was described against a wide range of disorders such as against nasal congestion, toothache, to stimulate menstruation and to promote lactation or as a diuretic. Its curative power was also described in the Bible. However, since Prophet Mohammad once stated that 'the black seed cures every disease, except death' (Saad and Said, 2011), most of the scientific investigations to prove its efficiency have been carried out by Muslim scientists. The scientific evidence has shown that the seeds possess significant antioxidant, anti-inflammatory, immune-modulator, anticancer, antinociceptive, antiallergic, hypoglycaemic and antimicrobial (against bacterial, yeast, viral and helminthic infections) activities (Salem, 2005).

## 30.4 Ethnobotany and ethnopharmacology in Turkey

As pointed out by Pieroni and Privitera (2014), with regard to the number of ethnobotanical field surveys conducted during the last four decades and published in international scientific journals in European countries, reports on Turkish local medicine have the first rank. This is clearly linked to the richness of the Turkish flora and cultural heritage. The history of current medicine was first written on the Anatolian peninsula and on Aegean Islands by Hippocrates, Dioscorides, Galen, etc. Most of the 600 plants recorded in Dioscorides' *Materia Medica* were from the Anatolian peninsula (Yesilada, 2005). During the following periods this information was enriched thanks to the influence of cultural links from east and west.

Similarly to neighbouring countries, the traditional healing system in Turkey may be categorized into two main groups:

- healing practices applied by using the plant materials of Unani medicine
- healing practices applied by using the plants gathered from the vicinity of villages.

In addition, recently popularized medicinal plants like *Echinacea* sp. flowers (Asteraceae), Ginkgo leaves (*Ginkgo biloba* L.; Ginkgoaceae) and Maté leaves (*Ilex paraguariensis* A. St. Hil.; Aquifoliaceae) have become available in herbalist shops (spice shops and *attars*) in cities and towns.

However, since the traditional practitioners' system (herbalists, healers, midwives, etc.) has been prohibited legally by the competent national authority (Ministry of Health), the materials sold in the herbalist shops are purchased by people in cities or towns to prepare these preparations themselves. People use recipes from old books (e.g. the Turkish translation of *Canon of Medicine* or other books on Islamic medicine) or information from more unreliable sources such as the internet or popular media. It should be noted that due to recently increased popular interest in natural medicines, in Turkey also an increasing number of fraudulent healers (without any qualification and certification) promote healing recipes in the tabloid media, which should not be considered as being a part of the traditional healing system.

Since publication of the first structured ethnobotanical survey on Turkish local medicine in 1991 (Sezik *et al.*, 1991), more than 50 research papers have been published reporting the present situation of local medicine in the various regions of Turkey (SCOPUS). Despite of a high rate of erosion in traditional knowledge due to modernization, i.e. easier access to modern health facilities, and expanded health insurance, the number of medicinal plants in use is expected to be over 1700 (based on the information input in the Turkish Databank of Folk Medicines).

## 30.5   Concluding remarks

In addition to a rich historical and cultural background, the rich flora (at least on the Balkan and Anatolian peninsulas) indicates accumulation of a rich repository of information in the eastern Mediterranean region. In other words, it is a region with enormous biocultural diversity.

As exemplified above, increasing numbers of ethnobotanical field surveys and ethnopharmacological investigations, i.e. *in vitro*, *in vivo* and clinical, would augment the chance for discovery of new drug candidates and diversify the number of therapeutic approaches in current medical therapy. Detailed investigations to evaluate the safety profile and possible risks, and to better understand the mechanisms of activity on of the herbal remedies used by the people should therefore be the primary task of the ethnopharmacologists in the region, while, if possible, identification of active ingredients for developing new drug molecules would highly be appreciated.

## References

Aburjai, T., Hudaib, M., Tayyem, R., *et al.* (2007) Ethnopharmacological survey of medicinal herbs in Jordan, the Ajloun Heights region. *Journal of Ethnopharmacology*, **110**, 294–304.

Agil, A., Miro, M., Jimenez, J., *et al.* (1999) Isolation of anti-hepatotoxic principle from the juice of *Ecbalium elaterium*. *Planta Medica*, **65**, 673–675.

Al-Qura'n, S. (2009) Ethnopharmacological survey of wild medicinal plants in Showbak, Jordan. *Journal of Ethnopharmacology*, **123**, 45–50.

Eissa, T.A.F., Palomino, O.M., Carretero, M.E. and Gómez-Serranillos, M.P. (2014) Ethnopharmacological study of medicinal plants used in the treatment of CNS disorders in Sinai Peninsula, Egypt. *Journal of Ethnopharmacology*, **151**, 317–332.

El-Beyrouthy, M., Arnold, N., Delelis-Dusollier, A. and Dupont, F. (2008) Plants used as remedies antirheumatic and antineuralgic in the traditional medicine of Lebanon. *Journal of Ethnopharmacology*, **120**, 315–334.

Erdemoglu, N., Küpeli, E. and Yesilada, E. (2003) Anti-inflammatory and antinociceptive activity assessment of plants used as remedy in Turkish folk medicine. *Journal of Ethnopharmacology*, **89**, 123–129.

Hadjichambis, A.Ch., Paraskeva-Hadjichambi, D., Della, A., *et al.* (2008) Wild and semi-domesticated food plant consumption in seven circum-Mediterranean areas. *International Journal of Food Sciences and Nutrition*, **59**, 383–414.

Hanlidou, E., Karousou, R., Kleftoyanni, V. and Kokkini, S. (2004) The herbal market of Thessaloniki (N. Greece) and its relation to the ethnobotanical tradition. *Journal of Ethnopharmacology*, **91**, 281–299.

Jarić, S., Popović, Z., Mačukanović-Jocić, M., *et al.* (2007) An ethnobotanical study on the usage of wild medicinal herbs from Kopaonik Mountain (Central Serbia). *Journal of Ethnopharmacology*, **111**, 160–175.

Karousou, R. and Deirmentzoglou, S. (2011) The herbal market of Cyprus: Traditional links and cultural exchanges. *Journal of Ethnopharmacology*, **133**, 191–203.

Lev, E. and Amar, Z. (2000) Ethnopharmacological survey of traditional drugs sold in Israel at the end of the 20th century. *Journal of Ethnopharmacology*, **72**, 191–205.

Lev, E. and Amar, Z. (2002) Ethnopharmacological survey of traditional drugs sold in the Kingdom of Jordan. *Journal of Ethnopharmacology*, **82**, 131–145.

Mati, E. and de Boer, H. (2011) Ethnobotany and trade of medicinal plants in the Qaysari Market, Kurdish Autonomous Region, Iraq. *Journal of Ethnopharmacology*, **133**, 490–510.

Menkovic, N., Savikin, K., Tasic, S., *et al.* (2011) Ethnobotanical study on traditional uses of wild medicinal plants in Prokletije Mountains (Montenegro). *Journal of Ethnopharmacology*, **133**, 97–107.

Mustafa B., Hajdari A., Pajazita Q., *et al.* (2012a) An ethnobotanical survey of the Gollak region, Kosovo. *Genetic Resources and Crop Evolution*, **59**, 739–754.

Mustafa, B., Hajdari, A., Krasniqi, F., *et al.* (2012b) Medical ethnobotany of the Albanian Alps in Kosovo. *Journal of Ethnobiology and Ethnomedicine*, **8**, 6.

Núñez, D.R., Seiquer, G.M., de Castro, C.O. and Ariza, F.A. (2011) *Plants and Humans in the Near East and the Caucasus, Vol. 2, The Plants: Angiosperms*, Editum, Murcia.

Pieroni, A. and Privitera, S. (2014) Ethnobotany and its links to medical sciences and public health: quo vadis? *Zeischrift für Phytotherapie*, **35**, 58–62.

Pieroni, A., Giusti, M.E. and Quave, C.L. (2011) Cross-cultural ethnobiology in the western Balkans: Medical ethnobotany and ethnozoology among albanians and serbs in the Pešter Plateau, Sandžak, south-western Serbia. *Human Ecology*, **39**, 333–349.

Pieroni, A., Rexhepi, B., Nedelcheva, A., *et al.* (2013) One century later: The folk botanical knowledge of the last remaining Albanians of the upper Reka Valley, Mount Korab, Western Macedonia. *Journal of Ethnobiology and Ethnomedicine*, **9**, article number 22.

Pieroni, A., Cianfaglione, K., Nedelcheva, A., *et al.* (2014) Resilience at the border: Traditional botanical knowledge among Macedonians and Albanians living in Gollobordo, Eastern Albania. *Journal of Ethnobiology and Ethnomedicine*, **10**, article number 31.

Rexhepi, B., Mustafa, B., Hajdari, A., *et al.* (2013) Traditional medicinal plant knowledge among Albanians, Macedonians and Gorani in the Sharr Mountains (Republic of Macedonia). *Genetic Resources and Crop Evolution*, **60**, 2055–2080.

Saad, B. and Said, O. (2011) *Greco-Arab and Islamic Herbal Medicine: Traditional system, ethics, safety, efficacy and regulatory issues*, John Wiley & Sons, Hoboken, New Jersey, p. 135.

Saad, B., Azaizeh, H. and Said, O. (2005) Tradition and perspectives of Arab herbal medicine: A review. *Evidence-Based Complementary and Alternative Medicine*, **2**, 475–479.

Salem, M.L. (2005) Immunomodulatory and therapeutic properties of the *Nigella sativa* L. seed. *International Immunopharmacology*, **5**, 1749–1770.

Sezik, E. and Yesilada, E. (1995) Clinical effects of the fruit juice of *Ecballium elaterium* in the treatment of sinusitis. *Journal of Toxicology and Clinical Toxicology*, **33**, 381–383.

Sezik, E., Tabata, M., Yesilada, E., *et al.* (1991) Traditional medicine in Turkey I. Folk medicine in Northeast Anatolia. *Journal of Ethnopharmacology*, **35**, 191–196.

Touwaide, A. and Appetiti, E. (2013) Knowledge of Eastern *materia medica* (Indian and Chinese) in pre-modern Mediterranean medical traditions: A study in comparative historical ethnopharmacology. *Journal of Ethnopharmacology*, **148**, 361–378.

Turrill, W.B. (1929) *The plant-life of the Balkan Peninsula*, Oxford Press, Leipzig.

Yesilada, E. (2005) Past and future contributions to traditional medicine in the health care system of the Middle-east. *Journal of Ethnopharmacology*, **100**, 135–137.

Yesilada, E., Tanaka, S., Sezik, E. and Tabata, M. (1988) Isolation of an anti-inflammatory principle from the fruit juice of *Ecbalium elaterium*. *Journal of Natural Products*, **51**, 504–508.

Zlatkovic, B.K., Bogosavljevic, S.S., Radivojevic, A.R. and Pavlovic, M.A. (2014) Traditional use of the native medicinal plant resource of Mt. Rtanj (Eastern Serbia): Ethnobotanical evaluation and comparison. *Journal of Ethnopharmacology*, **151**, 704–713.

# 31
# Ethnopharmacology in Australia and Oceania

Graham Lloyd Jones[1] and Nicholas J. Sadgrove[2]

[1]*Pharmaceuticals and Nutraceuticals Group, Centre for Bioactive Discovery in Health and Ageing, University of New England Armidale, Australia*
[2]*Pharmaceuticals and Nutraceuticals Group, Centre for Bioactive Discovery in Health and Ageing, University of New England Armidale, New South Wales, Australia*

## 31.1 Introduction

### 31.1.1 Australian ethnobotany

'Bioprospecting has gained much recent popular attention, particularly spurred by the apocryphal image of adventurous ethnobotanists penetrating at considerable peril the darkest recesses of the jungle at the behest of rich pharmaceutical firms'.

(Cox, 2008, p. 270)

As Cox (2008) describes above, the discipline of bioprospecting often evokes images of brilliant but erratic ethnopharmacologists, as portrayed, for example, by Harrison Ford (Indiana Jones) and Sean Connery (Medicine Man); battling through thick jungles or mountainous terrain in search of an infallible panacea, used for millennia by indigenous people. However, by contrast with the Amazonian rainforest or the Himalayas, the Australian landmass is predominantly arid with deserts and temperate grasslands predominating. Such arid flat landscapes are where most of the recorded ethnopharmacologically significant Australian plants are found.

Selective pressures in this geographically isolated arid land have nonetheless produced a higher proportion of total endemic flora, by comparison with the tropical or wet temperate islands of Oceania or indeed the rest of the world. Evolutionary biologists suggest that during prehistoric cycles of aridity, Australia's rich assortment of high secondary metabolite yielding flora emerged. This flora includes commercially important essential oil yielding species, such as *Eucalyptus*, *Melaleuca* and *Leptospermum* spp. Specific evolutionary advantages conferred on

*Ethnopharmacology*, First Edition. Edited by Michael Heinrich and Anna K. Jäger.
© 2015 John Wiley & Sons, Ltd. Published 2015 by John Wiley & Sons, Ltd.

plants by characteristic secondary metabolites remain contentious. However, their contribution to the *materia medica* of prehistoric Aboriginal people is beyond doubt.

In many cases, the plethora of plants with potentially therapeutic secondary metabolites has been subject to a process of iterative trial and error selection by human beings over the past 40,000 years. At the time of European colonization an indigenous *materia medica* had been developed empirically by the Aboriginal people, using successively iterated positive outcomes, passed on in the oral tradition of medicine men and women. The breadth and depth of this knowledge eventually became evident to the European colonizers, who initially imagined the indigenous inhabitants culturally poor because they lacked a written language. In early colonial times Europeans demonstrated a greater interest in botanical medicines that resembled those from their own homelands. For example, because of the odorous resemblance to English *Mentha piperita* (Lamiaceae), the piperitone rich essential oil from *Eucalyptus piperita* (Myrtaceae) (Sydney Peppermint) became Australia's first recorded medicinal export (Lassak and McCarthy, 2011).

A most unfortunate consequence of European colonization and altered land management practices was the decline of transfer of spiritual and medicinal knowledge to successive generations. Commenting on indigenous *materia medica*, Gould (1972) emphasizes the interconnectedness between land and botanical lore in traditional Aboriginal societies:

'Knowledge of this kind is precisely what the Aborigines possess in abundance, and the mechanisms for transmitting this knowledge from one generation to the next form an important part of traditional Aboriginal culture. More than their technology or their great physical endurance, it is this complex system of knowledge – what anthropologists sometimes call 'cognitive map' of both the terrain and the resources of their environment – that stands as the key to adaptive success of the Aborigines in this harsh region.'

While the botanical lore of the original inhabitants waned over time, interest in this ethnobotanical richness waxed increasingly in the minds of European Australians. Thus, a century after colonization, works describing indigenous *materia medica* were produced and may be considered 'Aboriginal pharmacopoeias' (Low, 1988). However, a large part of the cultural tradition of Aboriginal people had already disappeared prior to the appearance of these first written pharmacopoeias. This fragmentation of traditional knowledge has undercut the specific degree of recorded details involving the exacting therapeutic use of Aboriginal *materia medica*.

In traditional Aboriginal society, healers used plants in various ways together with precise ritual to achieve the desired healing outcome. The brilliance of the traditional healers, regarded as 'Aboriginal men of high degree' is described by Elkin (1946). Elkin describes how in Aboriginal societies these traditional healers or 'medicine men' had previously demonstrated a degree of aptitude for medicinal practice in their childhood, at which time they were adopted into decades of mentorship by the then current healers. During mentorship these young protégés graduated through various initiation rites and rituals, each signifying receipt of newer knowledge or skills that were otherwise guarded as 'secrets' from their family members (Elkin, 1946).

Traditional Aboriginal society is rigidly divided along gender lines. Medicinal plants were usually collected and prepared by women, although a recognition of men's plants and women's plants existed. 'Medicine men' also utilized a range of subtle approaches that were not immediately obvious. Elkin (1946) states:

'Such men understand quite well the power of faith and the influence which can be exercised by the mind over the body. They realize that their manipulation of a patient's body (sucking, extracting bones and stones) is only the external means of gaining the patient's confidence and restoring his faith in life. The final test is often a command to the sick person to get up at a certain time and go somewhere (perhaps down to the creek for water); if he obeys, he will get better; if not, then there is no hope.'

Ethnopharmacological discovery often depends on the translation of indigenous paradigms into the language of modern science, or 'building intellectual bridges' by linking ancient wisdom with modern science, acknowledging thereby the complex cognitive mapping used by Aboriginal people involving myth or 'dreamtime stories' (Isaacs, 1995). Such acknowledgement involves giving parity to both ontologies (scientist and autochthonous) and access-benefit sharing. These basic human rights are now protected by intellectual property rights law for traditional knowledge and the Nagoya protocol for genetic resources.

It is the expressed wish of Aboriginal people all over the world that their traditional knowledge systems be respected, promoted and protected. For Australian Aboriginal people the transfer of knowledge to their youth is hindered by an increasing preference for 'the busy world' and/ or by the expansion of mining companies (Edwards and Heinrich, 2006; Packer *et al.*, 2012). In such cases, profound social benefits may flow from a respectful confluence of science and traditional knowledge providing a source of pride and hope in marginalized communities and paving the way for meaningful employment in new healthcare industries.

## 31.1.2  Ethnobotany in Oceania

The islands of Oceania constitute a large number of smaller landmasses spread over a vast area of the Pacific Ocean. Since, compared with Australia, most of these islands are of very recent geological origin, the plant diversity is generally much diminished. Nonetheless, some of the plants endemic in Australia have found a foothold in these islands and diverged to produce characteristic plants of medicinal use. Most of the islands also demonstrate flora not represented on the Australian landmass. Some of this flora was established very recently by successive waves of predominantly Polynesian colonizers. However, most of the flora travelled across the sea as seed from Indo-Malaysia.

# 31.2  Ethnopharmacological 'classics'

## 31.2.1  Scopolamine from the Australian *Duboisia*

Perhaps the best known natural product success story in Australia is the development and commercialization of *Duboisia* alkaloids as stomach relaxants for use in motion sickness and as antispasmodics. In Aboriginal *materia medica* the lesser known species *D. hopwoodii* F.Muell (Solanaceae) is not used for such purposes, but was called *pituri*, made into a bolus, chewed as needed and placed behind the ear when not in use. Indeed, *pituri* from New South Wales and Queensland is considered by some to be the most highly valued trading commodity in traditional Aboriginal commerce.

Trade of *D. hopwoodii* was necessary because central Australian specimens were toxic and therefore not suitable for human use. Subsequently these types have been found to have the world's highest concentrations of nicotine and nornicotine. In traditional society this chemotype was used to poison animals by soaking the leaves in their drinking water. The stupefied animals were easily hunted and safely eaten afterwards (Latz, 2004).

Aboriginal people also exploited the related *D. myoporoides* R.Br for uses consistent with its subsequently demonstrated cholinergic activity. The German-Australian colonial botanist Ferdinand von Müller encouraged a comprehensive examination of the intoxicating drink produced from the plant by Aboriginal people. The psychoactive principles have been subsequently identified as the tropane alkaloids scopolamine (hyoscine) (**1**) and hyoscyamine (**2**), which are antagonists of the muscarinic acetylcholine receptors. Several years after scopolamine was first described it was used in the Second World War to treat sea sickness and shell shock, albeit with undesirable psychoactive side effects (Foley, 2006).

Today scopolamine is used as a chemical precursor for hyoscine hydrobromide (**3**) (motion sickness) or hyoscine butylbromide (**4**) (antispasmodic). These derivatives have substantially reduced unwanted side effects whilst maintaining specific therapeutic activity. The cultivar grown as feedstock for this industry is a hybrid of the two species *D. myoporoides* and *D. leichhardtii* F.Muell, which produces scopolamine in abundance (Foley, 2006).

Hyoscine (**1**)          Hyoscyamine (**2**)          Hyoscine hydrobromide (**3**)          Hyoscine butylbromide (**4**)

## 31.2.2   Polynesian breadfruit and kava used throughout Oceania

Perhaps the two best known plants of Polynesian origin are kava and breadfruit. Kava is known botanically as *Piper methysticum* G.Forst (Piperaceae) meaning 'intoxicating pepper'. An aqueous extract is produced from crushed lateral roots, stem or stem nodes and drunk ceremonially as a mild narcotic with sedative or soporific effects. By contrast, the medicinal and nutritious breadfruit plant *Artocarpus altilis* Fosberg (Moraceae) is better known as a food source.

Breadfruit was popularized in later colonial times after members of the crew of HMB *Endeavour* led by Captain James Cook observed it as a dietary staple on the Tahitian islands. Such was the popularity of breadfruit among the British sailors that Captain Bligh made an ill-fated journey to Tahiti in HMS *Bounty* specifically to collect the fruit for transport and subsequent cultivation in the West Indies. Although breadfruit was well known at the time from Tahiti it is found throughout most of Polynesia, including Hawaii, but not in colder areas such as New Zealand or Easter Island (Cox and Balick, 1996; Cox and Banack, 2003).

In the Marquesan islands, pit fermentation of breadfruit was developed for preservation. The Marquesan people called the subsequent sour pudding *ma* in their language, and the Samoans called it *masi*. Construction of a masi pit required perfect sealing to prevent spoilage. Allegedly the masi pits ensure preservation for several years (Cox and Balick, 1996; Cox and Banack, 2003).

Breadfruit is also used medicinally throughout Polynesia and Asia for various conditions, such as poisoning from the puffer fish, respiratory and other complaints. Although the evidence base is patchy at best, several novel compounds have been identified, including the triterpenoids cycloartenol (**5**), cycloartenone and cycloartenyl acetate (Cambie and Ash, 1994), and the novel prenylflavones isocyclomorusin, isocyclomulberrin and cycloaltilisin (**6**) (Chen *et al.*, 1993).

Every culture has at least one staple recreational drug. Kava fulfilled this role in much of Oceania. It is believed that the Polynesian species *P. methysticum* is a sterile cultivar derived from the species *P. wichmannii* C.DC, which has the same bioactivities and active kavalactones and is used for the same purpose as *P. methysticum* in its endemic areas, such as Vanuatu, the Solomon Islands and Papua New Guinea (Cambie and Ash, 1994).

Although better known for its ceremonial usage, kava is often used medicinally in the Fijian, Tongan and Samoan archipelagos. It is used for bladder or kidney troubles, as a diuretic, for filariasis and for other more general complaints such as coughs and colds or sore throat. Three kavalactone α-pyrone derivatives are believed to be the active components. These are dihydrokawain, dihydromethysticin (**7**) and the alkaloid pipermethystine. Together with the other α-pyrones, such as yangonin (**8**), kavain, desmethoxyyangonin and others, these kavalactones demonstrate *in vitro* activities consistent with anaesthetic, antifungal, sleep-producing, anti-convulsive and spasmolytic activities (Cambie and Ash, 1994; Mathews *et al.*, 2002). When kava did eventually become a licensed medicine, controversy continued to surround its use.

Cycloartenol (**5**)

Cycloaltilisin (**6**)

Dihydromethysticin (**7**)

Yangonin (**8**)

# 31.3  Australian aromatic plants

Australia has an abundance of endemic aromatic plants yielding significant levels of essential oil on hydrodistillation. Even though Aboriginal Australians did not have the technology to extract essential oils they were acutely responsive to olfactory cues and did use the particular properties of aromatic plants in various healing modalities, including 'smoking ceremonies' (Latz, 2004). Importantly, Aborigines were hunter gatherers and not cultivators; therefore there was little intentional interference with the process of natural selection of native plants, comparable with the process of cultivar selection familiar to Europeans. The extreme chemovariability within and between species of aromatic Australian plants must be seen within this context. This was first noted in the 1920s by Penfold and Morrison in respect of *Eucalyptus dives* Schauer (Myrtaceae), when the 1,8-cineole chemotype was first observed, differing from the better known piperitone/thymol chemotype (Lassak and McCarthy, 2011). With respect to the higher occurrence of chemovariation in Australian plants, it is very important to pay attention to the different regionally specific names and uses of aromatic plants in traditional Aboriginal *materia medica*.

## 31.3.1   Eucalyptus

Surprisingly, *Eucaluptus* does not often appear in written records of Australian Aboriginal medicine, although eucalyptus oil features prominently as *Oleum Eucalypti* in the British pharmacopoeia. Following European settlement in Australia, hundreds of species of eucalyptus have been described, displaying multiple chemotypes with usually only a few distinct molecular species constituting the bulk of any given oil (Lassak and McCarthy, 2011). Such predominating constituents include 1,8-cineol (**9**), globulol (**10**), citronellal (**11**) and piperitone (**12**).

1,8-cineole (**9**)    Globulol (**10**)                                    Piperitone (**12**)   Terpinen-4-ol (**13**)

Whether the first to distil eucalyptus oil and suggest its usefulness was the surgeon-general to the colony of New South Wales, John White, or the surgeon of the First Fleet, Dennis Considen, it was the aforementioned Baron Ferdinand von Müller who made the qualities of eucalyptus oil known throughout the world (Lassak and McCarthy, 2011).

The medicinal type of oil (ISO, 1974a) is commonly sold as such in pharmacies and general retail outlets or in the form of sprays, cough lollies and ointments, or in formulations with other oils as a general purpose liniment. It may be used as an inhalant or chest rub to ease breathing difficulties, as a disinfecting and soothing mouthwash in water, and as mentioned previously as a component of liniments designed to provide relief from muscular aches and pains. Eucalyptus oil is also used by itself or incorporated into household products as a general disinfectant, cleaner and domestic deodorizer.

## 31.3.2   *Melaleuca alternifolia* (tea tree oil)

By far the most important development from a commercial perspective is the essential oil from *Melaleuca alternifolia* Cheel (Myrtaceae), which in recent times has spawned an industry of global proportions. The tree is a paperbark shrub whose native habitat is swampy coastal regions of northern New South Wales. The local Bundjalung tribe inhaled the vapours emitted from heated leaves for the treatment of coughs and colds, and additionally applied a poultice from the leaves topically for the treatment of wounds and infections (Carson *et al.*, 2006).

The essential oil from the terpinen-4-ol (**13**) chemotype has a long history as a disinfectant. Thus, during the Second World War it was used as a surface disinfectant in machine oil in munitions factories. Additionally, Australian soldiers in the Second World War were issued with tea tree oil in their first-aid kits (Carson *et al.*, 2006).

The mechanism of action is relatively non-specific, which underlies its demonstrated activity against antibiotic-resistant bacteria. This feature combined with the non-irritant nature of the neat oil has led to its use in the antibacterial treatment of acne and as a suggested topical antifungal in the treatment of onychomycosis, candiasis and tinea. Its value as a mouthwash has been emphasized by recent studies on the susceptibility of oral bacteria, while its value as an inhalant is indicated in studies on antibacterial activity against respiratory tract pathogens. The oil also shows promise as a topical anti-inflammatory which, combined with its strong topical bactericidal and fungicidal activity, recommends it as an aid to accelerated wound healing (Carson *et al.*, 2006).

# 31.4   Recent developments: aromatic plants

*Eremophila species* (Scrophulariaceae) are regarded by many Aboriginal groups as their 'number one medicine' (Latz, 2004). Most *Eremophila* species have characteristic odours which were used by Aboriginal healers as key to their selection. In such cases therapeutic activity is probably partly mediated by small volatile compounds. This is particularly true where smoke fumigation rituals were performed using such species as *E. bignoniiflora*, *E. freelingii*, *E. gilesii*, *E. latrobei*, *E. longifolia* (all F.Muell) and *E. sturtii* R.Br (Latz, 2004). In this regard Aboriginal informants have routinely advised that they select for the most aromatic specimens when foraging for medicines (D. Murray (of Kamilaroi, an indigenous Australian Murri people), pers. comm.).

Although Aboriginal Australians lacked the technology to produce essential oils *per se*, the chemical character of such oils gives an indication of the range and proportion of volatile components produced during smoke fumigation modalities. Of course the range of molecules produced during smoke fumigation is no doubt wider than that produced in the hydrodistilled essential oil, therefore several studies have focused on simulating the traditional smoking process itself (Sadgrove and Jones, 2013b; Sadgrove *et al.*, 2014b).

With regard to the identification of essential oil chemotypes of *Eremophila longifolia*, 12 have been identified. In far western New South Wales two ketone-rich chemotypes were discovered, with significantly high yields of essential oils, making them potentially suitable for commercial development (Sadgrove *et al.*, 2011; Sadgrove and Jones, 2014a). These two chemotypes were previously known to Aboriginal groups by the name 'kaltika'. The other chemotypes found throughout Australia are listed in Table 31.1.

**Table 31.1**   Listed chemotypes of *Eremophila longifolia* (Sadgrove and Jones, 2014a).

| Chemotype | Principal compound(s) | Yield g/100g | Ploidy | Genifuranal |
|---|---|---|---|---|
| E-4n | *p*-Cymen-8-ol | 0.01–0.2 | 4n | Yes |
| F-4n | α-Pinene/limonene | 0.01–0.2 | 4n | Yes |
| D-4n | α-Pinene/sabinene/limonene/α-terpinolene | 0.01–0.2 | 4n | Yes |
| A-4n | Isomenthone/menthone | 0.1–0.4 | 4n | Yes |
| A-2n | Isomenthone/menthone | 3.5–8 | 2n | No |
| B-4n | Karahanaenone | 0.1–0.2 | 4n | Yes |
| B-2n | Karahanaenone | 0.4–5.5 | 2n | No |
| G-2n | Safrole/methyl eugenol | 2–5.5 | 2n | No |
| H-4n | Fenchone/camphor (2-bornanone) | 0.3–1 | 4n | Yes |
| I-4n | Fenchyl-/bornyl-acetate | 0.2–1 | 4n | Yes |
| C-4n | Borneol/fenchol | 0.4–0.7 | 4n | Yes |
| J-4n | α-Pinene/α-bisabolol | 0.1 | 4n | Yes |

One of these new essential oils, with dominant components of bornyl- (**14**) and fenchyl-acetate (**15**), is similar in composition to the antimicrobial essential oil produced from *Eremophila bignoniiflora* (Sadgrove *et al.*, 2013). Traditional ethnomedicinal use of *E. bignoniiflora* by Australian Aboriginal people involved applications consistent with antispasmodic activity and headache therapy. Essential oils rich in esters are often associated with antispasmodic and nervous calming activity, and so the ester-rich vapours utilized by Aboriginal people from *E. bignoniiflora* may have contributed to this effect.

The *E. longifolia* essential oils dominated by the alcohols borneol (**16**) and fenchol (**17**) demonstrated high antimicrobial activity against the yeast *C. albicans*, bacterial species, such as *Staphylococcus aureus*, *S. epidermidis*, and the human pathogenic fungal species *Trichophyton rubrum*, *T. mentagrophytes* and *T. interdigitalis*. Similar activity was demonstrated by the fenchyl- and bornyl acetate oils against *C. albicans* and *S. epidermidis* (Sadgrove *et al.*, 2011, 2013). The ketone analogues camphor (2-bornanone) (**18**) and fenchone (**19**) were never tested.

Bornyl acetate (**14**)          Borneol (**16**)          Camphor (**18**)

Fenchyl acetate (**15**)          Fenchol (**17**)          Fenchone (**19**)

It is relevant to note that the leaves of *E. longifolia* were placed on hot embers for traditional therapeutic use involving the resultant wet steamy smoke, possibly inhibiting bacterial or fungal pathogens, as well as stimulating lactagogue activity (Latz, 2004). The same smoking procedure was used to prepare surgical tools for circumcision, no doubt for sterilization but conceptualized as a type of purification ritual (Sadgrove and Jones, 2013b). In such fumigation rituals the recently identified compound (–)-genifuranal (**20**) may have been involved.

The heat-derived genifuranal was detected only after simulation of fumigation rituals (Sadgrove *et al.*, 2014b). It probably results from heat cleavage of geniposidic acid (**21**), producing genifuranal and a sugar moiety. Genifuranal itself exhibited significant antimicrobial activities, with mean inhibitory concentrations as low as 100 μg/ml against some species. Interestingly, genifuranal was produced by simulated smoking of all essential oil chemotypes, except the high-yielding diploid specimens.

During traditional fumigation rituals, antimicrobial activity would be enhanced by warm air delivery of genifuranal, essential oils and lignin decomposition products (Sadgrove and Jones, 2013b). *Eremophila* species are not only known for volatiles utilized in traditional fumigation rituals, but have also been shown to possess non-volatile highly antimicrobial compounds that may complement volatiles where lipophilic extraction into animal fat is used as the therapeutic modality. The previously mentioned iridoid glycoside geniposidic acid, together with verbascoside (**22**), is able to produce cardioactivity (Pennacchio *et al.*, 1996). Both of these iridoids occur in *E. longifolia* and *E. alternifolia* R.Br.

Geniposidic acid (**21**)

Genifuranal (**20**)

Verbascoside (**22**)

A class of resinous compounds called serrulatanes have been characterized in several species, after the first were found in *Eremophila serrulata* Druce (Croft *et al.*, 1977). In species such as *E. duttonii* F.Muell and *E. neglecta* J.M.Black, the character and bioactivity of the essential oil is relatively unknown, but serrulatanes have been implicated in significant antimicrobial activities, particularly serrulat-14-en-7,8,20-triol (**23**) and serrulat-14-en-3,7,8,20-tetraol (**24**) from *E. duttonii* (Smith *et al.*, 2007) and 8-hydroxyserrulat-14-en-19-oic acid (**25**), and biflorin (**26**) from *E. neglecta* (Ndi *et al.*, 2007).

Serrulat-14-en-3,7,8,20-tetraol (**24**)

Serrulat-14-en-7,8,20-triol (**23**)

8-Hydroxyserrulat-14-en-19-oic acid (**25**)

Biflorin (**26**)

In further experiments simulating traditional fumigation or smoke inhalation modalities, smoke condensates were produced from *Callitris endlicheri* F.M.Bailey and *C. glaucophylla* Joy Thomps. and L.A.S Johnson (Cupressaceae) (Sadgrove and Jones, 2014b). The latter species was shown to contain γ-lactones ferruginol (**27**) and pisiferal (**28**)/pisiferol, together with lignin decomposition products in the smoke condensate. Further experiments were carried out with select chemotypes of *Geijera parviflora* Lindl. (Rutaceae) (Sadgrove *et al.*, 2014a). A phase-separated solvent partition of the hydrosol produced after hydrodistillation of a sesquiterpene-rich essential oil chemotype of *G. parviflora* produced the coumarins xanthyletin (**29**), isopsoralen (**30**) and osthole (**31**).

Ferruginol (**27**)          Pisiferal (**28**)

The coumarin xanthyletin and the taraxerene myricadiol (**32**) have been characterized in *Scaevola spinescens* R.Br (Goodeniaceae) and are believed to be involved in cytotoxicity against cancer cell lines (Kerr *et al.*, 1996; Crago, 2011). Larger molecular mass compounds, such as xanthyletin from *Geijera* or *Scaevola*, or the γ-lactones from *Callitris*, are expected to be produced in higher abundances when smoking modalities of the three species are used, but are generally absent or in trace amounts in the hydrodistilled essential oils from untreated leaves.

Xanthyletin (**29**)          Isopsoralen (**30**)

Osthole (**31**)          Myricadiol (**32**)

*Geijera parviflora* occurs in a range of essential oil chemotypes with interesting antimicrobial and insecticidal activity, including the green essential oil made up of geijerene/pregeijerene (**33**), linalool (**34**) and germacrene D (**35**) (Sadgrove *et al.*, 2014a). These components are not, *prima facie,* expected to produce the psychoactivity purportedly achieved in traditional smoke inhalation modalities. Perhaps volatile alkaloid derivatives can be formed from precursor compounds such as the coumarin alkaloids parvifloranines A (**36**) and B, identified from a specimen growing in New South Wales (Shou *et al.*, 2013).

Pregeijerene (**33**)          Linalool (**34**)          Germacrene D (**35**)

*Pittosporum angustifolium* Lodd. (Pittosporaceae) was involved in a significant number of traditional medicinal applications. The most common of these are related to the treatment of coughs and colds, for lactagogue activity and in the treatment of eczema. More recently, a number of anecdotal reports have surfaced related to, among others, cancer inhibition and autoimmune conditions of the intestines. As yet no studies have comprehensively examined these reported activities.

Characterization of volatiles from *P. angustifolium* demonstrated compounds with structural similarities to previously described chemosemiotic compounds identified in mother–infant bonding, including acetic acid decyl ester or 1-dodecanol (Sadgrove and Jones, 2013a). Perhaps these compounds are involved in the traditional use as a lactagogue, particularly because the usage modality involved heating a compress of leaves to produce such volatiles to fumigate the breasts of the nursing woman. Another study has identified several novel triterpenoid glycosides, with pittangretoside A (**37**) as the most abundant (Bäcker *et al.*, 2013).

Parvifloranine A (**36**)

Pittangretoside A (**37**)

## 31.5  Recent developments: cancer and HIV

Cox started his search for a chemotherapeutic agent in the treatment of cancers in the Samoan archipelago. Cox observed the Samoan healers using the inner bark of *Homalanthus nutans* Guill. (Euphorbiaceae) for the treatment of yellow fever, suggesting possible anti-viral activity. Analysis of material from *H. nutans* demonstrated an abundance of a phorbol ester, prostratin (**38**). At first it was doubtful that prostratin could be used in humans because phorbol esters are generally tumour promoting. Informed by its existing traditional use in Samoa, Cox had prostratin examined for tumour-promoting activity, which tested negative. Subsequently prostratin was examined for *in vitro* anti-HIV activity in infected cells and tested positive. This has led to world-wide interest in both *H. nutans* and preservation of its endemic forest (Heinrich *et al.*, 2004).

An Australian native, *Castanospermum australe* A.Cunn. ex Mudie (Fabaceae), also produced an antiviral alkaloid castanospermine (**39**), which demonstrated significant inhibition of HIV (Duke, 1989). In traditional times Aboriginal Australians leached castanospermine out of the seed into a running stream before processing into food (Low, 1989) without which the seeds would be hepatotoxic.

In the search for anticancer products from the Australian endemic flora, a number of compounds have now been identified that are not yet available to the general public. Several novel spiroacetals named EBC-23 to EBC-25 and EBC-72 to EBC-76 have been isolated from *Cinnamomum laubatii* F.Muell (Lauraceae), most importantly EBC-23 (**40**), which was the least toxic to normal fibroblasts but among the most cytotoxic to melanoma, breast carcinoma and prostate cancer (Dong *et al.*, 2008, 2009). More recently another compound, a tiglien-3-one derivative called EBC-46 (**41**), has been discovered in abundance in *Hylandia dockrillii* Airy Shaw (Euphorbiaceae), also with significant anticancer activity. Surprisingly, for all the above-mentioned species there are no records of medicinal use by Aboriginal people, but a similar species, *Cinnamomum tamala* T.Nees and C.H.Eberm., was used as a carminative, stimulant, diuretic, diaphoretic, lactagogue and deobstruent in India (Lassak and McCarthy, 2011).

Prostratin (**38**)

Castanospermine (**39**)

EBC-23 (**40**)

EBC-46 (**41**)

## 31.6  Conclusion

With the wealth of potentially therapeutic natural products available from Australian or Oceanic flora, it is surprising that such a small number have found their way into the global or national market. Indeed the utilization of such products in the wider community could be seen as a way to preserve the cultural heritage of indigenous people, whilst also providing an improved range of healthcare products to the wider society.

With the dawning of the 21st century conventional medicine had reached a high degree of clinically proven safety and efficacy. With this came the expectation that 'natural' medicines be exhaustively validated in the same way. Although this task may seem daunting given the constant problem of inadequate funding, many ethnopharmacologists are now pursuing laboratory research followed by clinical trials in an attempt to bring the richness and diversity of traditional medicines into the international marketplace.

# References

Bäcker, C., Jenett-Siems, K., Siems, K., *et al.* (2013) Triterpene glycosides from the leaves of *Pittosporum angustifolium*. *Planta Medica*, **79**, 1461–1469.

Cambie, R. C. and Ash, J. (1994) *Fijian Medicinal Plants*, CSIRO, Auckland.

Carson, C.F., Hammer, K.A. and Riley, T.V. (2006) *Melaleuca alternifolia* (tea tree) oil: a review of antimicrobial and other medicinal properties. *Clinical Microbiology Reviews*, **19**, 50–62.

Chen, C.-C., Huang, Y.-L. and Ou, J.-C. (1993) Three new prenylflavones from *Artocarpus altilis*. *Journal of Natural Products*, **56**, 1594–1597.

Cox, P.A. (2008) Biodiversity and the search for new medicines, in *Biodiversity Change and Human Health. From ecosystem services to spread of disease* (eds O.E. Sala, L.A. Meyerson and C. Parmesan), Scope report No. 69., Island Press, Washington, DC.

Cox, P. A. and Balick, M. (1996) *Plants, People, and Culture: The science of ethnobotany*, New York Botanical Garden Press, New York.

Cox, P.A. and Banack, S.A. (2003) *Islands, Plants, and Polynesians: An introduction to Polynesian ethnobotany*, Dioscorides Press, Hong Kong.

Crago, J. (2011) *The Maroon Bush story: Nature's helping hand – Scaevola spinescens, history and use in Western Australia*, Aussie Outback Books, Bayswater.

Croft, K.D., Ghisalberti, E.L., Jefferies, P.R., *et al.* (1977) The chemistry of *Eremophila spp* – VI: Stereochemistry and crystal structure of dihydroxyserrulatic acid. *Tetrahedron*, **33**, 1475–1480.

Dong, L., Gordon, V.A., Grange, R.L., *et al.* (2008) Structure and absolute stereochemistry of the anticancer agent EBC-23 from the Australian rainforest. *Journal of The American Chemical Society*, **130**, 15262–15263.

Dong, L., Schill, H., Grange, R.L., *et al.* (2009) Anticancer agents from the Australain tropical rainforest: Spiroacetals EBC-23, 24, 25, 72, 73, 75 and 76. *Chemistry – A European Journal*, **15**, 11307–113018.

Duke, J.A. (1989) Castanospermum and anti-AIDS activity. *Journal of Ethnopharmacology*, **25**, 227–228.

Edwards, S.E. and Heinrich, M. (2006) Redressing cultural erosion and ecological decline in a far North Queensland Aboriginal community (Australia): the Aurukun ethnobiology database project. *Environmental Development and Sustainability*, **8**, 569–583.

Elkin, A.P. (1946) *Aboriginal Men of High Degree: Initiation and Sorcery in the Worlds Oldest Tradition*, Queensland University Press, St Lucia.

Foley, P. (2006) *Duboisia myoporoides*: the medical career of a native Australian plant. *Historical Records of Australian Science*, **17**, 31–69.

Gould, R. A. (1972) Progress to oblivion. *The Ecologist*, **2** (9), 17–22.

Heinrich, M., Barnes, J., Gibbons, S. and Williamson, E.M. (2004) *Fundamentals of Pharmacognosy and Phytotherapy, Churchill Livingstone (Elsevier)*, Budapest.

Isaacs, J. (1995) *Australian Dreaming: 40,000 years of Aboriginal History*, Lansdowne Press, Sydney.

Kerr, P.G., Longmore, R.B. and Betts, J.T. (1996) Myricadiol and other taraxerenes from Scaevola spinescens. *Planta Medica*, **62**, 519–522.

Lassak, E.V. and McCarthy, T. (2011) *Australian Medicinal Plants*, Methuen Australia Pty Ltd, North Rhyde.

Latz, P. (2004) *Bushfires and Bushtucker: Aboriginal plant use in central Australia*, IAD Press, Alice Springs.

Low, T. (1988) *Bush Medicine: A pharmacopoeia of natural remedies*, Greenhouse Publications Pty Ltd, Richmond.

Low, T. (1989) *Bush Tucker: Australia's wild food harvest*, Angus and Robertson Publishers, Sydney.

Mathews, J.M., Etheridge, A.S. and Black, S.P. (2002) Inhibition of human cytochrome P450 activities by kava extract and kavalactones. *Drug Metabolism and Disposition*, **30**, 1153–1157.

Ndi, C.P., Semple, S.J., Griesser, H.J., *et al.* (2007) Antimicrobial compounds from the Australian desert plant *Eremophila neglecta. Journal of Natural Products*, **70**, 1439–1443.

Packer, J., Brouwer, N., Harrington, D., *et al.* (2012) An ethnobotanical study of medicinal plants used by the Yaegl Aboriginal community in northern New South Wales, Australia. *Journal of Ethnopharmacology*, **139**, 244–255.

Pennacchio, M., Syah, Y. M., Ghisalberti, E. L. and Alexander, E. (1996) Cardioactive compounds from *Eremophila* species. *Journal of Ethnopharmacology*, **53**, 21–27.

Sadgrove, N. and Jones, G.L. (2013a) Chemical and biological characterisation of solvent extracts and essential oils from leaves and fruit of two Australian species of *Pittosporum* (Pittosporaceae) used in aboriginal medicinal practice. *Journal of Ethnopharmacology*, **145**, 813–821.

Sadgrove, N. and Jones, G.L. (2013b) A possible role of partially pyrolysed essential oils in Australian Aboriginal traditional ceremonial and medicinal smoking applications of *Eremophila longifolia* (R. Br.) F. Muell (*Scrophulariaceae*). *Journal of Ethnopharmacology*, **147**, 638–644.

Sadgrove, N. and Jones, G.L. (2014a) Cytogeography of essential oil chemotypes of *Eremophila longifolia* F. Muell (Schrophulariaceae). *Phytochemistry*, **105**, 43–51.

Sadgrove, N. and Jones, G.L. (2014b) Medicinal compounds, chemically and biologically characterised from extracts of Australian *Callitris endlicheri* and *C. glaucophylla* (Cupressaceae): used traditionally in Aboriginal and colonial pharmacopoeia. *Journal of Ethnopharmacology*, **153**, 872–883.

Sadgrove, N., Mijajlovic, S., Tucker, D.J., *et al.* (2011) Characterization and bioactivity of essential oils from novel chemotypes of *Eremophila longifolia* (F. Muell) (Myoporaceae): a highly valued traditional Australian medicine. *Flavour and Fragrance Journal*, **26**, 341–350.

Sadgrove, N., Hitchock, M., Watson, K. and Jones, G.L. (2013) Chemical and biological characterization of novel essential oils from *Eremophila bignoniiflora* (F. Muell) (Myoporaceae): a traditional Aboriginal Australian bush medicine. *Phytotherapy Research*, **27**, 1508–1516.

Sadgrove, N., Gonçalves-Martins, M. and Jones, G.L. (2014a) Chemogeography and antimicrobial activity of essential oils from *Geijera parviflora* and *Geijera salicifolia* (Rutaceae): Two traditional Australian medicinal plants. *Phytochemistry*, **104**, 60–71.

Sadgrove, N., Jones, G.L. and Greatrex, B.W. (2014b) Isolation and characterisation of (–)-genifuranal: The principal antimicrobial component in traditional smoking applications of *Eremophila longifolia* (Scrophulariaceae) by Australian Aboriginal peoples. *Journal of Ethnopharmacology*, **154**, 758–766.

Shou, Q., Banbury, L.K., Renshaw, D.E., *et al.* (2013) Parvifloranines A and B, two 11-carbon alkaloids from *Geijera parviflora. Journal of Natural Products*, **76**, 1384–1387.

Smith, J.E., Tucker, D., Watson, K. and Jones, G.L. (2007) Identification of antibacterial constituents from the indigenous Australian medicinal plant *Eremophila duttonii* F. Muell. (Myoporaceae). *Journal of Ethnopharmacology*, **112**, 386–393.

# 32
# Ethnopharmacology in Central and South America

Salvador Cañigueral[1] and Jaume Sanz-Biset[1]

*Unitat de Farmacologia i Farmacognòsia, Facultat de Farmàcia, Universitat de Barcelona, Catalonia, Spain*

## 32.1   Introduction

America was the last habitable continent settled by humans, since obviously this required crossing either the sea or large masses of ice. Although the timing and the routes used are uncertain, it is thought that the Americas had been initially colonized between about 35,000 and 14,000 years ago (Stanford and Bradley, 2012). Hunter-gatherers spread across the continent and appeared to reach the southernmost part, Patagonia, around 12,500 and 10,000 years ago (Borrero, 2001). The rise in sea level that took place during deglaciation between 11,000 and 7,000 years ago flooded the land bridges and melted ice sheets previously used to enter North America (Smith *et al.*, 2011). Apart from a very few exceptions, Native American societies seemed to have developed initially in complete isolation from those of the Old World. Advanced agricultural societies flourished, particularly in parts of Central and South America.

The arrival of Christopher Columbus in the West Indies in 1492 marked the end of the isolation between the societies of the Americas and other continents. By the late 15th century Central and South America harboured multiple indigenous groups with different levels of organization, many at a tribal level. It also had various chiefdoms and two well-recognized empires, the Incas and the Aztecs. Although these two complex societies were highly organized politically, in most cases they had not developed technology as advanced as their Eurasian peers. For example, the use of complex writing in the New World is considered to have been restricted to the hierarchies of some groups in Mesoamerica most notably Mayan groups (Diamond, 1997). This must have reduced the possibility of further exchanging ethnopharmacological knowledge between distant populations and generations. The writing

*Ethnopharmacology*, First Edition. Edited by Michael Heinrich and Anna K. Jäger.
© 2015 John Wiley & Sons, Ltd. Published 2015 by John Wiley & Sons, Ltd.

system known to have been developed by the Incas, the khipus (Urton and Brezine, 2005), is unlikely to have been able to transmit detailed information.

Thus, until very recently, the empirical knowledge accumulated by indigenous groups seemed to have been passed on nearly exclusively by oral traditions, even in empires such as the Aztec and the Inca. However, oral transmission in Native American groups must have been substantially truncated by the sudden and dramatic events that followed European colonization in the late 15th century. Within 100 years of the arrival of Columbus in 1492, a huge collapse in the demography of Native Americans occurred, which is thought to have been mainly caused by infectious diseases introduced by Europeans (Ramenofsky, 1993). Based on different reviews, Montenegro and Stephens (2006) have estimated that the indigenous population in Central and South America was diminished by more than 90% during that period. Despite the massive demographic fall, 10% of today's Central and South America's population is considered indigenous, but percentages differ substantially between countries (Table 32.1).

At present, most indigenous groups in this region are vulnerable due to their very poor socio-economic situation, a low and often fragmented demography, invading pressures, poor healthcare, insufficient organization and consequently a high rate of migration. Even in countries with the largest Native American populations, indigenous people tend to be the most marginalized groups (Lopez and Maloney, 2006).

Indigenous groups are particularly interesting as collaborators for ethnopharmacological research, as the use of medicinal plants is an essential component of indigenous medical practice. These groups inhabit highly diverse ecosystems, with a rich flora much differentiated from other continents.

For centuries, indigenous groups of Central and South America accumulated substantial knowledge on the bioactivity of a great number of plant species. It is not strange then, that shortly after the Europeans discovered the continent, some American plants began to be used as medicines worldwide.

**Table 32.1** Percentage of indigenous population by country in Central and South America (end 1990s to the beginning of 2000s).

| | |
|---|---|
| Bolivia | 71% |
| Guatemala | 66% |
| Peru | 47% |
| Ecuador | 43% |
| Belize | 19% |
| Honduras | 15% |
| Mexico | 14% |
| Chile | 8% |
| El Salvador | 7% |
| Suriname | 6% |
| Guyana | 6% |
| Panama | 6% |
| Nicaragua | 5% |

Only those countries with estimated percentages of 5% or higher are shown. Data from Montenegro and Stephens (2006).

In the following sections some of the most relevant medicinal and hallucinogenic plants of the region and their bioactive substances and derived medicinal products are described. Furthemore, the integration of indigenous and western medicinal knowledge is discussed.

## 32.2 The development of drugs

One of the most remarkable examples of drugs developed from South American plants is quinine, an active alkaloid found in *Cinchona* trees bark. In the early 17th century Jesuit missionaries in Peru became aware of the medicinal properties of this herbal drug, which was used by the Quechuas against shivering caused by chills (Guerra, 1977). The remedy was reported to have been used first in Europe to treat malaria in Rome in 1631, thereafter quickly becoming popular in most other European nations (Rocco, 2004). Until the 1940s quinine remained the drug of choice against malaria and it is still used today. Low-dose treatment with quinine is also used nowadays for restless leg syndrome. Moreover, hydroquinidine, a derivative of quinidine (a second alkaloid found in the same herbal drug and an optical isomer of quinine), is used for the treatment of cardiac arrhythmias. Furthermore, in the 1940s, the introduction of the skeletal muscle relaxant alkaloid (+)-tubocurarine adjunctively in anaesthesia represented an important clinical improvement. It was discovered in a type of curare, the arrow poison made from *Chondrodendron tomentosum* Ruiz & Pav. by Amazonian Indians (Nedergaard, 2003).

Other alkaloids that became medically relevant worldwide are pilocarpin, obtained from Brazilian species of *Pilocarpus*, and emetine from Central American and Brazilian species of the genus *Cephaelis* (ipecacuanha). Well-known compounds from Central and South American plants are still leading to new developments. The fruits of the capsaicinoid-rich varieties of *Capsicum annuum* L. (capsicum, chilli) are now used around the world to spice up food. Their extracts and capsaicin, the major compound of the group, are used as analgesic active ingredients of medicinal products for external use in the treatment of muscle pain, pain from osteoarthritis and rheumatoid arthritis, as well as neuralgias. The new derivative zucapsaicin ((Z)-capsaicin) was developed by Winston Pharmaceuticals and approved in Canada in July 2010 for the treatment of severe pain in adults with osteoarthritis of the knee (Butler *et al.*, 2014).

Many other plants, marketed as herbal medicinal products or dietary supplements, have gained widespread reputation for health care. South America has provided important caffeine-containing herbal drugs, such as mate (the leaf of *Ilex paraguariensis* A.St.-Hil.) and guarana seeds (*Paullinia cupana* Kunth H.B.K. var. *sorbilis* (Mart.) Ducke). Other herbal drugs traditionally used in the region are well established in phythotherapy, such as ratanhia root (*Krameria triandra* Ruiz & Pav.), passionflower (*Passiflora incarnata* L.) and boldo leaf (*Peumus boldus* L.). Others have been introduced more recently. This is the case for açai (*Euterpe oleracea* Mart.), the fruit of an Amazonian species used as antioxidant, and maca (*Lepidium meyenii* Walp.), native to the highlands of the Andes, whose rhizome is claimed to improve human fertility and enhance sexual drive (Wang *et al.*, 2007). Developed in Cuba, the aqueous extract of the bark of mango tree (*Mangifera indica* L.) (Vimang®) has shown immunomodulatory, antioxidant, analgesic and anti-inflammatory properties. Based on preclinical studies and clinical case reports in complex regional pain syndrome and zoster-associated pain, Garrido-Suárez *et al.* (2010) suggest that Vimag® could be useful for neuropathic pain, even though evidence from clinical trials is still pending. Cat's claw, the internal bark of *Uncaria tomentosa* (Willd. ex Schult.) DC., is mainly used as anti-inflammatory agent in arthritis (Quintela and Lock de Ugaz, 2000) and more recently has been proposed for the reduction of adverse effects of chemotherapy in breast cancer treatment (Santos Araujo *et al.*, 2012).

In addition, dragon's blood (the latex of *Croton lechleri* Muell. Arg.) and the essential oil of *Cordia verbenacea* DC. have given particularly interesting developments in the field of medicinal products. These are shown below.

## 32.2.1  The case of dragon's blood

*Sangre de drago* (dragon's blood), also known as *sangre de grado*, is the blood-red latex obtained from the bark of several species of *Croton* (Euphorbiaceae), mainly *C. lechleri* Muell. Arg. It is a medium-sized tree that occurs in the Amazonian regions of Peru, Ecuador, Colombia and Bolivia. The latex is widely used in traditional medicine in South America both internally (haemorrhages, stomach discomfort, ulcers, diarrhoeas, cough, flu, colds, respiratory ailments or rheumatic disorders) and externally (for healing and cicatrizing wounds, cuts and other skin injuries, and against herpes, bleeding gums or mouth ulcers) (Ubillas *et al.*, 1994; Risco *et al.*, 2005).

Several compounds have been isolated from *sangre de drago* (Risco *et al.*, 2005). The major constituents are monomeric flavan-3-ols (catechin, epicatechin, gallocatechin, epigallocatechin) and oligomeric proanthocyanidins of varying molecular size. It also contains the alkaloid taspine, 3'-4-O-dimethylcedrusin (dihydrobenzofuran lignan), and several diterpenes.

The beneficial effect of *sangre de drago* on wound healing was confirmed by Pieters *et al.* (1995) in rats. This activity was attributed to the lignan 3',4-O-dimethylcedrusin and to proanthocyanidins. The former seemed to stimulate the formation of fibroblasts and collagen, whereas the proanthocyanidins may contract the skin around the injury and contribute to the formation of a crust covering the wound by precipitating proteins. In addition, *sangre de drago* showed, *in vitro*, potent inhibitor effects on cutaneous neurogenic inflammation through the direct inhibition of substance P release by sensory afferent nerves (Pereira *et al.*, 2010).

Orally, in a dilute form, the latex was able to facilitate the healing of gastric ulcers by reducing their size and decreasing the bacterial content in experimental animals (Miller *et al.*, 2000).

The latex from *C. lechleri* also showed immunomodulatory activity *in vitro* through a potent inhibitory activity on classical and alternate pathways of the complement system, the inhibition of the proliferation of activated T-cells and free radical scavenging capacity. Depending on the concentration, it showed antioxidant or prooxidant properties, and the stimulation or inhibition of phagocytosis (Risco *et al.*, 2003). Moreover, the latex has shown anti-inflammatory, antibacterial and antiviral activities (Ubillas *et al.*, 1994; Jones, 2003; Risco *et al.*, 2003, 2005).

Among the proanthocyanidin preparations of *sangre de drago*, crofelemer has gained special relevance since, in December 2012, it obtained the US FDA approval as an anti-diarrheal indicated for the symptomatic relief of non-infectious diarrhea in adult patients with HIV/AIDS on anti-retroviral therapy (ART) (Salix Pharmaceuticals, 2014). Its development was started in the 1990s by the company Shaman Pharmaceuticals Inc. and continued by Napo Pharmaceuticals Inc. Crofelemer is marketed by Salix Pharmaceuticals Inc. as delayed-release tablets of 125 mg, under the brand name of Fulyzaq®.

Crofelemer (Figure 32.1), formerly known as SP-303, is an oligomeric proanthocyanidin mixture obtained from the latex of *C. lechleri* harvested from the wild and with an average

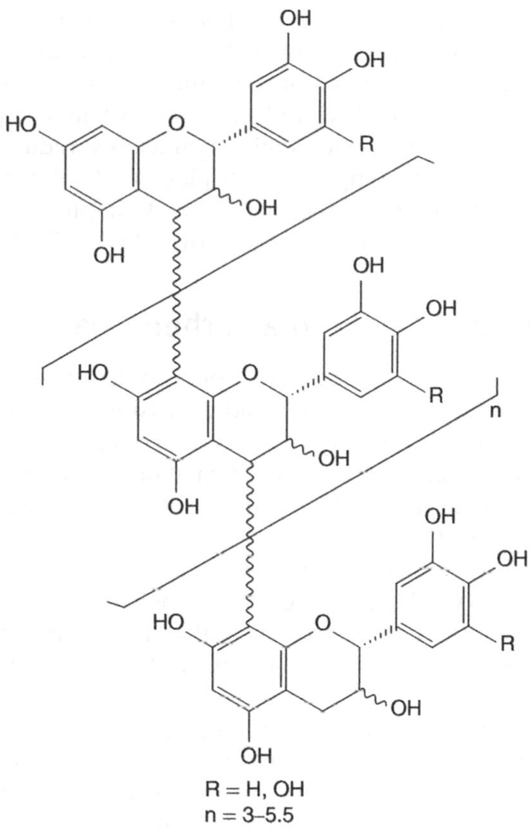

**Figure 32.1** Proposed structure of crofelemer, proanthocyanidin oligomer from the latex of *Croton lechleri*.

molecular weight of 2100 Da. It is composed of (+)-catechin, (–)-epicatechin, (+)-gallocatechin and (–)-epigallocatechin units, and has an average degree of polymerization ranging from 5 to 7.5.

In the 1990s the antiviral activity of SP-303 was confirmed against both HSV-1 and HSV-2, as well as its ability to inhibit aciclovir-resistant HSV. Mechanistic studies showed that SP-303 blocks viral infection of cells (Ubillas *et al.*, 1994).

In a multicentre, double-blind, placebo-controlled phase II study a topical preparation of SP-303 was evaluated against recurrent genital herpes lesions in patients with AIDS (Orozco-Topete *et al.*, 1997). It showed superiority compared to placebo: 41% of patients treated with SP-303 experienced complete healing of their lesions compared to 14% in the placebo group.

Crofelemer has also shown antidiarrheal activity, acting locally in the gastrointestinal tract. It inhibits cholera toxin-induced fluid secretion in mice, and decreases stool weight, abnormal stool frequency and chloride secretion in patients with HIV/AIDS and chronic diarrhoea. The mechanism of action is related to the inhibition of two distinct pro-secretory chloride channels in the luminal membrane of enterocytes (CFTR and CaCC) (Tradtrantip *et al.*, 2010; Frampton, 2013). Several clinical trials showed the beneficial effect of crofelemer in different types of secretory diarrhoea, such as AIDS-associated diarrhoea, traveller's diarrhoea, infectious diarrhoea including cholera, and diarrhoea-prominent irritable bowel syndrome (Crutchley *et al.*, 2010). The FDA approval of crofelemer was mainly based on the results of the ADVENT study, a large ($n = 376$ randomized patients), multicentre, phase III trial, with a 4-week assessment period controlled with placebo and a 5-month placebo-free extension phase. Results showed that 125 mg twice daily significantly reduced secretory diarrhoea in HIV-positive patients on ART compared with placebo. Crofelemer was generally well tolerated, both in the short term and in the long term (Frampton, 2013). Crofelemer is the second plant-derived complex active ingredient approved by the FDA.

## 32.2.2    *The essential oil of* Cordia verbenacea

*Cordia verbenacea* DC (Boraginaceae) is a native plant of the coastal of Brazil. It is used in traditional medicine to treat arthritis, wounds and contusions. Based on its leaves' essential oil, the Brazilian pharmaceutical company Aché, in collaboration with several Brazilian universities, developed a herbal medicinal product (Acheflan®, containing 0.5% of essential oil of *C. verbenacea*) applied topically for the treatment of chronic tendonitis, myofascial pain, muscular traumas and injuries. The essential oil is mainly composed of terpene hydrocarbons, both of monoterpene and sesquiterpene types, and each of these two groups may represent more than 40% of the oil. Oxygen-containing monoterpenes and sesquiterpenes usually represent less than 4% each. The major constituents of the oil are α-pinene, β-caryophyllene and α-santalene, but it also contains significant amounts of *allo*-aromadendrene and α-humulene (Vila *et al.*, 2009).

The oil has shown anti-inflammatory and anti-allergic activities in animals. Administered orally, it reduced carrageenan-induced rat paw oedema, myeloperoxidase activity and the mouse oedema provoked by carrageenan, bradykinin, substance P, histamine and platelet-activating factor. It also showed anti-inflammatory activity in carrageenan-induced pleurisy in rat and the carrageenan-induced air pouch in mouse. The oil also inhibited the oedema caused by *Apis mellifera* venom or ovalbumin in sensitized rats and ovalbumin-induced allergic pleurisy (Passos *et al.*, 2007).

The sesquiterpenes α-humulene and *trans*-caryophyllene (Figure 32.2) were identified as the key bioactive constituents of the oil. Oral treatment with both compounds produced marked inhibitory effects in several experimental models of inflammation in mice and rats. Both compounds reduced the production of tumor necrosis factor-α (TNFα) and prostaglandin E2 (PGE2), as well as the expression of inducible nitric oxide synthase (iNOS) and cyclooxygenase (COX-2) expression. In addition, α-humulene inhibited the production of interleukin-1β

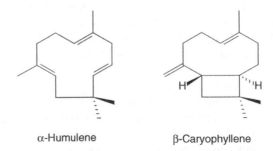

α-Humulene                β-Caryophyllene

**Figure 32.2**  α-Humulene and β-caryophyllene are the constituents considered responsible for the anti-inflammatory activity of the essential oil of *Cordia verbenacea* DC.

(IL-1β). Furthermore, α-humulene and *trans*-caryophyllene prevented lipopolysaccharide (LPS)-induced inflammation through NF-kB inhibition. (Fernandes *et al.*, 2007; Medeiros *et al.*, 2007).

The cream containing 0.5% of the essential oil of *C. verbenacea* was assessed clinically in phases I to III. In a phase III, double-blind, randomized, comparative study against a topical preparation with 1% of diethylammonium diclofenac, efficacy and tolerability were evaluated in patients within the first 24 hours of suffering from bruises, sprains, muscular traumas and injuries. In both groups, patients were administered the corresponding drug three times a day during 10 days. More than 90% of the patients treated with the oil of *C. verbenacea* showed a good or very good improvement, slightly higher than in the positive control group treated with diethylammonium diclofenac. In addition, the tolerability was found to be very good and similar to the control group (Brandao *et al.*, 2006). In another clinical trial, with an analogous design, the efficacy of the oil of *C. verbenacea* was demonstrated in patients suffering from chronic tendonitis and myofascial pain (Refsio *et al.*, 2005).

After marketing authorization by the Brazilian medicines agency (ANVISA), Acheflan® was launched in 2005. It has been the first innovative medicine introduced to the market by a Brazilian company. It received considerable acceptance by patients and medical doctors, reaching by 2007 a market share of more than 40% for topical non-steroidal anti-inflammatories in Brazil (Zwahlen, 2012).

## 32.2.3 The example of developing ethnopharmacological-based herbal medicinal products in Guatemala

In the mid-1970s the Mesoamerican Centre of Appropriate Technology Studies (CEMAT) carried out a number of ethnobotanical surveys in several regions of Guatemala. About 700 medicinal plants were recorded, 250 of which were used against infections (Cáceres *et al.*, 1987; Giron *et al.*, 1991; Cáceres and Girón, 2002). Given that infectious diseases are among the main health problems in the country, research was focused on developing products for treating these ailments. By the mid-1980s the company Laboratorio Farmaya had been established. Nine herbal drugs were selected in order to validate their traditional medicinal uses and to produce herbal medicinal products out of them. These were the bark of *Byrsonima crassifolia* HBK, the flowerheads of *Pseudognaphalium stramineum* (Kunth) Anderb., the flower of *Jacaranda mimosifolia* D.Don, the leaf of *Plantago major* L., the leaf of *Psidium guajava* L., the leaf of *Simarouba glauca* DC, the leaf of *Solanum americanum* Miller, the leaf and flower of *Tagetes lucida* Cav., and the rhizome of *Smilax domingensis* Willd. Pharmacological, phytochemical, agronomical and microbiological research was carried out. *In vitro, in vivo* and clinical research tested antibacterial, antifungal, antiparasitic and anti-inflammatory activities. From those plants showing higher antimicrobial activity and lower toxicity profiles three herbal formulations were developed and registered in Guatemala as herbal medicinal products: a hydroalcoholic liquid preparation (Antibactol®), an elixir (Jacameb®) and a gel (Mayaderm®).

Besides the development of medicinal products through Laboratorio Farmaya, the project initiated by CEMAT also had other objectives (Cáceres and Girón, 2002). Through the compilation of medicinal plant knowledge, the use of plants in traditional medicine was actively promoted across Guatemala. Groups of farmers in different regions of the country were trained in the cultivation, post-harvest handling and processing of medicinal plants, with emphasis on quality, a key factor for the use of the plants in manufacturing herbal preparations.

## 32.2.4  The Farmacias Vivas programme

Similar to the Guatemalan project, in Brazil the so-called Farmacias Vivas aimed to produce herbal products with guaranteed quality, safety and efficacy from validated medicinal plants, in order to offer a therapeutic option for local users as well as to educate the general population on the rational use of medicinal plants (Matos, 2002).

Farmacias Vivas was initiated in 1991 by Professor Francisco José de Abreu Matos from the Federal University of Ceará, in collaboration with agronomists, pharmacists, medical doctors and other health practitioners. This allowed the monitoring of all stages, from cultivation and manufacturing to prescription and administration in primary care. Farmacias Vivas is a non-profit project, organized at three levels of activities: the cultivation of medicinal plants, the production/dispensation of dried herbal drugs and the manufacture of standardized herbal products in agreement with GMP for the preparation of herbal medicines (Matos, 2002).

The Farmacias Vivas project was created partly as a way to return to local communities the scientific knowledge on medicinal plants gained by scientists such as Professor Matos. Educational activities to foster a better use of herbal medicinal products are provided (see Chapter 10), as well as cost-effective herbal products of good quality. Many similar socially oriented initiatives exist in Central and South America, where ethnopharmacological research encompasses activities other than the development of new drugs.

## 32.3  Beyond the development of new drugs

Although many medicines have been developed from indigenous knowledge, arguably most of these advances have had little if any impact on the health care of indigenous people. Although current international laws call for the protection and promotion of indigenous medical knowledge, health regulations often shift traditional medicine practices out of legal frameworks, making it sometimes illegal. However, it is well known that traditional medicine plays a major role, particularly in the primary health care of populations in developing countries (Robinson and Zhang, 2011). Therefore, by investigating the remedies used in traditional medicine ethnopharmacological research should also aim to improve the health of those communities being studied. This requires the integration of indigenous and western medicine through mutual respect and equal recognition. At present, in various parts of Central and South America it is possible to find different intercultural health programmes that support the local use of traditional medicines, which may be included satisfactorily into local health systems. However, this is still very marginal compared with countries in other regions of the world where, for instance, traditional medicinal systems are well established (e.g. China) or actively promoted by governments (e.g. South Africa).

For example, in Chile various intercultural health projects focusing on Mapuche indigenous medical knowledge have been carried out for some decades now. Today, some Chilean medical schools include courses on Mapuche health. One of the first intercultural health programmes in Chile was the Makewe Hospital, a clinic funded by the state and administered by a Mapuche association. The same indigenous association operates a pharmacy that offers both Mapuche herbal medicines and western drugs under the supervision of a pharmacist who is knowledgeable about indigenous medicine (Torri, 2012).

Since 1982 in the Caribbean the Traditional Medicine in the Islands (TRAMIL) scheme has identified, endorsed and disseminated information on the medicinal plants that are used in traditional medicine (Boulogne et al., 2011). From ethnopharmacological field surveys to laboratory studies, the TRAMIL programme releases a series of recommendations concerning the use of medicinal plants in public health, providing information on bioactivity and toxicity. Although there are concerns about issuing clinical practice advice based on preclinical study data of medicinal plants, the TRAMIL project provides initial scientific validations of some of the traditional medicinal plant uses of the region. This information is published and diffused to populations where the original knowledge came from through a number of educational programmes.

In some villages in southern Suriname regular workshops on medicinal plants are also held involving indigenous, national (western) health workers and scientists. Few of these villages have a clinic that provides traditional medicine, where indigenous healers can see patients and young apprentices learn from elder healers. Apprentices and scientists record the treatments given to patients, and voucher specimens are collected for the medicinal plants used in the clinics (Herndon, 2009).

The Brazilian Articulação Pacari network produces traditional medicines based on plants from the Cerrado. Accounting for about 20% of the country's area, the Cerrado is the largest savannah in South America. Articulação Pacari is organized by several communities that arrange the exchange of ethnopharmacological knowledge between collectors of medicinal plants, technicians, scientists and more than 260 traditional healers. Traditional knowledge on the use of medicinal plants is registered and published in a number of texts. Furthermore, about 40 different herbal preparations using 65 different plant species are sold through more than 30 small community-based pharmacies (Lal and Sorte-Junior, 2011). Educational courses for local practitioners are also organized, which draw on the knowledge of traditional healers as well as technicians. As a result, the quality of the preparation of traditional medicines is promoted and basic hygiene guidelines for traditional practitioners are given, such as the appropriate storage of herbal medicines in order to avoid contamination.

## 32.4   Bridging indigenous and western knowledge

It is crucial that research is based on a precise and culturally informed understanding of traditional uses and of the plants's roles within indigenous groups. This is a challenging issue for ethnopharmacological research in Central and South America. The many indigenous groups found in the region result in the existence of differentiated traditional medicinal systems, where medicinal plants are used in diverse therapeutic contexts.

For example, our investigations among the San Martín Quechuas of the Peruvian Amazon found that often medicinal plants were taken together with dietary norms, mostly restricting the consumption of some types of food, thus reducing the calorie intake and decreasing certain physical activities (Sanz-Biset et al., 2009). Also, it was found that an important number of medicinal plants were used for their emetic effects. According to local concepts a therapeutic 'depurative effect' might be induced by calorie restriction and emesis. This is thought to enhance health broadly speaking through a 'general cleansing effect'.

In the context of their traditional medicine, the San Martin Quechuas reported using medicinal plants in depurative practices against different ailments. Particularly when used against inflammatory diseases and infections, we found some correlation concerning the available bibliographic data on plant bioactivity and/or active compounds (Sanz-Biset and Cañigueral, 2011). For many other depurative practices observed in Chazuta, a high number of unspecific medicinal uses were recorded. For example, depurative practices were used as tonics, to augment work performance, to enhance physical endurance, to increase weight carrying, to extend cold resistance, to sharpen the senses, to lessen sluggishness or to improve sexual function. The fact that the induction of emesis was a common factor for the plants used led us to consider the emetic effect with a key medicinal role within the depurative practices observed in Chazuta. In addition, we suggested that in these cases the medicinal uses cannot be only explained by the bioactivity of plants alone, as the calorie restriction is likely to have an impact (Sanz-Biset and Cañigueral, 2013).

In indigenous medical systems it is often not straightforward to associate a medicinal effect that informants describe for a herbal preparation with an active compound found in the corresponding plant, or with a bioactivity entirely originating from the consequent herbal preparation. Frequently in traditional medicine, plants are used together with other elements relevant from a pharmacological and/or physiologic point of view. In the case presented about the San Martin Quechuas, just a simple emetic activity is not likely to cause the broad array of effects that informants describe, but instead it may trigger them in conjunction with the prescription of dietary restrictions and other norms.

## 32.5  Hallucinogens

Arguably, the 1960s fascination with psychoactive drugs, many of these of Central and South American origin, gave rise to what now is known as ethnopharmacology. Obviously, the medicinal uses of plants have been described for centuries with the aim of developing new or existing drugs. However, it is true that the term ethnopharmacology was coined in the context of hallucinogenic plants (Heinrich, 2014). At the time, this neologism provided a clear notion for an academic field concerned with the bioactivity of indigenous medicinal and toxic plants. Unsurprisingly, some of the most prolific ethnopharmacologists of the end of the last century were involved with the study of hallucinogens, and particularly with the hallucinogens of Central and South America, such as some of the extensive work by Richard Evans Schultes and collaborators.

Schultes and Hofmann (1992) estimated that nearly 130 species are known to be used as hallucinogens in the New World, whereas there are only 50 in the Old World. The number and significance of hallucinogenic plants in Central and South America is particularly overwhelming. Mesoamerica has by far the richest diversity, with the peyote cactus (*Lophophora williamsii* (Lem. ex Salm-Dyck) J.M. Coult.) one of the most important religious hallucinogens. Also of sacred importance are the different fungi species, known by the Aztecs as teonanácatl (*Psilocybe* spp.), the seeds of ololiuqui (*Turbina corymbosa* (L.) Raf.) and the leaves of *Salvia divinorum* Epling and Játiva. South America also harbours a diverse and large number of hallucinogenic plants, most notably the San Pedro cactus (*Trichocereus pachanoi* Britton and Rose), the Yopo snuff made from seeds of *Anadenanthera peregrina* (L.) Speg. or the famous ayahuasca (*Banisteriopsis caapi* (Spruce ex Griseb.) C.V. Morton), common to the lowlands of north-western Amazonia.

During the 1950s and 1960s, hundreds of studies on hallucinogens were published, indicating that some of these drugs are useful in treating substance misuse and relieving different types of psychological distress. However, illicit use of hallucinogens resulted in outlawing such drugs and a drop in research activity. It was not for some decades afterwards that attitudes blocking research on hallucinogens subsided and allowed new investigations. A new surge of more carefully carried out research on hallucinogens has begun to address whether these substances may have a therapeutic role in modern medicine. Results from new investigations seem to confirm the effectiveness of hallucinogens to treat the addictive habits and anxiety in patients with advance-stage cancer (Grob *et al.*, 2011). Some research also points out that in some patients significant spiritual experiences occur under the effects of these substances, which may have the capacity to trigger important life changes (Griffiths *et al.*, 2006). This is receiving special attention from some academics as with orthodox psychological therapy these changes may be achieved after many years. Not surprisingly, medicinal effects of this kind are closer to the common sacred-type use that indigenous populations seem to have made of hallucinogens.

Today, however, hallucinogens remain a highly controversial subject of scientific study, and confront Central and South American nations with a diverse range of legal and public health issues.

## 32.6  Conclusion

A rich bio- and ethno-diversity makes Central and South America attractive for ethnopharmacological research. As a result, the region has provided important therapeutic agents in recent years. Nevertheless, the number of innovative drugs reaching the market is small in comparison with the large number of publications of ethnopharmacological field surveys or plant bioactivity screenings. An effort should be made to enhance pre-clinical and particularly clinical research.

Ethnopharmacological research should not, however, be limited to the development of medicines but should include the improvement of the health care of those indigenous groups from where the original use of medicinal plants comes. The region shows some interesting experiences in that regard.

Whether aiming at the development of new drugs or improving the health care of indigenous people, it is crucial that ethnopharmacologically driven research is based on a precise and culturally informed understanding of traditional uses of medicinal plants. Because of the many indigenous groups found in Central and South America, this can be a challenging issue.

## References

Borrero, L.A. (2001) *El poblamiento de la Patagonia. Toldos, milodones y volcanes.* Emecé Editores, Buenos Aires.

Boulogne, I., Germosén-Robineau, L., Ozier-Lafontaine, H., *et al.* (2011) TRAMIL ethnopharmalogical survey in Les Saintes (Guadeloupe, French West Indies): A comparative study. *Journal of Ethnopharmacology,* **133** (3), 1039–1050.

Brandão, D.C., Brandão, G.D.C. and Miranda, J.B. (2006) Estudo fase III, duplo-cego, aleatório, comparativo para avaliar a eficácia e tolerabilidade da *Cordia verbenacea* e do diclofenaco dietilamônio em pacientes portadores de contusões, entorses, traumas e lesões musculares, com início inferior a 24 horas. *Revista Brasileira de Medicina,* **63** (8), 408–415.

Butler, M.S., Robertson A.A.B. and Cooper, M.A. (2014) Natural product and natural product derived drugs in clinical trials. *Natural Products Reports,* **31**, 1612–1661.

Cáceres, A. and Girón, L.M. (2002) Desarrollo de medicamentos fitoterápicos a partir de plantas medicinales en Guatemala. *Revista de Fitoterapia,* **2**, 41–46.

Cáceres, A., Girón, L.M., Alvarado, S.R. and Torres, M.F. (1987) Screening of antimicrobial activity of plants popularly used in Guatemala for the treatment of dermatomucosal diseases. *Journal of Ethnopharmacology,* **20** (3), 223–237.

Crutchley, R.D., Miller, J. and Garey, K.W. (2010) Crofelemer, a novel agent for treatment of secretory diarrhea. *Annals of Pharmacotherapy,* **44** (5), 878–884.

Diamond, J. (1997) *Guns, germs and steel: the fates of human societies,* W.W. Norton and Company, New York.

Fernandes, E.S., Passos, G.F., Medeiros, R., *et al.* (2007) Anti-inflammatory effects of compounds alpha-humulene and (−)-*trans*-caryophyllene isolated from the essential oil of *Cordia verbenacea*. *European Journal of Pharmacology,* **569** (3), 228–236.

Frampton, J.E. (2013) Crofelemer: A review of its use in the management of non-infectious diarrhoea in adult patients with HIV/AIDS on antiretroviral therapy. *Drugs*, **73** (10), 1121–1129.

Garrido-Suárez, B.B., Garrido, G., Delgado, R., *et al.* (2010) A *Mangifera indica* L. extract could be used to treat neuropathic pain and implication of mangiferin. *Molecules*, **15** (12), 9035–9045.

Girón, L.M., Freire, V., Alonzo, A. and Cáceres, A. (1991) Ethnobotanical survey of the medicinal flora used by the Caribs of Guatemala. *Journal of Ethnopharmacology*, **34** (2), 173–187.

Griffiths, R.R., Richards, W.A., McCann, U. and Jesse, R. (2006) Psylocibin can occasion mystical-type experiences having substantial and sustained personal meaning and spiritual significance. *Psychopharmacology*, **187** (3), 268–283.

Grob, C.S., Danforth, A.L., Chopra, G.S., *et al.* (2011) Pilot study of psilocybin treatment for anxiety in patients with advanced-stage cancer. *Archives of General Psychiatry*, **68**(1): 71-78.

Guerra, F. (1977). The introduction of Cinchona in the treatment of malaria. *Journal of Tropical Medicine and Hygiene*, **80** (6), 112–118.

Heinrich, M. (2014) Ethnopharmacology: quo vadis? Challenges for the future. *Revista Brasileira de Farmacognosia*, **24** (2), 99–102.

Herndon, C. N., Uiterloo, M., Uremaru, A., *et al.* (2009) Disease concepts and treatment by tribal healers of an Amazonian forest culture. *Journal of Ethnobiology and Ethnomedicine*, **5**, 27.

Jones, K. (2003) Review of Sangre de Drago (*Croton lechleri*) – a South American tree sap in the treatment of diarrhea, inflammation, insect bites, viral infections, and wounds: traditional uses to clinical research. *Journal of Alternative and Complementary Medicine*, **9** (6), 877–896.

Lal, R. and Sorte-Junior, W.F. (2011) Where biodiversity, traditional knowledge, health and livelihoods meet: Institutional pillars for the productive inclusion of local communities (Brazil case study), *Working Paper*, International Policy Centre for Inclusive Growth, Brasilia, p. 81.

Lopez, H. and Maloney, W. (2006) *Poverty reduction and growth – virtuous and vicious circles*, The World Bank, Washington.

Matos, F.J.A. (2002) *Farmácias vivas: sistema de utilização de plantas medicinais projetado para pequenas comunidades*, 4th edn, Editora UFC, Fortaleza.

Medeiros, R., Passos, G.F., Vitor, C.E., *et al.* (2007) Effect of two active compounds obtained from the essential oil of *Cordia verbenacea* on the acute inflammatory responses elicited by LPS in the rat paw. *British Journal of Pharmacology*, **151** (5), 618–627.

Miller, M.J., MacNaughton, W.K., Zhang, X.J., *et al.* (2000) Treatment of gastric ulcers and diarrhea with the Amazonian herbal medicine *sangre de grado*. *American Journal of Physiology – Gastrointestinal and Liver Physiology*, **279** (1), G192–G200.

Montenegro, R.A. and Stephens, C. (2006) Indigenous health in Latin America and the Caribbean. *The Lancet*, **367** (9525), 1859–1869.

Nedergaard, O.A. (2003) Curare: The flying death. *Pharmacology and Toxicology*, **92** (4), 154–155.

Orozco-Topete, R., Sierra-Madero, J., Cano-Dominguez, C., *et al.* (1997) Safety and efficacy of Virend® for topical treatment of genital and anal herpes simplex lesions in patients with AIDS. *Antiviral Research*, **35** (2), 91–103.

Passos, G.F., Fernandes, E.S., da Cunha, F.M., *et al.* (2007) Anti-inflammatory and anti-allergic properties of the essential oil and active compounds from *Cordia verbenacea*. *Journal of Ethnopharmacology*, **110** (2), 323–333.

Pereira, U., Garcia-Le Gal, C., Le Gal, G., *et al.* (2010) Effects of *sangre de drago* in an *in vitro* model of cutaneous neurogenic inflammation. *Experimental Dermatology*, **19** (9), 796–799.

Pieters, L., De Bruyne, T., van Poel, B., *et al.* (1995) *In vivo* wound healing activity of Dragon's Blood (Croton spp.), a traditional South American drug, and its constituents. *Phytomedicine*, **2** (1), 17–22.

Quintela, J.C. and Lock de Ugaz, O. (2003) Uña de gato, *Uncaria tomentosa* (Wild.) DC. *Revista de Fitoterapia*, **3** (1), 5–16.

Ramenofsky, A. (1993) *The Cambridge World History of Human Disease*, Cambridge University Press, Cambridge.

Refsio, C., Brandão, D.C., Brandão, G.C., *et al.* (2005) Avaliação clínica da eficácia e segurança do uso de extrato padronizado da *Cordia verbenacea* em pacientes portadores de tendinite e dor miofascial. *Revista Brasileira de Medicina*, **62** (1/2), 40–46.

Risco, E., Ghia, F., Vila, R., *et al.* (2003) Immunomodulatory activity and chemical characterisation of *Sangre de Drago* (Dragon's Blood) from *Croton lechleri*. *Planta Medica,* **69** (9), 785–794.

Risco, E., Vila, R., Henriques, A. and Cañigueral, S. (2005) Bases químicas y farmacológicas de la utilización de la *sangre de drago. Revista de Fitoterapia,* **5** (2), 101–114.

Robinson, M.M. and Zhang, X. (2011) *The world medicines situation 2011, traditional medicines: Global situation, issues and challenges,* World Health Organization, Geneva.

Rocco, F. (2004) *Quinine: malaria and the quest for a cure that changed the world,* Harper Collins Pub. Ltd, New York.

Salix Pharmaceuticals Inc. (2013) *Fulyzak® patient information leaflet,* retrieved from http://cdn.salix .com/shared/pi/fulyzaq-pi.pdf, accessed 10 October 2014.

Santos Araújo, M.C., Farias, I.L., Gutierres, J., *et al.* (2012) *Uncaria tomentosa* -adjuvant treatment for breast cancer: clinical trial. *Evidence-Based Complementary and Alternative Medicine,* article ID676984.

Sanz-Biset, J. and Cañigueral, S. (2011) Plant use in the medicinal practices known as 'strict diets' in Chazuta valley (PeruvianAmazon). *Journal of Ethnopharmacology,* **137**, 271–288.

Sanz-Biset, J. and Cañigueral, S. (2013) Plants as medicinal stressors, the case of depurative practices in Chazuta valley (Peruvian Amazonia). *Journal of Ethnopharmacology,* **145**, 67–76.

Sanz-Biset, J., Campos de la Cruz, J., Epiquién Rivera, M.A. and Cañigueral, S. (2009) A first survey on the medicinal plants of the Chazuta valley (Peruvian Amazon). *Journal of Ethnopharmacology,* **122**, 333–362.

Schultes, R.E. and Hofmann, A. (1992) *Plants of the Gods: their sacred, healing, and hallucinogenic powers,* Healing Arts Press, Rochester.

Smith D.E., Harrison, S., Firth, C.R. and Jordan, J.T. (2011) The early Holocene sea level rise. *Quaternary Science Reviews,* **30** (15–16), 1846–1860.

Stanford, D.J. and Bradley, B.A. (2012) *Across Atlantic ice: the origin of America's Clovis culture,* University of California Press, Berkeley and Los Angeles.

Torri, M.C. (2012) Intercultural Health Practices: Towards an Equal Recognition Between Indigenous Medicine and Biomedicine? A Case Study from Chile. *Health Care Analysis,* **20**, 31–49.

Tradtrantip, L., Namkung, W. and Verkman, A.S. (2010) Crofelemer, an antisecretory antidiarrheal proanthocyanidin oligomer extracted from *Croton lechleri,* targets two distinct intestinal chloride channels. *Molecular Pharmacology,* **77** (1), 69–78.

Ubillas, R., Jolad, S.D., Bruening, R.C., *et al.* (1994) SP-303, an antiviral oligomeric proanthocyanidin from the latex of *Croton lechleri* (sangre de drago). *Phytomedicine,* **1**, 77–106.

Urton, G. and Brezine, C.J. (2005) Khipu accounting in ancient Peru. *Science,* **309** (5737), 1065–1067.

Vila, R., Queiroz, E.F. and Cañigueral, S. (2009) Composition of the essential oil of the leaves of *Cordia verbenacea. Planta Medica,* **75**, PG17.

Wang, Y., Wang, Y., McNeil, B. and Harvey, L.M. (2007) Maca: An Andean crop with multi-pharmacological functions. *Food Research International,* **40** (7), 783–792.

Zwahlen, R. (2012) *Brazilian innovation: a patent success,* BioTechNow, retrieved from http://www .biotech-now.org/public-policy/patently-biotech/2012/01/brazilian-innovation-a-patent-success#, accessed 10 October 2014.

# 33
# Perspectives on Ethnopharmacology in Mexico

Robert Bye and Edelmira Linares

*Jardín Botánico del Instituto de Biología, Universidad Nacional Autónoma de México, 04510 México DF, Mexico*

## 33.1 Introduction

Ethnopharmacology is the scientific discipline concerned with the field observation, description, documentation and experimental investigation of indigenous vegetal medicines and their biological activities. Even though the term is relatively recent, these pursuits have been part of Mexico's history for almost five centuries. The conceptual basis and methodology have evolved rapidly such that minimum standards are drawn from the fields of biology, anthropology and ethnomedicine, as well as information quantification and analysis (Heinrich *et al.*, 2009). Standardization of data fields and characteristics has led to advances in comparative ethnobotanical studies (Cook, 1995). In Mexico, however, there has been reluctance to fully apply these normalized parameters because of the weakness of culturally bound concepts and nomenclature. With the proposal of new categories for the Economic Botany Data Collection Standard (Gruca *et al.*, 2014), it is anticipated that Mexican ethnopharmacological data will be incorporated into the global comparative data set.

The key linkage between western and indigenous knowledge in ethnopharmacological studies is the identification of the plants of interest in both the western scientific domain and the indigenous culture. Voucher specimens must meet the criteria of ethnopharmacological study as well as the contemporary practices of occidental scientific herbaria, including updated, precise taxonomic identification (Bye, 1986; Rivera *et al.*, 2014). Herbarium specimens that meet taxonomic standards may not reflect the phenological state in which the plant is employed for medicinal purposes. Hence the voucher requires dual components: (i) a voucher specimen representing the analysed sample with the appropriate plant part and in the state in which it is employed, and (ii) a corroborative specimen related to the plant which gave rise to the analysed sample and which includes the taxonomically diagnostic characters necessary to confirm

*Ethnopharmacology*, First Edition. Edited by Michael Heinrich and Anna K. Jäger.

the botanical identification according to western science nomenclature. These vouchers may form part of a conventional herbarium or be integrated into biocultural collections (Salick *et al.*, 2014). The voucher specimens are unique opportunities to ensure the identity authentication of plant materials obtained in field studies as well as analysed in laboratories (Rivera *et al.*, 2014).

Over 3000 botanical species have been documented as medicinal plants in Mexico (Argueta *et al.*, 1994; Bye *et al.*, 1995), which ranks as the fifth largest mega-diverse country of the world with 23,424 vascular plant species (CONABIO, 2014). The principal plant families (in descending order of numerical importance) are Astertaceae, Fabaceae, Euphorbiaceae, Lamiaceae and Solanaceae. Since the Mexican revolution, institutional research on medicinal plants has grown immensely. Public health services, such as the Instituto Mexicano de Seguro Social (IMSS, the Mexican Social Security Service), have promoted traditional health centres alongside conventional allopathic clinics in indigenous communities. IMSS also maintains the largest national herbarium dedicated to medicinal plants, which documents its research programme as well as training institutional and traditional health practitioners. It also maintains the Biomedical Research Center in Xochitepec, Morelos, where phytopharmaceutical research is carried out. Recently the Health Secretariat of the Federal District inaugurated an integrated medicine clinic in Mexico City, which includes a phytotherapy clinic.

Universities at national and state levels as well as specialized universities and professional schools have been centres for ethnopharmacological research throughout Mexico. Up until the last decade, much of the research carried out by students has been hidden away in unpublished theses on library shelves. The Instituto Nacional Indigenista's Biblioteca de la Medicina Tradicional Mexicana project has provided a great service by including references to theses in their bibliography (Argueta and Zolla, 1994). Today, original contributions derived from Mexican graduate studies are published in professional journals and many theses are available online from universities.

The future for ethnopharmacological research in Mexico is promising. Local indigenous clinics and social networks are associating themselves with academic and governmental institutions that share common interests in the promotion and documentation of Mexican *herbolaria*. Nonetheless, certain limitations need to be addressed to achieve greater benefits. For instance, the newly formed network of intercultural universities established in regions with a high density of indigenous populations have incorporated ethnopharmacological field studies in their academic curricula but their results have been published in institutional newsletters and social network pages; their contributions should be available in indexed scientific journals. With more clinics offering herbal medicine as part of their treatment programme, the opportunity to move ethnopharmacological research beyond *in vitro* and *in vivo* laboratory experiments and into clinical trials will soon be a reality, a goal promoted by Sociedad Mexicana de Fitoterapia Clinica, A.C. The measure of the effectiveness of medicinal plants in contemporary ethnopharmacological research is based on models of western science's allopathic medicine. There are few studies such as those of Ortiz de Montellano (1990) which evaluate a herbal remedy's therapeutic effectiveness based on the indigenous cultural concepts of a disease's etiology, which is based on magic, religion and indigenous science.

## 33.2   Mexican tradition

Shortly after the Spanish conquest of Mexico, the documentation and appropriation of the medicinal plants of New Spain began and it continued for three centuries. Three basic references generated during the 16th century established the basis for the Spanish crown's inventory and control of remedial plants in hospitals and for commerce.

*Libellus de Medicinalibus Indorum Herbis – Tratado sobre hierbas medicinales indias*, produced in 1552, represents the first book written by indigenous people about their curative plants and produced in the western hemisphere. This *Libellus* documents the meeting of native Mesoamerican remedies with European medicine. Martín de la Cruz, an indigenous healer, transmitted his experiences with 227 plants (185 of which are illustrated) to Juan Badiano, a Indian with formal education in Latin and Spanish. The objectives of the New Spain Viceroy's gift of the *Libellus* were to demonstrate the level of indigenous knowledge, request support to improve the school for indigenous students and obtain concessions to commercialize American medicinal plants. After being lost for almost four centuries, the *Libellus* was rediscovered in 1929. A recent multidisciplinary study of the *Libellus* is that of Kumate (1992). Isolated treatments of various topics continually appear, such as the etymological analysis of indigenous names (Clayton and de Avila, 2009) and the re-evaluation of the taxonomic identities of the plants and their phytogeography (Bye and Linares, 2013).

*Historia general de las cosas de Nueva España*, or Florentine Codex, represents 50 years of careful ethnographic studies by Bernardino de Sahagún. The Franciscan friar's work, which was sent to Spain between 1577 and 1580, included data on the diversity and use of 382 plants of central Mexico; about three-quarters of the ethnobotanical data are found in Book 11, entitled *Earthly Things*, which describes the properties of animals, birds, fish, trees, herbs, flowers, metals, stones and colours. Data from the Spanish-Nahuatl version may have been incorporated in later works of Mexican chroniclers such as Francisco Javier Clavijero. The classic multidisciplinary study (including the only translation of the complete Nahuatl text, which is more detailed than the Spanish text) is that of Anderson and Dibble (1950–1982). An analysis of the ethnobotanical information based on the 1979 facsimile edition is available (Estrada Lugo, 1989).

*Historia Natural de las Plantas de Nueva España* compiles the surviving fragments of the first formal inventory of biotic resources of New Spain sanctioned by the Spanish Crown. Between 1571 and 1577, Francisco Hernández, as the court physician of King Philip II, documented the plants, animals and minerals of this Viceroyalty with texts, dried specimens, seeds, live plants and drawings. Although some of the esculent and medicinal properties are derived from indigenous informants, the therapeutic properties are often based on Galenic principles of medicine, suggesting that his work reflects more an etic perspective. Various versions were produced during the 17th and 18th centuries. The first major interdisciplinary examination of the works of Hernandez was conducted by the Comisión Editora de las Obras de Francisco Hernández of the Universidad Nacional de Mexico (1959–1985). Descriptions of 3076 plants are presented, of which only 667 botanical species are identified taxonomically (Valdés and Flores, 1985). Contemporary multidisciplinary studies on the importance of Hernandez's contributions can be found in Chabrán *et al.* (2000) and Varey *et al.* (2000).

Throughout the Viceroyalty Period, various chroniclers recorded medicinal plants used by both indigenous peoples and mestizos. *Florilegio Medicinal de todas las enfermedades sacado de varios y clásicos autores para bien de los pobres y de los que tienen falta de medicos* is the most important document dealing with medicinal plants because it was used throughout New Spain and continued to be consulted by traditional Mexican healers into the 20th century (Kay, 1977). First published in 1712, Juan de Esteyneffer, a German Jesuit who dedicated much of his life to working in mission hospitals, compiled various treatments for illnesses, including formulations based on almost 300 different plants or plant derivatives and founded on European and indigenous medical concepts (Esteyneffer, 1978; orig. 1712).

At the end of the Viceroyalty Period, botanical documentation gained a solid footing as part of the Spanish Age of Enlightenment, which attempted to develop the Spanish Empire based on science, in part through the reevaluation of the 16th century work of Francisco Hernández. The Royal Botanical Expedition of 1787–1803 (also known as the Sessé and Mociño Expedition) not only established the medical botany curriculum in Mexico's university but also carried out botanical exploration throughout New Spain and Central America. The expedition's botanists and their students reported in *Anales de Historia Natural de Madrid* only the medicinal plants that exhibited curative effects in their experiments and clinical trials; there was no place for reporting on indigenous 'superstitions' about plants that did not pass their tests.

After Mexico's independence from Spain, scientific studies of Mexican medicinal plants advanced little until the Porfiriato Period (1876–1910). Towards the end of the 19th century, the modernizing government established a national institute for the study of public health that included the re-evaluation of medicinal plants. Between 1888 and 1915, the Instituto Médico Nacional developed the Materia Médica Mexicana (Guerra, 1950) and was recognized worldwide as the most profuse and studied in all the Americas (Fernández, 1961). The results were incorporated into various editions of the *Nueva Farmacopea Mexicana* and of the classic book *Plantas Medicinales de México* (Martínez, 1933). After the Mexican revolution, the number of vegetal species in the official Mexican pharmacopeias plummeted drastically to 5% of that of 1904 (Hersh, 2013); not until the early 21st century was *Farmacopea Herbolaria de los Estados Unidos Mexicanos* published (Comisión Permanente de la Farmacopea de los Estados Unidos Mexicanos, 2001). This new effort of Mexico's Secretary of Health officially accepted 41 plant species and appended an *ExtraFarmacopeia* of 19 botanical drugs recognized as being of national importance. A total of 17 of these are native to Mexico. The second edition increased the official botanicals by 52 and added four plants to the *ExtraFarmacopea* (Comisión Permanente de la Farmacopea de los Estados Unidos Mexicanos, 2013). The number of species native to Mexico increased to a total of 27. To promote scientific recognition of Mexico's therapeutic flora based on national research, a team at UNAM has initiated a series titled *Plantas Medicinales de México – Monografía Científica* (e.g. Mata *et al.*, 2009).

## 33.3  Compilation of medicinal plants

Given the richness of Mexico's medicinal flora and the nearly five centuries of its study, the compilation of this information during the last century has been a priority. However, one should be aware of that each collation varies in terms of the critieria employed, hence certain problems exist, such as the lack of taxonomic verification, outdated botanical nomenclature, inappropriate interpretation of illnesses and antiquated pharmacological experiments, among others. The appropriate use of these secondary sources requires consultation of the orignal sources from which the data were derived.

The classic book of Maximino Martínez entitled *Plantas Medicinales de México* condensed much of the study by the Instituto Médico Nacional along with information from historical sources and local inventories. With the encouragement of the non-governmental Instituto Mexicano para el Estudio de las Plantas Medicinales (IMEPLAM), a cross-index of scientific and common names was generated (Diáz, 1976a) and each botanical species classified as to its medicinal application, preparation and part utilized (Diáz, 1976b). The next major effort was the compilation of botanical, phytochemical and pharmacological data on 1000 medicinal plants in *Atlas de las Plantas de la Medicina Tradicional Mexicana* by the government's

Instituto Nacional Indigenista (Argueta *et al.*, 1994). Building on this work, a modified digital version has been made available by UNAM (http://www.medicinatradicionalmexicana.unam.mx/atlas.php.) In the near future, UNAM will bring online two databases derived from national surveys related to medicinal plants: *Base de Datos Etnobotánicos de Plantas Mexicanas* (BADEPLAM, http://unibio.unam.mx/html/proyectos/badeplam.htm) and *Unidad de Informática del Instituto de Química* (UNIIQUIM, http://uniiquim.iquimica.unam.mx/). The latter expands on an earlier series dedicated to detailing the composition, uses and biological activities of plants studied in that institute (Lara and Márquez, 1996; Márquez *et al.*, 1999). In addition to the national surveys, medicinal plant inventories have been developed for certain Mexican states (Table 33.1).

Given the 67 recognized linguistic groups in Mexico, the documentation of indigenous knowledge and use of medicinal plants is of interest (see also above). Since 1981, the national

**Table 33.1**  Examples of state inventories of medicinal plants in Mexico.

| State or region | Bibliography | Year |
| --- | --- | --- |
| Aguascalientes | García Regalado, G. *Plantas Medicinales de Aguascalientes*, Universidad Autónoma de Aguascalientes, Aguascalientes, 109 pp. | 1989 |
| Chihuahua | Olivas Sánchez, M.P. *Plantas Medicinales del Estado de Chihuahua*, Universidad Autónoma de Ciudad Juárez, Cd. Juárez, Chih, 127 pp. | 1999 |
| Distrito Federal and adjacent states | Linares, E., Flores Peñafiel, B. and Bye, R. *Selección de Plantas Medicinales de México*, Editorial LIMUSA, México, DF, 125 pp. | 1994 |
| Distrito Federal and adjacent states | Linares, E., Bye, R. and Flores, B. *Plantas Medicinales de México/Medicinal Plants of México*, Universidad Nacional Autónoma de México & Sistema de Información Geográfica, SA de CV, México, DF, 155 pp. | 1999 |
| Distrito Federal and adjacent states | Jimenéz Merino, F. *Alberto. Herbolaria Mexicana*, Colegio de Postgraduados, Montecillos, 531 pp. | 2011 |
| Durango | González Elizondo, M., López Enríquez, I.L. González Elizondo, S. and Tena Flores, J.A. *Plantas Medicinales del Estado de Durango y Zonas Aledañas*, Instituto Politécnico Nacional, México, DF, 209 pp. | 2004 |
| Morelos | Monroy-Ortiz, C. and Castillo-España, P. *Plantas Medicinales Utilizadas en el Estado de Morelos*, Universidad Autónoma del Estado de Morelos, Cuernavaca, Morelos, 405 pp. | 2007 |
| Oaxaca | Méndez Hernández, Á., Hernández Hernández, A.A., del Carmen López Santiago, M. and Morales López, J. *Herbolaria Oaxaqueña para la Salud*, Instituto Nacional de las Mujeres, México, DF, 143 pp. | 2011 |
| Quintana Roo | Pulido Salas, M.T. and Serralta Peraza, L. *Lista anotada de las plantas medicinales de uso actual en el Estado de Quintana Roo, México*, Centro de Investigaciones de Quintana Roo, Chetumal, QR, v + 105 pp. | 1993 |
| Sonora | López Estudillo, R. and Hinojosa García, A. *Catálogo de Plantas Medicinales Sonorenses*, Universidad de Sonora, Hermosillo, SON, 133 pp. | 1988 |
| Veracruz | Cano, L. and Leticia, M. (Vázquez Torres, M., Jácome Castillo, E., colaboradores). *Flora Medicinal de Veracruz. I. Inventario etnobotánico*, Universidad Veracruzana, Xalapa, Ver., 606 pp. (921 especies medicinales) | 1997 |
| Veracruz | Del Amo, R.S. *Plantas Medicinales del Estado de Veracruz*, Instituto Nacional de Investigaciones sobre Recursos Bióticos, Xalapa, VER, ix + 279 pp. | 1979 |
| Yucatán | Mendieta, R.M. and del Amo, S.R. *Plantas Medicinales del Estado de Yucatán*, Instituto Nacional de Investigaciones sobre Recursos Bióticos, Xalapa, Ver., xxv + 428 pp. | 1981 |

medicinal plant herbarium of the IMSS has vouchered plants used in indigenous curing practices, principally in central and southern Mexico (Aguilar *et al.*, 1994). The Instituto Nacional Indigenista conducted a parallel programme to that of the *Atlas* in which 29 native peoples recorded in their respective languages along with Spanish texts and drawings the important remedial plants in their cultures (Torres and Rodarte, 1994). In recent years, representatives of native communities have begun to record their traditional knowledge for the benefit of future generations (e.g. Méndez *et al.*, 2011). One region of Mexico participates in a multinational ethnopharmacological programme. The Mexican states of Yucatán and Quintana Roo contribute to TRAMIL, a programme of applied research focused on popular medicine in the Caribbean basin. Its principal aim is to validate scientifically the traditional uses of medicinal plants for primary health care in the participating countries through various workshops and publications, the key one being the *Caribbean Herbal Pharmacopoeia* (Germosén-Robineau, 2014).

These compilations of Mexican medicinal flora provide a bountiful background for the academic growth of quantitative ethnopharmacology to examine intercultural and intracultural knowledge transmission, assessment of plant remedy consensus within and among groups, and factors that influence variation in plant use (Heinrich *et al.*, 2014). Initial studies at a regional or national level have focused on specific ailments such as diabetes (Andrade and Heinrich, 2005; Mata *et al.*, 2013) and gastrointestinal illnesses (Heinrich *et al.*, 2014) as well as on plant families (e.g. Asteraceae, Heinrich, 1998; Lamiaceae, Heinrich, 1992).

## 33.4  Medicinal plant complex

When Francisco Hernández surveyed medicinal plants throughout central New Spain, he encountered different plants with a similar name. These he organized in the same books of his *Historia Natural de la Nueva España* but he distinguished them geographically or morphologically (Hernández, 1959). Acknowledging these historical similarities and integrating them with the diversity of medicinal plants traded nationally in the markets, the concept of a medicinal plant complex emerged (Linares and Bye, 1987). Such a complex is defined as an assemblage of taxonomically distinct plants (usually at the specific level, but may also be placed in different botanical families) that share certain features, in particular the local or trade name. In addition, the plants may hold in common medicinal uses, morphological features of the utilized part, organoleptic properties and phytochemical composition or pharmacological assets. Usually in each complex, there is a dominant or signature species that is commercialized beyond its natural phytogeographic range (and often with early historical references) while the subordinate species tend to be used within their respective natural phytogeographic ranges or as a substitute for the signature taxon. It is hypothesized that the signature species has a greater demand because it is considered to be more effective.

One of the first medicinal plant complexes defined was that of *matarique*, which includes various species of the genera *Psacalium* and *Acourtia* employed in the treatment of diabetes in Mexico. In a study utilizing laboratory mice treated with extracts from three members of the matarique complex, the signature species, *P. decompositum* (A. Gray) H. Rob. and Brettell, exhibited the greatest decrease in blood glucose level (Alarcón *et al.*, 1997). The original paper focused on only four medicinal plant complexes even though many more exist in Mexico, such as *árnica*, *contrayerba*, *jalapa*, *quina*, *toronjil* and *yerba de víbora*, among others. This concept has been applied to the European *árnica* complex with 32 species of Asteraceae (Obón *et al.*, 2012) and to American *mirto*, *ñucchu*, *cantueso* and *manga-paqui* complexes with 17 species in *Salvia* subgenus *Calosphace* (Jenks and Kim, 2013).

## 33.5   Markets and medicinal plants

Markets have played a dominant political and economic role in Mexico's history, even prior to the Spanish Conquest. Many products encountered in the markets, including medicinal plants, were drawn from across the Aztec Empire and concentrated in Tenochtitlán for tribute payments as well as for sale in the central marketplaces. The diversity of plants and the spatial extension of the Mexica markets surpassed those known to the conquistadors in Europe. Hence the movement of medicinal plants, the transmission of knowledge related to their properties and employment, and their role in health of the indigenous communities depended, in part, upon the market. The continuity of medicinal plants via the markets extends into present-day Mexico (Bye and Linares, 1987). Consequently, Mexican local, regional and national markets are an essential element in contemporary ethnopharmacological research (Bye and Linares, 1983; Hernández *et al.*, 1983).

The markets are also good indicators of the social well-being and conservation status of medicinal plants. Throughout Mexico environmental degradation of source areas is linked strongly with socioeconomic marginalization of the human populations who inhabit those areas. In Puebla, as in many other areas throughout the country, the local herbal collector receives about 7% of the consumer retail price of the herbal products and each year must seek the plants at greater distances from home (Hersch, 1995, 1997). This reduction in the availability of medicinal plants is reflected in a recent study of markets in Chiapas, where 5% of the plants sold to the public are listed in the categorie of extinction danger in Mexico's Environmental Protection law NOM-059 SEMARNAT (Díaz *et al.*, 2011).

In Mexico, the principal medicinal plant market is the Mercado de Sonora in México, D.F., where over 290 species of fresh plants are available and even more in dried form (Mendoza *et al.*, 1997). More research is need on medicinal plants in the markets. Recent studies in regional markets, such as Puebla, reveal that half of the medicinal plants recorded had not been reported earlier (Martínez *et al.*, 2006). Factors such as time of day, seasonality, religious feasts days and spatial-temporal partitioning of plant production among multiple source areas influence the availability and quantity of medicinal plants present in the market at any given time (Linares and Bye, 2010).

## 33.6   Bioprospection and conservation

The Convention on Biological Diversity (CBD) of 1992 has become a milestone for biological research around the world. Ethnopharmacology has played a central role in its implementation at the international level as well as generating controversy at the local level. Even though the USA has failed to ratify the CBD to date, various sectors of the US government have supported the implementation trails of the CBD through the International Cooperative Biodiversity Group (ICBG), in which US academic institutions partner foreign counterparts and the productive sector (Rosenthal, 1999). The objectives of ICBG parallel those of the CBD (Table 33.2), with an emphasis on medicinal plants.

Mexico participated initially with two programmes: Agents from Dryland Biodiversity of Latin America and Maya ICBG. These projects built on established research platforms: in the former case, a collaborative ethnopharmacological investigation between the Facultad de Química and the Instituto de Biología of Universidad Nacional Autónoma de México (UNAM) and in the latter case, the ethnoscientific principles of the cultural and linguistic research of Brent and Eloise Berlin (initiated at the University of California Berkeley and

**Table 33.2**   Comparative table of the objectives of the CBD and the ICBG.

| Convention on Biological Diversity | International Cooperative Biodiversity Group |
| --- | --- |
| 1. Conservation of biological diversity | 1. Conservation of biological diversity |
| 2. Sustainable use of its components | 2. Pharmaceutical discovery from natural sources for both developed and developing country diseases |
| 3. Just and equitable participation in the benefits derived from the utilization of genetic resources | 3. Promote sustained economic activity in developing countries for the communities |

continued at the University of Georgia) with the Tzeltal and Tzotzil populations and El Colegio de la Frontera Sur in Chiapas.

In the case of the first programme, botanical, phytochemical and preliminary pharmacological analyses were conducted on vegetal samples at UNAM. Bioactive fractions were coded to safeguard their taxonomic identity. ICBG-supported contracts with commercial and institutional laboratories in the USA supported high-through-put bioanalysis related to 40 health issues of interest (cancer, diabetes, tuberculosis, women's health, etc.). The Dryland project focused on traditional medicine information or *herbolaria* circulated in the public domain of herbal markets around the country. Emphasis was placed on local medicinal plants at each site and selected native plants that were widely traded as well as on certain illnesses, the fluctuations in the plants' availability and price over time, and the customers' preference based on personal satisfaction relative to other plants employed similarly. In selected cases, 'upstreaming' retraced the marketing chain to the geographic source area and the local collectors to evaluate the ecological status of the source populations (Hutchinson *et al.*, 2001).

In contrast, the latter project focused on local plants in the Chiapas highlands that the indigenous peoples proposed for analysis and development. The explanation and negotiation were carried out in the native language and traditional story telling to communicate the objectives of the project and negotiate the agreements.

Appropriate national and local permits were obtained. Botanical samples were acquired for phytochemical and pharmacological analyses. The benefits were of two types. The short-term benefits focused on the requests of the communities' civil and educational leaders and the institutional capabilities. The long-term benefits derived from royalties from any resulting commercial products, which would be shared through a trust fund established by the academic institutions' policies. For the most part, participating communities requested capacity-building workshops for students, teachers and inhabitants that dealt with curriculum enhancement, plant propagation, conservation and value-added productive projects that were supplemented by external support (e.g. Hutchinson *et al.*, 2001; Linares *et al.*, 2004; Mendoza *et al.*, 2009). Initially, these benefits were belittled by critics (e.g. Hayden, 2003) but recent international clarification of the access and benefit-sharing policies of the CBD through the Nagoya Protocol (Secretariat of the Convention on Biological Diversity, 2011) has highlighted the significance of such actions.

As ICBG evolved, in particular with its expansion to include marine organisms, which was not compatible with land-based ethnopharmacological studies with benefits for communties of plant collectors and cultivators, ICBG funding for Mexico's projects was not renewed.

Even though to date these ICBG projects have not developed a commercial product, they have generated benefits for ethnopharmacological documentation and plant resource conservation. One example is that of *copalquin o copalchi*, *Hintonia latiflora* (Sessé and Moc. ex DC.) Bullock, the signature species of the *quina* medicinal plant complex. Its bark is widely appreciated for its antimalarial, antifebrifugic and antidiabetic properties, and it is intensely commercialized in the national and international markets (Mata *et al.*, 2009). The increased demand in recent years has drastically reduced the natural populations due to the indiscriminant tree felling in order to completely remove the bark (rather than periodically shimmying cortical segments on different sides of the standing trunks). The antihyperglycemic properties of the bark (found in commercial antidiabetic medications such as Sucontral®) are due to 4-phenylcoumarins, ursolic acid and chlorogenic acid. Recent studies have also shown their presence in the leaves, the extracts of which have hypoglycemic activity in streptozotozin (STZ)-induced diabetic mice (Christian *et al.*, 2009). Consequently, ethnopharmacological research not only demonstrated the pharmacological basis of *Hintonia* in the treatment of diabetes but also the presence of similar bioactivity in the leaves (a renewable alternative source of *materia prima*), which can be incorporated into a sustainable exploitation programme for this Mexican dry tropical tree.

## 33.7 Conclusions

The scientific and cultural basis of medicinal plants in the maintenance of peoples' well-being continues to be the focus of basic and applied research in Mexico after nearly five centuries. Today's endeavours have become complicated by political debate. Nonetheless, ethnopharmacological research has identified potential bioactive natural products for the treatment of common illnesses such as gastrointestinal disorders as well as emerging metabolic disorders such as diabetes. The integration of ethnopharmacological results into the public health system and social-economic development programmes strengthens biodiversity conservation for the benefit of local inhabitants as well as the global community (as outlined in the CBD).

## Acknowledgements

The authors appreciate the support from collegaues in our academic circles and in the Mexican *herbolaria* networks. This chapter benefited from the library support provided by Georgina Ortega Leite and the constructive suggestions of Miguel Heinrich and Anna Jäger.

## References

Aguilar, A., Camacho, J.R., Chino, S., *et al.* (1994) *Herbario Medicinal del Instituto Mexicano del Seguro Social – Información Etnobotánica*, Instituto Mexicano del Seguro Social, México, DF, 253 p.

Alarcón-Aguilar, F.J., Roman-Ramos, R., Jimenez-Estrada, M. *et al.* (1997) Effects of three Mexican medicinal plants (Asteraceae) on blood glucose levels in healthy mice and rabbits. *Journal of Ethnopharmacology*, **55**, 171–177.

Anderson, A.J.O. and Dibble, C.E. (eds) (1950–1982) *Bernardino de Sahagún, General history of the things of New Spain*, Florentine Codex, **13** volumes, University of Utah Press, Salt Lake City.

Andrade-Cetto, A. and Heinrich, M. 2005. Mexican plants with hypoglycaemic effect used in the treatment of diabetes. *Journal of Ethnopharmacology*, **99**, 325–348.

Argueta, A. and Zolla, C. (1994) *Nueva Bibliography de la Medicina Tradicional Mexicana*, Instituto Nacional Indigenista, México, DF, 450 pp.

Argueta Villamar, A., Cano Asseleih, L.M. and Rodarte, M.E. (eds) (1994) *Atlas de las Plantas de la Medicina Tradicional Mexicana*, Instituto Nacional Indigenista, México, DF, 1786 pp., http://www.medicinatradicionalmexicana.unam.mx/atlas.php.

Bye, R. 1(986) Voucher specimens in ethnobiological studies and publications. *Journal of Ethnobiology*, **6**, 1–8.

Bye, R. and Linares, E. (1983) The role of plants found in the Mexican markets and their importance in ethnobotanical studies. *Journal of Ethnobiology*, **3**, 1–13.

Bye, R. and Linares, E. (1987) Usos pasados y presentes de algunas plantas medicinales econtradas en los mercados mexicanos. *América Indígena*, **47**, 199–230.

Bye, R. and Linares, E. (2013) Códice De la Cruz–Badiano. *Arqueología Mexicana (Edición Especial)*, **50**, 8–91, **51**, 9–93.

Bye, R., Linares, E. and Estrada, E. (1995) Biological diversity of medicinal plants in Mexico. *Recent Advances in Phytochemistry*, **29**, 65–82.

Chabran, R., Chamberlin, C. and Varey, S. (2000) *The Mexican Treasury: The Writings of Dr Francisco Hernández*, Stanford University Press.

Comisión Editora de las Obras de Francisco Hernández (1959–1985) *Obras Completas de Francisco Hernández*, Tomos *I–VII*, Universidad Nacional Autónoma de México, México, DF.

Comisión Nacional para el Conocimiento y Uso de la Biodiversidad (CONABIO) (2014) Biodiversidad Mexicana, http://www.biodiversidad.gob.mx/.

Comisión Permanente de la Farmacopea de los Estados Unidos Mexicanos (2001) Farmacopea Herbolaria de los Estados Unidos Mexicanos, Secretaría de Salud, México, DF, 177 + 51 pp.

Comisión Permanente de la Farmacopea de los Estados Unidos Mexicanos (2013) *Farmacopea Herbolaria de los Estados Unidos Mexicanos*, segunda edición, Secretaria de Salud, Comisión Permanente de la Farmacopea de los Estados Unidos Mexicanos, México, DF, 371 pp.

Cook, F.E.M. (1995) Economic Botany Data Collection Standard *(Prepared for the International Working Group on Taxonomic Databases for Plant Sciences (TDWG))*, Royal Botanic Gardens Kew, Richmond, 146 pp.

Cristians, S., Guerrero-Analco, J.A., Pérez-Vásquez, A., *et al.* (2009) Hypoglycemic activity of extracts and compounds from the leaves of *Hintonia standleyana* and *H. latiflora*: potential alternatives to the use of the stem bark of these species. *Journal of Natural Products*, **72** (3), 408–414.

de la Cruz, M. (1964) *Libellus de Medicinalibus Indorum Herbis*, manuscrito azteca de 1552 según traducción latina de Juan Badiano, versión española con estudios y comentarios por diversos autores, Instituto Mexicano del Seguro Social, México, DF, 394 pp.

Díaz, J.L. (ed.) (1976a) *Índice y Sinonimia de las Plantas Medicinales de México. Monografías Científicas I*, Instituto Mexicano para el Estudio de las Plantas Medicinales, México, DF, 358 pp.

Díaz, J.L. (ed.) (1976b) *Usos de las Plantas Medicinales de México. Monografías Científicas II*, Instituto Mexicano para el Estudio de las Plantas Medicinales, México, DF, 345 pp.

Díaz Montesinos, M.G., Farrera Sarmiento, O. and Isidro Vázquez, M.A. (2011) Estudio etnobotánico de los principales mercados de Tuxtla Gutiérrez, Chiapas, México. *Lacandonia*, **5**, 21–42.

Esteyneffer, J. de. (1978) *Florilegio Medicinal de todas las enfermedades sacado de varios y clásicos autores para bien de los pobres y de los que tienen falta de médicos; orig. 1712* (Edición, estudio preliminar, notas, glosario e índice analítico por Ma. De C. Anzures y Bolaños), Academia Nacional de Medicina, México, DF, 973 pp.

Estrada Lugo, E.I.J. (1989) *El Códice Florentino – su información etnobotánica*, Colegio de Postgraduados, Chapingo, Estado de México, 399 pp.

Fernández del Castillo, F. (1961) *Historia bibliográfica del Instituto Médico Nacional de México – 1888–1915*, Imprenta Universitaria, México, DF, 209 pp.

Germosén-Robineau, L. (ed.) (2014) *Caribbean Herbal Phramacopoeia*, 3rd edn, TRAMIL, Centro de Investigación Científica de Yucatán, A.C. Mérida, Yucatán, México, 400 pp.

Gruca, M., Cámara-Leret, R., Macía, M.J. and Balslev, H. (2014) New categories for traditional medicine in the Economic Botany Data Collection Standard. *Journal of Ethnopharmacology*, **155**, 1388–1392.

Guerra, F. (1950) *Bibliografía del a Materia Medica Mexicana*, La Prensa Medica Mexicana, México, DF, 423 pp.

Hayden, C. (2003) *When Nature Goes Public: The Making and Unmaking of Bioprospecting in Mexico*, Princeton University Press, Princeton, NJ, 312 pp.

Heinrich, M. (1992) Economic Botany of American Labiatae, in *Advances in Labiatae Science* (eds R.M. Harley and T. Reynolds), Kew Botanical Gardens, Richmond, pp. 475–488.

Heinrich, M. (1998) Ethnopharmacology of Mexican Asteraceae (Compositae). *Annual Review of Pharmacology and Toxicology*, **38**, 539–565.

Heinrich, M., Edwards, S., Moerman, D.E. and Leonti, M. (2009) Ethnopharmacological field studies: A critical assessment of their conceptual basis and methods. *Journal of Ethnopharmacology*, **124**, 1–17.

Heinrich, M., Leonti, M. and Frei Haller, B. (2014) A perspective on natural products research and ethnopharmacology in México. The eagle and the serpent on the prickly pear cactus. *Journal of Natural Products*, **77**, 678–689.

Hernández, F. (1959) Historia Natural de Nueva España, *Volúmenes 1 y 2, Obras Completas, Tomos II y III*, Universidad Nacional Autónoma de México, México, DF.

Hernández Xolocotzi, E., Vargas, N., Gómez Hernández, A.T. *et al.* (1983) Consideraciones etnobotánicas de los mercados en México. *Revista Geografía Agrícola*, **4**, 13–28.

Herrera, T., Ortega, M.M., Godínez, J.L. and Butanda, A. (1998) *Breve Historia de la Botánica en Mexico*, Fondo de Cultura Economica, México, DF, 167 pp.

Hersch-Martínez, P. (1996) Destino común: Los recolectores y su flora medicinal, *Instituto Nacional de Antropología e Historia*, México, DF, ISBN: 9682990521.

Hersch-Martinez, P. (1995) Commercialization of wild medicinal plants from Southwest Puebla, Mexico. *Economic Botany*, **49**,197–206.

Hersch-Martínez, P. (1997) Medicinal plants and regional traders in Mexico: physiographic differences and conservational challenge. *Economic Botany*, **51**, 107–120.

Hersch-Martínez, P. (2011) *Integración de Saberes y Poderes – Plantas medicinales y servicios públicos de atención en la Ciudad de México*, Instituto de Ciencia y Tecnología del Distrito Federal. México, DF, 107 pp.

Hersch-Martínez, P. (2013) *Historia, in Comisión Permanente de la Farmacopea de los Estados Unidos Mexicanos, Farmacopea Herbolaria de los Estados Unidos Mexicanos*, segunda edición, Secretaria de Salud, Comisión Permanente de la Farmacopea de los Estados Unidos Mexicanos, México, DF, pp. 336–346.

Hutchinson, B., Suarez, E., Fortunato, R., *et al.* (2001) Consservation and ethnobotanical programs of the bioactive agents from Dryland Biodiversity of Latin America Project. *Arid Lands Newsletter*, **48**, http://ag.arizona.edu/oals/ALN/aln48/hutchinsonetal.html.

Jenks, A.A. and Kim, S.C. (2013) Medicinal plant complexes of *Salvia* subgenus *Calosphace*: An ethnobotanical study of new world sages. *Journal of Ethnopharmacology*, **146**, 214–224.

Kay, M.A. (1977) The Florilegio Medicinal: Source of southwest ethnomedicine. *Ethnohistory*, **24**, 251–259.

Kumate, J. (ed.) (1992) Estudios Actuales sobre el Libellus de Medicinalibus Indorum Herbis, *Secretaria de Salud*, México, DF, 202 pp.

Lara Ochoa, F. and Márquez Alonso, C. (1996) *Plantas Medicinales de México I. Composición, Usos y Actividad Biológica*, Universidad Nacional Autónoma de México, México, DF, 137 pp.

Linares, E. and Bye, R. (1987) A study of four medicinal plant complexes of México and adjacent United States. *Journal of Ethnopharmacology*, **19**, 153–183.

Linares, E. and Bye, R. (2010) La dinámica de un mercado periférico de plantas medicinales en México: el Mercado de Ozumba, Estado de México, como centro acopiador para el Mercado Sonora, in *Caminos y Mercados de México* (eds J. Long and A. Attolini), Universidad Nacional Autónoma de México – Instituto de Investigaciones Históricas, pp. 631–663.

Márquez Alonso, C., Lara Ochoa, F., Esquivel Rodríguez, B. and Mata Essayag, R. (1999) Plantas Medicinales de México II. Composición, Usos y Actividad Biológica, Universidad Nacional Autónoma de México, México, DF, 178 pp.

Martínez, M. (1933) *Plantas Medicinales de México*, edn. Botas , México, DF, 657 pp.

Martínez Moreno, D., Alvarado Flores, R., Mendoza Cruz, M. and Basurto Peña, F. (2006) Plantas medicinales de cuatro mercados del estado de Puebla, México. *Boletín de la Sociedad Botánica de México*, **79**, 79–87.

Mata, R., Navarrete, A., Cristians, S., *et al.* (2009) *Plantas Medicinales de México*, Monografía científica – pruebas de control de calidad (identidad y composición), eficacia y seguridad. Copalchi – *Hintonia latiflora* (Sessé et Mociño ex DC.) Bullock (Rubiaceae), Sentido Giratorio Ediciones, S.C., México, DF, 32 pp.

Mata, R., Cristians, S., Escandón-Rivera, S. *et al.* (2013) Mexican antidiabetic herbs: valuable source of inhibitors of α-glycosidases. *Journal of Natural Products*, **76**, 468–483.

Méndez Hernández, Á., Hernández Hernández, A.A., López Santiago, M.C. and Morales López, J. (2011) Herbolaria Oaxaqueña para la Salud, *Instituto Nacional de las Mujeres*, México, DF, 143 pp.

Mendoza Castelán, G., García Pérez, J. and Estrada Lugo, E. (1997) *Catalogo y usos terapéuticos de plantas medicinales que se comercializan en fresco en el Mercado Sonora*, Universidad Autónoma Chapingo, Chapingo, Estado de México, 137 pp.

Obón, C., Rivera, D., Verde, A., *et al.* (2012) Árnica: A multivariate analysis of the botany and ethnopharmacology of a medicinal plant complex in the Iberian Peninsula and the Balearic Islands. *Journal of Ethnopharmacology*, **144**, 44–56.

Ortiz de Montellano, B.R. (1990) *Aztec Medicine, Health, and Nutrition*, Rutgers University Press, New Brunswick, NJ, 308 pp.

Rivera Morales, I. (1941) Ensayo de interpretacion botanica del libro X de la historia de Sahagún. *Anales del Instituto de Biología de la Universidad Nacional Autónoma de México [Serie botánica]*, **12**, 439–488.

Rivera, D., Allkin, R., Obón, C., *et al.* (2014) What is in a name? The need for accurate scientific nomenclature for plants. *Journal of Ethnopharmacology*, **152**, 393–402.

Sahagún, B. (1979) *Historia General de las cosas de Nueva España*, Manuscrito 218-20 de la Colección Palatina de la Biblioteca Medicea Laurenziana, Florencia [reproducción facsimilar: Códice Florentino], Archivo General de la Nación,México, DF.

Salick, J., Konchar, K. and Nesbitt, M. (eds) (2014) *Curating Biocultural Collections: A Handbook*, Royal Botanic Gardens, Kew, Richmond, 250 pp.

Secretariat of the Convention on Biological Diversity (2011) *Nagoya Protocol on Access to Genetic Resources and the Fair and Equitable Sharing of Benefits Arising from their Utilization (ABS) to the Convention on Biological Diversity*, United Nations Environmental Programme, Nairobi, Kenya.

Torres, G. and Rodarte, M.E. (eds) (1994) *Flora Medicinal Indígena de México, 3 volumes*, Instituto Nacional Indigenista, México, DF.

Valdés, J. and Flores, H. (1985) *Historia de las plantas de Nueva España, in Comentarios a la Obra de Francisco Hernández, Obras Completas, Tomo VII*, Universidad Nacional Autónoma de México, México, DF, pp. 7–222.

Varey, S., Chabrán, R. and Weiner, D.B. (2000) *Searching for the Secrets of Nature: The Life and Works of Dr Francisco Hernández*, Stanford University Press, Stanford, CA, 229 pp.

# 34

# Encounters with Elephants: A Personal Perspective on Ethnopharmacology

Peter J. Houghton

*Department of Pharmacy and Forensic Science, Institute of Pharmaceutical Sciences, King's College London, London, UK*

## 34.1    Introduction

A few years ago I published a paper (Houghton *et al.*, 2007a) which attracted some degree of interest. This was probably due to part of its title, *Visualising an Elephant*, as much as its content[1]. The title arose from the originally Indian story of several blind men describing an elephant in different ways, according to the part of the elephant they handled, and the aim of the paper was to highlight the fact that, in a similar fashion, several bioassays are usually needed to construct a meaningful profile of the biological activity of a traditional remedy, to help explain its reputed 'clinical' use.

The same paradigm could be applied to how ethnopharmacology is described, since it is a multidisciplinary and interdisciplinary subject (Etkin and Elisabetsky, 2005), and displays a range of features which I, amongst many others, have 'handled' during my scientific career. In addition, its more prominent features have changed during the almost 50 years since 'ethnopharmacology' arrived as a neologism,[2] so that the following account of my interactions with the subject over the last 40 years could be described as the visualization of a four-dimensional elephant!

Although an anecdotal approach is frowned upon as rigorous in some contexts, it has its place as a springboard for further investigations. In fact, most cultures and societies have a

[1] The paper was based on a plenary lecture given at the 9th Congress of the International Society for Ethnopharmacology in Nanning, PR China, August 2006.
[2] Efron *et al.* (1970) and Holmstedt (1967) are usually credited with introducing the term (Heinrich, 2014).

*Ethnopharmacology*, First Edition. Edited by Michael Heinrich and Anna K. Jäger.
© 2015 John Wiley & Sons, Ltd. Published 2015 by John Wiley & Sons, Ltd.

collection of stories that help them define their history and characteristics, and so I am using this approach to outline how ethnopharmacology has woven itself into my life.

## 34.2   The primacy of plants

It should be noted that most ethnopharmacological research undertaken has concentrated on flowering plants and their products. This is not surprising since traditional *material medica* in most cultures is composed mainly of plants. However, TCM and the Ayurvedic and Siddha systems from South Asia make use of minerals, and TCM utilizes a variety of macrofungal species and animals, either entire or in part. Although investigations of fungi have not come into my orbit, research into TCM materials used traditionally to treat cancer and memory loss in old age has encompassed animals as diverse as earthworms, geckos, beetles and centipedes (Fang and Houghton, 2004; Ren *et al.*, 2006; Houghton *et al.*, 2007b). However, most of my research has been concerned with flowering plants.

## 34.3   Sources: dirty hands and databases

Every researcher needs to select a topic for their studies and, in ethnopharmacology perhaps more than some subjects, it is important to select a topic and mode of investigation which encompasses both ethnography (or anthropology) and some experimental testing connected with medicinal use. Etkin (2001) deplored the lack of much evidence of a 'bridge' between the social and experimental sciences in many ethnopharmacological papers, a situation which was soon apparent when in 1994 I started editorial work with the *Journal of Ethnopharmacology*. Owen *et al.* (2011) also pleaded for a greater integration of disciplines by researchers, acknowledging that it was the constraints imposed by academia which often compromised the feasibility of true interdisciplinary study, making it the exception rather than the rule that the researcher who gathered data in the field also carried out laboratory studies. An established researcher in the UK, especially in a teaching-intensive course such as pharmacy, finds it very difficult to have any prolonged spell 'getting their hands dirty' in the lab, but even more so 'in the field'.

The subject of field research also raises the question of the 'purity' of knowledge of a particular culture. Migration, conquest and trade have a profound effect on what 'alien' materials and species are used, even in quite isolated situations, e.g. the use of 'western' medicines in Oaxaca, Mexico (Giovanni and Heinrich, 2009), so an introduced species may well be incorporated as a valuable part of the local *materia medica*, e.g. *Argemone mexicana* L. as an antimalarial in Mali (Willcox *et al.*, 2007).

My personal experience of 'field studies' has been limited to informal conversations when travelling overseas and highlighted for me the difficulties of botanical identification, language generally and translating local ideas about disease into western medical concepts which occur in short-term field work. However, my experiences had their lighter side, such as when I spent two hours in a big market in Cairo trying, unsuccessfully, to find asafoetida (a resin produced from some *Ferula* species) for a project I was working on at the time. I did not know the Arabic name, so had to describe it, and I was offered a wide variety of substances (many unlike what I had described!), and every seller was convinced he had what I wanted!

However, a considerable amount of my research was done by PhD students who had previously carried out well-designed ethnopharmacological field work in their home countries, and who came to me to do the relevant laboratory work. This resulted in publications encompassing both disciplines mentioned above, e.g. Laupattarakesem (2003) for Thai plants used to treat arthritis, Itharat *et al.* (2004) for Thai anticancer plants, Ashidi *et al.* (2010)

for Nigerian anticancer plants, and Annan and Houghton (2008), Dickson *et al.* (2006) and Mensah *et al.* (2006) for Ghanaian plants used for wound healing.

In the absence of time, resources and ability to carry out field research, much information can be gained from databases. The advent of electronic databases and the translation of printed material into electronic form have revolutionized the speed of information retrieval, although many older printed (and also written) documents containing ethnopharmacological information have not yet been reduced to this form. It should not be forgotten that a huge amount of information, of various levels of reliability, is stored in archives, libraries and similar reference collections, whence information on a particular ethnopharmacological topic can be collected and collated, providing a platform whereby workers in that area can select plants or other organisms for their studies. The series of papers in *Lloydia* (now *Journal of Natural Products*) in the 1960s by Hartwell on plants used traditionally against cancer is a case in point.

London is endowed with a wealth of libraries and museums, so enabling me to make modest contributions of this type for plants used to treat snakebite (Houghton and Osibogun, 1993), scorpion envenomation (Hutt and Houghton, 1998) and memory-deficient states similar to Alzheimer's disease (Howes *et al.*, 2003). It is perhaps regrettable that papers consisting only of such lists are much less welcomed by journals than formerly, since they are often cited by subsequent workers.

## 34.4   From cultural use to chemistry

In common with many who have become prominent figures in ethnopharmacological research, my original expertise was in phytochemistry of medicinal plants, many species investigated having some reputation as a poison or a medicine. By the 1970s many common potent examples of this type used in Europe, or which had attracted the attention of European colonialists, had already been investigated. In some instances compounds isolated and determined were brought into clinical use, the opium alkaloids and *Digitalis* cardenolides being classic examples from Europe and physostigmine from *Physostigma venenosum* Balfour a good example from the second category (Proudfoot, 2006).

Consequently there was an increasing amount of research into plants with less well-known uses, especially those from other cultures not used in European–North American pharmacy and medicine.

I spent almost all my working life in the Department of Pharmacy, Chelsea College, which became part of King's College London in 1984. A considerable amount of phytochemical work had been performed there on the alkaloids of *Mitragyna* (Rubiaceae) because of the use of the leaves of *M. speciosa* Korth. in Thailand and Malaysia as a stimulant but also because it has opiate-like properties. No pharmacological studies were undertaken, but many alkaloids were isolated from most of the nine *Mitragyna* species then recognized (Shellard, 1974). My PhD thesis was even further away from any ethnopharmacological aspect of the alkaloids since it concentrated on their biogenesis and interconversion (Shellard and Houghton, 1972, 1974). It is only since the Chelsea studies terminated that others have published work on their pharmacology, especially that of mitragynine, the major alkaloid in *M. speciosa* Korth. (Adkins *et al.*, 2011; Raffa *et al.*, 2013; Ulbricht *et al.*, 2013).

## 34.5   Chemistry as a starter

By definition, ethnopharmacological research on a particular species should start with a defined medical application, but sometimes a species is known, at least to western science, only as a 'medicinal plant'. Chemical studies occasionally reveal a novel or unusual chemical structure and this stimulates interest in traditional uses of the plant in question, as well as investigation into the biological activity of the compounds. My work on *Schumanniophyton magnificum* Harms. (Rubiaceae) is an example of this. Bark of this species had lain for several years in our laboratory after being collected from a former colleague who had worked in Nigeria. When the bark was finally investigated chemically, chromone alkaloids, an uncommon type, were isolated. A literature search revealed that the plant was widely used by local healers in south-eastern Nigeria, especially for snakebite, but exploration of the anti-snakebite properties showed that peptides present, not the alkaloids, were responsible for its action (Houghton *et al.*, 1992).

## 34.6   Botany as a basis

It would probably be true to say that the heyday of phytochemistry was the latter half of the 20th century as advances in chromatographic and spectroscopic techniques enabled the separation, isolation and structural elucidation of a large number of secondary metabolites. This facilitated the rise of chemosystematics and the subsequent chemical study of plant taxa previously little investigated, but of interest in clarifying systematic relationships rather than because of biological activities.

A case in point is the genus *Buddleja*, which had been placed within the Loganiaceae, a family of chemotaxonomic interest since some genera, notably *Strychnos*, produced indole alkaloids of pharmacological interest such as strychnine. My interest in indole alkaloids from *Mitragyna* stimulated chemical exploration of *Buddleja*, but I considered that such work, undertaken in a school of pharmacy, necessitated also exploration of any medicinal uses of *Buddleja*. A literature search revealed that indeed many of the 100 species of *Buddleja* did have uses in traditional medicine in many parts of the world where they were endemic (Houghton, 1984). Of particular interest was that many of these uses, e.g. for liver complaints, for healing wounds and for treating inflammation of the eyes and skin, were common, even from geographically-distinct areas, e.g. China, Mexico, Chile. Thus the *Buddleja* project moved from a purely chemical investigation to studies involving biological testing for relevant activities, particularly those related to wound-healing (Mensah *et al.*, 2001). Interestingly an ecological observation that newly dug roots of *Buddleja* had a fairly strong odour led to the isolation of fungicidal terpenoids from the roots (Mensah *et al.*, 2000), thus illustrating the complex chemical interplay between ecology, biological activity and systematics that may arise originally from botanical investigations.

## 34.7   Of mice and men and microwell plates

The experimental pharmacological dimension of ethnopharmacological research, especially *in vivo* studies, did not feature strongly until fairly recently, partly because of ethical and financial considerations. The strongest validation of the traditional use of a substance for treating a human condition is achieved when properly designed and properly analysed clinical trials are carried out and show significant improvement when the test substance is used. Two colleagues of mine published one of the first papers of this type on the use of the leaves of feverfew (*Tanacetum parthenium* (L.) Sch. Bip.) for treating migraine (Johnson *et al.*, 1985), but good examples are uncommon in the ethnopharmacological literature. Common reasons for poor-quality studies are that many clinicians do not realize the importance of establishing botanical authenticity and/or a chemical profile for the material they use. Low numbers, a lack of controls, blinding and randomization, as well inadequate markers and endpoints in the design and execution of the study also are features of papers with low value. Funding of clinical trials is extremely costly and difficult to acquire, even for treatments of serious disease, so to find funds to carry out trials for efficacy in minor conditions, such as for diuretics or laxatives, is impossible, at least in western countries.

Even with these considerations, it is frustrating to see the lack of clinical studies on several widely used traditional remedies for serious diseases. The use of extracts of *Cryptolepis sanguinolenta* (Lindl.) Schltr. roots in Ghana for malaria is a case in point. A considerable amount of chemistry and many *in vitro* tests have been carried out, including some from my group, e.g Paulo *et al.* (1995, 2000), but the only refereed clinical studies published have been in a local journal (Bugyei *et al.*, 2010; Tempesta, 2010).

The next best thing to human studies is to use animal models of disease. In many countries, including the UK, a strong case has to be made on ethical grounds to justify the use of animals, and fees and time spent in compulsory training and acquiring a licence. This acted as a deterrent in performing any such experiments in my laboratory, although it enabled cooperation with groups having such facilities, e.g. Mukherjee *et al.* (2007) and Govindarajan *et al.* (2007). Similar cooperation using *ex vivo* 'classical' pharmacological 'gut bath' techniques was also used in anti-snake venom studies (Houghton and Harvey, 1989).

The introduction of microtitre well plates in the last two decades of the 20th century for rapid testing of biological activity using small amounts revolutionized ethnopharmacological studies, along with the much wider drug discovery process. Tests were devised, often employing some form of rapid spectrophotometry using a plate reader for *in vitro* activities such as cell viability, incorporation and release of substances in living cells and enzyme inhibition. Because of these new techniques, ethnopharmacologists were able to use bioassay-guided fractionation to investigate the chemical basis for the activity observed, rather than making conjectures that compounds easily isolated because of their abundance or their ease of crystallization had some link to the activity.

This shift in focus also applied to my research and it features prominently in my papers published after 1993. My experience of applying such techniques to several different biological activities relevant to traditional treatments for cancer, diabetes, wound-healing and inflammatory conditions enabled appraisal of their advantages and limitations. In particular caution was advised against proposing that an activity shown in a microwell plate would automatically be seen *in vivo*, since efficacy clinically depends on several features that are not always possible to determine from *in vitro* tests (Houghton, 2000; Houghton *et al.*, 2005, 2007a). Another negative aspect of bioassay-guided fractionation as a discovery route to novel active compounds is that much work might be carried out before final structural elucidation of the active substance, only to find that its identity and activity were previously known, but reported from another botanical source. The approach which minimizes this occurring is known as dereplication, and usually monitors the crude extract for known compounds by techniques such as LC-MS (liquid chromatography linked with mass spectrometry).

## 34.8   Aims and ethics

The diversity of human culture, the range of habitats in which humans manage to survive and the breadth of accompanying biodiversity, of flowering plants in particular, are a source of wonder and fascination, so it is not surprising that curiosity alone often drove early ethnopharmacological research.

However, the days when scientists could do research only for this reason have largely passed. Very few have private means and resources, and most have to rely on external funding, whether from governments, charitable foundations or industry. Such donors usually look for a short- or long-term return on the funds provided and so any application has to be prepared with this in mind.

Ethnopharmacology research is often promoted as a method of discovering new drugs, or other substances such as pesticides and cosmetics, and has a long history of providing useful medicines. The work involved in selecting suitable plants for study is usually too intensive for industrial research, which tends to favour 'random screening' from a geographical area or from extreme living conditions, so most ethnopharmacological research occurs in universities and research-based institutions. If any interesting leads are found, industry is then approached to develop the substance in question commercially.

However, a less well promoted result of ethnopharmacological studies might be to provide scientific support for the adoption of a local medically applicable product in some countries, as a substitute for expensive imported drugs. Such medicines are often not geographically or economically available to a large proportion of the population, and well-researched, standardized ethnopharmacological material could be adopted.

In my research lifetime, the ethical dimension of ethnopharmacology has caused a significant change to the ease of obtaining materials for research. 'Biopiracy', the exploitation of natural resources without any recognition of the intellectual property rights of the people who originally held the relevant knowledge, was one target of the CBD, which arose from the 1992 Rio Earth Summit. This was unquestionably a move in the right direction, although at times the difficulties in obtaining the desired material for research have been rather frustrating.

## 34.9  Molecules and mixtures

In drug discovery, the classic approach has been to isolate one active compound, which is then used as a 'lead' develop novel drugs. Although this approach yielded some useful drugs from ethnopharmacological sources, in many cases more than one compound, or even several compound classes, appear to contribute to the overall effect (Houghton *et al.*, 2007a). In many cases polyvalence, or multiple functions, with a variety of relevant activities, can be demonstrated. Several examples are seen in my research, e.g. in Malaysian plants used to treat cancer (Houghton *et al.*, 2007b) and Ghanaian wound-healing plants (Annan and Houghton, 2008).

In some instances synergistic effects may be observed and it is not unusual for bioassay guided fractionation to result in the activity of any of the fractions being much less than the extract as a whole, as seen in cytotoxicity studies on *Kigelia* (Houghton, 2000).

Thus many traditional remedies do not easily fit the single-chemical entity drug approach favoured by western regulatory and medical agencies, and this affects their acceptance into orthodox medicine and consequent development. One cannot help speculate how many potentially useful medicinal treatments may have been discarded because of this.

## 34.10  Tales of the unexpected

The discovery of the anticancer compounds vincristine and vinblastine from *Catharanthus roseus* G. Don as a result of its originally being investigated as an antidiabetic remedy is the classic example of interesting information arising which is unrelated to the initial investigation. It is a salutary reminder that investigators should be vigilant and observant of unexpected results.

In my research there have been similar instances. Publication of the structures of some alkaloids of *Schumanniophyton magnificum* Harms. led to a request to submit them for testing against HIV, with ensuing positive results and eventually the determination of schumannificine as the most active compound (Houghton *et al.*, 1994a), although it was not taken up for commercial development. The fruits of *Kigelia pinnata* (Jacq.) DC. were originally investigated because of their antibacterial use (Akunyili *et al.*, 1991) but later reports of their use in cancerous skin conditions led to the discovery of cytotoxic compounds (Houghton *et al.*, 1994b), which have also been shown to have anti-protozoal properties (Moideen *et al.*, 1999; Weiss *et al.*, 2000).

## 34.11    The end of the matter

My ethnopharmacological studies were aimed at improving health for all. It would probably be true to say that the possibility of finding a novel therapeutic agent was the Holy Grail, but anything that was carried out was done with a clear understanding that the likelihood of finding anything useful in the clinic was very small. However, perhaps personal satisfaction was greater when my findings gave some scientific support to the traditional use of natural materials, since this honours the culture in question and demonstrates that knowledge acquired down the ages demands more than a cursory glance from western science. Another important dimension, which in my opinion is generally not investigated as much as it ought to have be, is the way in which good ethnopharmacological research may facilitate replacement of expensive imported 'conventional' medicines by locally available products. It is true that this has been introduced to some extent in countries such as China and India, but globally recognized regulatory processes, geared very much towards single-chemical entity medicines, militate against this in most of the world. Positive ethnopharmacological findings are a first, but important, step in the process of introducing traditionally based extracts and similar medicines into standard health care but the role of testing for safety and efficacy by clinical trials are even more important and it is encouraging to see that more such work is now being carried on in the Far East and some countries in other parts of the world.

Last but not least, ethnopharmacology is fascinating. It not only demonstrates the ingenuity of humankind in making use of a particular environment to meet health needs, but when pursued it often opens new vistas of usefulness, not only in the therapeutic and other applications of the original culture, but in unrelated areas.

## References

Adkins, J.E., Boyer, E.W. and McCurdy, C.R. (2011) *Mitragyna speciosa*, a psychoactive tree from southeast Asia with opioid activity. *Current Topics in Medicinal Chemistry*, **11**, 1165–1175.

Akunyili, D.N., Houghton, P.J. and Raman, A. (1991) Investigation of the antimicrobial activity of extracts of *Kigelia pinnata*. *Journal of Ethnopharmacology*, **35**, 173–177.

Annan, K. and Houghton, P.J. (2008) Antibacterial, antioxidant and fibroblast growth stimulation of aqueous extracts of *Ficus asperifolia* Miq. and *Gossypium arboreum* L., wound-healing plants of Ghana. *Journal of Ethnopharmacology*, **119**, 141–144.

Ashidi, J.S., Houghton, P.J., Hylands, P.J. and Efferth, T. (2010) Ethnobotanical survey and cytotoxicity testing of plants of South-western Nigeria used to treat cancer, with isolation of cytotoxic constituents from *Cajanus cajan* Millsp leaves. *Journal of Ethnopharmacology*, **128**, 501–512.

Bugyei, K.A., Boye, G.L. and Addy, M.E. (2010) Clinical efficacy of a tea-bag formulation of Cryptolepis sanguinolenta root in the treatment of acute uncomplicated falciparum malaria. *Ghana Medical Journal*, **44**, 3–9.

Dickson, R.A., Houghton, P.J., Hylands, P.J. and Gibbons, S. (2006) Antimicrobial, resistance-modifying effects, antioxidant and free radical scavenging activities of *Mezoneuron benthamianum* Baill., *Securinega virosa* Roxb. & Wlld. and *Microglossa pyrifolia* Lam. *Phytotherapy Research*, **20**, 41–45.

Efron, D., Holmstedt, B. and Kline, N.L. (1970) *Ethnopharmacologic Search for Psychoactive Drugs*, Government Printing Office, Public Health Service Publications No. 1645 (originally 1967).

Etkin, N.L. (2001) Perspectives in ethnopharmacology: forging a closer link between bioscience and traditional empirical knowledge. *Journal of Ethnopharmacology*, **76**, 177–182.

Etkin, N.L. and Elisabetsky, E. (2005) Seeking a transdisciplinary and culturally germane science: The future of ethnopharmacology. *Journal of Ethnopharmacology*, **100**, 23–26.

Fang, R. and Houghton, P.J. (2004) Investigation of some Chinese traditional medicines used to treat cancer. *Journal of Pharmacy and Pharmacology*, **56**, S79.

Giovannini, P. and Heinrich, M. (2009) Xki yoma' (our medicine) and xki tienda (patent medicine) – Interface between traditional and modern medicine among the Mazatecs of Oaxaca, Mexico. *Journal of Ethnopharmacology*, **121**, 383–399.

Govindarajan, R., Asare-Anane, H., Persaud, S., *et al.* (2007) Effect of *Desmodium gangeticum* extract on blood glucose in rats and on insulin secretion in vitro. *Planta Medica*, **73**, 427–432.

Heinrich, M. (2014) Ethnopharmacology: quo vadis? Challenges for the future. *Revista Brasileira de Farmacognosia*, **24**, 99–102.

Holmstedt, B. (1967) An overview of ethnopharmacology. Historical survey. *Psychopharmacology Bulletin*, **4**, 2–3.

Houghton, P.J. (1984) Ethnopharmacology of some *Buddleja* species. *Journal of Ethnopharmacology*, **11**, 293–308.

Houghton, P.J. (2000) Use of small scale bioassays in the discovery of novel drugs from natural sources. *Phytotherapy Research*, **14**, 419–423.

Houghton, P.J. and Harvey, A.L. (1989) Investigation of the anti-snake venom activity of *Schumanniophyton magnificum*. *Planta Medica*, **55**, 273–276.

Houghton, P.J. and Osibogun, I.M. (1993) Flowering plants used against snakebite. *Journal of Ethnopharmacology*, **39**, 1–30.

Houghton, P.J., Osibogun, I.M. and Bansal, S. (1992) A peptide from *Schumanniophyton magnificum* with anti-Cobra venom activity. *Planta Medica*, **58**, 263–265.

Houghton, P.J., Jackson, S.J., Browning, M., *et al.* (1994a) Activity of extracts of *Kigelia pinnata* against melanoma and renal carcinoma cells. *Planta Medica*, **60**, 430–433.

Houghton, P.J., Woldemariam, T.Z., Khan, A.I., *et al.* (1994b) Antiviral activity of natural and semi-synthetic chromone alkaloids. *Antiviral Research*, **25**, 235–244.

Houghton, P.J., Hylands, P.J., Mensah, A.Y., *et al.* (2005) In vitro tests and ethnopharmacological investigations: Wound healing as an example. *Journal of Ethnopharmacology*, **100**, 100–107.

Houghton, P.J., Howes, M.-J., Lee, C.C. and Steventon, G. (2007a) Uses and abuses of in vitro tests in ethnopharmacology: Visualising an elephant. *Journal of Ethnopharmacology*, **110**, 391-400.

Houghton, P., Fang, R., Techatanawat, I., *et al.* (2007b) The sulphorhodamine (SRB) assay and other approaches to testing plant extracts and derived compounds for activities related to reputed anticancer activity. *Methods*, **42**, 377–387.

Howes, M.-J.R., Perry, N.S.L. and Houghton, P.J. (2003) Plants with traditional uses and activities, relevant to the management of Alzheimer's disease and other cognitive disorders. *Phytotherapy Research*, **17**, 1–18.

Hutt, M.J. and Houghton, P.J. (1998) A literature survey of plants used to treat scorpion envenomation. *Journal of Ethnopharmacology*, **60**, 97–110.

Itharat, A., Houghton, P.J., Eno-Amooquaye, E., *et al.* (2004) In vitro cytotoxic activity of Thai medicinal plants used traditionally to treat cancer. *Journal of Ethnopharmacology*, **90**, 33–38.

Johnson, E.S., Kadam, N.P., Hylands, D.M. and Hylands, P.J. (1985) Efficacy of feverfew as prophylactic treatment of migraine. *British Medical Journal*, **291**, 569–573.

Laupattarakasem, P., Houghton, P.J., Hoult, J.R.S. and Itharat, A. (2003) An evaluation of the activity related to inflammation of four plants used in Thailand to treat arthritis. *Journal of Ethnopharmacology*, **85**, 207–215.

Mensah, A.Y., Houghton, P.J., Bloomfield, S., *et al.* (2000) Known and novel terpenes from *Buddleja globosa* displaying selective antifungal activity against dermatophytes. *Journal of Natural Products*, **63**, 1210–1213.

Mensah, A.Y., Sampson, J., Houghton, P.J., *et al.* (2001) Effects of *Buddleja globosa* leaf and its constituents relevant to wound healing. *Journal of Ethnopharmacology*, **77**, 219–226.

Mensah, A.Y., Houghton, P.J., Dickson, R.A., *et al.* (2006) In vitro evaluation of effects of two Ghanaian plants relevant to wound healing. *Phytotherapy Research*, **20**, 941–944.

Moideen, S.V.K., Houghton, P.J., Rock, P., *et al.* (1999) Activity of extracts and naphthoquinones from *Kigelia pinnata* against *Trypanosoma brucei brucei* and *Trypanosoma brucei rhodiesiense*. *Planta Medica*, **65**, 493–588.

Mukherjee, P.K., Nazeer Ahamed, K.F.H., Kumar, V., *et al.* (2007) Protective effect of biflavones from *Araucaria bidwillii* Hook in rat cerebral ischemia/perfusion induced oxidative stress. *Behavioural Brain Research*, **178**, 221–228.

Owen, P.L., Johns, T. and Etkin, N.L. (2011) Bridging the 'two cultures' in ethnopharmacology: Barriers against interdisciplinarity in postgraduate education. *Journal of Ethnopharmacology*, **134**, 999–1005.

Paulo, M.A., Gomes, E.T. and Houghton, P.J. (1995) New alkaloids from *Cryptolepis sanguinolenta*. *Journal of Natural Products*, **58**, 1485–1491.

Paulo, A., Gomes, E.T., Steele, J., *et al.* (2000) Antiplasmodial activity of *Cryptolepis sanguinolenta* alkaloids from leaves and roots. *Planta Medica*, **66**, 30–34.

Proudfoot, A. (2006) The early toxicology of physostigmine: a tale of beans, great men and egos. *Toxicology Review*, **25**, 99–138.

Raffa, R.B., Beckett, J.R., Brahmbhatt, V.N., *et al.* (2013) Orally active opioid compounds from a non-Poppy source. *Journal of Medical Chemistry*, **56**, 4840–4848.

Ren, Y., Houghton, P.J. and Hider, R.C. (2006) Relevant activities of extracts and constituents of animals used in traditional Chinese medicine for central nervous system effects associated with Alzheimer's disease. *Journal of Pharmacy and Pharmacology*, **58**, 989–996.

Shellard, E.J. (1974) Alkaloids of *Mitragyna* with special reference to those of *Mitragyna speciosa* Korth. *Bulletin of Narcotics*, **26**, 41–55.

Shellard, E.J. and Houghton, P.J. (1972) The *Mitragyna* species of Asia part XXI. The distribution of alkaloids in young plants of *Mitragyna parvifolia* grown from seed obtained from Ceylon. *Planta Medica*, **21**, 382–392.

Shellard, E.J. and Houghton, P.J. (1974) The *Mitragyna* species of Asia part XXVI. Further *in vivo* studies, using ¹⁴C-alkaloids, in the alkaloidal pattern in young plants of *Mitragyna parvifolia* grown from seed obtained from Sri Lanka (Ceylon). *Planta Medica*, **25**, 80–87.

Tempesta, M.S. (2010) The clinical efficacy of *Cryptolepis sanguinolenta* in the treatment of malaria. *Ghana Medical Journal*, **44**, 1–2.

Ulbricht, C., Costa, D., Dao, J., *et al.* (2013) An evidence-based systematic review of kratom (*Mitragyna speciosa*) by the Natural Standard Research Collaboration. *Journal of Dietary Supplements*, **10**, 152–170.

Weiss, C.R., Moideen, S.V.K., Croft, S.L. and Houghton, P.J. (2000) Activity of extracts and isolated naphthoquinones from *Kigelia pinnata* against *Plasmodium falciparum*. *Journal of Natural Products*, **63**, 1306–1309.

Willcox, M.L., Graz, B., Falquet, J., *et al.* (2007) *Argemone mexicana* decoction for the treatment of uncomplicated falciparum malaria. *Transactions of the Royal Society for Tropical Medicine and Hygiene*, **101**, 1190–1198.

# Index

*Italics* are used to indicate tables or figures

Binomial (Latin) nomenclature is used for species names

---

*Ethnopharmacology*, First Edition. Edited by Michael Heinrich and Anna K. Jäger.
© 2015 John Wiley & Sons, Ltd. Published 2015 by John Wiley & Sons, Ltd.

Printed and bound by CPI Group (UK) Ltd, Croydon, CR0 4YY

09/10/2024

14571435-0004